Anatomy for Diagnostic Imaging

Anatomy for Diagnostic Imaging

FOURTH EDITION

Stephanie Ryan FRCSI FFR(RCSI)

Consultant Paediatric Radiologist (Retd.), Children's Health Ireland, Temple Street, and Rotunda Hospital, Dublin
Associate Professor, University College Dublin

Michelle McNicholas FRCPI FFR(RCSI) FRCR

Consultant Radiologist, Mater Misericordiae University Hospital, Dublin, and National Breast Screening Programme, Ireland
Associate Professor, University College Dublin

Stephen Eustace MSc(RadSci) MRCPI FFR(RCSI) FRCR

Consultant Radiologist, Mater Misericordiae University Hospital and Cappagh National Orthopaedic Hospitals, Dublin
Newman Professor of Radiology, University College Dublin

ELSEVIER

ISBN: 978-0-443-10560-9

Content Strategist: Trinity Hutton
Content Project Manager: Taranpreet Kaur
Design: Patrick Ferguson
Illustration Manager: Akshaya Mohan
Marketing Manager: Deborah Watkins

Printed in India

Last digit is the print number: 9 8 7 6 5 4 3 2 1

Working together
to grow libraries in
developing countries

www.elsevier.com • www.bookaid.org

This book is dedicated to:

Tom, Stephen, Ellen, Niamh, Sarah, Conor and Alex Ryan (SR)
Billy, Barry, Jack, Sam, Michael, Georgina, Isabelle and Sienna Power (MMcN)
Nicola, Sarah, Emma, Jack and Nick Eustace (SE)

Contents

Contributors, viii
Preface, x
Acknowledgements, xi

1 Head and Neck, 1
DANIELLE BYRNE
EDITED BY STEPHANIE RYAN
The Skull and Facial Bones, 1
The Nasal Cavity and Paranasal Sinuses, 12
The Mandible and Teeth, 14
The Orbital Contents, 18
The Ear, 22
The Upper Aerodigestive Tract, 23
The Neck Lymph Node Levels, 38
Layers of the Deep Cervical Fascia, 41
Deep Spaces of the Head and Neck, 42
The Salivary Glands, 45
Radiology of the Salivary Glands, 47
The Thyroid and Parathyroid Glands, 48
The Neck Vessels, 50
The Brachial Plexus, 56

2 The Central Nervous System, 58
TERENCE FARRELL
EDITED BY STEPHANIE RYAN
Cerebral Hemispheres, 58
Cerebral Cortex, 58
White Matter of the Hemispheres, 60
Basal Ganglia, 66
Thalamus, Hypothalamus and Pineal Gland, 69
Pituitary Gland, 71
The Limbic Lobe System, 73
The Brainstem, 74
Cerebellum, 78
Ventricles, Cisterns, CSF Production and Flow, 80
Meninges, 87
Arterial Supply of the CNS, 90
Venous Drainage of the Brain, 95

3 The Spinal Column and Its Contents, 101
TERENCE FARRELL AND JOHN HYNES
EDITED BY STEPHEN EUSTACE AND STEPHANIE RYAN
The Vertebral Column, 101
Joints of the Vertebral Column, 109
Ligaments of the Vertebral Column, 111
The Intervertebral Discs, 113
Blood Supply of the Vertebral Column, 114
The Spinal Cord, 114
The Spinal Meninges, 118
Blood Supply of the Spinal Cord, 118

4 The Thorax, 123
PHILIP DEMPSEY AND BARRY HUTCHINSON
EDITED BY MICHELLE McNICHOLAS
The Thoracic Cage, 123
The Diaphragm, 129

The Pleura, 135
The Extrapleural Space, 138
The Trachea and Bronchi, 138
The Lungs, 143
The Mediastinum, 152
The Heart, 153
The Great Vessels, 167
The Oesophagus, 170
The Thoracic Duct and Mediastinal Lymphatics, 172
The Thymus, 173
The Azygos System, 174
Important Nerves of the Mediastinum, 175
The Mediastinum on the Chest Radiograph, 177
Cross-Sectional Anatomy, 179

5 The Abdomen, 184
EMMA DUNNE
EDITED BY MICHELLE McNICHOLAS
Anterior Abdominal Wall, 184
The Stomach, 185
The Duodenum, 189
The Small Intestine, 193
The Ileocaecal Valve, 196
The Appendix, 197
The Large Intestine, 198
The Liver, 201
The Biliary System, 208
The Pancreas, 212
The Spleen, 218
The Portal Venous System, 219
The Kidneys, 222
The Ureter, 226
The Adrenal Glands, 229
The Abdominal Aorta, 230
The Inferior Vena Cava, 231
Veins of the Posterior Abdominal Wall, 232
Peritoneal Spaces of the Abdomen, 235
Cross-Sectional Anatomy of the Upper Abdomen, 239

6 The Pelvis, 245
JACK POWER
EDITED BY MICHELLE McNICHOLAS
The Bony Pelvis, Muscles and Ligaments, 245
The Pelvic Floor, 248
The Sigmoid Colon, Rectum and Anal Canal, 250
Blood Vessels, Lymphatics and Nerves of the Pelvis, 258
The Lower Urinary Tract, 261
The Male Urethra, 263
The Female Urethra, 264
The Male Reproductive Organs, 264
The Female Reproductive Tract, 272
Cross-Sectional Anatomy, 281

7 *The Upper Limb,* 284
JOHN HYNES
EDITED BY STEPHEN EUSTACE
The Bones of the Upper Limb,   284
The Joints of the Upper Limb,   290
The Muscles of the Upper Limb,   308
The Arterial Supply of the Upper Limb,   309
The Veins of the Upper Limb,   310

8 *The Lower Limb,* 312
JOHN HYNES
EDITED BY STEPHEN EUSTACE
The Bones of the Lower Limb,   312
The Joints of the Lower Limb,   318
The Muscles of the Lower Limb,   337
The Arteries of the Lower Limb,   340
The Veins of the Lower Limb,   343

9 *The Breast,* 345
MICHELLE McNICHOLAS
General Anatomy,   345
Lobular Structure,   345
Blood Supply,   345
Lymphatic Drainage,   345
Axillary Lymph Nodes,   346
Lymph Node Imaging,   346
Radiology of the Breast,   347
Radiological Significance of Breast Density and
Parenchymal Pattern,   350
Age Changes in the Breast,   353

Index,   355

Contributors

Danielle Byrne, MRCP MD FFR(RCSI)
Danielle is a consultant radiologist at St James's University Hospital, Dublin, and a clinical senior lecturer at Trinity College Dublin, since 2020. She did her radiology training at Mater Misericordiae University Hospital, Dublin, before completing fellowships in neuroradiology at Vancouver General Hospital, and in cardiothoracic radiology at the University of British Columbia. She runs revision days in head and neck imaging for radiology registrars.

Philip Dempsey, MRCPI FFR(RCSI)
Philip is a fellow in musculoskeletal radiology at Cappagh National Orthopaedic Hospital, having completed his radiology training at Mater Misericordiae University Hospital, Dublin. He plans to undertake a further fellowship in abdominal imaging and intervention at Brigham and Women's Hospital, Boston in 2025.

Emma Dunne, MRCSI FFR(RCSI)
Emma is a fellow in interventional radiology at Mater Misericordiae University Hospital, Dublin, having recently completed her radiology specialist training there. She is interested in clinical education and plans to pursue a career in interventional radiology and abdominal imaging.

Stephen Eustace, MSc(RadSci) MRCPI FFR(RCSI) FRCR
Stephen is Newman Professor of Radiology at University College Dublin, Director of Radiology Cappagh National Orthopaedic Hospital and consultant radiologist at the Mater Misericordiae University Hospital, Dublin. He is an inaugural founder fellow and former board member of the faculty of sports medicine (RCPI, RCSI) and a fellow of the faculty of radiologists (RCSI) with special interests in imaging in orthopaedics and sports medicine and image-guided intervention, particularly of the spine. Having trained in radiology at Mater Misericordiae University Hospital, he completed fellowships at Boston University and Harvard before returning to his current position. Reflecting his interest in sports imaging, Stephen has been chairperson of the medical committee of the Football Association of Ireland, chairperson of the medical committee of the Irish Rugby Football Union and has served as support radiologist for the Irish Olympic Team. He is committed to teaching and education for the next generation.

Terence Farrell, MRCPI FFR(RCSI) FRCR
Terrence is a consultant neuroradiologist at Beaumont Hospital, Dublin, since 2021. He completed his radiology training at St James's Hospital, Dublin, and a fellowship in emergency radiology at Mater Misericordiae University Hospital, Dublin. He subsequently completed further fellowship training in neuroradiology and musculoskeletal radiology at Thomas Jefferson University Hospital in Philadelphia, USA. He has a strong academic and teaching background and is interested in all aspects of neuroradiology including spinal imaging and intervention.

Barry Hutchinson, MRCS FFR(RCSI) FRCR
Barry did his radiology training at University Hospital, Galway, before completing a fellowship in thoracic imaging at NYU Langone Hospital, New York. He subsequently worked at NYU as a consultant thoracic radiologist before returning to Mater Misericordiae University Hospital, Dublin, in 2019 as a consultant with a special interest in cardiothoracic imaging and intervention. He has a particular interest in teaching. He is national coordinator of the RCSI Faculty of Radiologists training scheme. He is also a faculty examiner.

John Hynes, MRCS FFR(RCSI)
John completed his radiology training at Mater Misericordiae University Hospital, Dublin, and a fellowship in musculoskeletal radiology at Cappagh National Orthopaedic Hospital, Dublin. He now works as a consultant with a special interest in musculoskeletal radiology and intervention at St Vincent's University and Cappagh National Orthopaedic Hospital.

Michelle McNicholas, FRCPI FFR(RCSI) FRCR

Michelle did her radiology training at St Vincent's University Hospital, Dublin, before undertaking a fellowship in abdominal imaging and interventional radiology at Massachusetts General Hospital, Boston. She subsequently worked as a consultant at the Beth Israel Deaconess Medical Centre Boston, leading GU imaging, for a number of years. During that time, she was an Assistant Professor at Harvard Medical School, involved in teaching radiology residents and medical students. She returned to Dublin's Mater Misericordiae University Hospital as a consultant radiologist in 2000 and has maintained her interest in teaching, lecturing at the Faculty of Radiologists RCSI Dublin throughout her career, and been invited faculty at many national and international refresher courses including RSNA. Her main interests are GU, gynaecological and prostate imaging and intervention. She is also a consultant in the national breast screening programme.

Jack Power, MRCPI FFR(RCSI)

Jack completed his radiology training at Mater Misericordiae University Hospital, Dublin, and is currently a fellow in abdominal imaging and intervention at Brigham and Women's Hospital, Boston. He is interested in GU and prostate imaging and intervention, and plans to do a further fellowship in nuclear radiology at Massachusetts General Hospital in 2025.

Stephanie Ryan, FRCSI FFR(RCSI)

Stephanie was a Paediatric Radiologist at Temple Street Children's Hospital and at the Neonatal Radiology Department of the Rotunda Hospital in Dublin for nearly 25 years. Having completed her radiology training at St James's Hospital, Dublin, she undertook fellowships in paediatric radiology in Seattle, Washington, and in interventional radiology at the Mayo Clinic, USA. In addition to this textbook on imaging anatomy, she has written several papers and book chapters on paediatric imaging. She is a regular invited speaker at national and international radiology meetings. She has a special interest in neonatal radiology, neuroradiology and in the imaging of metabolic disorders. Stephanie is an enthusiastic teacher of anatomy and of paediatric radiology and is a mentor of several generations of paediatric radiologists.

Preface

The first edition of this book (at that time, just 'Ryan and McNicholas') was published in 1994 in response to the lack of a succinct imaging-focused anatomy book for radiologists. At that time, studying anatomy for Part I of our Radiology Fellowship exams, we found ourselves studying out of an array of books and atlases, then distilling the information for ourselves into notes and diagrams to keep for revision. This gave us the idea of creating what was missing from the market at the time—an imaging-focused anatomy textbook that covered pretty much all the radiologist in training needed to know. We wanted it to be of a manageable length with simple diagrams and typical exam focussed imaging examples. That undertaking was a phenomenal amount of work; all images were from photographed radiographs, painstakingly labelled by hand with sticky arrows! The project took us over two years to complete, taking us from our radiology registrar training in Dublin through our fellowship training in the USA, with X-ray films, drawings and text being couriered over and back across the Atlantic Ocean. With young families and busy fellowships at the time we vowed 'never again!' When invited to do a second edition some ten years later, life was still very busy, families had grown further, and 'what the radiologist needed to know' had also increased. Musculoskeletal imaging had grown hugely with the evolution of MRI. At this point, having forgotten our 'never again' declaration, we invited our colleague and internationally recognised MSK expert, Stephen Eustace, to update the MSK sections for the second edition. 'Ryan, McNicholas and Eustace' became a very successful reference book for radiologists and sold thousands of copies. The book was translated into Spanish, Greek and Russian and we met radiologists from round the world who knew us from using our textbook. When we were invited to do a third edition in 2010, our family commitments had abated somewhat, and we were at the peaks of our radiology careers. With plenty of radiology and life experience under our belts, and all of us still very involved in teaching, we were delighted to draw on our collective learned experiences for the third edition. The job of updating the book a third time round, though still a lot of work, was probably more enjoyable than previous editions had been, and it was easier to collect good quality images from a national PACS (although it is still astonishingly difficult to get that 'perfect one'!). We have gotten immeasurable satisfaction over the years from seeing our colleagues use our textbook and continue to find it helpful.

Being asked to do a fourth edition 30 years after our first edition did catch us somewhat off guard. The authors were beginning to consider a chapter of life that had more to do with hiking, fishing and golf rather than writing new anatomy chapters. We decided to invite some new blood on board to freshen up the book. For the fourth edition, we have had the benefit of input from colleagues who are earlier in their careers and have more recently completed the subspecialist fellowships in areas such as neuroradiology, head and neck imaging and thoracic imaging at internationally recognised academic centres. We have also gone 'back to the beginning' and invited some of our very recently trained colleagues to help update several chapters. The result is a collaboration of the young and enthusiastic radiologists who very much understand what is required by examiners, and the recently highly trained subspecialists in their early careers as consultants, with the original experienced radiology teachers at the editorial helm.

Since the first edition 30 years ago, there has been an explosion in imaging, both anatomic and functional. Interventional radiology continues to forge ahead in importance and scope, daring to go where no person has gone before! Techniques have come and gone and come back again. We stated that lymphography was 'long since' gone in the preface to the last edition. Now we have added a new section on lymphatic anatomy, as interest in lymphography has been reborn following new interventional radiology possibilities. Of course, the anatomy will always stay the same, but how imagers and interventionalists interact with it, and even how they understand it, continually evolves.

This latest edition has over 200 new images and diagrams and a new all colour format. There is emphasis on important anatomic detail by subspecialist authors bringing the latest edition completely up to date. *Anatomy for Diagnostic Imaging* has been a labour of love that has bookended radiology careers of its original authors and is something that we have been hugely proud of. With the new crew on board, we hope that there will be enthusiasm to continue to keep the book up to date as imaging continues to evolve over the next decade and beyond. It will certainly be in the best of hands. It has been fun. For me anyway!

Michelle McNicholas

Acknowledgements

As for the first three editions, we would like to acknowledge the help of many people in collecting the images for the new edition. In particular, we are grateful to our radiology and radiography colleagues at Mater Misericordiae University Hospital, Temple Street Hospital/Children's Health Ireland, Beaumont Hospital, St James's Hospital, Cappagh National Orthopaedic Hospital and St Vincent's University Hospital.

We continue to be grateful to the legendary late Professor JB Coakley, Professor Emeritus of Anatomy at Trinity College Dublin, whose simple but excellent line drawings live on in our textbook, now with added colour!

Professor Calvin Coffey of University Hospital Limerick was generous in sharing his work on a new understanding of the development of the mesentery, now included in *Gray's Anatomy 42e*, Elsevier, 2023.

A huge 'thank you' to our new contributors, Terence, Danielle, Barry, John, Emma, Jack and Phil.

We are grateful to our editors Taranpreet Kaur and Trinity Hutton of Elsevier who supported us throughout the project.

Finally, we are grateful to our families, who are very important to us all. They will be very happy that we are finally finished with 'The Book' again.

1 *Head and Neck*

DANIELLE BYRNE
EDITED BY STEPHANIE RYAN

CHAPTER CONTENTS

The Skull and Facial Bones 1
The Nasal Cavity and Paranasal
Sinuses 12
The Mandible and Teeth 14
The Orbital Contents 18
The Ear 22
The Upper Aerodigestive Tract 23
The Neck Lymph Node Levels 38

Layers of the Deep Cervical Fascia 41
Deep Spaces of the Head and Neck 42
The Salivary Glands 45
Radiology of the Salivary Glands 47
The Thyroid and Parathyroid Glands 48
The Neck Vessels 50
The Brachial Plexus 56

The Skull and Facial Bones

The skull consists of the calvarium, facial bones and mandible. The calvarium is the brain case and comprises the skull vault and skull base. The bones of the calvarium and face are joined at immovable fibrous joints, except for the temporomandibular joint, which is a movable cartilaginous joint.

THE SKULL VAULT (FIGS. 1.1–1.4)

The skull vault is made up of several flat bones, joined at sutures, which can be recognized on skull radiographs. The bones consist of the diploic space – a cancellous layer containing vascular spaces – sandwiched between the inner and outer tables of cortical bone. The skull is covered by periosteum, which is continuous with the fibrous tissue in the sutures. The periosteum is called the pericranium externally and on the deep surface of the skull it is called the endosteum. The endosteum is the outer layer of the dura. The diploic veins within the skull are large, valveless vessels with thin walls. They communicate with the meningeal veins, the dural sinuses and the scalp veins.

The paired parietal bones form much of the side and the roof of the skull and are joined in the midline at the sagittal suture. Parietal foramina are paired foramina or areas of thin bone close to the midline in the parietal bones. They are often visible on a radiograph, may be big and may even be palpable. They may transmit emissary veins from the sagittal sinus. The frontal bone forms the front of the skull vault. It is formed by two frontal bones that unite at the metopic suture. The frontal bones join the parietal bones at the coronal suture. The junction of coronal and sagittal sutures is known as the **bregma**. The occipital bone forms the back of the skull vault and is joined to the parietal bones at the lambdoid suture. The lambdoid and sagittal sutures join at a point known as the **lambda**.

The greater wing of sphenoid and the squamous part of the temporal bone form the side of the skull vault below the frontal and parietal bones. The sutures formed here are: (1) the sphenosquamosal suture between the sphenoid and temporal bones; (2) the sphenofrontal and sphenoparietal sutures between the greater wing of the sphenoid and frontal and parietal bones; and (3) the squamosal suture between the temporal and parietal bones. The sphenofrontal, sphenoparietal and squamosal sutures form a continuous curved line (see Fig. 1.1). The intersection of the sutures between the frontal, sphenoidal, parietal and temporal bones is termed the **pterion** and provides a surface marking for the anterior branch of the middle meningeal artery on the lateral skull radiograph. The **asterion** is the point where the squamosal suture meets the lambdoid suture.

The parietal and occipital bones develop from multiple ossification centres and may have **accessory sutures**, particularly in childhood, that can persist into adulthood. An accessory intraparietal suture may extend superolaterally from the lambdoid suture into the parietal bone. Mendosal sutures in the occipital bone extend for a variable distance superomedially from the inferior part of the lambdoid sutures. An intraoccipital accessory suture may be seen crossing horizontally just above the foramen magnum.

RADIOLOGY PEARL

Accessory sutures, more common in children, should not be mistaken for skull fractures. Accessory sutures, compared with fractures, can be seen on computed tomography (CT) to have a zig-zag configuration with sclerotic borders, to arise from but not cross suture lines, and are often bilateral and symmetrical.

THE SKULL BASE (FIGS. 1.5, 1.6)

The inner aspect of the skull base is made up of the following bones from anterior to posterior:
- The orbital plates of the frontal bone, with the cribriform plate of the ethmoid bone and crista galli in the midline
- The sphenoid bone with its lesser wings anteriorly forming the posterior part of the floor of the anterior cranial fossa, the greater wings posteriorly forming the anterior part of the floor of the middle cranial fossa. The body of the sphenoid bone with the elevated sella turcica is in the midline

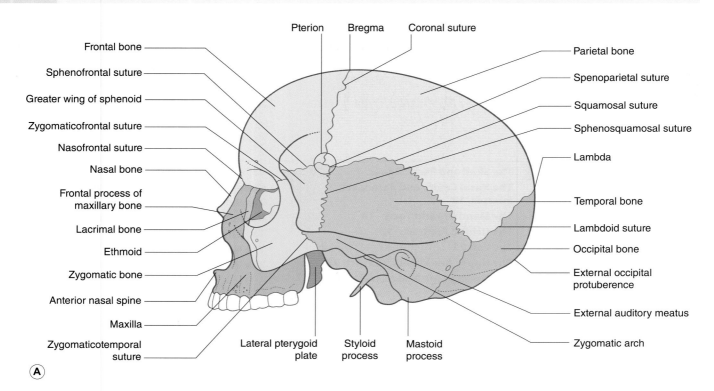

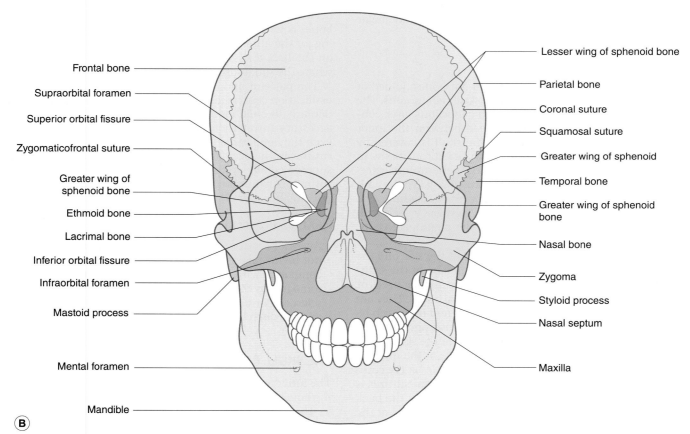

Fig. 1.1 (A) Lateral view of the skull. (B) Frontal view of the skull.

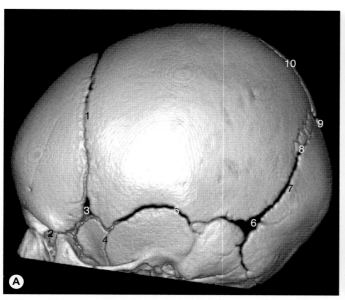 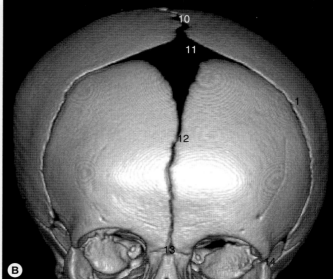

Fig. 1.2 Three-dimensional computed tomography scan of the skull of a 2-month-old infant to show sutures. (A) Lateral and (B) anterior views.

1. Coronal suture
2. Zygomaticofrontal suture
3. Pterion
4. Sphenotemporal (sphenosquamosal) suture
5. Temporoparietal (squamosal) suture
6. Asterion
7. Lambdoid suture

8. Wormian bones
9. Lambda
10. Sagittal suture
11. Anterior fontanelle
12. Metopic suture
13. Nasofrontal suture
14. Zygomaticofrontal suture

- Part of the squamous temporal bone and the petrous temporal bone, and
- The occipital bone

INDIVIDUAL BONES OF THE SKULL BASE

The **orbital plates of the frontal bones** are thin and irregular, and separate the anterior cranial fossa from the orbital cavity.

The **cribriform plate** of the ethmoid bone is a thin, depressed bone separating the anterior cranial fossa from the nasal cavity. It has a superior perpendicular projection, the crista galli, which is continuous below with the nasal septum on the frontal skull radiograph (see Fig. 1.4).

The sphenoid bone consists of a body and greater and lesser wings, which curve laterally from the body and join at the sharply posteriorly angulated sphenoid ridge. The body houses the sphenoid sinuses and is grooved laterally by the carotid sulcus, in which the cavernous sinus and carotid artery run. The sphenoid body has a deep fossa superiorly (Figs. 1.7 and 2.14) known as the **sella turcica** or **pituitary fossa**, which houses the pituitary gland. On the anterior part of the sella is a prominence known as the **tuberculum sellae**; anterior to this is a groove called the **sulcus chiasmaticus**, which leads to the optic canal on each side. The optic chiasm lies over this sulcus. Two bony projections on either side of the front of the sella are called the **anterior clinoid processes**. The posterior part of the sella is called the **dorsum sellae**, and this is continuous posteriorly with

the **clivus**. Two posterior projections of the dorsum sellae form the **posterior clinoid processes**. The floor of the sella is formed by a thin bone known as the **lamina dura**, which may be eroded by raised intracranial pressure or tumours of the pituitary.

The **temporal bone** consists of four parts:
- A flat **squamous** part, which forms part of the vault and part of the skull base
- A pyramidal **petrous** part, which houses the middle and inner ears and forms part the boundary between the middle and posterior cranial fossae
- An aerated **mastoid** part, and
- An inferior projection known as the **styloid process**

The **zygomatic process** projects from the outer side of the squamous temporal bone and is continuous with the zygomatic process of the zygoma to form the zygomatic arch.

The curved occipital bone forms part of the skull vault and posterior part of the skull base. It has the **foramen magnum** in the midline, through which the cranial cavity is continuous with the spinal canal. Anterolaterally it is continuous with the posterior part of the petrous bones on each side, and anterior to the foramen magnum it forms the clivus. The clivus is continuous anteriorly with the dorsum sellae. Thus the occipital bone articulates with both the temporal and sphenoid bones. The occipital condyles for articulation with the atlas vertebra project from the inferior surface of the occipital bone lateral to the anterior half of the foramen magnum.

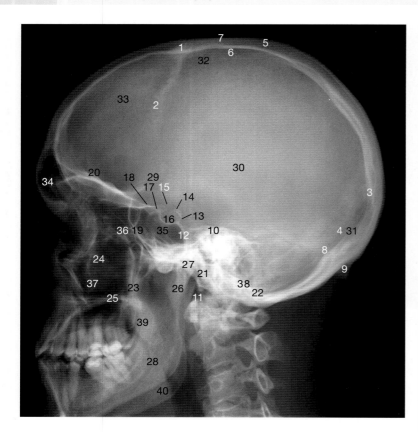

Fig. 1.3 Lateral skull radiograph.

Bony landmarks
1. Bregma
2. Coronal suture
3. Lambda
4. Lambdoid suture
5. Vertex
6. Inner skull table
7. Outer skull table
8. Internal occipital protuberance
9. External occipital protuberance
10. External auditory meatus
11. Styloid process
12. Clivus
13. Dorsum sellae
14. Posterior clinoid process
15. Anterior clinoid process
16. Pituitary fossa (sella turcica)
17. Tuberculum sellae
18. Planum sphenoidale
19. Greater wings of sphenoid
20. Undulating floor of anterior cranial fossa (roof of orbit)
21. Anterior limit of foramen magnum
22. Posterior limit of foramen magnum
23. Posterior wall of maxillary sinus
24. Floor of orbit
25. Hard palate
26. Neck of mandible
27. Temporomandibular joint
28. Condylar (mandibular) canal

Vascular markings
29. Middle meningeal vessels: anterior branches
30. Middle meningeal vessels: posterior branches
31. Transverse sinus
32. Diploic vein
33. Diploic venous confl uence: parietal star

Sinuses/air cells
34. Frontal sinus
35. Sphenoid sinus
36. Posterior ethmoidal cells
37. Maxillary sinus
38. Mastoid air cells

Soft tissues
39. Soft palate
40. Base of tongue

CRANIAL FOSSAE (SEE FIG. 1.5)

The anterior cranial fossa is limited posteriorly by the sphenoid ridge and anterior clinoid processes, and supports the frontal lobes of the brain.

The middle cranial fossa is limited anteriorly by the sphenoid ridge and anterior clinoid processes. Its posterior boundary is formed laterally by the petrous ridges and in the midline by the posterior clinoid processes and dorsum sellae. It contains the temporal lobes of the brain, the pituitary gland and most of the foramina of the skull base.

The posterior cranial fossa is the largest and deepest fossa. Anteriorly it is limited by the dorsum sellae and the petrous ridge, and it is demarcated posteriorly on the skull radiograph by the groove for the transverse sinus. It contains the cerebellum posteriorly, and anteriorly the pons and medulla lie on the clivus and are continuous, through the foramen magnum, with the spinal cord.

FORAMINA OF THE SKULL BASE (SEE FIGS. 1.5, 1.6; TABLE 1.1)

The **optic canals** run from the sulcus chiasmaticus anterior to the tuberculum sellae, anteroinferolaterally to the orbital apex. They transmit the optic nerves and ophthalmic arteries. The optic canals are wider posteriorly than anteriorly.

> **RADIOLOGY PEARL**
>
> The close proximity of the optic canal to the sphenoid sinus is important in planning paranasal sinus surgery.

The **superior orbital fissure** is a triangular defect between the greater and lesser wings of the sphenoid. It transmits the first (orbital) division of the fifth cranial nerve, and the third, fourth and sixth cranial nerves, along with

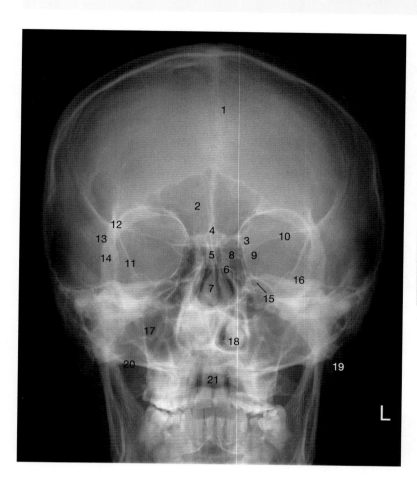

Fig. 1.4 Occipitofrontal (OF) 20 skull radiograph.

1. Sagittal suture
2. Frontal sinus
3. Planum sphenoidale
4. Crista galli
5. Perpendicular plate of ethmoid
6. Floor of pituitary fossa
7. Nasal septum
8. Ethmoid air cells
9. Superior orbital fissure
10. Lesser wing of sphenoid
11. Innominate line
12. Zygomatic process of frontal bone
13. Zygomaticofrontal suture
14. Frontal process of zygomatic bone
15. Foramen rotundum
16. Petrous ridge
17. Maxillary sinus
18. Inferior nasal turbinate
19. Mastoid process
20. Occipital bone
21. Dens of atlas

the superior orbital vein and a branch of the middle meningeal artery from the middle cranial fossa to the orbital apex. This fissure is best seen on the OF20 view (occipitofrontal view with 20 degrees caudal angulation) and on CTs of the orbit (see Fig. 1.4 and later Fig. 1.10).

The **foramen rotundum** is posterior to the superior orbital fissure in the greater wing of the sphenoid. It runs from the middle cranial fossa to the pterygopalatine fossa and transmits the second (maxillary) division of the fifth cranial nerve. It is seen on the OF20 view (see Fig. 1.4) and also on CT scans (see Fig. 1.6). See also 'The infratemporal space and the pterygopalatine fossa' section (see later Fig. 1.36) for this and **sphenopalatine foramen** and **greater palatine foramen**.

The **foramen ovale** is posterolateral to the foramen rotundum in the greater wing of the sphenoid. It runs from the middle cranial fossa to the infratemporal fossa and transmits the third (mandibular) division of the fifth cranial nerve and the accessory meningeal artery.

The **foramen spinosum**, posterolateral to the foramen rotundum, is a small foramen and transmits the middle meningeal artery from the infratemporal to the middle cranial fossa.

The **foramen lacerum** is a ragged bony canal posteromedial to the foramen ovale at the apex of the petrous bone. The internal carotid artery passes through its posterior wall, having emerged from the carotid canal (which runs in the petrous bone), before turning upwards to run in the carotid sulcus.

The **internal auditory meatus (IAM) and canal** run from the posterior cranial fossa through the posterior wall of the petrous bone into the inner ear. They transmit the seventh and eighth cranial nerves and the internal auditory artery. The **jugular foramen** is an irregular opening situated at the posterior end of the junction of the occipital and petrous bones. It runs downward and medially from the posterior cranial fossa and transmits the internal jugular vein lateral to the ninth, tenth and eleventh cranial nerves. It also transmits the inferior petrosal sinus (which drains into the internal jugular vein), and ascending occipital and pharyngeal arterial branches.

The **hypoglossal canal** is anterior to the foramen magnum and medial to the jugular fossa and transmits the twelfth (hypoglossal) cranial nerve.

The **foramen magnum** runs from the posterior cranial fossa to the spinal canal and transmits the medulla oblongata, which is continuous with the spinal cord, along with the vertebral and spinal arteries and veins and the spinal root of the eleventh cranial nerve.

THE NEONATAL AND GROWING SKULL (SEE FIG. 1.2)

At birth there may be overlapping of the cranial bones due to moulding; this disappears over several days. The diploic space is not developed, vascular markings are not visible and the sinuses are not aerated. The sutures are straight lines, the fontanelles are open and multiple small Wormian bones may be

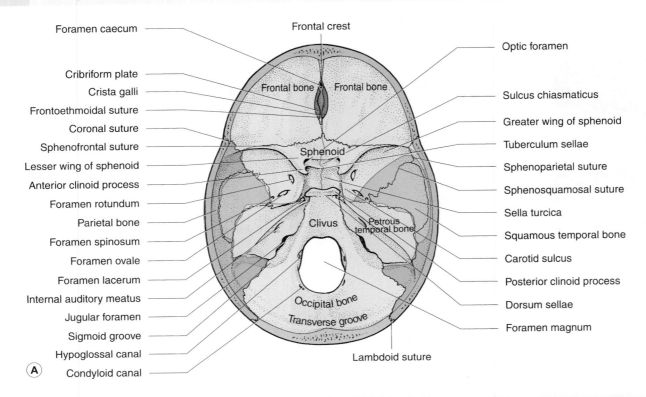

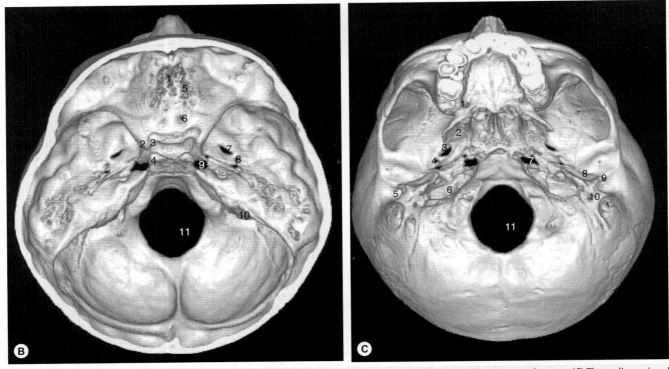

Fig. 1.5 (A) The skull base: internal aspect. (B) Three-dimensional computed tomography scan of the skull base, internal aspect. (C) Three-dimensional computed tomography of the skull base, inferior view.

(B)
1. Crista galli
2. Anterior clinoid process
3. Optic canal
4. Posterior clinoid process
5. Cribriform plate
6. Posterior ethmoidal foramen
7. Foramen ovale
8. Foramen spinosum
9. Foramen lacerum
10. Jugular foramen
11. Foramen magnum

(C)
1. Greater palatine foramen
2. Pterygoid plate
3. Foramen ovale
4. Foramen spinosum
5. External acoustic foramen
6. Jugular fossa
7. Foramen lacerum
8. Groove for pharyngotympanic tube
9. Styloid process
10. Stylomastoid foramen
11. Foramen magnum

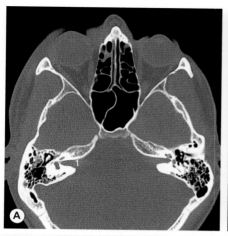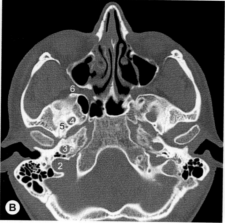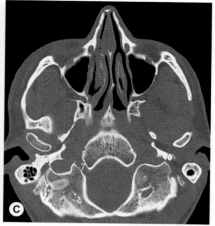

Fig. 1.6 Skull base foramina. (A) At the level of the internal auditory foramina. (B) At the level of the jugular foramen. (C) At the level of the foramen magnum.

1. Right internal auditory meatus
2. Right jugular foramen
3. Right carotid canal
4. Right foramen ovale

5. Right foramen spinosum
6. Right pterygopalatine fossa
7. Right hypoglossal canal

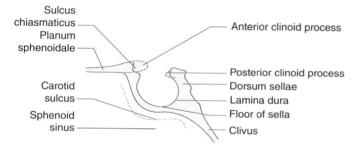

Fig. 1.7 The pituitary fossa: lateral view.

seen. The skull vault is approximately eight times the size of the facial bones on the lateral skull radiograph in a newborn compared with a ratio of 2.5 to 1 in an adult.

The posterior fontanelle closes by 6–8 months of age and the anterior fontanelle is usually closed by 15–18 months. Two pairs of lateral fontanelles close in the second or third month.

RADIOLOGY PEARL

Lateral and posterior fontanelles offer alternative access points for ultrasound of the infant brain in the first few months of life.

By 6 months the sutures have narrowed to 3 mm or less. They begin to interlock in the first year and have begun to assume the serrated appearance of the adult sutures by 2 years of age. By this time the diploic space has begun to develop and the middle meningeal and convolutional markings start to appear. The convolutional markings may be very prominent but become less so after the age of 10 years and eventually disappear in early adulthood.

The fastest period of growth of the skull vault is the first year, and adult proportions are almost attained by the age of 7

years. Growth of the facial bones is more rapid than that of the skull vault, being fastest during the first 7 years with a further growth spurt at puberty. Thereafter growth is slower until the facial bones occupy a similar volume to the cranium.

Sutures are essentially fused in the second decade, but complete bony fusion occurs in the third decade.

In old age the cranium becomes thinner, and the maxilla and mandible shrink with the loss of dentition and the resorption of the alveolar processes.

CALCIFICATION ON THE SKULL RADIOGRAPH IN THE NORMAL PERSON (SEE ALSO CHAPTER 2)

The **pineal gland** is a midline structure situated behind the third ventricle and is calcified in 50% of adults over 20 years and in most elderly subjects.

The **habenular commissure**, just anterior to the pineal gland, often calcifies in association with it, in a C-shaped curve with its concavity towards the pineal gland.

The **glomus of the choroid plexus** in the atria of the lateral ventricles is frequently calcified. The degree of calcification is variable, but calcification is usually symmetrical and bilateral.

Dural calcification may occur anywhere but is frequently seen in the falx and tentorium cerebelli. The petroclinoid and interclinoid ligaments are dural reflections that run from the petrous apex to the dorsum sellae and between the anterior and posterior clinoid processes. These may also calcify, especially in the elderly.

The **arachnoid granulations** may also calcify, usually close to the vault along the line of the superior longitudinal venous sinus.

The **basal ganglia** and **dentate nucleus** may show punctate calcification in asymptomatic individuals; again this is more frequent with increasing age.

The **internal carotid artery** may be calcified in the elderly, especially in the region of the siphon.

The **lens of the eye** may be calcified in the elderly.

Table 1.1   Foramina of the Skull Base

		Comment	Transmits
Optic canals	Sphenoid bone	Middle cranial fossa to orbital apex	Optic nerves and ophthalmic arteries
Superior orbital fissure	Sphenoid bone	From the middle cranial fossa to the orbital apex	First (orbital) division of the fifth, and the third, fourth and sixth cranial nerves, superior orbital vein and a branch of the middle meningeal artery
Inferior orbital fissure	Between maxilla and sphenoid bones	At its posterior part it forms an opening between the orbit and the pterygopalatine fossa, and more anteriorly between the orbital cavity and the infratemporal fossa	Infraorbital nerve and infraorbital artery and the inferior ophthalmic veins
Foramen rotundum	Sphenoid bone	From the middle cranial fossa to the pterygopalatine fossa	Second (maxillary) division of the fifth cranial nerve
Foramen ovale	Sphenoid bone	From the middle cranial fossa to the infratemporal fossa	Third (mandibular) division of the fifth cranial nerve and the accessory meningeal artery
Foramen spinosum	Sphenoid bone	From the infratemporal to the middle cranial fossa	The middle meningeal artery
Foramen lacerum	Apex of temporal bone		Carotid artery passes through its posterior wall
IAM	Petrous temporal bone	From the posterior cranial fossa to inner ear	Seventh and eighth cranial nerves and the internal auditory artery
Jugular foramen	Junction of occipital and petrous temporal bones	Not visible on SMV	Internal jugular vein, ninth, tenth and eleventh cranial nerves. Inferior petrosal sinus (which drains into the internal jugular vein), and ascending occipital and pharyngeal arterial branches
Hypoglossal canal	Occipital bone		12th (hypoglossal) cranial nerve
Foramen magnum	Occipital bone	From the posterior cranial fossa to the spinal canal	Medulla oblongata/spinal cord, along vertebral and spinal arteries and veins, and the spinal root of the 11th cranial nerve

SMV, Submentovertical.

RADIOLOGICAL FEATURES OF THE SKULL BASE AND VAULT (SEE FIGS. 1.2–1.6)

Plain Films

Several radiographic projections can be used to assess the skull vault. The standard projections are lateral, occipitofrontal view with 20-degree caudal angulation (OF20) and Towne's projections (fronto-occipital projection with 30-degree caudal angulation). The submentovertical projection is a view of the skull base. Views for facial bones and sinuses also include occipitomental (OM) and OM with 30-degree cranial angulation (OM30) views. Skull and sinus radiographs are seldom used now outside of paediatric practice and have been widely replaced by CT. Skull X-rays still have a role in paediatrics for assessment of the skull configuration; for example in craniosynostosis – abnormal fusion of some of the skull sutures – and in assessment of bone dysplasias that affect the skull.

> **RADIOLOGY PEARL**
>
> Sphenoidal electrodes used in electroencephalogram (EEG) for better recording of activity in the temporal lobe are inserted between the zygoma and the mandibular notch of the mandible and advanced until the tip lies just lateral to the foramen ovale. Its position here is checked by SMV view of the skull.

> **RADIOLOGY PEARL**
>
> The degree of pneumatization of sphenoid sinus has implications for trans-sphenoidal pituitary surgery.

> **RADIOLOGY PEARL**
>
> Elongation of the pituitary fossa with a prominent sulcus chiasmaticus is variously known as a 'J-shaped', 'omega' or 'hour-glass' sella and is a normal variant in 5% of children.

Computed Tomography

CT provides excellent visualization of the skull vault, the skull base and foramina. The **middle meningeal vessels** form a prominent groove on the inner table of the skull vault, running superiorly from the foramen spinosum across the squamous temporal bone before dividing into anterior and posterior branches.

The **diploic markings** are larger irregular less well-defined venous channels running in the diploic space. They are very variable in appearance, but a stellate confluence is often seen on the parietal bone.

The **dural sinuses** are wide channels, many of which groove the inner table of the skull vault.

The **supraorbital artery** grooves the outer table of the frontal bone as it runs superiorly from the orbit, and the **superficial temporal artery** grooves the outer table of the temporal and parietal bones, running superiorly from the region of the external auditory meatus on the lateral projection.

The **arachnoid granulation pits** are small irregular impressions on the inner table related to the superior sagittal sinus (see Chapter 2).

The major **sutures** have been described. The **metopic suture** between the two halves of the frontal bone normally disappears by 2 years of age, but persists into adulthood in approximately 10% of people and may be incomplete. If the metopic suture persists the frontal sinuses are not developed. The **spheno-occipital synchondrosis** is the suture between the anterior part of the occipital bone and the sphenoid body. This usually fuses at puberty but may persist into adulthood and be mistaken for a fracture of the skull base on the lateral skull radiograph. An **intraoccipital** suture or **mendosal suture (accessory occipital suture)** are often seen extending from the lambdoid suture and should not be mistaken for fractures.

Wormian bones are small bony islands that may be seen in suture lines and at sutural junctions, particularly in relation to the lambdoid suture. These are greater in number in infants and reduce in number as they become incorporated into adjacent bone.

The thickness of the skull vault is not uniform. The parietal convexities may be markedly thinned and appear radiolucent. Also, marked focal thickening may be seen, particularly in the region of the frontal bone in the normal person. The inner and outer tables are thickened at the internal and external occipital protuberances. The external protuberance and muscular attachments of the occipital bone may be very prominent in the male skull.

Magnetic Resonance Imaging

Magnetic resonance imaging (MRI) with narrow section thickness slices is excellent for demonstration of the soft-tissue contents of the foramina of the skull, in particular the cranial nerves. The plane of imaging can be chosen to demonstrate the structure of interest: for example, imaging in several planes is necessary to demonstrate the course of the facial nerve through the skull base from its entry into the internal auditory canal to its exit through the stylomastoid foramen. Visualization of the optic foramen and its contained optic nerve is best done by coronal T2 fat-saturated images.

THE FACIAL BONES (SEE FIGS. 1.1, 1.8)

Several bones contribute to the bony skeleton of the face, including the mandible, which forms the only freely mobile joint of the skull. The maxillae, zygomata and mandible contribute most to the shape of the face, and the orbits, nose and paranasal sinuses form bony cavities contained by the facial skeleton. The individual components of the face will be described separately with reference to their radiological assessment.

THE ZYGOMA

This forms the eminence of the cheek and is also known as the malar bone. It is a thin, bony bar that articulates with the frontal, maxillary and temporal bones at the zygomaticofrontal, zygomaticomaxillary and zygomaticotemporal

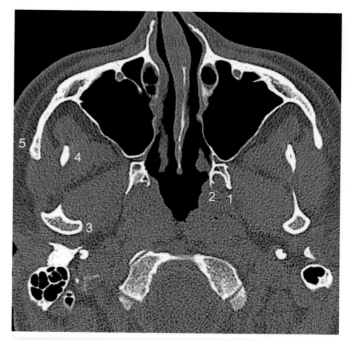

Fig. 1.8 Axial computed tomography scan of the facial bones through the maxillary sinuses.

1. Left lateral pterygoid plate
2. Left medial pterygoid plate
3. Right mandibular condyle
4. Coronoid process of the right mandible
5. Right zygomatic arch

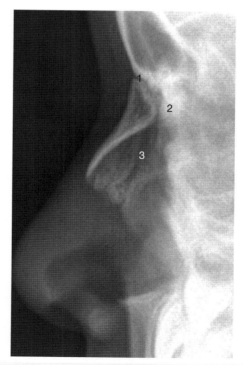

Fig. 1.9 Lateral radiograph of the nasal bones.

1. Frontonasal synchondrosis
2. Nasal spine of frontal bone
3. Groove for anterior ethmoidal nerve

sutures. Its anterior end reinforces the lateral and inferior margins of the orbital rim. The zygoma forms the lateral boundary of the **temporal fossa** above and the **infra-temporal fossa** below.

The zygoma is prone to trauma and may be assessed readily by CT.

THE NASAL BONES

The paired nasal bones are attached to each other and to the nasal spine of the frontal bone. They are grooved on their deep surface by one or more anterior ethmoidal nerves. These vertically orientated grooves can be seen on a radiograph and should not be mistaken for fractures (Fig. 1.9).

> **RADIOLOGY PEARL**
>
> Linear lucencies in the nasal bones that run vertically are grooves for the ethmoidal nerves. Horizontally orientated lucencies are likely to be fractures.

THE BONY ORBIT (FIG. 1.10)

The orbit is a four-sided pyramidal bony cavity whose skeleton is contributed to by several bones of the skull. The base of the pyramid is open and points anteriorly to form the orbital rim. Lateral, superior, medial and inferior walls converge posteromedially to an **apex**, onto which the **optic foramen** opens, transmitting the **optic nerve** and **ophthalmic artery** from the **optic canal**.

The lateral orbital wall is strong and is formed by the zygomatic bone in front and the greater wing of the sphenoid behind. It separates the orbital cavity from the temporal fossa.

The superior wall, or roof, is thin and undulating and separates the orbit from the anterior cranial fossa. It is formed by the orbital plate of the frontal bone in front and the lesser wing of the sphenoid behind.

The medial orbital wall is a thin bone contributed to by maxillary, lacrimal and ethmoid bones, with a small contribution from the sphenoid bone at the apex. It separates the orbit from the nasal cavity, ethmoid air cells and anterior part of sphenoid. The bone between the orbit and ethmoids is paper thin and is known as the **lamina papyracea**.

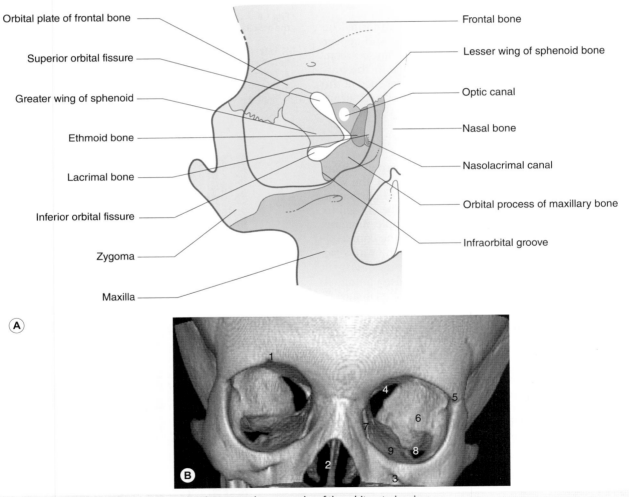

Fig. 1.10 (A) The bony orbit. (B) Three-dimensional computed tomography of the orbit, anterior view.

1. Supraorbital notch
2. Nasal septum
3. Infraorbital foramen
4. Superior orbital fissure
5. Zygomaticofrontal suture
6. Greater wing of sphenoid
7. Nasolacrimal canal
8. Lateral aspect of inferior orbital fissure
9. Orbital process of maxillary bone

The inferior wall, or floor, is formed by the orbital process of the maxillary bone, separating the orbit from the cavity of the maxillary sinus. The orbital process of the maxillary bone also extends superomedially to contribute to the medial part of the orbital rim, and the zygoma contributes to the orbital floor laterally. Near the apex there is a tiny bit of palatine bone in the orbital floor.

The orbit has a superolateral depression for the **lacrimal gland** (see later Fig. 1.24A and B) and a medial groove for the **lacrimal sac** and its **duct**. It also bears the optic foramen, two fissures and a groove in its floor to house the infraorbital nerve.

The **superior orbital fissure** is a triangular slit between the greater and lesser wings of the sphenoid. Its medial end is wider than its lateral end and is very close to the optic foramen in the apex of the cavity. It transmits the first division of the fifth, and the third, fourth and sixth cranial nerves, as well as the superior ophthalmic veins and a branch of the middle meningeal artery. The middle meningeal artery may communicate with the ophthalmic artery, forming one of the anastomotic connections between internal and external carotid systems.

The **inferior orbital** fissure is a slit between the lateral and inferior walls of the orbit as they converge on the apex. It runs downward and laterally, and its posteromedial end is close to the medial end of the superior fissure. In its posterior part it forms an opening between the orbit and the pterygopalatine fossa, and more anteriorly it forms an opening between the orbital cavity and the infratemporal fossa. It transmits the infraorbital nerve, which is a branch of the maxillary division of the fifth cranial nerve after it has passed from the middle cranial fossa into the pterygopalatine fossa via the foramen rotundum. It also transmits the infraorbital artery, a branch of the maxillary artery and the inferior ophthalmic veins.

The **infraorbital groove** runs from the inferior orbital fissure in the floor of the orbit before dipping down to become the infraorbital canal (Fig. 1.11). The nerve emerges from the canal onto the anterior surface of the maxillary bone through the infraorbital foramen.

The **periorbita** is a fibrous covering that lines the bony cavity of the orbit. It is continuous with the dura through the optic canal and superior orbital fissure. It closes over the inferior orbital fissure, separating the orbit from the infratemporal and pterygopalatine fossae.

RADIOLOGY OF THE BONY ORBIT

Plain Films

The orbits may be assessed on OF20 and OM projections (see Fig. 1.4). Asymmetry between the superior orbital fissures is common.

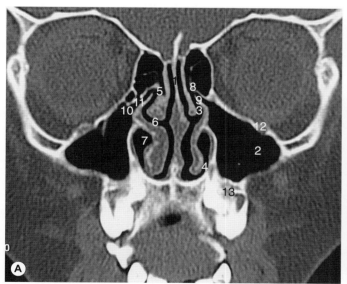 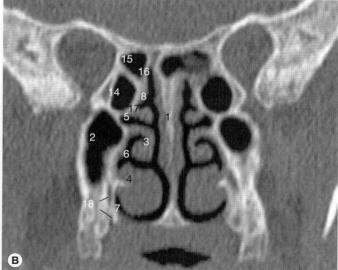

Fig. 1.11 Coronal computed tomography scan of the sinuses. (A) Coronal view at the level of the ostiomeatal complex and (B) posterior view at the level of the sphenoethmoidal recess.

1. Nasal septum
2. Maxillary sinus
3. Middle nasal turbinate
4. Inferior nasal turbinate
5. Superior meatus
6. Middle meatus
7. Inferior meatus
8. Ethmoid infundibulum
9. Uncinate process
10. Maxillary ostium
11. Maxillary infundibulum
12. Infraorbital nerve
13. Alveolar process of maxilla
14. Ethmoid sinus
15. Sphenoid sinus
16. Sphenoethmoidal recess
17. Superior turbinate
18. Greater palatine canal

A straight line is seen running through the orbit from the superolateral part of the rim inferiorly and medially. This is caused by the X-ray beam hitting the curving greater wing of the sphenoid at a tangent and is known as the **innominate line**.

Computed Tomography

The bony orbit and its soft-tissue contents are demonstrated very well by CT (see Figs. 1.10B and 1.11A). Axial or coronal images may be obtained. Coronal imaging shows the floor of the orbit and is useful for the assessment of trauma where a fracture is suspected.

Magnetic Resonance Imaging

MRI (see later Fig. 1.23) is more valuable for demonstration of the soft-tissue contents of the orbit than the bone.

The Nasal Cavity and Paranasal Sinuses (see Figs. 1.8, 1.11)

The nasal cavity is a passage from the external nose anteriorly to the nasopharynx posteriorly. The frontal, ethmoid, sphenoid and maxillary sinuses form the paired paranasal sinuses and are situated around, and drain into, the nasal cavity. The entire complex is lined by mucus-secreting epithelium.

THE NASAL CAVITY

This is divided in two by the nasal septum in the sagittal plane. The nasal septum is part bony and part cartilaginous. The floor of the nasal cavity is the roof of the oral cavity and is formed by the palatine process of the maxilla, with the palatine bone posteriorly. The lateral walls of the cavity are formed by contributions from the maxillary, palatine, lacrimal and ethmoid bones. These walls bear three curved extensions known as **turbinates** or **conchae**, which divide the cavity into inferior, middle and superior **meati**, each lying beneath the turbinate of the corresponding name. The space above the superior turbinate is the **sphenoethmoidal recess**.

- The sphenoid air cells drain into the sphenoethmoidal recess.
- The posterior group of ethmoidal air cells drain into the superior meatus.
- The frontal sinus opens in the most anterior opening of the middle meatus. The anterior ethmoidal air cells and maxillary sinus drain into the middle meatus at the hiatus semilunaris, below the ethmoid bulla.
- The nasolacrimal duct opens into the inferior meatus, draining the lacrimal secretions.

Blood Supply of the Nasal Cavity

The **sphenopalatine artery** is the terminal part of the maxillary artery. It passes with its associated nerves through the sphenopalatine foramen from the pterygopalatine fossa to the nasal cavity posterior to the superior meatus. It has medial branches to the nasal septum and lateral branches to the lateral wall of the nose and turbinates.

The **greater palatine artery** supplies some of the lower part of the nasal cavity by branches that pass through the incisive foramen in the anterior part of the hard palate.

The **superior labial branch of the facial artery** supplies some branches to the anteroinferior part of the nasal septum and the nasal alae.

Anterior and posterior ethmoidal branches of the ophthalmic artery from the internal carotid artery pass through the cribriform plate to supply the superior part of the nasal cavity.

THE PARANASAL SINUSES

The Frontal Sinuses

These lie between the inner and outer tables of the frontal bone above the nose and medial part of the orbits; they vary greatly in size and are often asymmetrical. They may extend into the orbital plate of the frontal bone.

The Ethmoid Sinuses

These consist of a labyrinth of bony cavities or cells situated between the medial walls of the orbit and the lateral walls of the upper nasal cavity. Enlargements of anterior cells towards the frontal bone are called agger nasi cells, and enlargements of posterior cells below the apex of the orbit are known as Haller's cells.

The Sphenoid Sinuses

These paired cavities in the body of the sphenoid are often incompletely separated from each other or may be subdivided further into smaller bony cells. They are so closely related to the ethmoid air cell anteriorly that it may be difficult to distinguish a boundary. The anatomical relationships of the sphenoid sinus are of considerable importance. The sella turcica, bearing the pituitary gland with the optic chiasm anteriorly, is superior. The cavernous sinus and contents run along its lateral walls. The floor of the sphenoid sinus forms the roof of the nasopharynx (see also Chapter 2, Pituitary Gland).

The Maxillary Sinuses

The maxillary sinuses, or antra, are the largest of the paranasal sinuses. They are sometimes described as having a body and four processes.

The processes comprise: (1) the **orbital process**, which extends superomedially to contribute to the medial rim of the orbit; (2) the **zygomatic process**, which is continuous with the zygomatic arch; (3) the **alveolar process**, which bears the teeth; and (4) the **palatine process**, which forms the roof of the mouth and floor of the nasal cavity.

RADIOLOGY PEARL

Little's area is a vascular region of mucosa in the anterior and inferior part of the nasal septum supplied by branches of the sphenopalatine, greater palatine and facial arteries. This is a common site of anterior epistaxis.

The body of the maxilla is roughly pyramidal in shape, with its apex projecting superomedially between the orbit and nasal cavity. It houses the maxillary sinus. It has an anterior surface that is directed downward and laterally and forms part of the contour of the cheek. It has a curved infratemporal or posterior surface, and this also forms the anterior wall of the infratemporal fossa. Its orbital or superior surface is smooth and triangular and separates the sinus from the orbital cavity. The nasal or medial surface forms the lateral wall of the lower part of the nasal cavity, onto whose middle meatus the sinus drains. The medial wall of the sinus is continued superiorly as a bony projection known as the **uncinate process**. The maxillary **ostium** opens superiorly into the **infundibulum**, which is the channel between the inferomedial aspect of the orbit laterally and the uncinate process medially. The region of the ostium, infundibulum and middle meatus is important clinically and is known as the **ostiomeatal complex**.

Development of the Paranasal Sinuses in Infants and Children

The **maxillary sinuses** are the first to appear and are visible radiologically from a few weeks after birth. They continue to grow and develop throughout childhood. The tooth-bearing alveolar process does not begin to develop until the age of 6 years. Full pneumatization of the maxillary sinus is not achieved until there has been complete eruption of the permanent dentition in early adulthood.

The **frontal sinuses** are not visible on the skull radiograph until the age of 2 years and achieve adult proportions by the age of 14 years. Asymmetry is common, and one or both may fail to develop. Absence of both may be associated with persistence of the metopic suture between the two halves of the frontal bone.

Development of the **ethmoids** occurs parallel to that of the frontal sinuses.

Pneumatization of the **sphenoid sinus** commences at 3 years of age and may extend into the greater wings of the sphenoid or clinoid processes. The degree of pneumatization is variable and relevant to trans-sphenoidal hypophysectomy.

> **RADIOLOGY PEARL**
>
> During fundoscopic ethmoidal sinus surgery (FESS) the anterior ethmoidal artery is considered unprotected and at risk of injury if there are pneumatized supraorbital anterior ethmoid air cells. The anterior ethmoidal arteries are considered protected if adjacent to the lateral lamella or fovea ethmoidalis in the absence of supraorbital pneumatized anterior ethmoid air cells (see Fig. 1.12A and B).

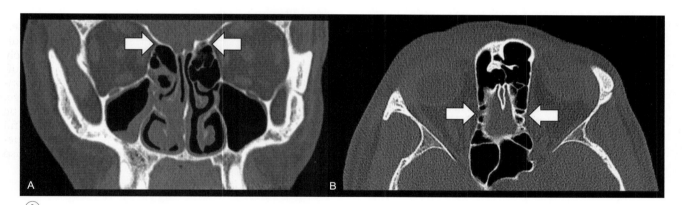

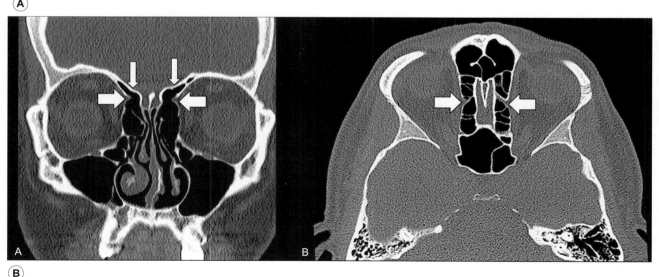

Fig. 1.12 A, Protected anterior ethmoidal arteries. Axial (A) and coronal (B) images in a patient with bilateral protected anterior ethmoidal arteries showing the anterior ethmoidal notch (thick white arrows). The anterior ethmoidal arteries are considered protected if adjacent to the lateral lamella or fovea ethmoidalis in the absence of supra-orbital pneumatized anterior ethmoid air cells. B, Unprotected anterior ethmoidal arteries Axial (A) and coronal (B) images in a patient with bilateral unprotected anterior ethmoidal arteries showing the anterior ethmoidal notch (thick white arrows) and pneumatized supra-orbital anterior ethmoid cells (thin white arrows). During fundoscopic ethmoidal sinus surgery (FESS) the anterior ethmoidal artery is considered unprotected and at risk of injury if there are pneumatized supra-orbital anterior ethmoid air cells.

RADIOLOGY OF THE NASAL CAVITY AND PARANASAL SINUSES

Computed Tomography (see Figs. 1.8, 1.11)

CT scanning in axial and, more importantly, coronal planes provides excellent visualization of the paranasal sinuses (see Fig. 1.11). Particular attention is paid to the region of the ostiomeatal complex, where the maxillary, frontal and anterior ethmoidal sinuses drain, and the sphenoethmoid recess and superior meatus, into which the sphenoid and posterior ethmoid sinuses drain. The pneumatized sinuses should contain nothing but air.

Magnetic Resonance Imaging

MRI is good at demonstrating the sinuses, as the bony septa, which have no signal themselves, are lined by high-signal mucosa on T_2 scans.

RADIOLOGY PEARL

Embolization for epistaxis: When cautery of the bleeding area and nasal packing and other surgical methods fail to control epistaxis, embolization may be successful. Angiographic assessment of the facial, sphenopalatine and greater palatine branches of the external carotid circulation is most likely to identify the source of bleeding. The ethmoidal branches of the ophthalmic artery may also need to be visualized and embolized. In all vessels, the microcatheter to be used for embolization must be advanced distal to branches with a high potential for dangerous anastomotic collaterals, such as the middle meningeal or ophthalmic arteries. Embolization of the superior labial branch of the facial artery may be associated with necrosis of the nasal alae.

The Mandible and Teeth (see Figs. 1.13–1.19)

THE MANDIBLE (SEE FIG. 1.13)

The mandible is composed of two halves united at the **symphysis menti**. Each half comprises a horizontal body and a vertical ramus joined at the **angle** of the mandible. The ramus has two superior projections, the **coronoid process** anteriorly and the **condylar process** posteriorly, separated by the **mandibular** (or **condylar**) **notch**. The coronoid process gives attachment to the temporalis muscle, and the condylar process (or head of mandible) articulates with the base of the skull at the temporomandibular joint. The body of the mandible bears the **alveolar border** with its 16 tooth sockets.

The **mandibular canal** runs in the ramus and body of the bone, transmitting the inferior alveolar artery (branch of the maxillary artery) and nerve (branch of the mandibular division of the trigeminal nerve). The mandibular canal opens proximally as the **mandibular foramen** on the inner surface of the upper ramus, and its distal opening is the **mental foramen** on the external surface of the body below and between the two premolars.

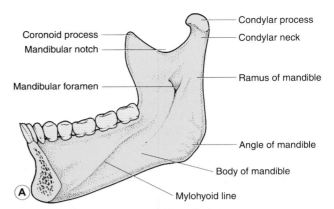

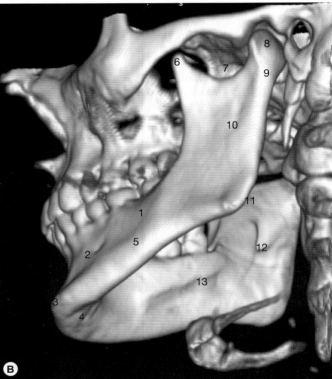

Fig. 1.13 The mandible. (A) Inner aspect. (B) Three-dimensional computed tomography scan.

(B)
1. Oblique line
2. Mental foramen
3. Mental protuberance
4. Mental tubercle
5. Body of mandible
6. Coronoid process
7. Mandibular notch
8. Condylar process
9. Neck
10. Ramus
11. Angle
12. Mandibular foramen
13. Mylohyoid line

The muscles of the floor of the mouth, including the medial pterygoid muscles, are attached to the inner surface of the mandible and the muscles of mastication are attached to its outer surface.

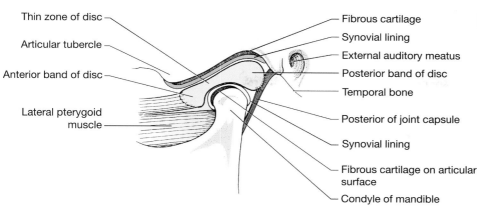

Thin zone of disc

Articular tubercle

Anterior band of disc

Lateral pterygoid muscle

Fibrous cartilage

Synovial lining

External auditory meatus

Posterior band of disc

Temporal bone

Posterior of joint capsule

Synovial lining

Fibrous cartilage on articular surface

Condyle of mandible

Fig. 1.14 The temporomandibular joint.

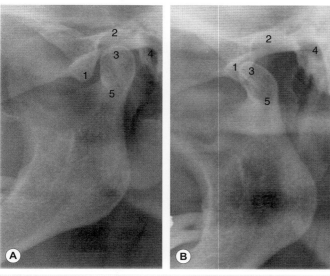

Fig. 1.15 Radiographs of the temporomandibular joint. (A) Closed mouth and (B) open mouth views.

1. Articular tubercle
2. Temporomandibular fossa
3. Head
4. External auditory meatus
5. Neck

THE TEMPOROMANDIBULAR JOINT (SEE FIGS. 1.14–1.16)

This is a synovial joint between the condyle of the mandible and the temporal bone. The temporal articular surface consists of a fossa posteriorly, the **temporomandibular fossa**, and a prominence anteriorly, the **articular tubercle**. The head of the mandible sits in the fossa at rest and glides anteriorly on to the articular tubercle when fully open. The joint is least stable during occlusion.

The articular surfaces are covered with fibrous cartilage. In addition, a fibrocartilaginous disc divides the joint into separate smaller upper and larger lower compartments, each lined by a synovial membrane. The disc is described as having **anterior** and **posterior bands** with a **thin zone** in the middle and is attached to the joint capsule. The anterior band is also attached to the lateral pterygoid muscle. The posterior band is attached to the temporal bone by bands of fibres called the translational zone. No communication between joint compartments is possible unless the disc is damaged. The upper compartment is involved in translational movements and the lower in rotational movements.

THE TEETH: NOMENCLATURE AND ANATOMY (SEE FIGS. 1.17–1.19)

There are 20 deciduous or milk teeth; in the adult these are replaced by 32 permanent teeth. The complement of teeth in each quadrant is as follows:

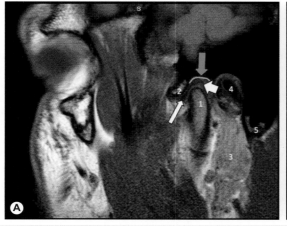
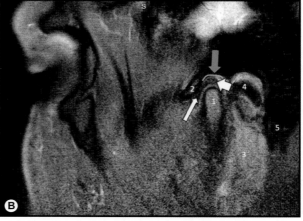

Fig. 1.16 (A) Sagittal T1 and (B) PD images of the left TMJ (closed). Thin white arrow: Anterior band of disc. Block white arrow: Posterior band of disc. Green arrow and line: Mandibular fossa of the temporal bone.

1. Mandibular condyle
2. Articular tubercle/eminence
3. Parotid gland
4. External auditory canal
5. Mastoid process of the temporal bone

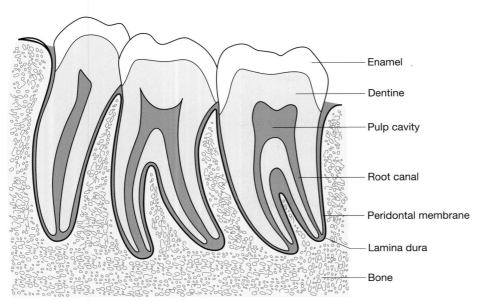

Enamel

Dentine

Pulp cavity

Root canal

Peridontal membrane

Lamina dura

Bone

Fig. 1.17 (A) The structure of teeth, adult.
(B) A radiograph of the teeth, adult.

1. Bone
2. Lamina dura
3. Periodontal membrane
4. Root canal
5. Pulp cavity
6. Dentine
7. Enamel

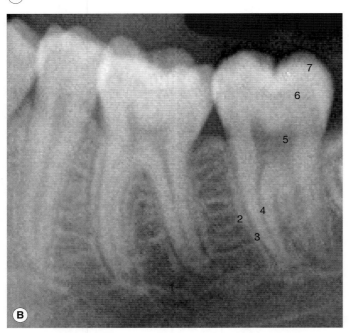

- In the child: two incisors, one canine, two molars and
- In the adult: two incisors, one canine, two premolars, three molars

The teeth are referred to by their position in each of the four quadrants. The relevant quadrant is designated by two arms of a cross, and the tooth by its position relative to the midline. The permanent teeth are referred to by number and the milk teeth by capital letter. Thus the second right lower premolar in the adult is designated 5 and the second left upper molar in a child's milk dentition is designated E.

Each tooth has its own **root** embedded in a separate socket. The **neck** of the tooth is covered by the firm fibrous tissue of the gum, and this is covered by the mucous membrane of the mouth. The exposed intraoral part of the tooth is the **crown**, and this is covered by enamel, which is the hardest and most radio-opaque substance in the body. The remainder of the tooth is composed mostly of dentine, which is of a radiographic density similar to compact bone. A radiolucent **pulp cavity** occupies the middle of the tooth and is continuous with the **root canal**, which transmits the nerves and vessels from the supporting bone. The root and neck of the tooth are surrounded by the **periodontal membrane**, which forms a radiolucent line around them on the radiograph. A dense white line of bone surrounds this and is known as the **lamina dura**. This surrounds the root of each tooth and is continuous with the lamina dura of the adjacent teeth around the margin of the alveolar crest.

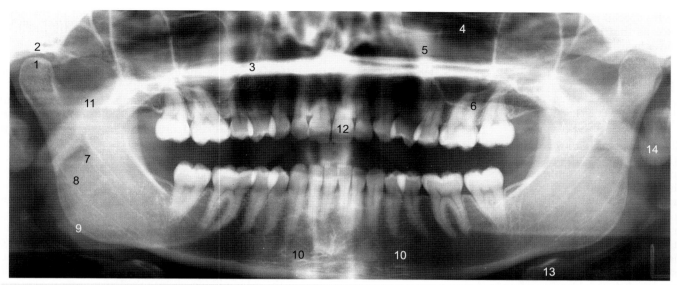

Fig. 1.18 Dental pantomogram. The third molars have been extracted.

1. Condylar process of mandible
2. Temporomandibular fossa
3. Hard palate
4. Maxillary sinus
5. Medial wall of maxillary sinus
6. Floor of maxillary sinus
7. Condylar canal
8. Ramus of mandible
9. Angle of mandible
10. Body of mandible
11. Mandibular notch
12. Upper left incisor
13. Hyoid bone (projected laterally)
14. Ear lobe

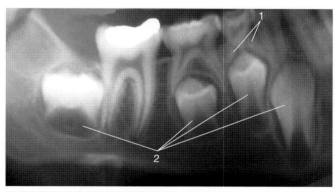

Fig. 1.19 Radiograph of the teeth of a 9-year-old child.

1. Resorbing roots of a deciduous tooth
2. Unerupted teeth

RADIOLOGY OF THE MANDIBLE, TEMPOROMANDIBULAR JOINTS AND TEETH (SEE FIGS. 1.13–1.19)

Plain Films

The mandible may be seen on skull radiographs and dedicated oblique views of the mandible. The mandibular canal and mandibular and mental foramina may be identified on radiographs of the mandible.

There are also special views for the temporomandibular joints, and a full radiographic study of these includes images of each joint with the mouth open and closed. The teeth can be radiographed on small films, occlusal films, placed close up against them inside the mouth, which provide excellent detail.

The symphysis menti fuses at 2 years of age. Eruption of the milk dentition is normally complete by this time. The permanent dentition develops in the mandible and maxilla during childhood and can be identified radiographically. Most have calcified by 3 years of age. The roots of the milk teeth are resorbed as the permanent teeth erupt. The medial teeth erupt before the lateral teeth, and lower teeth erupt approximately 6–12 months before the upper teeth. The first permanent molar erupts at 6 years of age, and all the permanent dentition is present by the age of 12 or 13 years except the third molar (wisdom tooth), which does not appear until early adulthood.

The mandibular canal and mandibular and mental foramina may be identified on radiographs of the mandible.

Computed Tomography (see Fig. 1.13)

High-resolution CT is used in the assessment of fractures or bony abnormalities of the mandible.

Magnetic Resonance Imaging (see Fig. 1.16)

MRI is excellent for the demonstration of the internal temporomandibular joint anatomy. The anterior and posterior bands and the thin zone of the disc are identifiable, as are the disc attachments. Cine MRI studies can also be performed with sagittal images of the joint that show the meniscoligamentous complex in varying degrees of mouth opening and closing.

Dental Pantomography (see Fig. 1.18)

The **dental pantomogram** gives a panoramic image of both dental arches, as well as the mandible, temporomandibular joints and lower maxilla. This study is obtained using special equipment that moves around the patient's face as the radiograph is being taken, mapping out the lower face and jaw in a straight line.

The Orbital Contents (Figs. 1.20–1.24)

The orbit contains the globe, the extraocular muscles (including levator palpebrae), the lacrimal gland, the optic nerve and the ophthalmic vessels. The whole is embedded in fat. The orbit is limited anteriorly by the **orbital septum**. This is a thin layer of fascia that extends from the orbital rim to the superior and inferior tarsal plates, separating the orbital contents from the eyelids. A fascial layer, the **periorbita**, lines the bony cavity of the orbit and this is continuous with the dura mater of the brain through the superior orbital fissure and optic canal.

The **globe** of the eye is composed of a transparent anterior part covered by the **cornea**, and an opaque posterior part covered by the **sclera**. These are joined at the corneoscleral junction, known as the **limbus**. The anterior and posterior extremities of the globe are known as the anterior and posterior **poles**. The midcoronal plane of the globe is the **equator**. A further layer of fascia, **Tenon's capsule**, covers the sclera from the limbus to the exit of the optic nerve from the eye. This facial layer fuses with the fascia of the extrinsic ocular muscles at their insertions. Anteriorly, a mucous membrane known as the **conjunctiva** covers the anterior aspect of the eye. It is reflected from the inner surface of the eyelids and fuses with the limbus.

There are six extrinsic ocular muscles that insert into the sclera. The four rectus muscles, the **superior, inferior, medial** and **lateral recti**, arise from a common tendinous ring called the **annulus of Zinn**. This is attached to the lower border of the superior orbital fissure. These muscles insert into the corresponding aspects of the globe, anterior to its equator. The **superior oblique** arises from the sphenoid bone superomedial to the optic foramen. It passes through a tendinous ring, the **trochlea**, which is attached to the frontal bone in the superolateral part of the orbit, acting as a pulley. It then passes posteriorly to insert into the upper outer surface of the globe, posterior to the equator. The inferior oblique arises from the anterior part of the floor of the orbit and inserts into the lower outer part of the globe, behind the equator.

The **levator palpebrae superioris** is also within the anterior fascial limit of the orbit, arising from the inferior surface of the lesser wing of sphenoid (see Fig. 1.10) and inserting into the tarsal plate of the upper eyelid behind the orbital septum (see Fig. 1.20).

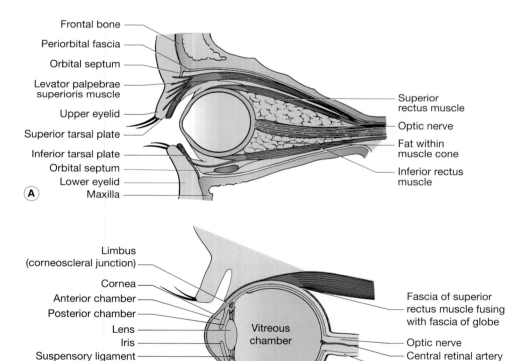

Fig. 1.20 (A) The orbit: sagittal section. (B) The eye: internal anatomy; sagittal section.

Frontal bone
Periorbital fascia
Orbital septum
Levator palpebrae superioris muscle
Upper eyelid
Superior tarsal plate
Inferior tarsal plate
Orbital septum
Lower eyelid
Maxilla

Superior rectus muscle
Optic nerve
Fat within muscle cone
Inferior rectus muscle

(A)

Limbus (corneoscleral junction)
Cornea
Anterior chamber
Posterior chamber
Lens
Iris
Suspensory ligament
Ciliary body
Conjunctival membrane
Ora serrata of retina

Vitreous chamber

Fascia of superior rectus muscle fusing with fascia of globe
Optic nerve
Central retinal artery
Subarachnoid space
Layers of globe:
Retina
Choroid
Sclera
Fascia (Tenon's capsule)

(B)

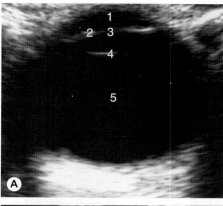

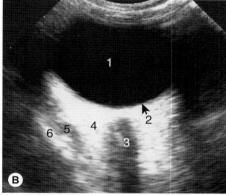

Fig. 1.21 Ultrasound of the eye. (A) Transverse image showing anterior structures. (B) Longitudinal image showing posterior structures.

(A)
1. Anterior chamber
2. Iris
3. Anterior aspect of lens
4. Posterior aspect of lens
5. Vitreous body

(B)
1. Vitreous body
2. Retinal surface
3. Optic nerve
4. Retrobulbar fat
5. Lateral rectus muscle
6. Lateral wall of bony orbit

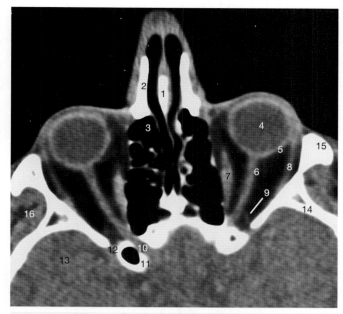

Fig. 1.22 Computed tomography scan of the orbit: axial section through the optic nerve.

1. Nasal septum
2. Nasal bone
3. Ethmoid air cells
4. Globe of left eye
5. Sclera
6. Optic nerve
7. Medial rectus muscle
8. Lateral rectus muscle
9. Superior ophthalmic vein
10. Optic canal
11. Anterior clinoid process (pneumatized)
12. Superior orbital fissure
13. Middle cranial fossa
14. Greater wing of sphenoid
15. Frontal process of zygomatic bone
16. Temporal fossa/temporalis muscle

RADIOLOGY PEARL

The orbital veins drain the periorbital skin and thus provide a possible pathway for infection, causing potentially lethal cavernous sinus thrombosis.

The arterial supply of the orbit is from the **ophthalmic artery**. This enters the orbit through the optic canal and gives rise to the **central retinal artery**, which runs in the optic nerve into the back of the eye. It supplies the orbital contents and its anterior branches anastomose with branches of the external carotid in the eyelids.

The venous drainage of the orbit is through the **superior** and **inferior ophthalmic veins** into the **cavernous sinus**. The superior ophthalmic vein is formed by the union of the **angular vein** and the **supraorbital vein** at the superomedial angle of the orbit.

The superior ophthalmic vein runs posterolaterally, then medially, and drains to the cavernous sinus via the superior orbital fissure. The inferior ophthalmic vein passes posteriorly and may join the cavernous sinus alone or with the superior vein.

The optic nerve is a direct extension of the brain. It is myelinated and has external coverings of dura, arachnoid and pia, forming its own subarachnoid space continuous with that of the brain. It is 4 mm thick and has four parts. The **intraocular** part begins at the optic disc. The **intraorbital part** runs posteriorly within the muscle cone formed by the four recti and is lax to allow movement of the globe. The **intracanalicular part** lies in the narrow optic canal with the ophthalmic artery, and the **intracranial part** is between the intracranial opening of the optic canal and the optic chiasm.

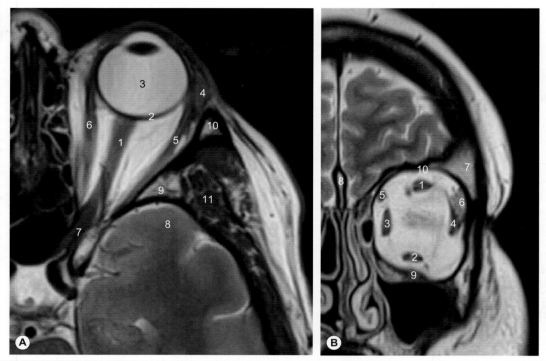

Fig. 1.23 Magnetic resonance image of the orbit. (A) Axial and (B) coronal T2-weighted images of the left orbit.

(A)
1. Optic nerve
2. Sclera
3. Globe
4. Lacrimal gland
5. Lateral rectus muscle
6. Medial rectus muscle
7. Optic canal
8. Temporal lobe
9. Greater wing of sphenoid
10. Frontal process of zygomatic bone
11. Temporalis muscle

(B)
1. Superior rectus muscle
2. Inferior rectus muscle
3. Medial rectus muscle
4. Lateral rectus muscle
5. Superior oblique muscle
6. Lacrimal gland
7. Frontal bone
8. Crista galli
9. Infra-orbital foramen/nerve
10. Roof of orbit

INTERNAL ANATOMY AND COVERINGS OF THE EYE (FIG. 1.20)

The globe of the eye is composed of three layers. The outermost consists of the tough white **sclera** posteriorly and the transparent **cornea** anteriorly. The junction of the sclera and cornea is called the **limbus**.

The middle layer is a vascular layer known as the **uveal tract**. It consists of **choroid** posteriorly, and the **ciliary body** and **iris** anteriorly. The ciliary body is a fibrous ring continuous with both the choroid and iris, and gives rise to the **ciliary muscle**, which alters the shape of the lens of the eye, allowing accommodation.

The innermost layer is the **retina**, which contains the rods and cones. The retina ends anteriorly a short distance behind the ciliary body, and its anterior limit is known as the **ora serrata**. Posteriorly, nerve fibres converge to form the optic nerve at the **optic disc**. The nerve pierces both the choroid and sclera as it passes posteriorly. The sclera is continuous with the dural covering of the optic nerve. The **macula**, which has the greatest concentration of cones and is responsible for central vision, lies temporal to the optic disc.

The **anterior segment** of the eye is that part anterior to the lens. It is divided into two chambers. The **anterior chamber** is between the cornea and iris, and the **posterior chamber** is between the iris and lens. The two chambers are filled with **aqueous humour** and are continuous through the aperture of the iris (the **pupil**).

The **posterior segment** is behind the lens and is filled with a gelatinous fluid known as the **vitreous body**. The outer part of the vitreous is condensed to form the so-called **vitreous** or **hyaline membrane**. A potential space exists between the vitreous and the retina known as the **subhyaloid space**. In pathological conditions fluid or blood may accumulate in this space.

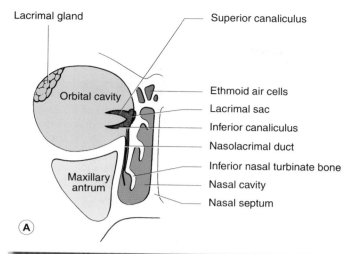

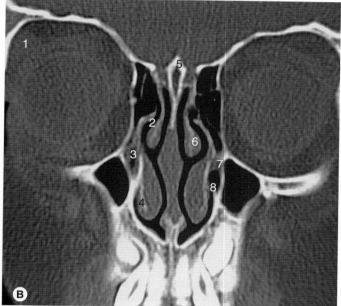

Fig. 1.24 (A) The lacrimal apparatus: coronal section. (B) The nasolacrimal duct. Coronal computed tomography scan through the anterior nose.

1. Lacrimal gland
2. Ethmoid infundibulum draining to middle meatus
3. Upper end of right nasolacrimal duct
4. Inferior turbinate
5. Crista galli
6. Middle turbinate
7. Inferior part of left nasolacrimal duct
8. Opening of nasolacrimal duct

RADIOLOGY OF THE ORBIT AND EYE (SEE FIGS. 1.21–1.24)

Plain Films

The orbital margins may be assessed by plain radiography of the skull and facial bones. The floor of the orbit is undulating and not well defined on radiographs.

RADIOLOGY PEARL

Fracture of the floor of the orbit may be associated with entrapment of the inferior rectus muscle associated with restriction of movement of the eye. The entrapped muscle may give rise to an apparent mass in the roof of the maxillary sinus on plain radiographs or CT, called the teardrop sign.

Ultrasound (see Fig. 1.21)

Ultrasound of the eye using high-frequency transducers (5–20 MHz) can demonstrate its internal anatomy (see Fig. 1.21). The higher frequency transducer visualizes the anterior segment and the lower frequency transducers (5–10 MHz) image the posterior segment. Scans may be performed in any plane, but are usually obtained in transverse (axial) and longitudinal (sagittal) planes. The aqueous and vitreous chambers are anechoic spaces. The cornea and lens are echogenic and easily defined. The inner walls of the eye – the choroid, retina and sclera – are not distinguishable from each other and are seen as a line of low-amplitude echoes. The retrobulbar fat is also echogenic, and the extraocular muscles and optic nerve appear as echo-free structures within it.

Computed Tomography (see Fig. 1.22)

CT is an excellent modality for demonstrating the extraocular contents of the orbit. The lacrimal gland, extraocular muscles, globe, optic nerve and superior ophthalmic vein are routinely seen. The lens has a low water content and is dense on CT. The bony walls of the orbit are demonstrated, and the foramina of the orbit and related anatomy are readily assessed. Coronal images are best for assessment of the orbital floor, especially in trauma.

Magnetic Resonance Imaging (see Fig. 1.23)

MRI demonstrates the soft tissues of the orbit. It is of particular value in demonstrating the optic nerve, allowing excellent visualization of the entire nerve, including the intracanalicular segment on sagittal oblique images along the nerve's long axis. On coronal images the third, fourth and sixth nerves and the first division of the fifth can be seen just below the anterior clinoid process. Much of the internal anatomy of the eye can also be distinguished, as can the orbital septum, extraocular muscles, nerves and vessels. Images of the intraorbital part of the optic nerve are performed with T2 fat-saturation pulses to help distinguish the optic nerve and its sleeve of dura and cerebrospinal fluid (CSF) from the surrounding high-signal fat.

The Lacrimal Apparatus (Fig. 1.24)

This consists of the **lacrimal gland**, which lies in the superolateral part of the orbit and produces the tears, and the lacrimal **canaliculi**, **lacrimal sac** and **nasolacrimal duct**, which drain the secretions to the nose.

The lacrimal gland lies lateral to the levator palpebrae. This muscle grooves the gland, dividing it into an almond-sized **orbital lobe** posteriorly and a smaller **palpebral lobe**, which extends anteriorly under the lateral part of the upper eyelid. The orbital lobe lies in a bony depression called the **lacrimal fossa**. The gland secretes tears into the space between the upper eyelid and eye (the **upper fornix**) through several small ducts.

On the medial margins of each eyelid are openings known as the **lacrimal puncta**. Tears drain through these openings into the superior and inferior lacrimal canaliculi. The canaliculi drain into the lacrimal sac, which is situated in a bony groove in the medial wall of the orbit but outside the fascial plane, which limits the orbit proper. This drains via the nasolacrimal duct, which runs in its own bony canal to the inferior meatus of the nasal cavity. A mucosal fold at its inferior end, the plica lacrimalis, acts as a valve, the valve of Hasner, to prevent reflux into the duct.

RADIOLOGY OF THE LACRIMAL GLAND

Dacryocystography

The canaliculi may be cannulated and injected with radio-opaque contrast to outline the drainage system of the lacrimal apparatus. Patency of the duct can also be established by nuclear dacryocystography without cannulation of the duct. Drops containing radionuclide are dropped onto the conjunctiva and the path of the duct is imaged by gamma camera.

CT (see Fig. 1.24B) and MRI

These imaging techniques may be used to study the lacrimal gland and orbital contents. The bony canal of the nasolacrimal duct may be identified on axial and coronal CT images.

The Ear (see Figs. 1.25–1.28)

THE EXTERNAL EAR

The external ear consists of the **pinna** and the **external auditory meatus**. The external meatus is 3.5 cm long and runs medially to the ear drum or **tympanic membrane**. The outer part of the canal is cartilaginous and the medial two-thirds is bony. The entire canal is lined by skin.

THE MIDDLE EAR (SEE FIGS. 1.26, 1.27)

The middle ear is a slit-like cavity housed in the petrous bone. It lies between the tympanic membrane laterally and the inner ear medially. A tiny spur of bone, the **scutum**, where the tympanic membrane is attached, is seen between the external auditory canal and the middle ear (see Figs. 1.26 and 1.27). The middle ear has an upper part, which is recessed superiorly into the petrous bone and is known as the **epitympanic recess** or **attic**, as it lies at a higher level than the tympanic membrane. The roof of the cavity is formed by a thin layer of bone called the **tegmen tympani**, separating it from the middle cranial fossa and temporal lobe of the brain. The attic communicates with the mastoid air cells through a narrow posterior opening called the **aditus ad antrum**. The lower part of the middle ear contains the **ossicles**, and is

continuous inferiorly with the **Eustachian tube**, which opens into the lateral wall of the nasopharynx. This tube is 3.5 cm long, bony at first, and cartilaginous in its lower portion.

RADIOLOGY PEARL

Erosion of the scutum is a sensitive marker for erosion by middle-ear disease states, including cholesteatoma. Infection may spread from the middle ear to the mastoid air cells, which are related posteriorly to the sigmoid sinus and cerebellum in the posterior cranial fossa. Infection may erode directly through the thin tegmen tympani to the middle cranial fossa.

The floor of the middle ear is a thin plate of bone separating the cavity from the bulb of the jugular vein.

The lateral wall of the cavity is the tympanic membrane and the ring of bone to which it is attached.

The medial wall of the middle ear also forms the lateral wall of the inner ear, and its middle-ear surface is shaped by the contents of the inner ear. The lateral semicircular canal causes a prominence in the wall superiorly. Below this is a bulge caused by the cochlea called the **promontory**. The **oval window**, into which the base of the stapes inserts, is above and behind the promontory. The **round window**, covered by a membrane, is below and behind. The bony canal of the **third part of the facial nerve** also causes a prominence on the medial wall of the cavity. This runs from front to back, between the prominence of the lateral semicircular canal and the promontory, before turning down in the posterior wall of the cavity to emerge through the stylomastoid foramen (fourth part).

The ossicles traverse the middle-ear cavity. The **malleus** has a handle that is attached to the tympanic membrane, and a rounded head that articulates with the body of the **incus** at the **incudomallear joint**. This joint is orientated superiorly and projects into the epitympanic recess. The incus has a long process that articulates with the head of the **stapes**, the base of which is firmly fixed in the oval window. The joints between the ossicles are synovial.

THE INNER EAR

This is a membranous system of fluid-filled sacs concerned with hearing and balance. It is housed in a protective labyrinth of dense bone and lies in the petrous bone medial to the middle ear.

The **bony labyrinth** consists of a **vestibule**, which communicates posteriorly with the three **semicircular canals**, and anteriorly with the spiral **cochlea**. The bony covering of the lateral semicircular canal bulges into the medial wall of the middle-ear cavity as the promontory and that of the superior semicircular canal forms the **arcuate eminence** on the superior aspect of the petrous bone. The **vestibular aqueduct** passes from the vestibule to open in the posterior fossa midway between the IAM and the groove for the jugular vein. The **cochlear aqueduct** extends from the cochlea to a slit-like opening in the posterior fossa inferior – although parallel – to the IAM (see Fig. 1.27).

Within the bony labyrinth is the **membranous labyrinth**, which comprises the **utricle**, which is connected to the semicircular canals, and the **saccule**, which is connected with the cochlear canal. A utriculosaccular duct connects these two. The **endolymphatic duct** arises from this connecting duct and passes in the vestibular aqueduct to end in a blind dilatation, the **endolymphatic sac**. The membranous labyrinth is filled with endolymph and is surrounded by perilymph. The perilymph is continuous with CSF in the subarachnoid space at the vestibular aqueduct (see Fig. 1.28).

The **cochlea** has between $2\frac{1}{2}$ and $2\frac{3}{4}$ turns, and its apex points anterolaterally so that the axis of the cochlea is perpendicular to the axis of the petrous bone. The bony cochlea has a central modiolus from which a shelf-like spiral lamina projects.

The Internal Auditory Meatus (see Fig. 1.27)

This bony canal is about 1 cm long and transmits the seventh and eighth cranial nerves from the posterior cranial fossa. Its lateral extent is separated from the inner ear by a perforated plate of bone. A crest on this bone, the **crista falciformis**, divides the canal into upper and lower compartments. The upper compartment contains the **facial nerve** and the superior vestibular branch of the eighth cranial nerve, and the lower compartment contains the acoustic and inferior vestibular branches of the eighth cranial nerve. The vestibular and acoustic nerves pass through the perforated plate of bone into the inner ear. The facial nerve turns anteriorly through the anterior wall of the lateral part of the canal into its own bony canal. The first part of the facial nerve runs in the IAM. The second part runs anteriorly from this in its bony canal, then curves laterally and posteriorly around the cochlea to the anterior part of the medial wall of the middle-ear cavity. This U-bend around the cochlea is known as the **genu** of the nerve. The third and fourth parts have been described in the section on the middle ear.

The posterior lip of the medial end of the IAM is called the **porus acousticus** and is normally sharply defined. It may be eroded by pathology in this region.

DEVELOPMENT OF THE EAR

The external and middle ear develop from the first and second branchial arches. The inner ear develops from the otic capsule.

RADIOLOGY OF THE MIDDLE AND INNER EAR

Plain Films

The internal acoustic meati and parts of the bony labyrinth of the inner ear may be identified on a straight OF skull projection.

Computed Tomography (see Figs. 1.26, 1.27)

Images may be obtained in both axial and coronal planes. The internal auditory meati are readily assessed and the extent of any pathology and its relationship to other important intracranial structures may be determined. High-resolution scanning of the temporal bone can image the cochlea, vestibule, semicircular canals, ossicles and bony canal of the facial nerve in axial or coronal planes.

On high cuts through the petrous bone the two limbs of the superior semicircular canal may be seen as two round bony defects.

At lower levels, the vestibule, with the horizontal semicircular canal projecting posteriorly in an arc, is seen. The entire horizontal semicircular canal may be seen as it lies in the plane of section. The internal auditory canal is seen medially, running laterally from the posterior cranial fossa to the cochlea. The vestibule is posterolateral. The posterior semicircular canal projects posteriorly from the vestibule. The malleus and incus are seen laterally in the epitympanic recess. The bony canal of the facial nerve passes from front to back, medial to the middle-ear cavity, lateral to the vestibule and just below the level of the horizontal semicircular canal.

Scans at a slightly lower level pass through the external auditory canal and middle-ear cavity. The ossicles are seen traversing the middle-ear cavity. An ice cream cone sign describes the normal appearance of the middle ear ossicles on axial CT scan. The ball of the ice cream is formed by the head of the malleus and cone is formed by the body of the incus, with lowest tip formed by the short process of the incus pointing towards the aditus ad antrum.

The basal turn of the cochlea is seen anteriorly. The lower part of the posterior semicircular canal and vestibule are posterolateral. The facial nerve in its bony canal may be seen in cross-section as a circular structure laterally running down to the stylomastoid foramen.

Magnetic Resonance Imaging (see Fig. 1.28)

MRI may also be used to study the contents of the temporal bone. Coronal images demonstrate the contents of the internal auditory canal to advantage, showing the facial and cochlear nerves separated by a signal void caused by the falciform crest. The loop of the **anterior inferior cerebellar artery** as it coils near the IAM is often visible and should not be mistaken for pathology. The cochlea and vestibule may also be identified. These are fluid-filled and of high signal intensity (and thus easier to see) on T_2-weighted images. Neither CT nor MRI can distinguish the membranous labyrinth from the fluid in the bony labyrinth in which it lies.

RADIOLOGY PEARL

CT and MRI are important prior to placement of a cochlear implant. An intact cochlea with normal turns and intact vestibulocochlear nerves are requirements of a successful implant.

The Upper Aerodigestive Tract (Fig. 1.29)

The upper aerodigestive tract includes the oral cavity, the pharynx including the nasopharynx and the oropharynx, as well as the larynx and the hypopharynx (see Fig. 1.29).

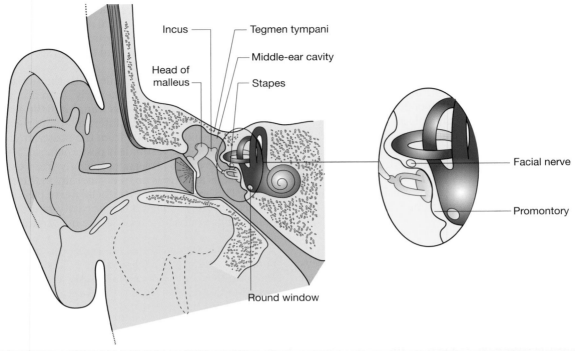

Fig. 1.25 Ear: coronal section showing the outer, middle and inner ear.

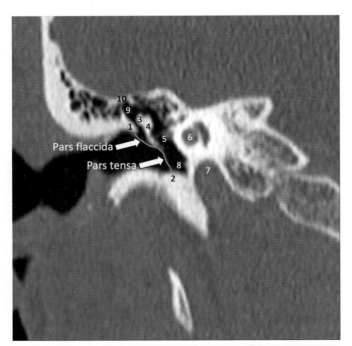

Fig. 1.26 Coronal computed tomography scan of the middle ear and ossicles.

1. Scutum
2. Tympanic annulus
3. Head of malleus
4. Incus
5. Stapes
6. Cochlea
7. Carotid canal
8. Hypotympanum
9. Epitympanum
10. Tegmen tympani

THE ORAL CAVITY (FIGS. 1.30, 1.31)

This forms a passage from the lips to the oropharynx. It is largely filled by the tongue and teeth and is lined by a mucous membrane. The parotid gland opens onto its lateral wall, and the submandibular and sublingual glands open onto its floor. The roof is formed by the hard palate anteriorly and the soft palate posteriorly. The soft palate is a mobile flap that hangs posteroinferiorly at rest, separating the oro- from the nasopharynx. Two muscles insert into it from the lateral wall of the pharynx – the **levator** and the **tensor veli palatini**. These elevate the soft palate during swallowing to prevent reflux into the nose. The **uvula** hangs from the middle of the soft palate, and two pairs of muscles, the **palatoglossus** and the **palatopharyngeus**, run from its base to the tongue and pharynx. These muscles and their overlying mucosa form the anterior and posterior **fauces**, in whose concavity the **palatine tonsils** lie.

The muscles of the tongue form two groups. The **intrinsic** group are arranged in various planes and alter the shape of the tongue. The **extrinsic** group are paired muscles that move the tongue and have attachments outside it. The **genioglossus** arises from the inner surface of the symphysis menti and fans out to form the ventral surface of the tongue. Its inferior fibres form a tendon that attaches to the hyoid bone. The **hyoglossus** and **chondroglossus** are thin sheets of muscle that arise from the hyoid bone and insert into the side of the tongue. The **styloglossus** passes from the styloid process to the side of the tongue. A median **raphe** divides the tongue into two halves.

The floor of the mouth is formed by other muscles that also support the tongue. The most important is the **mylohyoid** muscle, which is slung from the **mylohyoid line** on the inner surface of the mandible to the hyoid bone on either side.

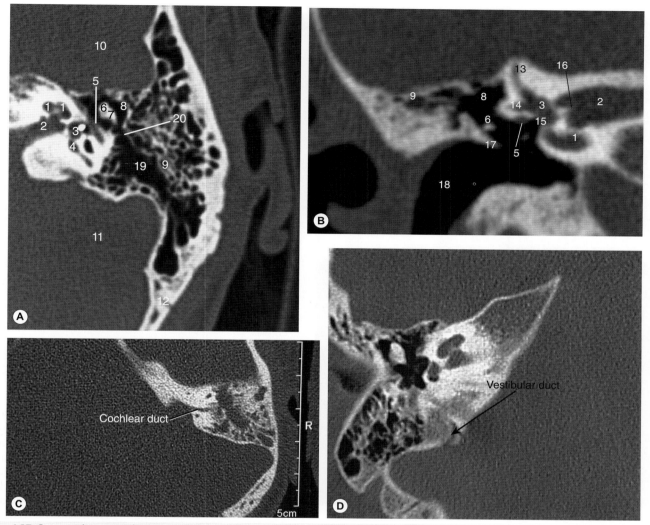

Fig. 1.27 Computed tomography (CT) scan of the inner ear. (A) Axial section at the mid-cochlear level. (B) Coronal section in the vestibular plane. (C) Axial CT to show the cochlear duct. (D) Axial CT to show the vestibular duct.

1. Cochlear turns
2. Internal auditory meatus
3. Vestibule
4. Posterior semicircular canal
5. Facial nerve in its bony canal
6. Malleus
7. Incus
8. Epitympanic recess
9. Mastoid air cells
10. Middle cranial fossa

11. Posterior cranial fossa
12. Lambdoid suture
13. Superior semicircular canal
14. Lateral semicircular canal
15. Oval window
16. Crista falciformis
17. Scutum
18. External auditory meatus
19. Mastoid antrum
20. Aditus ad antrum

The inferior fibres of **genioglossus** pass from the hyoid to the symphysis above the mylohyoid, and the **anterior belly of digastric** passes from the hyoid to the symphysis below the mylohyoid. The **stylohyoid** is lateral, passing from the styloid process to the hyoid. The **posterior belly of digastric** runs from the mastoid process to the lateral aspect of the hyoid bone. The **anterior belly** runs from here to the base of the anterior part of the mandible.

Lymphatic drainage of the oral cavity is to the submental and submandibular nodes, and to the retropharyngeal and deep cervical nodes.

Boundaries of the Oral Cavity

Superior: Hard palate.

Anterior: Lips (for oral cancer staging, the anterior border is defined by the opposing lips (wet mucosa) and excludes the dry lips).

Posterior: circumvallate papillae, anterior tonsillar pillars and junction of hard and soft palates that separates it from the oropharynx.

Inferior: floor of mouth.

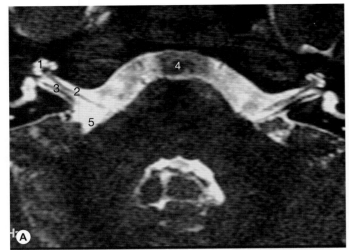

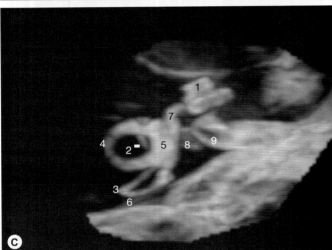

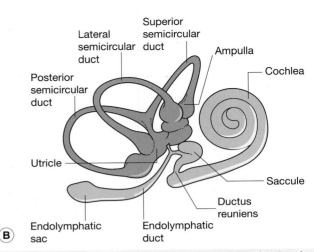

Fig. 1.28 (A) Axial T$_2$ magnetic resonance image (MRI) showing the internal auditory meatus and its contained nerves. (B) Diagram of the membranous labyrinth. (C) The membranous labyrinth as seen on three-dimensional MRI.

(A)
1. Cochlea
2. Vestibulocochlear nerve
3. Facial nerve
4. Basilar artery with flow artefact
5. Cerebellopontine angle cistern

(C)
1. Cochlear duct
2. Superior semicircular canal
3. Posterior semicircular canal
4. Lateral semicircular canal
5. Utricle
6. Endolymphatic duct
7. Utriculosaccular duct
8. Saccule
9. Internal auditory meatus

THE PHARYNX (FIG. 1.32)

The pharynx is a muscular tube extending from the base of the skull to the level of the cricoid cartilage, approximately C$_6$, where it is continuous with the oesophagus. It lies behind, and communicates with, the nasal and oral cavities, providing a common entrance to the respiratory and gastrointestinal tracts.

The pharynx has three coats. Innermost is the mucous coat, which is continuous with the mucosa of the oral and nasal cavities. The submucous layer is the **pharyngobasilar fascia** and forms a thick fibrous coat, which gives the pharynx its shape. It is attached superiorly to the base of the skull and is continuous with the fibrous material filling the foramen lacerum. It is pierced only by the Eustachian tube. The outermost coat is formed by the three **constrictor muscles**. These fan out laterally from their anterior attachments to insert into a posterior raphe, which is attached superiorly to the base of the skull anterior to the foramen magnum and is continuous with the oesophagus inferiorly.

The superior pharyngeal constrictor is attached anteriorly to the inferior extension of the medial pterygoid plate (the **pterygoid hamulus**), and to a raphe joining this to the inner surface of the mandible. The middle constrictor muscle is attached anteriorly to the hyoid bone and lower part of the stylohyoid ligament. Its upper fibres overlap the superior constrictor muscle superficially. The inferior constrictor muscle attaches anteriorly to cricoid and thyroid cartilages and overlaps the inferior part of the middle constrictor. Its lowermost fibres are horizontally orientated and merge with the circular fibres of the oesophagus. The constrictor muscles are covered by loose **buccopharyngeal fascia**, which is continuous with the fascia covering the buccinator muscle.

The pharynx lies behind the nasal and oral cavities and the larynx, and is divided accordingly into the nasopharynx, oropharynx and hypo- or laryngopharynx (see Fig. 1.29). Posteriorly it lies on the upper cervical vertebrae and their prevertebral muscles.

RADIOLOGY PEARL

A gap between the oblique and horizontal fibres of the inferior constrictor may become a weak spot known as **Killian's dehiscence**, through which a pharyngeal pouch may emerge.

THE NASOPHARYNX (FIG. 1.33)

The **nasopharynx** is that part of the pharynx between the posterior choanae anteriorly, the anterior border of the longus colli muscles posteriorly, the skull base superiorly and the lower limit of the soft palate inferiorly. It communicates anteriorly with the nasal cavity and inferiorly with the oropharynx. The roof of the nasopharynx is bound to the inferior surface of the sphenoid and clivus by the pharyngobasilar fascia. It has the parapharyngeal space and the deep soft tissues of the infratemporal space laterally. Posteriorly it lies on the upper cervical vertebrae and longus collis and capitus, and posterolaterally the styloid muscles separate it from the carotid sheath.

The Eustachian tube opens onto the lateral wall of the nasopharynx on either side, piercing the pharyngobasilar fascia. This opening has a posterior ridge formed by the cartilaginous end of the tube known as the **torus tubarius**. Behind these ridges are the paired **lateral pharyngeal recesses**, also known as the **fossae of Rosenmüller**.

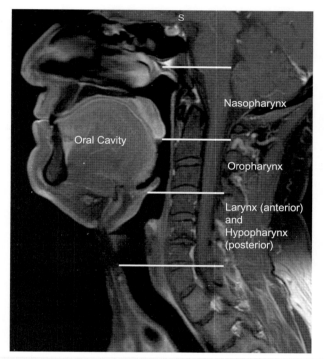

Fig. 1.29 Divisions of the pharynx on coronal magnetic resonance imaging.

S

Nasopharynx

Oral Cavity

Oropharynx

Larynx (anterior) and Hypopharynx (posterior)

> **RADIOLOGY PEARL**
>
> Many nasopharyngeal tumours start in the fossa of Rosenmüller and can push the torus tubarius anteriorly, blocking off the Eustachian tube and resulting in a unilateral mastoid effusion. It is therefore important to carefully inspect the ipsilateral fossa of Rosenmüller in the presence of a unilateral mastoid effusion.

The muscular layer of the nasopharynx is formed by the superior pharyngeal constrictor. The palatal muscles arise from the base of the skull on either side of the Eustachian tube. The **levator veli palatini** accompanies the Eustachian tube, piercing the pharyngobasilar fascia before inserting into the posterior part of the soft palate.

> **RADIOLOGY PEARL**
>
> There is a weak point in the buccopharyngeal fascia termed the sinus of Morgagni (between the upper border of the superior constrictor muscle, pharyngeal aponeurosis and skull base) which can allow nasopharyngeal tumours to spread laterally.

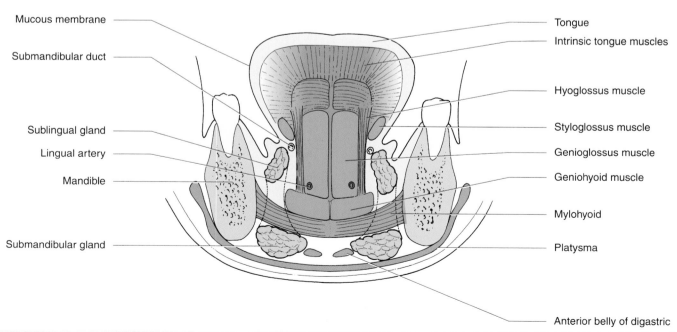

Mucous membrane

Submandibular duct

Sublingual gland

Lingual artery

Mandible

Submandibular gland

Tongue

Intrinsic tongue muscles

Hyoglossus muscle

Styloglossus muscle

Genioglossus muscle

Geniohyoid muscle

Mylohyoid

Platysma

Anterior belly of digastric

Fig. 1.30 Floor of the mouth coronal section.

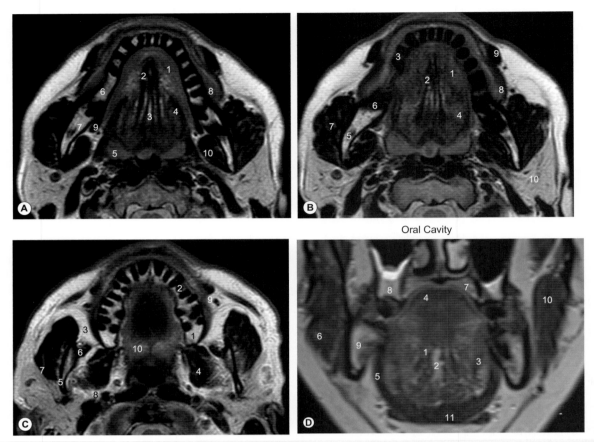

Oral Cavity

Fig. 1.31 Magnetic resonance image of the oral cavity. (A–C) Axial sections and (D) coronal magnetic resonance image.

(A)
1. Sublingual gland
2. Genioglossus
3. Lingual septum
4. Hyoglossus
5. Oropharyngeal tonsil
6. Body of mandible
7. Angle of mandible
8. Buccinator
9. Mylohyoid
10. Medial pterygoid

(B)
1. Sublingual gland
2. Genioglossus
3. Mandibular alveolus
4. Hyoglossus
5. Ramus of mandible
6. Region of retromolar trigone
7. Masseter
8. Buccinator
9. Depressor anguli oris
10. Parotid gland

(C)
1. Maxillary tuberosity
2. Maxillary alveolus
3. Retromaxillary fat pad
4. Medial pterygoid
5. Ramus of mandible
6. Temporalis tendon
7. Masseter muscle
8. Parapharyngeal fat
9. Buccinator
10. Soft palate

(D)
1. Genioglossus
2. Lingual septum
3. Hyoglossus
4. Superior longitudinal muscle
5. Mylohyoid
6. Anterior belly of digastric
7. Hard palate
8. Maxillary tuberosity
9. Body of mandible
10. Masseter
11. Geniohyoid

The **tensor veli palatini** runs around the nasopharynx and hooks around the pterygoid hamulus before inserting into the membranous part of the soft palate. These muscles, along with those in the palatopharyngeal arch, elevate the soft palate, closing it against a muscular ridge in the superior constrictor muscle (known as the Passavant ridge) during deglutition, thereby isolating the nasopharynx from the oropharynx.

Lymphoid tissue lines the nasopharynx, and this is prominent superiorly where it forms the nasopharyngeal tonsil - also known as **adenoids**.

The lymphatic drainage of the nasopharynx and related spaces is to the jugular chain of lymph nodes, especially the jugulodigastric node, which lies at the angle of the mandible.

Cross-Sectional Anatomy of the Nasopharynx (Figs. 1.33, 1.34)

At the level of the upper nasopharynx, the paired lateral pharyngeal recesses or fossae of Rosenmüller are posterolateral with the torus tubarius anteriorly. The

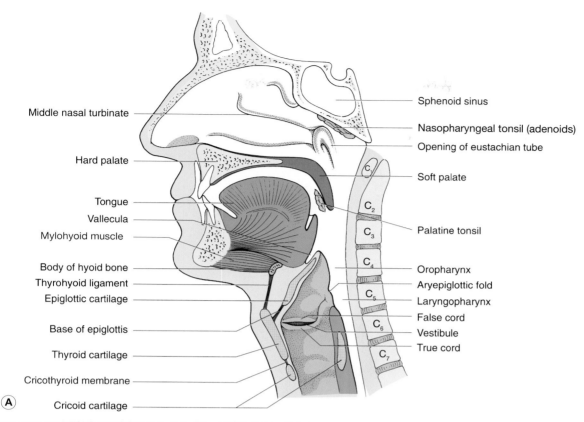

Middle nasal turbinate

Hard palate

Tongue
Vallecula
Mylohyoid muscle

Body of hyoid bone
Thyrohyoid ligament
Epiglottic cartilage

Base of epiglottis

Thyroid cartilage

Cricothyroid membrane

(A)   Cricoid cartilage

Sphenoid sinus

Nasopharyngeal tonsil (adenoids)
Opening of eustachian tube

Soft palate

Palatine tonsil

Oropharynx
Aryepiglottic fold
Laryngopharynx
False cord
Vestibule
True cord

C_1 C_2 C_3 C_4 C_5 C_6 C_7

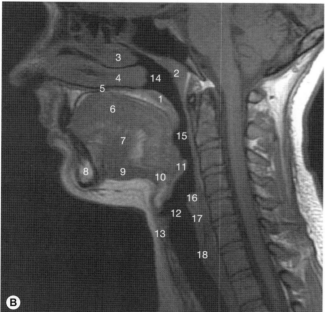

(B)

Fig. 1.32 Pharynx: sagittal section. (A) Diagram. (B) Sagittal T_1 MRI.

1. Soft palate
2. Adenoids
3. Middle turbinate
4. Inferior turbinate
5. Hard palate
6. Intrinsic muscle of tongue
7. Genioglossus
8. Mandible
9. Mylohyoid muscle
10. Hyoid bone
11. Epiglottis
12. Vocal cord
13. Thyroid cartilage
14. Nasopharynx
15. Oropharynx
16. Corniculate cartilage
17. Arytenoid cartilage
18. Cricoid cartilage

entrance to the Eustachian tube forms a recess anterior to the torus on either side. The medial and lateral pterygoid plates and their muscles are anterolateral to the nasopharynx. The lateral pterygoid muscle extends across the infratemporal space to the condyle and neck of the mandible. The parapharyngeal space is posterior to the infratemporal space, lying anterior to the carotid vessels and the styloid process and its muscles. The deep part of the parotid gland is lateral to the parapharyngeal space. The prevertebral muscles and upper cervical spine are posterior. Anteriorly are seen the maxillary antra, with the nasal cavity between.

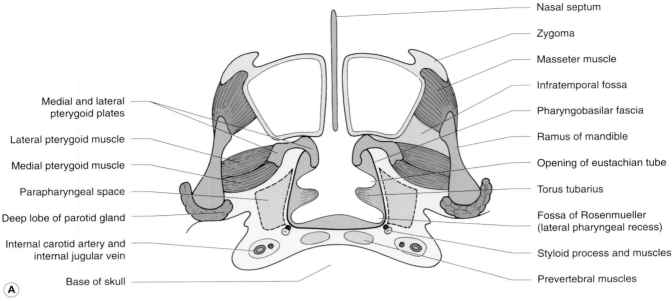

Nasal septum

Zygoma

Masseter muscle

Infratemporal fossa

Pharyngobasilar fascia

Ramus of mandible

Opening of eustachian tube

Torus tubarius

Fossa of Rosenmueller
(lateral pharyngeal recess)

Styloid process and muscles

Prevertebral muscles

Medial and lateral
pterygoid plates

Lateral pterygoid muscle

Medial pterygoid muscle

Parapharyngeal space

Deep lobe of parotid gland

Internal carotid artery and
internal jugular vein

Base of skull

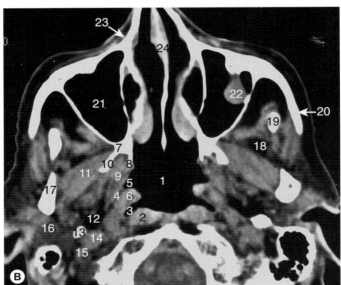

Fig. 1.33 Nasopharynx: axial section. (A) Diagram. (B) Axial computed tomography.

1. Nasopharyngeal space
2. Prevertebral muscle
3. Lateral pharyngeal recess, fossa of Rosenmüeller
4. Cartilaginous end of eustachian tube
5. Opening of eustachian tube
6. Torus tubarius
7. Pterygoid bone
8. Medial pterygoid plate
9. Medial pterygoid muscle
10. Lateral pterygoid plate
11. Lateral pterygoid muscle
12. Parapharyngeal space

13. Styloid process
14. Internal carotid artery
15. Internal jugular vein
16. Parotid gland
17. Ramus of mandible
18. Infratemporal space
19. Coronoid process of mandible and masseter muscle
20. Zygoma
21. Maxillary sinus
22. Polyp in left maxillary sinus
23. Nasal bone
24. Nasal septum

The Infratemporal Space and the Pterygopalatine Fossa (Figs. 1.35, 1.36)

The **infratemporal space** (see Fig. 1.35) lies lateral to the nasopharynx and behind the posterior wall of the maxilla. It extends from the base of the skull to the hyoid bone and contains the pterygoid muscles. It is continuous superiorly with the temporal fossa through the gap between the zygomatic arch and the side of the skull. Medial to this, the roof is formed by the inferior surface of the middle cranial fossa and is pierced by the foramen ovale and foramen spinosum. Laterally, the space is bounded by the zygomatic arch, temporalis muscle, ascending ramus of mandible and its coronoid process. Medially, the space is limited by the lateral pterygoid plate and nasopharynx. The space lies

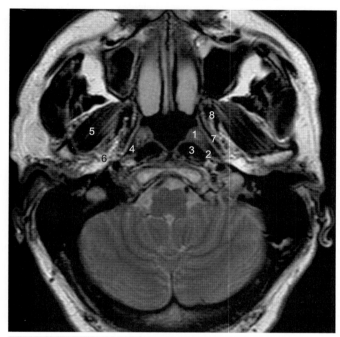

Fig. 1.34 The nasopharynx: axial magnetic resonance image.

1. Torus tubarius
2. Fossa of Rosenmüller
3. Longus capitis
4. Levator veli palatini
5. Lateral pterygoid
6. Parapharyngeal fat
7. Tensor veli palatini
8. Medial pterygoid

anterior to the deep part of the parotid, the styloid process and its muscles, and the carotid artery and jugular vein.

The anteromedial limit of the infratemporal space is formed by the junction of the lateral pterygoid plate with the posteromedial limit of the maxilla superiorly and the posterior border of the perpendicular plate of the palate inferiorly. The anterior and medial walls of the space meet inferiorly but are separated superiorly by the **pterygo-maxillary fissure**, where the pterygoid plates diverge from the posterior wall of the maxilla.

The **pterygopalatine fossa** (see Fig. 1.36) is a medial depression of the pterygomaxillary fissure lying just below the apex of the orbit between the pterygoid process and the posterior maxilla. Its medial margin is the perpendicular plate of the palatine bone. It is important as it connects several spaces and may facilitate the spread of pathology between them. It communicates superiorly with the orbit through the posterior part of the inferior orbital fissure. The foramen rotundum opens into it superiorly, connecting it with the middle cranial fossa. Laterally it communicates freely with the infratemporal fossa. Medially the space communicates with the nasal cavity via the **sphenopalatine foramen** in the perpendicular plate of the palatine bone, and with the oral cavity through the **greater palatine canal**, which runs inferiorly between the palatine bone and the maxilla. The fossa contains the maxillary division of the fifth cranial nerve, which runs through the foramen rotundum and into the orbit via the inferior orbital fissure. It also contains the pterygopalatine segment of the maxillary artery, which makes a characteristic loop and gives off branches to the middle cranial and masticator space and to the nasal cavity, palate and pharynx.

THE OROPHARYNX (FIG. 1.38)

The oropharynx is the part of the pharynx that extends from the lower part of the soft palate superiorly to the hyoid bone/tip of epiglottis inferiorly and is bounded anteriorly

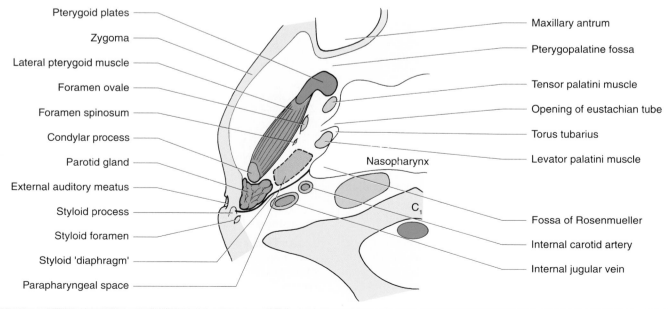

Fig. 1.35 Infratemporal fossa: axial section.

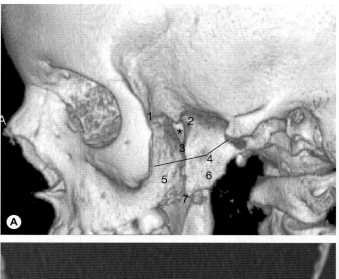

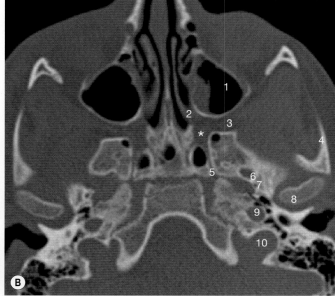

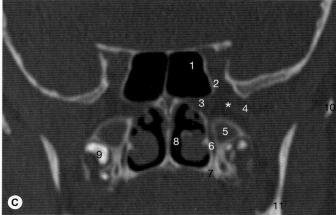

Fig. 1.36 Computed tomography of the pterygopalatine fossa. *Asterisk*, pterygopalatine fossa.

(A) 3D CT lateral view
1. Inferior orbital fissure
2. Foramen rotundum
3. Pterygomaxillary fissure
4. Cut ends of zygomatic arch
5. Maxilla
6. Lateral pterygoid plate
7. Greater palatine foramen

(B) Axial CT
1. Maxillary sinus
2. Sphenopalatine foramen
3. Pterygomaxillary fissure
4. Zygomatic arch
5. Vidian canal
6. Foramen ovale
7. Foramen spinosum

8. Mandibular head
9. Carotid foramen
10. Jugular foramen

(C) Coronal CT
1. Sphenoid sinus
2. Inferior orbital fissure
3. Sphenopalatine foramen
4. Pterygomaxillary fissure
5. Maxillary sinus
6. Greater palatine canal
7. Greater palatine foramen
8. Nares
9. Unerupted teeth
10. Zygomatic arch
11. Mandible

via a vertical plane defined by the junction of the hard and soft palate, anterior tonsillar pillars and circumvallate papillae, and posteriorly by the posterior wall of the pharynx. For oropharyngeal cancer staging, the lingual surface of the epiglottis is a subsite of the oropharynx.

It is continuous through the posterior fauces with the oral cavity and with the larynx and hypopharynx below. It is lined by mucosa that is continuous with that of the oral cavity and nasopharynx. Its submucosal layer is continuous with the pharyngobasilar fascia above, and its muscular layer has contributions from the superior constrictor,

some of the tongue muscles, and levator and tensor veli palatini.

Radiology of the Pharynx (see Figs. 1.32–1.38)

Plain Films (see Fig. 1.37). Lateral views of the skull and neck demonstrate the soft-tissue outlines of the pharynx. The posterior wall of the pharynx forms a soft-tissue shadow curving posteroinferiorly below the body of the sphenoid and anterior to the cervical vertebrae. This shadow thins as it passes down anterior to the

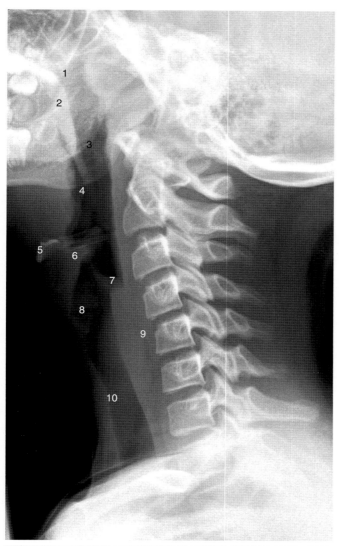

Fig. 1.37 Lateral radiograph of the neck: soft-tissue view showing the pharynx and larynx.

1. Nasopharynx
2. Soft palate
3. Oropharynx
4. Laryngopharynx
5. Hyoid bone
6. Epiglottis
7. Aryepiglottic fold
8. Laryngeal ventricle
9. Prevertebral space
10. Trachea

upper cervical vertebrae, measuring 3 mm anterior to C_4. Below this the wall is thicker but should not exceed the anteroposterior (AP) diameter of the cervical vertebrae. In children, lymphoid tissue results in a relatively thicker posterior wall, measuring up to 5 mm anterior to C_4 and up to 12 mm anterior to C_6. The lymphoid tissue in the upper posterior part of the nasopharynx (adenoids) may cause a large soft-tissue shadow. It tends to swell down towards the soft palate in young children and may be continuous with the pharyngeal tonsils on the lateral walls of the oropharynx and the lingual tonsils on the posterior surface

of the tongue, forming a ring of lymphoid tissue known as Waldeyer's ring.

The base of the tongue and the epiglottis, forming the anterior surface of the oropharynx, are also identifiable on lateral radiographs.

Palatal Studies and Videofluoroscopic Feeding Studies

The movement of the palate during phonation can be imaged by radiography in the lateral projection, where the position of the soft palate can be seen outlined by air. Movement of the palate during complex speech is studied by videofluoroscopy with or without coating the nasal and oral surfaces of the palate with barium.

Videofluoroscopy is also used to study the movement of the tongue, palate and pharynx during feeding by using foods and liquids of various consistencies mixed with radiopaque contrast.

RADIOLOGY PEARL

Coating or some filling of the valleculae and piriform sinuses during swallowing is normal. Excess filling is associated with a risk of aspiration, however.

Cross-Sectional Imaging

CT and MRI provide excellent detail of the pharynx, its fascial planes and its related spaces (see Figs. 1.32–1.34 and 1.38). Pathology in this region tends to cause asymmetry, which is readily detected.

RADIOLOGY PEARL

Pathology, especially carcinoma, of the nasopharynx spreads along the fascial planes and may extend intracranially through the many foramina described. For this reason, imaging in both axial and coronal planes is necessary to evaluate the base of the skull. CT yields excellent images of the base of the skull and provides good bone detail.

THE LARYNX (FIGS. 1.39–1.43)

The larynx forms the entrance to the airway and is responsible for voice production. It lies between the great vessels and is bound anteriorly by the strap muscles, posteriorly by the hypopharynx lying anterior to C_3–C_6, superiorly by the hyoid bone and inferiorly by the trachea. It is lined by mucosa, which is continuous with that of the pharynx above and the trachea below. Its framework is composed of three single and three paired cartilages, which articulate with each other and are joined by muscles, folds and connective tissue.

The anchor cartilage of the larynx is the **cricoid cartilage**. This is shaped like a signet ring, with a flat, wide lamina posteriorly and an arch anteriorly. It is joined to the thyroid cartilage above by the **cricothyroid membrane**, and to the trachea below by the **cricotracheal membrane**. The paired pyramidal **arytenoid cartilages** sit on the superolateral margin of the signet posteriorly. These bear anteroinferior vocal processes, which give rise to the **vocal ligaments** of the true vocal cords.

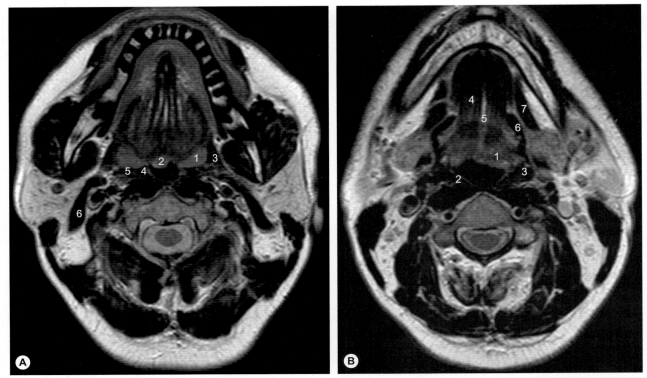

Fig. 1.38 Axial magnetic resonance image of the oropharynx. (A) At the level of the oropharyngeal tonsils and uvula. (B) At the level of the base of the tongue.

(A)
1. Oropharyngeal tonsil
2. Uvula
3. Styloglossus
4. Palatopharyngeus
5. Stylopharyngeus
6. Posterior belly of digastric

(B)
1. Base of tongue
2. Palatopharyngeus and middle constrictor
3. Stylopharyngeus
4. Genioglossus
5. Lingual septum
6. Hyoglossus
7. Mylohyoid

The **thyroid cartilage** forms the anterior and lateral boundary of the larynx. It is formed by a pair of laminae, which are joined anteriorly forming an angle and are separated above to form the **superior thyroid notch**. This notch is at approximately C_4 level. The posterior parts of the laminae have upper and lower projections known as the **superior** and **inferior horns** or **cornua**. The inferior horns project down posterolaterally to articulate with the signet of the cricoid cartilage with a synovial joint. The vocal ligaments are attached to the inner surface of the thyroid cartilage near its lower margin.

The **epiglottis** is a leaf-shaped cartilage whose narrow base or **petiole** is attached to the inner surface of the thyroid cartilage at the same point as the anterior extremity of the vocal cords. It projects up behind the base of the tongue and directs boluses laterally into the piriform fossae during deglutition, thus protecting the larynx. A pair of mucosal folds, called the **pharyngeal folds**, pass laterally from the epiglottis to the pharyngeal wall. Three mucosal folds, a central and two lateral folds (the **glossoepiglottic folds**), pass from the anterior surface of the epiglottis to the base of the tongue. These form paired recesses between the base of the tongue and the epiglottis known as the **valleculae**. A further pair of mucosal folds pass from the lateral margin of the epiglottis posteriorly to the arytenoid cartilages, separating the larynx from the piriform fossae. These are the **aryepiglottic folds** which, together with the epiglottis, define the entrance to the larynx.

Two further pairs of cartilages lie in the aryepiglottic folds. The **corniculate cartilages** sit on top of the arytenoid cartilages, and the **cuneiform cartilages** lie immediately laterally in the free margin of the fold.

The cavity of the larynx is divided into three parts by upper and lower pairs of mucosal folds. The upper pair of folds are the **vestibular** or **false cords**. The space between the laryngeal entrance and the false cords is known as the **vestibule** or the **sinus** of the larynx. The lower pair of folds are the **true cords** and contain the vocal ligaments, which are responsible for voice production. The space between the false and true vocal cords is the **laryngeal ventricle**. This space may extend anterosuperiorly, forming a small pouch known as the **saccule** of the larynx. The term **glottis** refers

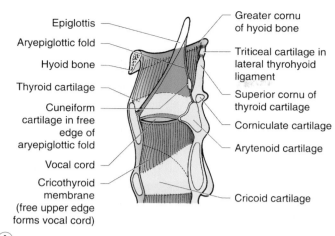

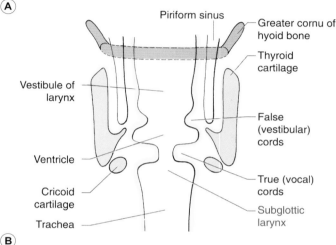

Fig. 1.39 The larynx. (A) Sagittal section showing cartilages. (B) Coronal section.

to the true vocal cords and the triangular space between them when open (**rima glottidis**). The lowest part of the larynx is the **subglottic larynx**, which lies between the true cords and the trachea. It is elliptical in cross-section superiorly, and circular inferiorly as it merges with the trachea.

The **hyoid bone** is a U-shaped bone between the mandible and the thyroid cartilage. It has a small central body and a long extension on each side called the **greater cornua** or horns. Smaller **lesser cornua** arise from its upper surface. The tip of each greater cornu is attached to the styloid process by the **stylohyoid ligament**.

The entire larynx is slung from the hyoid bone by the thyrohyoid **membrane** and **ligaments**. Anteriorly the thyrohyoid membrane arises from an oblique line on the thyroid cartilage and inserts into the inferior part of the hyoid bone. A midline thickening forms the thyrohyoid ligament. The thickened posterior part of the same membrane passes from the superior horns of the thyroid cartilage to the greater horns of the hyoid bone, forming the lateral thyrohyoid ligaments. The hyoid bone, in turn, is attached to the mandible, tongue and styloid process, and to the pharynx by the middle pharyngeal constrictor.

Cross-Sectional Anatomy of the Larynx (see Figs. 1.40–1.43)

For larynx cancer staging, the larynx is divided into three subsites:

Supraglottic Level (see Figs. 1.41A, 1.42)

The larynx is anterior to the piriform sinuses, separated from them by the aryepiglottic folds. At a higher level, the thyroid cartilage and the hyoid bone, with its greater horns laterally, may be seen. The epiglottis, pharyngoepiglottic folds, valleculae and base of tongue may also be identified posterior to the hyoid bone. The sternocleidomastoid

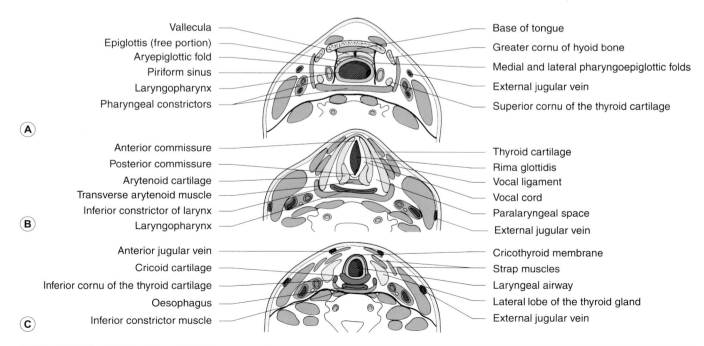

Fig. 1.40 The larynx. (A) Axial section, supraglottic level. (B) Axial section, glottic level. (C) Axial section, subglottic level.

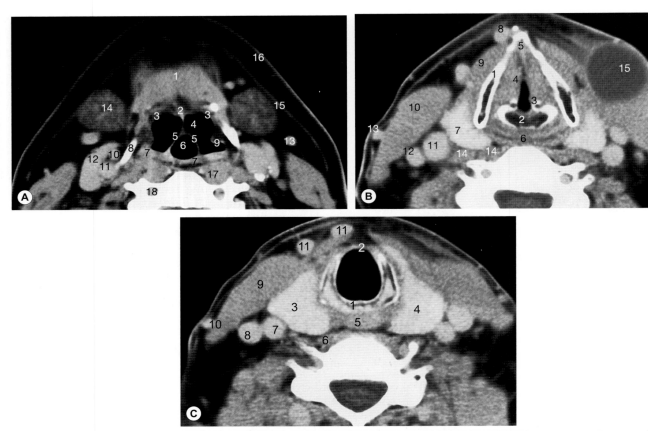

Fig. 1.41 Computed tomography scan of the larynx/neck. (A) Supraglottic level. (B) Glottic level. (C) infraglottic level.

(A)
1. Base of tongue
2. Median glossoepiglottic fold
3. Lateral glossoepiglottic fold
4. Vallecula
5. Epiglottis
6. Laryngopharynx
7. Pharyngeal constrictor muscle
8. Greater cornu of hyoid bone
9. Tip of piriform sinus (the sinus is separated from the laryngopharynx on lower cuts by the aryepiglottic fold)
10. Internal carotid artery
11. Internal jugular vein
12. Sternomastoid muscle
13. External jugular vein
14. Submandibular gland
15. Platysma muscle
16. Subcutaneous fat
17. Prevertebral muscle
18. Foramen transversarium

(B) (There is a pathological abscess in the left sternomastoid muscle.)
1. Thyroid cartilage
2. Cricoid cartilage
3. Vocal process of arytenoid cartilage
4. Vocal cord
5. Anterior commissure
6. Laryngopharynx
7. Upper pole of thyroid gland
8. Anterior jugular vein
9. Strap muscles
10. Sternomastoid muscle
11. Internal jugular vein
12. Common carotid artery
13. External jugular vein
14. Prevertebral muscle
15. Abscess in sternomastoid muscle

(C)
1. Cricoid cartilage
2. Cricothyroid membrane
3. Right lobe of thyroid gland
4. Left lobe of thyroid gland
5. Oesophagus (collapsed)
6. Prevertebral muscles
7. Common carotid artery
8. Internal jugular vein
9. Sternomastoid muscle
10. External jugular vein
11. Anterior jugular veins

muscles are seen posterolaterally with the carotid and internal jugular vessels medial to them. Contents of the supraglottic larynx include the epiglottis, pre-epiglottic space, aryepiglottic folds (excluding the posterior walls that belong to the piriform sinuses), paraglottic space, false vocal cords (at the level of the arytenoids) and other structures superior to an imaginary line drawn through the laryngeal ventricles. The false cords are at the level of the foot processes of the arytenoid cartilages and divide the laryngeal vestibule above from the laryngeal ventricle below. The larynx is triangular in shape at the level of the false cords.

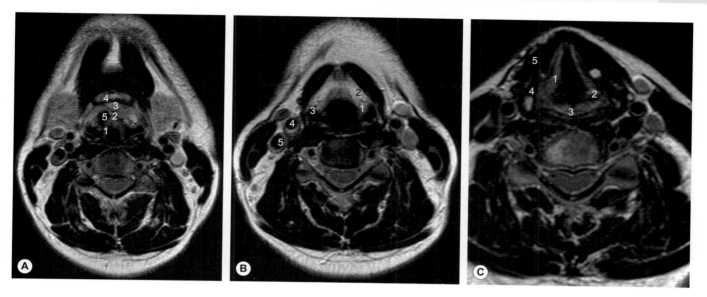

Fig. 1.42 Axial magnetic resonance images of the supraglottic larynx.

(A)
1. Epiglottis
2. Median Glosso-epiglottic fold
3. Pre-epiglottic space
4. Hyoid bone
5. Vallecula

(B)
1. Aryepiglottic fold
2. Paraglottic fat

3. Piriform fossa
4. Right common carotid artery
5. Right internal Jugular vein

(C)
1. False cord
2. Arytenoid
3. Cricoid cartilage
4. Thyroid cartilage
5. Strap muscles

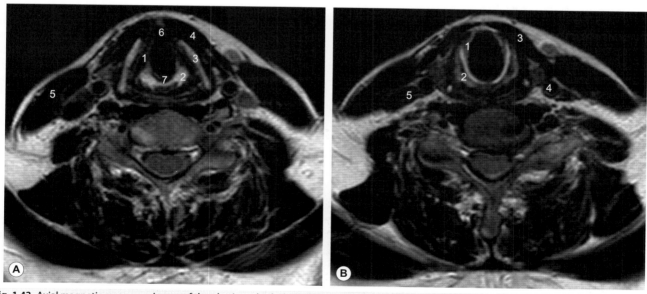

Fig. 1.43 Axial magnetic resonance image of the glottic and subglottic larynx. (A) Glottic larynx. (B) Subglottic larynx.

(A)
1. True cord
2. Cricoid cartilage
3. Thyroid cartilage
4. Strap muscles
5. Sternocleidomastoid muscle
6. Anterior Commissure
7. Posterior Commissure

(B)
1. Sub-glottis
2. Cricoid cartilage
3. Strap muscles
4. Left common carotid artery
5. Right internal jugular vein

Glottic Level (see Figs. 1.41B, 1.43A)

A complete ring of cartilage is seen at this level – the thyroid cartilage anteriorly and the lamina of the cricoid cartilage posteriorly. The vocal processes of the arytenoids may be identified giving attachment to the vocal ligaments and defining the level of the glottis.

The anterior fusion of the true vocal cords is known as the anterior **commissure** and is very thin when the cords are abducted. Similarly, the **posterior commissure**, which is seen between the arytenoids, is also thin in abduction of the cords. Both commissures may appear thickened during adduction of the cords (phonation). The larynx is elliptical in shape at the level of the true cords. The thyroid cartilage is anterior. The **paralaryngeal space** is between the larynx and the thyroid cartilage.

Subglottic Level (see Figs. 1.41C, 1.43B)

The subglottic larynx extends from the inferior margin of the true vocal cords to the inferior margin of the cricoid cartilage. Just below the true cords the larynx is elliptical. The lamina of the cricoid is posterior, with the cricothyroid membrane anterior. The inferior thyroid horns and part of the thyroid lamina are posterior and lateral to the cricoid. At a lower level the larynx is more circular and the cricoid forms a complete ring. Part of the lobes of the thyroid gland may be seen laterally, with the neck vessels situated posterolaterally. The external jugular vein may be seen anterior to the sternocleidomastoid muscle.

Radiology of the Larynx (see Figs. 1.37, 1.40–1.43)

Plain Radiography. This is a relatively simple method of demonstrating the anatomy of the larynx.

Lateral views are the most useful as the larynx is not obscured by the vertebrae. The air in the pharynx and larynx provides intrinsic contrast with the soft-tissue walls and mucosal folds (see Fig. 1.37).

On the lateral view, the hyoid bone and cartilages of the larynx are seen. The thyroid, cricoid and arytenoid cartilages are composed of hyaline cartilage and may calcify or undergo true ossification. Calcification is often irregular but may be homogeneous with a dense cortex and less dense medulla. The other cartilages are composed of yellow elastic fibrocartilage and do not calcify. The lateral thyrohyoid ligaments may contain **triticeal cartilages**, which can calcify and should not be mistaken for foreign bodies. The base of the tongue, vallecula, epiglottis, aryepiglottic folds, and true and false cords may be identified. The vestibule, ventricle and infraglottic larynx are those spaces above, between and below the cords.

CT and MRI. Cross-sectional imaging using CT (see Figs. 1.40–1.43) provides excellent anatomical detail of the larynx and surrounding structures. The cartilages are of low density on CT unless calcified, which occurs increasingly with age. They are of high signal intensity on MRI as they contain fatty marrow. The mucosa of the subglottic larynx and the anterior commissure should not be thicker than 1 mm on MRI. The true cords (ligament) are of low signal intensity and the false cords (fat containing) are of high signal intensity. Symmetry of the soft tissues is important.

RADIOLOGY PEARL

Medialization of an arytenoid cartilage can indicate the presence of an ipsilateral vocal cord paralysis most commonly due to recurrent laryngeal nerve (RLN) injury but can also be due to upstream injury of the vagus nerve (from which the RLN arises) or the brain. The RLN is longer on the left and therefore more prone to injury.

THE HYPOPHARYNX (FIG. 1.44)

The hypopharynx is the part of the pharynx that lies behind the larynx. It is bounded anteriorly by the postcricoid mucosa and posterior cricoarytenoid muscle, posteriorly by the mucosal wall, middle and inferior constrictor muscles, superiorly by the hyoid bone, glossoepiglottic and pharyngoepiglottic folds and inferiorly by the cricoid cartilage and cricopharyngeus muscle. Below the postcricoid region, it is continuous with the oesophagus from approximately the level of C6.

The upper hypopharynx is moulded around the proximal part of the larynx, forming two deep recesses on either side known as the **piriform fossae**. During deglutition the epiglottis helps conduct fluid and solid boluses along the piriform fossae from the oropharynx to the oesophagus, avoiding the entrance to the larynx.

For the purpose of hypopharyngeal cancer staging, there are three main subsites: piriform sinuses/fossae, the posterior wall of the hypopharynx and the postcricoid region.

The Neck Lymph Node Levels (Figs. 1.45, 1.46)

Cervical lymph node staging is particularly important for the management of patients with cancer of the head and neck. The nomenclature described below has been proposed by the American Academy of Otolaryngology-Head and Neck Surgery and the American Head and Neck Society. Important anatomical landmarks include the internal jugular vein, the carotid artery, the sternocleidomastoid muscle, the inferior border of the hyoid bone, the inferior border of the cricoid cartilage and the manubrium of the sternum. For clinical relevance, tumour sites at risk of metastasizing to the different lymph node levels are briefly mentioned.

Level 1: Submental and Submandibular

Bound superiorly by the mandible and mylohyoid muscle, inferiorly by the inferior border of the hyoid bone, anteriorly by the platysma muscle and posteriorly by the posterior border of the submandibular gland.

Level 1a (submental) lymph nodes are located close to the midline between the digastric muscle anterior bellies and level 1b (submandibular) lymph nodes are located posterolateral to the digastric muscle anterior bellies and medial to the mandible on either side.

Level 1 nodal metastases may result from cancers of the oral cavity, anterior nasal cavity, submandibular gland and soft tissue of the mid-face.

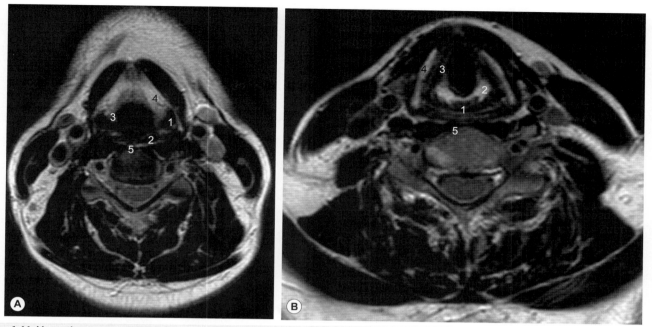

Fig. 1.44 Magnetic resonance image of the hypopharynx. (A) At the level of the piriform fossae. (B) At the level of the cricoid cartilage.

(A)
1. Piriform fossa
2. Posterior wall of the hypopharynx
3. Aryepiglottic fold
4. Paraglottic fat
5. Prevertebral fascia

(B)
1. Post-cricoid region
2. Cricoid cartilage
3. True cord
4. Thyroid cartilage
5. Prevertebral fascia

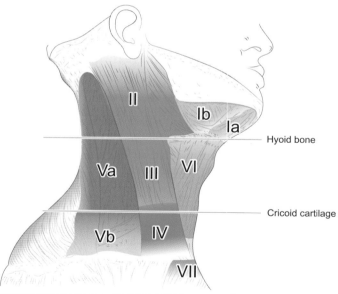

Fig. 1.45 Diagram of lymph node levels.

Level 2: Upper Internal Jugular (Deep Cervical) Chain

Bound superiorly by the base of the skull, inferiorly by the inferior border of the hyoid bone, anteriorly by the posterior border of the submandibular gland, posterolaterally by the posterior margin of the sternocleidomastoid muscle and medially by the medial border of the internal carotid artery. Level 2a anteriorly is separated from level 2b posteriorly by the posterior margin of the internal jugular vein.

Level 2 nodal metastases may result from cancers of the oral and nasal cavities, salivary glands, nasopharynx, oropharynx, hypopharynx and larynx.

Level 3: Middle Internal Jugular (Deep Cervical) Chain

Bound superiorly by the inferior border of the hyoid bone, inferiorly by the inferior border of the cricoid cartilage, anteriorly by the sternocleidomastoid muscle anterior border, posterolaterally by the sternocleidomastoid muscle posterior border and medially by the medial border of the common carotid artery.

Level 3 nodal metastases may result from cancers of the oral cavity, nasopharynx, oropharynx, hypopharynx and larynx.

Level 4: Lower Internal Jugular (Deep Cervical) and Medial Supraclavicular Chain

Bound superiorly by the inferior border of the cricoid cartilage, inferiorly by the level of the clavicle, anteriorly by the sternocleidomastoid muscle anterior border, posterolaterally by the posterolateral margin of the sternocleidomastoid muscle and the lateral edge of the anterior scalene muscle and medially by the medial border of the common carotid artery.

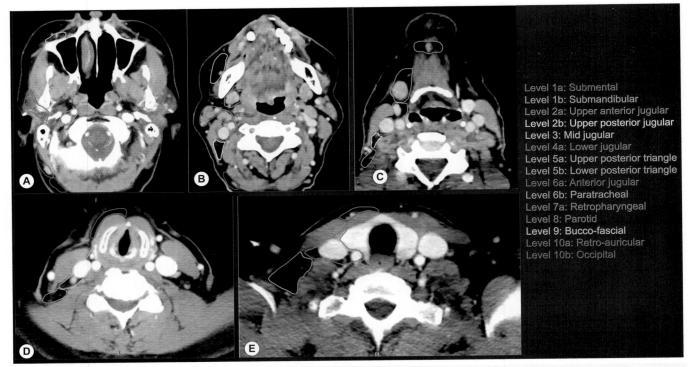

Level 1a: Submental
Level 1b: Submandibular
Level 2a: Upper anterior jugular
Level 2b: Upper posterior jugular
Level 3: Mid jugular
Level 4a: Lower jugular
Level 5a: Upper posterior triangle
Level 5b: Lower posterior triangle
Level 6a: Anterior jugular
Level 6b: Paratracheal
Level 7a: Retropharyngeal
Level 8: Parotid
Level 9: Bucco-fascial
Level 10a: Retro-auricular
Level 10b: Occipital

Fig. 1.46 Axial computed tomography showing lymph node levels A, B, C, D, E.

Level 4a lymph nodes are separated from level 4b lymph nodes inferiorly by a line drawn 2 cm superior to the sterno-clavicular joint.

Level 4a nodal metastases may result from cancers of the thyroid gland, cervical oesophagus, hypopharynx and larynx. Level 4b nodal metastases may result from the same cancers as level 4a and from cancers of the trachea.

Level 5: Posterior Triangle and Supraclavicular Chain

Bound superiorly by the skull base where the sternoclei-domastoid and trapezius muscles meet, inferiorly by the clavicle, anteromedially by the posterior border of the ster-nocleidomastoid muscle and posterolaterally by the ante-rior border of the trapezius muscle. Level 5a lymph nodes are posterior to levels 2 and 3, and are separated from level 5b inferiorly by the inferior border of the cricoid cartilage. Level 5b lymph nodes are posterior to level 4 nodes.

Level 5 nodal metastases may result from cancers of the nasopharynx, oropharynx, skin and soft tissue overlying the posterior scalp and the thyroid gland.

Level 6: Central Anterior Cervical Chain

Bound superiorly by the inferior border of hyoid bone, infe-riorly by the superior border of the manubrium (suprasternal notch), anteriorly by the platysma muscle, laterally by the medial borders of both common carotid arteries, posteromedially by the trachea and posterolaterally by the prevertebral space. Level 6a lymph nodes reflect the super-ficial anterior jugular nodes and level 6b nodes are between the medial borders of the common carotid arteries and comprise the prelaryngeal, pretracheal, paratracheal and recurrent laryngeal lymph nodes.

Level 6 nodal metastases may result from cancers of the larynx, trachea, lung and thyroid gland.

Level 7: Retropharyngeal and Retrostyloid Lymph Nodes

Retropharyngeal (level 7a) lymph nodes are bound superi-orly by the upper border of C1, inferiorly by the hyoid, lat-erally by the medial border of the internal carotid artery, posteriorly by the prevertebral muscles and anteriorly by the constrictor muscles.

Retrostyloid (level 7b) lymph nodes continue superiorly from the level 2 group bound superiorly by the skull base, medially by the internal carotid artery, laterally by the sty-loid process and deep lobe of the parotid, posteriorly by C1 and anteriorly by the parapharyngeal fat.

Level 7 nodal metastases may result from cancers of the nasopharynx and oropharynx.

Level 8: Parotid Lymph Nodes

Bound superiorly by the external auditory canal and zygo-matic arch, inferiorly by the mandible, laterally by the subcutaneous tissues, medially by the styloid process, pos-teriorly by the posterior belly of digastric and anteriorly by the posterior margin of the pterygoid muscles and mas-seter to the anterior margin of the sternocleidomastoid muscle.

Level 8 nodal metastases may result from cancers of the parotid gland, skin overlying the temporal and frontal bones, nasal cavity and external auditory canal.

Level 9: Bucco-Fascial Lymph Nodes

Bound posteriorly by the anterior wall of the maxilla, supe-riorly by the inferior margin of the orbit and inferiorly by the inferior border of the mandible.

Level 9 nodal metastases may result from cancers of the buccal mucosa, skin of the face, the nasal cavity and maxil-lary sinus.

Level 10a and 10b: Retro-Auricular and Occipital Lymph Nodes

Retro-auricular lymph nodes extend from the superior margin of the external auditory canal inferiorly to the mastoid tip. Occipital lymph nodes sit between the posterior margin of the sternocleidomastoid muscle and anterior margin of the trapezius and continue from the level 5a group up to the occipital protuberance.

Level 10 nodal metastases may result from regional skin cancers.

Layers of the Deep Cervical Fascia (Fig. 1.47)

The deep cervical fascia comprises three separate layers of fascia (superficial, middle and deep layers) that surround neck structures and anatomically delineate the deep spaces of the head and neck. All layers of deep cervical fascia contribute to the carotid sheath.

The **superficial fascia** (also known as the **investing layer**) is deep to the platysma and encases most of the neck structures, splitting to encase the submandibular glands, parotid glands, masticator space, sternocleidomastoid and trapezius muscles.

The **middle layer** of deep cervical fascia contains the infrahyoid strap muscles, visceral space and pharyngeal mucosal space. Anteriorly it is composed of the strap muscle fascia and posteriorly it is composed of the visceral fascia, also known as the **pharyngobasilar and buccopharyngeal fascia**. In the suprahyoid neck, the middle layer of deep cervical fascia which contributes to the carotid sheath is incomplete, allowing communication with the retropharyngeal space, jugular foramen, carotid canal and hypoglossal canal.

The **deep layer** of deep cervical fascia consists of the **perivertebral and alar fascia**. It contains the danger space (between the prevertebral and alar fascia), prevertebral space, vertebral column and paraspinal/paravertebral space.

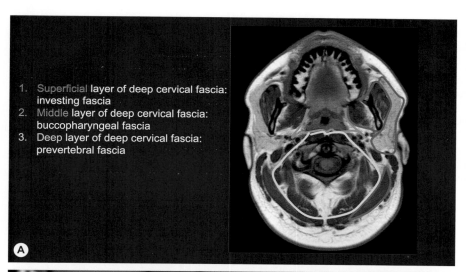

1. Superficial **layer** of deep cervical fascia: investing fascia
2. Middle **layer** of deep cervical fascia: buccopharyngeal fascia
3. Deep layer of deep cervical fascia: prevertebral fascia

A

S/A

Bucoopharyngeal fascia

Superficial Layer of deep cervical fascia

B

Fig. 1.47 (A) Deep cervical fascia layers. Three layers of deep cervical fascia that divide the neck into different spaces

1. Superficial layer of deep cervical fascia: investing fascia (Blue)
2. Middle layer of deep cervical fascia: buccopharyngeal fascia (Red)
3. Deep layer of deep cervical fascia: prevertebral fascia (Yellow)

(B) Coronal view of the parapharyngeal space The enclosing fascias insert on the skull base MEDIAL to the foramen ovale.

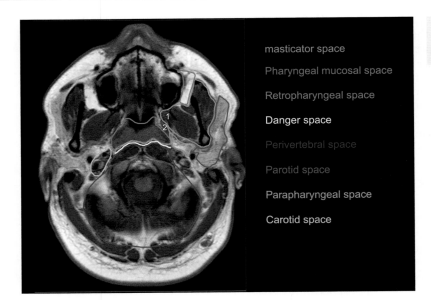

masticator space

Pharyngeal mucosal space

Retropharyngeal space

Danger space

Perivertebral space

Parotid space

Parapharyngeal space

Carotid space

Fig. 1.48 Deep spaces of the head and neck.

1. Medial pterygoid
2. Tensor veli palatini (attaches to medial pterygoid plate)

Deep Spaces of the Head and Neck (Figs. 1.48–1.52)

The deep spaces of the head and neck are delineated by the layers of deep cervical fascia. Spaces confined to the suprahyoid neck include the pharyngeal mucosal space, parapharyngeal space, submandibular space, sublingual space, parotid space and the masticator space.

Deep spaces that traverse both the supra- and infrahyoid neck include the perivertebral space, retropharyngeal space, danger space and carotid space.

Deep spaces confined to the infrahyoid neck include the visceral space (contiguous with the pharyngeal mucosal space), anterior cervical space and strap muscle compartment.

MASTICATOR SPACE

The masticator space is surrounded by the superficial layer of deep cervical fascia. It is bounded anteriorly by the buccal space, posterolaterally by the carotid space, medially by the parapharyngeal space and inferiorly by the submandibular space.

It contains the posterior body and ramus of mandible, muscles of mastication (temporalis, masseter, medial and lateral pterygoid muscles), the maxillary artery, pterygoid venous plexus, mandibular nerve which provides motor function to the muscles of mastication, tensor veli palatini, mylohyoid and anterior belly of digastric and sensation to lower face.

Infratemporal Fossa. Infratemporal fossa is a surgical term with predominantly bony landmarks including the floor of the middle cranial fossa superiorly, the zygomatic arch and mandibular ramus laterally, the lateral pterygoid plate medially, the mastoid portion of the temporal bone posteriorly, the posterior aspect of the maxilla anteriorly and the insertion of the medial pterygoid muscle inferiorly.

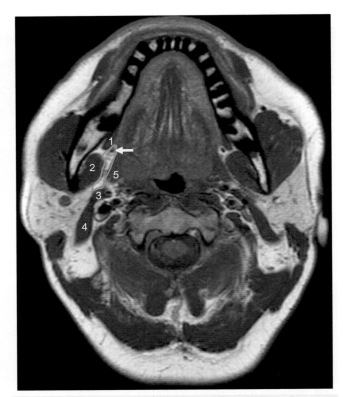

Fig. 1.49 Trigeminal fat pad in the parapharyngeal space.

1. Mylohyoid
2. Medial pterygoid
3. Stylohyoid
4. Posterior belly of digastric
5. Medial constrictor
Orange: Trigeminal fat pad. White arrow: Lingual nerve

PAROTID SPACE

It is enclosed by the superficial layer of deep cervical fascia. It is bound superiorly by the external auditory canal, inferiorly by the inferior margin of the mandible, anteriorly by the masticator space, medially by the parapharyngeal space and posteriorly by the parotid space. It contains the parotid glands, intraparotid lymph nodes, intraparotid facial nerve (adjacent to the retromandibular vein), retromandibular vein and branches of the eternal carotid artery.

PARAPHARYNGEAL SPACE

Extends from the skull base to the submandibular space with which it communicates and is between the tensor veli palatini muscle and medial pterygoid muscle and their fascias. In most people, the parapharyngeal space also communicates with the deep lobe of the parotid gland (i.e. the parotid space) as the fascia is incomplete here. It contains the trigeminal fat pad which houses the lingual nerve and sits on top of the submandibular space.

It is bound laterally by the medial pterygoid, medially by tensor veli palatini and the medial constrictor, and posteriorly by the styloid process, posterior belly of digastric and stylohyoid muscle.

RADIOLOGY PEARL	

If a tumour is truly in the parapharyngeal space, it is difficult for it to spread intracranially as the enclosing fascias are very tough and insert medial to the foramen ovale. If a tumour is in the masticator space, it is easier to spread to the foramen ovale and intracranially.

The main content of the parapharyngeal space is fat. It also contains branches of mandibular nerve (small branch of the mandibular division of the trigeminal nerve supplying the tensor veli palatini muscle and nerve to tensor tympani), vessels including the internal maxillary artery, ascending pharyngeal artery and part of the pterygoid venous plexus, and salivary tissue (minor or ectopic salivary gland/rests).

HOW THE PARAPHARYNGEAL FAT IS DISPLACED ACCORDING TO WHERE A LESION IS

The parapharyngeal fat will be laterally displaced by a mucosal space lesion, medially displaced by a masticator and parotid space lesion, posteriorly displaced by submandibular and masticator space lesions and anteriorly displaced by a carotid space (deep lobe) or carotid space lesion.

- Parotid space (deep lobe): widens the stylomandibular tunnel (space between the styloid process and mandible). Carotid space also displaced posteriorly.
- Carotid space: narrows the stylomandibular tunnel. Usually pushes the internal carotid artery anteriorly.

SUBLINGUAL SPACE (SEE FIG. 1.50)

The sublingual spaces form part of the anterior floor of mouth and communicate in the midline. As the sublingual space is not enclosed by fascia posteriorly, it is sometimes

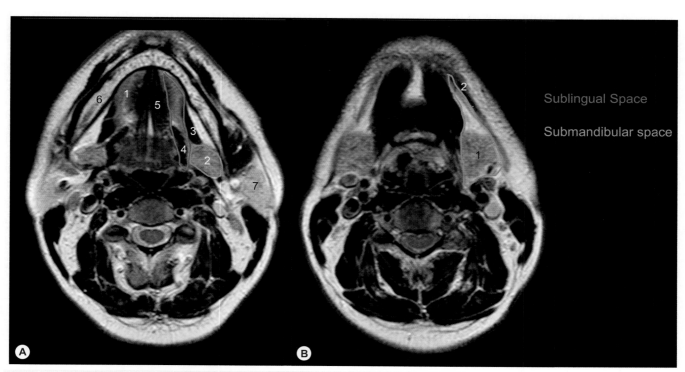

Fig. 1.50 Submandibular and sublingual spaces.

(A)
1. Right sublingual gland
2. Left submandibular gland
3. Left mylohyoid
4. Left hyoglossus
5. Left genioglossus
6. Right mandibular body
7. Left parotid gland

(B)
1. Left submandibular gland
2. Left platysma

considered part of the submandibular space. They are bound superiorly by the intrinsic tongue muscles, inferiorly by the mylohyoid muscles, anteriorly by the mandible and medially by the genioglossus and geniohyoid muscles. Posteriorly, the sublingual space communicates with the submandibular and parapharyngeal spaces along the posterior border of mylohyoid.

The sublingual space contains the sublingual gland and duct, lingual artery and vein, lingual nerve, hypoglossal and glossopharyngeal nerves and deep portion of the submandibular gland and duct.

SUBMANDIBULAR SPACE (SEE FIG. 1.50)

This is a suprahyoid deep neck space which is enclosed by the superficial layer of deep cervical fascia, superficially bound by the platysma muscle and contains the submandibular gland and surrounding structures. It communicates with the sublingual and parapharyngeal spaces. It is bound anteriorly by the mandible, posteriorly by the tongue muscles and parapharyngeal space posterosuperiorly, superiorly by the mylohyoid muscle and sublingual space (continuous posteriorly around the posterior edge of mylohyoid) and inferiorly by the hyoid bone.

It contains the superficial lobe of the submandibular gland, lymph nodes (level 1b), facial artery and vein and a branch of the hypoglossal nerve.

BUCCAL SPACE

The buccal space is bound anteriorly by the orbicularis muscle, superiorly by the zygoma, medially by the buccinator muscle, laterally by the platysma muscle and inferiorly by the depressor anguli oris muscle and fascia, which attaches to the mandible. It communicates with the submandibular space.

It contains buccal fat, the parotid duct, accessory parotid tissue (anatomical variant), facial and buccal vessels, branches of the facial and trigeminal nerves.

PHARYNGEAL MUCOSAL SPACE

This is not a true deep space as it is not entirely enclosed by fascia. It is the deepest neck compartment and is surrounded by the middle layer of deep cervical fascia.

It is bound laterally by the parapharyngeal space, posteriorly by the retropharyngeal space, superiorly by the merging of the superior pharyngeal constrictor muscle aponeurosis and middle layer of the deep cervical fascia and inferiorly by the cricoid cartilage.

It contains squamous mucosa, lymphoid tissue, the cartilaginous portion of the Eustachian tube, the superior pharyngeal constrictor, the middle pharyngeal constrictor and the levator veli palatini.

RETROPHARYNGEAL SPACE

It is a deep midline space that mainly consists of fatty tissue, small vessels and lymph nodes which drain the upper aerodigestive tract.

It is bound anteriorly by the middle layer of deep cervical fascia, posteriorly by the alar fascia (separates the retropharyngeal space from the danger space posteriorly), laterally

by the deep layer of deep cervical fascia, superiorly by the clivus and inferiorly by the fusion point of the middle layer of deep cervical fascia and alar fascia, usually at the level of T1.

DANGER SPACE

This contains a small volume of fatty connective tissue and extends from the skull base to the mediastinum. It is posterior to the retropharyngeal space, from which it is separated by the alar fascia which is not perceptible on imaging.

It is bound anteriorly by the alar fascia, posteriorly by the prevertebral layer of deep cervical fascia, superiorly by the clivus and inferiorly by the posterior mediastinum at the level of the diaphragm.

PERIVERTEBRAL SPACE

Extends from the skull base to the mediastinum and is surrounded by the deep layer of deep cervical fascia.

It is bound anteriorly by the danger space and retropharyngeal space, posteriorly by fascia attached to ligamentum nuchae and spinous processes, superiorly by the skull base and inferiorly by the superior mediastinum. A slip of fascia attached to the transverse processes divides the perivertebral space into prevertebral and paraspinal components.

The prevertebral component contains vertebral bodies and discs, prevertebral and scalene muscles, the vertebral artery and vein, the phrenic nerve and brachial plexus roots. The paraspinal component contains the cervical paraspinal muscles and neural arches of the cervical vertebrae.

> **RADIOLOGY PEARL**
>
> On plain radiographs, normal prevertebral soft-tissue thickness is <7 mm at C2 and <20 mm at C7.

CAROTID SPACE (SEE FIG. 1.51)

A poststyloid parapharyngeal space, the carotid space, is located in the supra- and infrahyoid neck and extends from the skull base to the aortic arch. The carotid space is

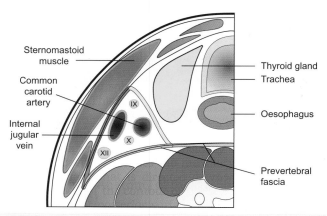

Fig. 1.51 The carotid space.

Labels: Sternomastoid muscle; Common carotid artery; Internal jugular vein; IX; X; XII; Thyroid gland; Trachea; Oesophagus; Prevertebral fascia

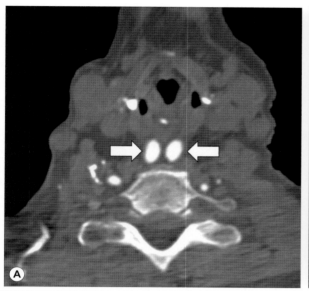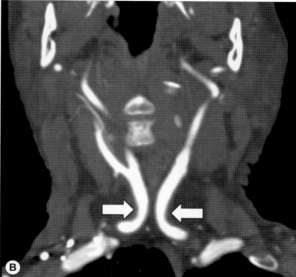

Fig. 1.52 Medial deviation of the carotid arteries. (A) Axial and (B) Coronal CT angiogram images illustrating the right and left common carotid arteries (white block arrows) almost touching in the midline, a term known as 'kissing carotids'.

bound anteriorly by the styloid process, posteriorly by the fascia of perivertebral space and prevertebral muscles and superiorly by the carotid and jugular foramina. The carotid space communicates with the retropharyngeal space, jugular foramen, carotid canal and hypoglossal canal because medially, the deep layer of enclosing fascia is incomplete.

The carotid space contains the carotid artery, jugular vein, the 9th–12th cranial nerves, some branches of the ansa cervicalis of the brachial plexus, some sympathetic nerves and lymph nodes.

RADIOLOGY PEARL

The layer of deep cervical fascia at the medial aspect of the carotid sheath is incomplete which can allow communication of pathology between both carotid spaces. If the carotid arteries are tortuous, they can touch in the midline, a term known as 'kissing carotids' (see Fig. 1.52). This can occur along the course of the common and internal carotid arteries with potentially catastrophic implications for surgery involving the pharynx if the medial position of the vessels is not appreciated.

POSTERIOR CERVICAL SPACE

The posterior cervical space extends from the skull base to the clavicles in the posterolateral aspect of the neck. It is bound by the superficial and deep layers of deep cervical fascia and contains fat, lymph nodes, part of the brachial plexus and the spinal accessory nerve.

VISCERAL SPACE

The visceral space is in the infrahyoid neck and extends superiorly from the hyoid bone to the superior mediastinum inferiorly and is surrounded by the middle layer of deep cervical fascia.

It contains the larynx, hypopharynx, trachea, oesophagus, thyroid and parathyroid glands, the recurrent laryngeal nerve and level 6 lymph nodes.

ANTERIOR CERVICAL SPACE

The anterior cervical space is not a true deep neck space as it is not entirely enclosed by fascia. It is located in the infrahyoid neck and is anterior to the carotid space, anterolateral to the strap muscles and lateral to the visceral space. It contains fat.

The Salivary Glands (Figs. 1.53–1.56)

These exocrine glands are situated symmetrically around the oral cavity and produce saliva.

THE PAROTID GLAND (SEE FIGS. 1.53–1.55)

This is the largest of the salivary glands and lies behind the angle of the jaw and in front of the ear. It is moulded against the adjacent bones and muscles. The gland has a smaller deep part and a larger superficial part, both of which are continuous around the posterior aspect of the ramus of the mandible via the **isthmus**.

The deep part of the gland extends medially to the carotid sheath and lateral wall of the pharynx, separated from these by the styloid process and muscles. The superficial part lies anterior to the tragus of the ear and is moulded to the mastoid process and sternomastoid muscle posteriorly, and to the posterior ramus of the mandible and masseter muscle anteriorly. It has an anteroinferior extension, or tail, which wraps around the angle of the mandible.

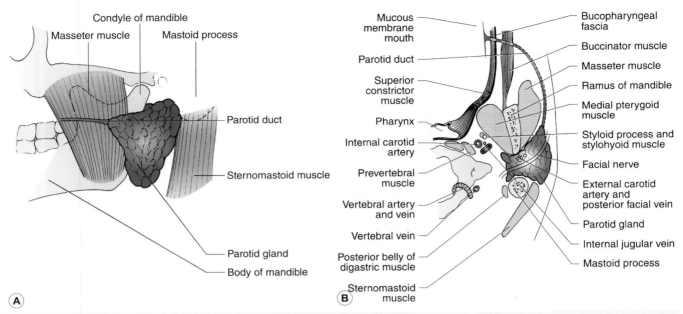

Fig. 1.53 Parotid gland. (A) Lateral view. (B) Transverse section.

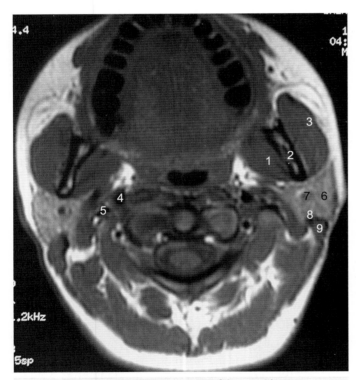

Fig. 1.54 Axial magnetic resonance image of the parotid.

1. Medial pterygoid muscle
2. Mandible
3. Masseter muscle
4. Internal carotid artery
5. Internal jugular vein
6. Parotid gland
7. External carotid artery and posterior facial vein
8. Mastoid process
9. Sternocleidomastoid muscle

The terminal part of the external carotid artery runs through the isthmus, dividing into superficial temporal and maxillary branches within the substance of the gland, and the confluence of the veins of the same name form the retromandibular vein just superficial to the artery. The facial nerve, having emerged from the stylomastoid foramen, runs through the deep part of the gland via the isthmus to the superficial part within which it branches into its five terminal divisions. It passes superficial to the internal carotid artery and retromandibular vein in the isthmus.

The parotid duct (**Stensen's duct**) begins as the confluence of two ducts in the superficial part of the gland and runs anteriorly deep to the gland. It arches over the masseter muscle before turning medially to pierce buccinator and drain into the mouth opposite the second upper molar. The duct is approximately 5 cm long. Small accessory parotid glands are common (20%), joining the duct along its length.

THE SUBMANDIBULAR GLAND (SEE FIGS. 1.55 AND 1.56)

This gland lies in the floor of the mouth medial to the angle of the mandible. It is a mixed mucinous and serous gland, hence its tendency to form calculi. It has a larger superficial lobe continuous around the posterior border of the mylohyoid muscle with a smaller deep lobe.

The submandibular (Wharton's) duct is about 5 cm long and commences as a confluence of several ducts in the superficial (lower) lobe. From here it runs superiorly through the deep (upper) lobe before running forward in the floor of the mouth to open at the side of the frenulum of the tongue. The facial artery passes over the superior surface of the gland to come to lie between the gland and the mandible. The facial vein grooves the posterior part of the gland.

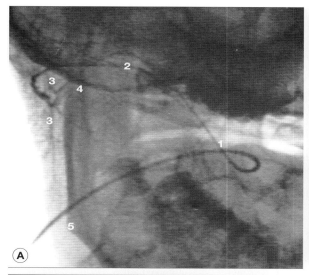

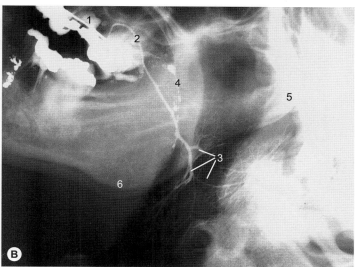

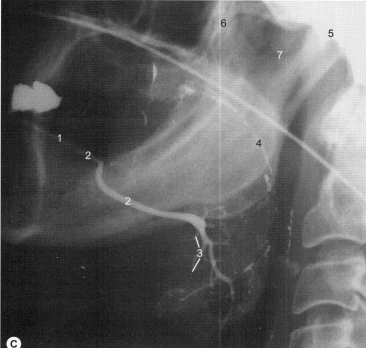

Fig. 1.55 Sialography. (A) Anteroposterior view parotid sialography. (B) Lateral view parotid sialography. (C) Lateral view submandibular sialography. Note how the duct and its branches are moulded around the body of the mandible.

(A)
1. Cannula in parotid duct
2. Parotid duct (Stensen's)
3. Normal branching ductules
4. Condylar process of mandible
5. Angle of mandible

(B)
1. Cannula in parotid orifice
2. Parotid duct
3. Secondary ductules
4. Contrast on surface of tongue
5. Condylar process of mandible
6. Angle of mandible

(C)
1. Cannula in orifice of submandibular duct
2. Submandibular duct
3. Secondary ductules
4. Contrast on superior surface of tongue
5. Condylar process of mandible
6. Coronoid process of mandible
7. Mandibular notch

THE SUBLINGUAL GLAND (SEE FIGS. 1.30, 1.31)

This small gland lies submucosally just anterior to the deep lobe of the submandibular gland and drains via several ducts (up to 20) directly into the floor of the mouth, posterior to the opening of the submandibular gland. Some of its ducts may unite and join the submandibular gland.

Radiology of the Salivary Glands

SIALOGRAPHY (SEE FIG. 1.55)

The ducts of the parotid and submandibular glands may be cannulated and injected with radio-opaque contrast to outline the ductal system. The ducts of the parotid gland arch around the mandible because of the way in which the gland is moulded to the adjacent structures. This is best seen on the AP view. The parotid duct is seen on the lateral view. The submandibular gland and duct system may be seen on the lateral projection. The ducts of the sublingual gland are not amenable to canalization.

CT and MRI (see Figs. 1.33, 1.38, 1.46, 1.54)

CT and MRI are of particular value for tumours of the glands, to assess involvement of surrounding structures. CT may be performed after sialography to improve visualization of the ducts.

MR images may demonstrate the facial nerve within the parotid gland. It is of slightly lower intensity than the surrounding gland on T_1-weighted images. MR sialography uses heavily T_2-weighted sequences to demonstrate the salivary ducts in an image like conventional sialography

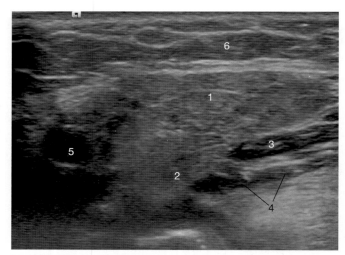

Fig. 1.56 Ultrasound of the submandibular gland.

1. Submandibular gland – superficial part
2. Submandibular gland – deep part
3. Mylohyoid muscle
4. Submandibular duct
5. Facial vein
6. Digastric muscle

without the need for canalization, contrast or radiation. The ducts are best seen if dilated by obstruction.

Ultrasound (see Fig. 1.56)

This may be performed through the skin or intraorally with high-frequency transducers.

> **RADIOLOGY PEARL**
>
> The submandibular gland may be injected with botulinum toxin using ultrasound guidance, for the treatment of sialorrhoea. One must be wary not to inject the adjacent mylohyoid muscle, paralysis of which could impair swallowing for several months. One must also identify and avoid the facial artery and the vein.

NUCLEAR IMAGING

Because the salivary gland accumulates and secretes technetium-99m (^{99m}Tc) used in nuclear imaging, this can be used to image several glands at once without cannulating the ducts. Graphs of uptake and excretion of the agent by individual glands may be computed.

The Thyroid and Parathyroid Glands

THE THYROID GLAND (FIGS. 1.57, 1.58)

The thyroid gland is derived from the first and second pharyngeal pouches. It consists of two lateral **lobes** joined by a midline **isthmus**, and lies anterior and lateral to the trachea. The lobes are approximately 4 cm in height, 3 cm in depth and 2 cm in width, and extend from the thyroid

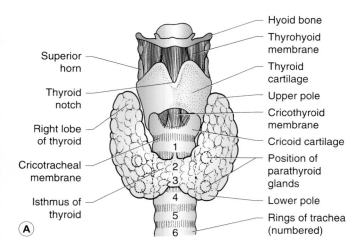

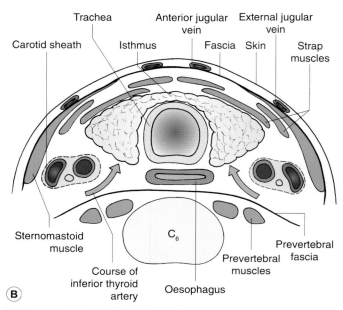

Fig. 1.57 Thyroid gland. (A) Gross anatomy. (B) Axial section.

cartilage of the trachea superiorly to the fourth or even the sixth tracheal ring inferiorly. The lobes are described as having upper and lower **poles**. The lobes are often asymmetrical, with the right being larger and more vascular than the left. The isthmus is draped across the second to fourth tracheal rings at the level of C_6. A small midline superior extension of the isthmus called a pyramidal lobe may be present. The gland is invested in the **pretracheal fascia**. This fascial layer also invests the larynx and trachea, and the pharynx and oesophagus. The deep surface of the gland lies on these structures. Posterolaterally are the neck vessels, invested in their own fascia, the **carotid sheath**. Behind these, on either side, are the prevertebral muscles and their fasciae.

Anterior to the gland are the strap muscles of the neck and the sternomastoid muscles invested in an outer layer of fascia. Superficially, the **anterior jugular vein** runs in the midline, and the **external jugular vein** runs inferiorly on either side. The **parathyroid glands** lie close to the deep surface of the gland and may be intracapsular.

Cross-Sectional Anatomy (see Fig. 1.57)

At the level of C_6 the gland appears as two triangles of tissue on each side of the trachea and connected across the trachea by the isthmus. Each triangular lobe measures approximately 3 cm in depth by 2 cm in width and has a convex anterior surface. The strap muscles of the neck, sternomastoid and the anterior jugular veins are anterior. The posterolateral surface is related to the carotid sheath. The posteromedial surface lies on the trachea and oesophagus and may be interposed between them.

Blood Supply and Lymph Drainage

Two constant pairs of arteries supply the thyroid gland. The **superior thyroid artery** is the first branch of the external carotid and supplies the upper pole. The **inferior thyroid artery** arises from the thyrocervical trunk, which is a branch of the subclavian artery. This passes behind the carotid sheath to gain access to the deep part of the gland. Both arteries anastomose freely with each other. A variable (3%) third artery, the **thyroidea ima**, may arise from the brachiocephalic artery or the aortic arch and ascends anterior to the trachea to join in the anastomotic plexus.

Three pairs of veins arise from a venous plexus on the surface of the gland. The **superior** and **middle thyroid veins** drain into the internal jugular vein. The **inferior thyroid veins** (often multiple) end in the left brachiocephalic vein. Lymph drainage is directly into the thoracic duct and the right lymphatic duct.

Development of the Thyroid Gland

The thyroid gland develops from an outpouching of the pharynx and descends into the neck, passing anterior to the hyoid bone and trachea.

RADIOLOGY PEARL

Maldevelopment may cause thyroid tissue to be found anywhere along a line from the base of the tongue to its normal position. Less commonly, thyroid tissue may migrate inferiorly to the mediastinum or even to the pericardium or myocardium. The **thyroglossal duct** may persist as a midline structure extending superiorly from the isthmus of the gland and a **thyroglossal cyst** may be found at any site related to this. More commonly (40%), part of the duct persists as the **pyramidal lobe** of the gland, extending superiorly from the isthmus or the medial part of either lobe more commonly the left.

RADIOLOGY OF THE THYROID GLAND

Ultrasound (see Fig. 1.58)

Ultrasound of the gland with a high-frequency transducer provides excellent detail. The normal thyroid gland has a homogeneous echotexture of medium echogenicity. The carotid vessels may be seen as anechoic structures on either side of the gland. The strap muscles are seen as structures of low echogenicity. Linear echogenic lines may be seen separating the muscles. The prevertebral muscles may be identified posteriorly. Numerous vascular structures may be

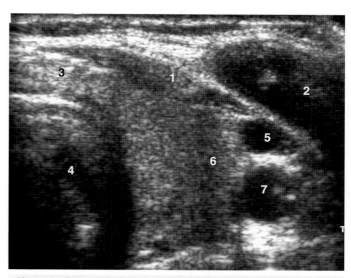

Fig. 1.58 Ultrasound of the thyroid gland showing the left lobe.

1. Strap muscle
2. Sternomastoid muscle
3. Isthmus
4. Trachea
5. Left common carotid artery
6. Left lobe of gland
7. Left internal jugular vein

seen surrounding the gland, and its extreme vascularity is readily appreciated with colour flow imaging.

Nuclear Medicine Studies

Isotope scanning provides functional rather than anatomical detail. Both lobes and the isthmus can be identified. It is useful for identifying ectopic thyroid tissue, which is most likely to be in the base of the tongue, reflecting its site of development.

Computed Tomography (see Figs. 1.41, 1.46)

CT may be used to assess the gland with or without contrast. It shows as soft-tissue areas of high attenuation because of the iodine content. The surrounding structures of the neck may also be imaged. Imaging with short scan times during dynamic infusion of contrast gives the best images and definition of the gland and surrounding structures.

Magnetic Resonance Imaging

The gland is of higher signal intensity than surrounding muscles on T_2-weighted MRIs. The use of surface coils improves detail.

THE PARATHYROID GLANDS

These endocrine glands are small lentiform structures measuring approximately 6 mm in length, 3–4 mm in transverse diameter and 1–2 mm in AP diameter. They usually number four – two superior and two inferior – but any number from two to six is possible. The glands lie posterior to the thyroid gland within its fascial sheath in 90% of cases. The superior glands lie on the posterior border of the middle third of the thyroid, and the inferior glands lie near the lower pole of the thyroid.

The superior gland develops from the fourth pharyngeal pouch and does not migrate. The inferior parathyroid gland develops from the third pharyngeal pouch with the thymus and migrates inferiorly. Maldescent may cause the inferior parathyroid gland to be found in ectopic sites, and this may be of clinical importance in the search for a parathyroid adenoma. The most common ectopic site is just below the inferior pole of the thyroid. Occasionally the gland descends into the superior mediastinum with the thymus. Less commonly it does not descend at all and remains above the superior parathyroid, or it may be found behind the oesophagus or in the posterior mediastinum. Most of the blood supply of the parathyroid glands is derived from the inferior thyroid artery.

RADIOLOGY OF THE PARATHYROID GLANDS

Cross-Sectional Imaging

On ultrasound the normal parathyroids are seen as hypoechoic structures lying posterior to the thyroid gland. On CT the parathyroids appear as structures of lower attenuation than thyroid tissue.

Nuclear Medicine Studies

The parathyroids may be imaged using a subtraction technique. Both the thyroid and the parathyroid glands take up thallium-201 (^{201}Tl) chloride. The thyroid (but not the parathyroids) takes up ^{99m}Tc pertechnetate. By computed subtraction of the technetium image from the thallium image, the parathyroids may be demonstrated.

The Neck Vessels (Figs. 1.59–1.66)

THE CAROTID ARTERIES IN THE NECK (SEE FIGS. 1.59–1.62)

The left common carotid artery arises from the aortic arch in front of the trachea and passes across the trachea to lie on its left side in the root of the neck. The right common carotid arises from the brachiocephalic trunk behind the right sternoclavicular joint. From this point the right and left common carotid arteries have a similar course. The common carotid artery passes upwards and slightly laterally. It is accompanied by the internal jugular vein on its lateral aspect, with the vagus nerve lying posteriorly between the two. All three structures are invested in the carotid sheath (see section on Deep Spaces of the Head and Neck, see Fig. 1.51). The common carotid artery bifurcates into internal and external branches at the level of C_4. The external carotid artery passes anteriorly and curves slightly posteriorly as it ascends to enter the substance of the parotid gland, where it terminates by dividing into maxillary and superficial temporal arteries. The internal carotid artery continues superiorly from its origin to the base of the skull, maintaining the relationship of the common carotid artery with the internal jugular vein and vagus nerve in the carotid sheath. It has a localized dilatation at its origin called the carotid sinus. This is a neurovascular structure innervated by the glossopharyngeal nerve that has a role in blood pressure regulation. The internal carotid artery has no branches in the neck.

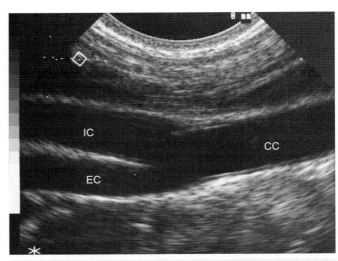
Fig. 1.59 Ultrasound of the carotid artery: longitudinal section. *CC*, Common carotid artery; *EC*, external carotid artery; *IC*, internal carotid artery.

Anatomical Relations of the Common Carotid Artery Within the Carotid Sheath

The anatomical relations are as follows:
- Posteriorly is the sympathetic trunk. It is separated from the transverse processes of C_4–C_6 by the prevertebral muscles.
- Medially are the trachea and oesophagus, with the RLN between them at first. At a higher level the larynx, pharynx and RLN are medial, with the thyroid gland lying anteromedially.
- Anterolaterally the artery is covered by sternomastoid and the strap muscles at first. Above the level of the cricoid cartilage it is covered only by skin and fascia.

Anatomical Relations of the Internal Carotid Artery Within the Carotid Sheath

These are as follows:
- Posteriorly is the sympathetic trunk, prevertebral muscles and transverse processes of C_1–C_3.
- Medially is the lateral wall of the pharynx.
- Anterolaterally it is covered throughout its length by sternomastoid muscle. The styloid process and muscles separate it from the external carotid artery in its upper part.

The artery becomes anterior to the internal jugular vein at the base of the skull and enters the carotid canal. The internal jugular vein and vagus nerve pass through the jugular foramen.

Anatomical Relations of the External Carotid Artery

At its origin the internal carotid artery is lateral. As the external carotid artery ascends in the neck, it comes to lie in a more lateral plane than the internal carotid artery.
- Medially is the lateral wall of the pharynx at first. At a higher level it is separated from the internal carotid artery by the styloid process and its muscles.

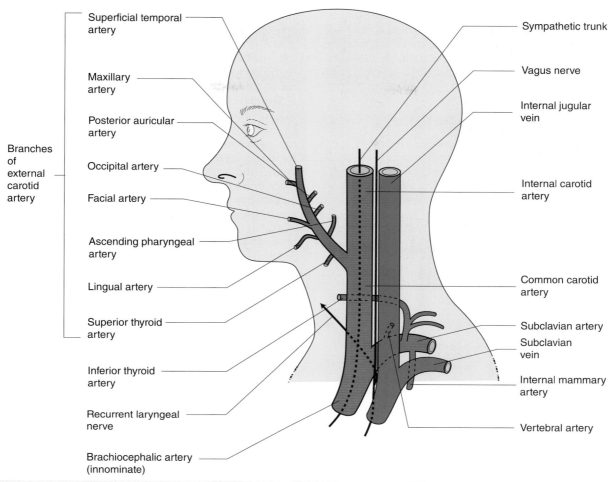

Fig. 1.60 Carotid artery in the neck.

- Anterolaterally is the anterior part of sternomastoid at first. It then passes deep to the posterior belly of the digastric and stylohyoid muscles before entering the substance of the parotid gland.

Branches of the External Carotid Artery (see Figs. 1.60–1.62)

The branches of the external carotid artery anastomose freely with each other and with their partners on the opposite side. There are also several points of anastomosis with the internal carotid circulation and with branches of the subclavian artery.

Superior thyroid artery. This branch arises anteriorly close to the origin and passes inferiorly to supply the thyroid gland, anastomosing with the inferior thyroid artery.

Ascending pharyngeal artery. This is a small branch that ascends deep to the external carotid on the lateral wall of the pharynx. It supplies the larynx and also gives rise to meningeal vessels, which pass through the foramen lacerum.

Lingual artery. This branch arises anteriorly and runs upwards and medially before curving downward and forward towards the hyoid bone in a characteristic loop. It then runs under muscles arising from that bone to supply the tongue and floor of the mouth. The lingual artery may arise with the facial artery as a common trunk, the linguofacial trunk.

Facial artery. This vessel arises from the anterior surface of the external carotid artery above the level of the hyoid bone. It passes upward deep to the ramus of the mandible, grooving the posterior part of the submandibular gland. It then curves downward under the ramus of the mandible and hooks around it to supply the muscles and tissues of the face with a tortuous course. Its terminal branch anastomoses with a branch of the ophthalmic artery. It also supplies the submandibular gland, soft palate and tonsil.

Occipital artery. This arises posteriorly opposite the origin of the facial artery. It runs to the posterior part of the scalp, crossing the internal carotid and jugular vessels, and terminates in tortuous occipital branches supplying the scalp. It gives off muscular branches in the neck. The stylomastoid artery arises from the vessel in two-thirds of people, passing superiorly through the stylomastoid foramen to supply the middle and inner ear. Meningeal branches enter the skull through the jugular foramen and condylar canal and supply the dura of the posterior cranial fossa.

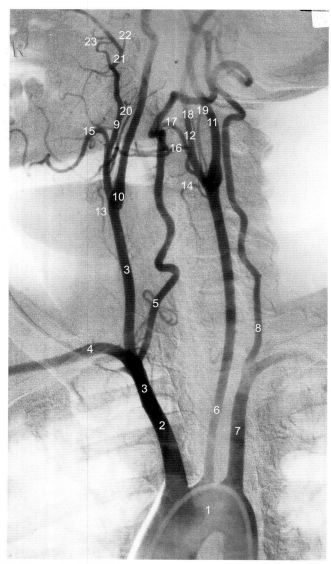

Fig. 1.61 Arch aortogram: subtraction film. The catheter is in the aortic arch. All branches of the external carotid are shown except the occipital artery. The facial artery is not filling on the right.

1. Arch of aorta
2. Brachiocephalic trunk
3. Right common carotid artery (superimposed upon the subclavian artery)
4. Right subclavian artery
5. Right vertebral artery
6. Left common carotid artery
7. Left subclavian artery
8. Left vertebral artery
9. Right external carotid artery
10. Sinus of right internal carotid artery
11. Left internal carotid artery
12. Left external carotid artery
13. Right superior thyroid artery (arising from the external carotid artery)
14. Left superior thyroid artery (arising from common carotid artery)
15. Right lingual artery
16. Left lingual artery
17. Left facial artery
18. Left ascending pharyngeal artery
19. Left posterior auricular artery
20. Right posterior auricular artery
21. Right maxillary artery
22. Middle meningeal artery (branch of right maxillary artery)
23. Right superfi cial temporal artery.

Posterior auricular artery. This vessel arises posteriorly and ascends between the styloid process and parotid gland. It has muscular branches in the neck and supplies the parotid, pinna and scalp, anastomosing with branches of the occipital artery. In one-third of people it gives rise to the stylomastoid artery.

Superficial temporal artery. This is the smaller of the two terminal branches. It arises within the parotid gland behind the neck of the mandible. It ascends over the posterior root of the zygomatic arch, dividing into tortuous anterior and posterior branches 5 cm above that point, and supplies the scalp and pericranium. It also gives branches to the parotid, temporomandibular joint, facial structures and the outer ear. One of its branches anastomoses with the lacrimal and palpebral branches of the ophthalmic artery in yet another communication between internal and external systems.

Maxillary artery. This is the larger of the two terminal branches. It arises within the parotid gland behind the neck of the mandible. It supplies the upper and lower jaws, muscles of mastication, palate, nose and cranial dura mater. It is divided into three parts by the lateral pterygoid muscle. Its first (mandibular) part passes deep to the neck of the mandible. Its second (pterygoid) part runs forward and upward between the temporalis and the lower head of the lateral pterygoid. Its third (pterygopalatine) part passes between the upper and lower heads of the lateral pterygoid through the pterygomaxillary fissure to enter the pterygopalatine fossa.

The maxillary artery has several important branches. Those of the first part are as follows:

- The middle meningeal artery enters the skull through the foramen spinosum and supplies the dura mater and bone of the cranium. This is a relatively straight artery compared with the tortuous overlying superficial temporal artery.
- The accessory meningeal artery may arise from this part or from the middle meningeal artery. It passes through the foramen ovale to supply dura mater and bone.
- The inferior dental artery descends to supply the structures of the lower jaw.

The branches of the second part are the branches to temporalis, pterygoid and masseter muscles.

The branches of the third part are as follows:

- The superior dental artery arises just as the artery enters the pterygopalatine fossa and supplies the structures of the upper jaw.
- The infraorbital artery enters the orbital cavity through the infraorbital fissure, running along the infraorbital groove to supply the contents of the orbit.
- The greater palatine artery descends from the pterygopalatine fossa through the palatine canal and through the greater palatine foramen of the hard palate. It supplies the tonsil, palate, gums and mucous membrane of the roof of the mouth.
- The sphenopalatine artery is the terminal part of the maxillary artery. It passes from the fossa through the sphenopalatine foramen into the cavity of the nose, branching to supply the nasal structures and the sinuses.

RADIOLOGY OF THE CAROTID VESSELS
(SEE FIGS. 1.59, 1.61, 1.62)

Ultrasound (see Fig. 1.59)

The common carotid artery and its bifurcation may be imaged using a high-frequency probe (7.5 or 10 MHz). The external carotid artery may be distinguished from the internal carotid artery by identifying the superior thyroid branch. The carotid sinus is seen as a localized dilation of the internal carotid artery close to the bifurcation. Ultrasound is most useful for assessment of the inner walls of the vessels, which should appear smooth in the normal patient.

Angiography

The carotid vessels may be demonstrated by injection of contrast through a catheter in the aortic arch, or by selective injection of the common carotid artery or of either carotid vessel. Selective injection of the common carotid artery is usually performed to assess this vessel and the cervical part of the internal carotid artery, which should be smooth and of even calibre. Selective injection of the external carotid may be necessary when demonstration of supply to vascular tumours or arteriovascular malformations is required. Both intracranial and extracranial pathology may cause pathological enlargement of external branches, owing to the numerous pathways of possible anastomosis. Selective injection of the internal carotid artery is performed to assess intracranial pathology.

Variations in the anatomy of the vessels may be seen. The left common carotid artery may arise with the brachiocephalic artery. This is the commonest variation of the aortic arch vessels and is seen in 27% of the population. The right common carotid artery may arise from the arch of the aorta. Occasionally, the common carotid arteries arise from a single trunk. Congenital absence of the internal or external carotid artery may occur rarely. The right subclavian artery may arise as the last branch of the arch in

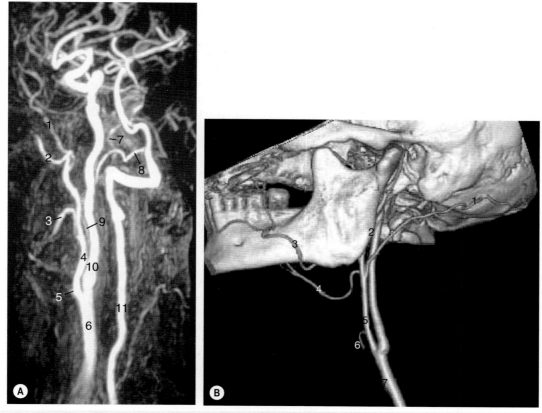

Fig. 1.62 Carotid arteries in the neck. (A) Magnetic resonance angiogram. (B) Computed tomography angiogram.

(A)
1. Superficial temporal artery
2. Maxillary artery
3. Lingual artery
4. External carotid artery
5. Origin of superior thyroid artery
6. Common carotid artery
7. Posterior auricular artery
8. Occipital artery
9. Ascending pharyngeal artery
10. Internal carotid artery
11. Vertebral artery

(B)
1. Occipital artery
2. Internal carotid artery
3. Facial artery
4. Lingual artery
5. External carotid artery
6. Superior thyroid artery
7. Common carotid artery

approximately 0.5% of people. In this situation it ascends to the right, passing behind the oesophagus, and causes an oblique posterior indentation, which can be seen on a barium-swallow examination.

CT and MRI

The carotid vessels may be imaged by CT or MR angiography (see Fig. 1.62). Pathology in the neck may displace or involve the vessels, and symmetry between the two sides should be evident in normal cases.

VENOUS DRAINAGE OF THE HEAD AND NECK (FIGS. 1.63, 1.66)

The **facial vein** drains the anterior part of the scalp and facial structures. It forms at the angle of the eye and runs posteroinferiorly to the angle of the mandible.

The **superficial temporal vein** (which also drains the scalp) joins with the **maxillary vein** (which drains the infratemporal area) to form the retromandibular vein behind the angle of the mandible.

The **retromandibular vein** descends through the parotid gland deep to the facial nerve and superficial to the external carotid artery. Below this, it divides in two. The anterior branch joins with the facial vein to join the **internal jugular vein**. The posterior branch joins with the **posterior auricular vein** (which drains the posterior scalp) to form the **external jugular vein**.

The internal jugular vein is formed at the jugular foramen, where it is a continuation of the sigmoid sinus. It descends in the carotid sheath lateral to its artery, then passes inferiorly to behind the medial end of the clavicle, where it is joined by the subclavian vein to become the **brachiocephalic vein**. It drains the petrosal sinus from within the cranium, as well as the facial vein. In addition, it receives the superior and middle thyroid veins as well as pharyngeal and lingual veins. The thoracic duct drains to the junction of the left internal jugular vein and the left subclavian vein. The right lymph duct usually drains into the junction of the right internal jugular vein and the right subclavian vein. These openings are variable and may also be into either vein or may be multiple.

The external jugular vein descends superficial to the sternomastoid muscle and pierces the cervical fascia above the midpoint of the clavicle to enter the subclavian vein.

The **anterior jugular vein** arises at the level of the hyoid bone near the midline. It passes downward and laterally, passing deep to the sternomastoid to enter the external jugular vein behind the clavicle.

The **jugular arch** is a U-shaped communication between the two anterior jugular veins above the manubrium sterni.

The **vertebral vein** exits from the transverse foramen of C_6 and runs down and forward to drain into the posterior aspect of the brachiocephalic vein.

RADIOLOGY OF THE VEINS OF THE HEAD AND NECK

The veins of the face and scalp are not usually imaged specifically. The neck veins are identified on cross-sectional imaging techniques such as ultrasound, CT (see Fig. 1.42) and MRI.

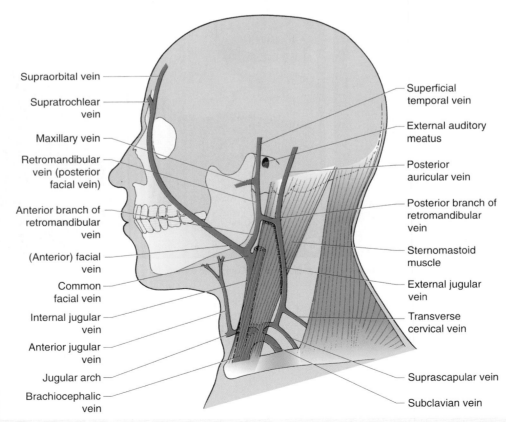

Fig. 1.63 Veins of the face and neck.

THE SUBCLAVIAN ARTERIES IN THE NECK (SEE FIGS. 1.64, 1.65)

The right subclavian artery arises from the bifurcation of the brachiocephalic trunk behind the right sternoclavicular joint. The left subclavian artery arises from the arch of the aorta in front of the trachea at the level of the T_3/T_4 disc space. It ascends on the left of the trachea to behind the left sternoclavicular joint. From this point, both arteries have a similar course. The scalenus anterior muscle (which passes from the transverse processes of the upper cervical vertebrae to the inner border of the first rib) divides the artery into three parts. The first part arches over the apex of the lung and lies deeply in the neck. The second part passes laterally behind the scalenus anterior muscle, which separates it from the subclavian vein. The third part passes to the lateral border of the first rib, where it becomes the axillary artery.

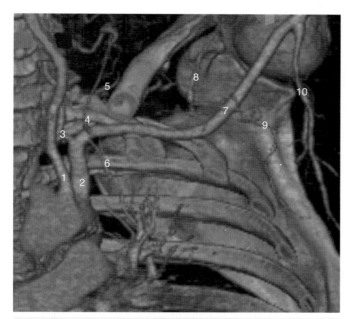

Fig. 1.64 Subclavian computed tomography angiogram.

1. Left common carotid artery
2. Left subclavian artery
3. Vertebral artery
4. Thyrocervical trunk
5. Transverse cervical artery
6. Internal thoracic artery
7. Thoracoacromial artery
8. Acromial artery
9. Lateral thoracic artery
10. Subscapular artery

Branches of the Subclavian Artery in the Neck

First part of the subclavian artery:

- **Vertebral artery**. This crosses the dome of the pleura to enter the transverse foramen of C_6. It passes through the transverse foramina of C_6–C_1 then arches medially, passing behind the lateral masses of C_1 before entering the cranial cavity through the foramen magnum. In the neck it supplies the vertebral muscles and the spinal cord. Within the vertebral transverse foramina, it is accompanied by the vertebral vein.
- **Internal mammary (thoracic) artery**. This arises from the inferior aspect of the subclavian artery and descends behind the costal cartilages of the ribs about 2 cm from the lateral border of the sternum. It supplies the anterior mediastinum, the anterior pericardium, the sternum and the anterior chest wall.
- **Thyrocervical trunk**. This arises close to the medial border of the scalenus and trifurcates almost immediately. Its branches are the inferior thyroid artery, which runs upwards and medially to enter the lower pole of the thyroid gland, and the suprascapular and transverse cervical arteries, which run laterally over the scalenus muscles to join in the scapular anastomosis and supply the muscles of the shoulder region.

Second part of the subclavian artery:

- **The costocervical artery** (this usually arises from the first part on the left). It divides into supreme intercostal artery, which supplies the first two intercostal spaces, and the deep cervical artery.

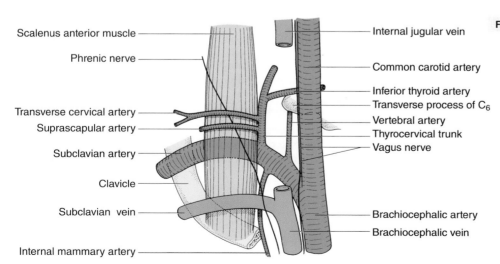

Fig. 1.65 Arteries in the root of the neck.

Scalenus anterior muscle

Phrenic nerve

Transverse cervical artery

Suprascapular artery

Subclavian artery

Clavicle

Subclavian vein

Internal mammary artery

Internal jugular vein

Common carotid artery

Inferior thyroid artery

Transverse process of C_6

Vertebral artery

Thyrocervical trunk

Vagus nerve

Brachiocephalic artery

Brachiocephalic vein

Third part of the subclavian artery:

- **The dorsal scapular artery**. This supplies the levator scapulae, rhomboids and trapezius. It may arise from the second part of the subclavian artery or even from the transverse cervical branch of the thyrocervical trunk from the first part of the subclavian artery.

THE SUBCLAVIAN VEINS IN THE NECK (SEE FIG. 1.66)

These are the continuation of the axillary veins from the outer border of the first rib to where they join with the internal jugular to form the brachiocephalic veins. As the vessel crosses the first rib, it grooves its superior surface. Anterior to the vein is the clavicle, and posteriorly it is separated from the subclavian artery by the scalenus anterior muscle. It receives the external jugular vein on both sides. On the left it receives the **thoracic duct** (which drains lymph from the body except for the right arm, the right side of the head and neck and the right lung) just at its union with the internal jugular vein to form the left brachiocephalic vein. On the right, the right lymphatic duct (often several small ducts) drains into it as it unites with the internal jugular to form the right brachiocephalic vein.

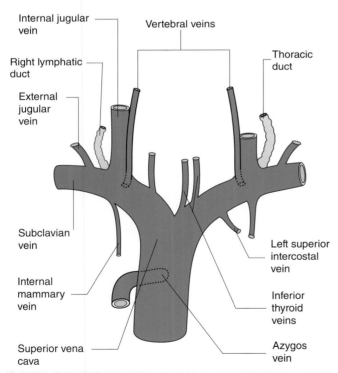

Internal jugular vein

Vertebral veins

Thoracic duct

Right lymphatic duct

External jugular vein

Subclavian vein

Left superior intercostal vein

Internal mammary vein

Inferior thyroid veins

Superior vena cava

Azygos vein

Fig. 1.66 Veins in the root of the neck.

RADIOLOGY OF THE SUBCLAVIAN VESSELS

Ultrasound

The subclavian vessels may be imaged at least in part by ultrasound. This is technically difficult, however, because of the overlying bone and adjacent lung, neither of which transmits sound.

Angiography, CT Angiography and MR Angiography

The subclavian arteries are best demonstrated by angiography or CT or MR arteriography (see Fig. 1.64).

The subclavian veins are best demonstrated by venography, with an injection into one of the veins in the arm, by CT venography with contrast or by MR venography with or without contrast.

The Brachial Plexus (see Figs. 1.67, 1.68)

This plexus of nerves is formed by five roots derived from the anterior primary rami of C_5–T1. The roots lie between the anterior and middle scalene muscles. These unite to form three trunks: $C_{5/6}$ to upper, C_7 to middle and C_8, T_1 to lower. The trunks traverse the posterior triangle of the neck. Each trunk divides to form three anterior and three posterior **divisions**. The anterior divisions supply the flexor and the posterior division supplies the extensor division of the arm. The divisions lie behind the clavicle. Three **cords** are formed in the axilla: the anterior divisions of the upper and lower cords form the lateral cord; the anterior division of the lower trunk forms the medial cord; the posterior divisions of all three trunks unite to form the posterior cord. The cords continue as the **main nerve trunks** of the arm. Lateral cord – **musculocutaneous nerve**; medial cord – the **ulnar nerve**; posterior cord – **axillary** and **radial nerves**; lateral and medial cords give fibres to the **median nerve**.

RADIOLOGY OF THE BRACHIAL PLEXUS

CT and MRI (see Fig. 1.68)

In traumatic plexopathy, the brachial plexus is imaged by CT or CT myelography. In all other circumstances the brachial plexus is imaged by MRI. On MRI the nerves are iso- or hypointense compared with muscle on T_1- or T_2-weighted images. T_1 is probably best, as nerves are surrounded by fat. Axial, coronal and sagittal planes are used for imaging.

RADIOLOGY PEARL

When assessing brachial plexus injury in an infant, MRI is focused on demonstrating a pseudomeningocele close to the cervical thecal sac at the site of the avulsed nerve root.

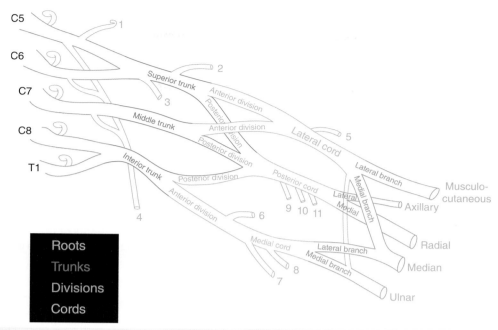

Fig. 1.67 Brachial Plexus: Locations of the roots, trunks, divisions and cords of the brachial plexus on coronal STIR imaging. 1. Scalenus anterior muscle. 2. Sternomastoid muscle.

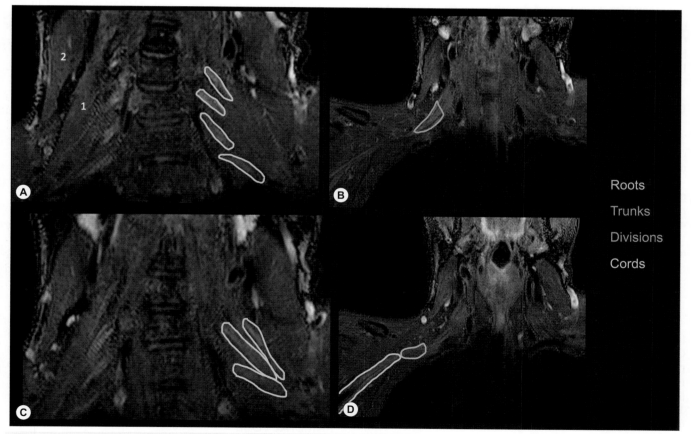

Fig. 1.68 Coronal magnetic resonance image of the brachial plexus.

1. Sternomastoid muscle
2. Roots of brachial plexus
3. Scalenus anterior muscle

2 | *The Central Nervous System*

TERENCE FARRELL
EDITED BY STEPHANIE RYAN

CHAPTER CONTENTS

Cerebral Hemispheres 58
Cerebral Cortex 58
White Matter of the Hemispheres 60
Basal Ganglia 66
Thalamus, Hypothalamus and Pineal Gland 69
Pituitary Gland 71
The Limbic Lobe System 73

The Brainstem 74
Cerebellum 78
Ventricles, Cisterns, CSF Production and Flow 80
Meninges 87
Arterial Supply of the CNS 90
Venous Drainage of the Brain 95

Cerebral Hemispheres

The cerebral hemispheres fill the cranial vault above the tentorium cerebelli. Right and left hemispheres are partly separated by the interhemispheric fissure. There are several white matter tracts connecting both hemispheres, the largest of which is the corpus callosum. The hemispheres consist of cortical grey matter, white matter, basal ganglia, thalamus, hypothalamus, pituitary gland and the limbic lobe. The lateral ventricles form a cavity within each hemisphere.

Cerebral Cortex (Figs. 2.1, 2.2)

The cerebral cortex is the superficial grey matter and is composed of neuronal cell bodies. There are four main subdivisions – the frontal, temporal, parietal and occipital lobes – which are delineated by sulci in the cortex. The superolateral surface of each cerebral hemisphere has two deep sulci; these are:

- The **lateral sulcus**, also known as the Sylvian fissure, which separates the frontal and temporal lobes.
- The **central sulcus** (of Rolando), which passes upwards from the lateral sulcus to the superior border of the hemisphere. This separates the frontal and parietal lobes.

The **parieto-occipital sulcus** on the medial surface of the hemisphere separates the parietal and occipital lobes. On the lateral surface of the hemispheres there is no complete sulcal separation of the parietal, temporal and occipital lobes. The boundary between the parietal and temporal lobes lies on a line extended back from the lateral sulcus. The boundary separating the parietal and temporal lobes from the occipital lobe is a line between the superior border of the parieto-occipital sulcus and the preoccipital notch (see Fig. 2.1).

Cortical regions within each lobe control different functions, some of which have been identified to date.

FRONTAL LOBE

The frontal lobe includes all of the cortex anterior to the central sulcus and superior to the lateral sulcus. The frontal cortex contains four main gyri, the precentral gyrus and the superior, middle and inferior frontal gyri. The motor cortex, premotor cortex and prefrontal area are some of the regions associated with known major functions.

Primary Motor Cortex

The motor cortex is centred on the precentral gyrus, which is immediately anterior to the central sulcus. It controls voluntary movement. Specific regions of the motor cortex control specific and predictable body parts. This can be displayed diagrammatically as the 'human homunculus'. The corticospinal and corticobulbar motor tracts emanate from the primary motor cortex.

Premotor Cortex

The premotor cortex is the anterior part of the precentral gyrus and adjoining gyri. Its function is less well understood but it is also associated with the control of voluntary movement. The posteroinferior part of the premotor area, on the inferior portion of the inferior frontal gyrus on the dominant hemisphere, is **Broca's area**, which is responsible for the production of speech.

Prefrontal Area

Anterior to the motor and premotor cortex, the frontal lobes are involved with intellectual, emotional and autonomic activity. On the medial surface of the frontal lobe, above and parallel to the corpus callosum, is the callosal sulcus. Above this, the cingulate gyrus extends posteriorly from the frontal lobe into the parietal lobe. This, in turn, is separated superiorly from the remainder of the medial surface by the cingulate sulcus.

PARIETAL LOBE

The parietal lobe is posterior to the central sulcus and superior to the lateral sulcus and a line drawn from its posterior end to the occipital lobe (see Fig. 2.1). Areas with known

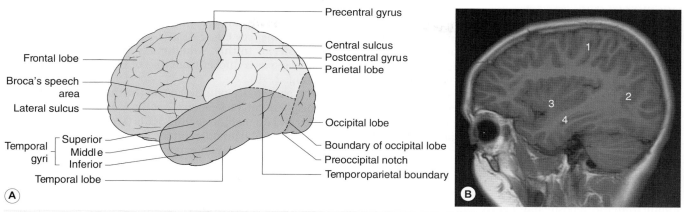

Fig. 2.1 (A) Superolateral surface of the cerebral hemisphere. (B) Sagittal magnetic resonance image of the brain lateral to midline.

(B)
1. Central sulcus
2. Parieto-occipital sulcus
3. Insula
4. Temporal horn of lateral ventricle and hippocampus

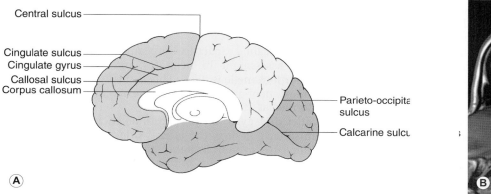
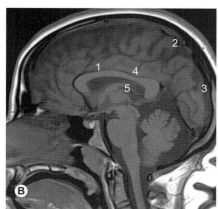

Fig. 2.2 (A) Medial surface of the cerebral hemisphere. (B) Midline sagittal magnetic resonance image of the brain.

(B)
1. Cingulate gyrus
2. Central sulcus
3. Parieto-occipital sulcus
4. Corpus callosum
5. Fornix

function include the primary somatosensory cortex and the parietal association cortex.

Primary Somatosensory Cortex

This is found on the gyrus posterior to the central sulcus and is known as the postcentral gyrus. This controls somatic sensations.

Parietal Association Cortex

This is posterior to the sensory cortex. This area is involved with recognition and integration of sensory stimuli.

TEMPORAL LOBE

The temporal lobe lies inferior to the lateral sulcus and anterior to the occipital lobe. Two horizontal gyri separate the superolateral surface into superior, middle and inferior temporal gyri. Areas associated with known function include the primary auditory cortex and the temporal association cortex.

Primary Auditory Cortex

Found on the superior temporal gyrus, the auditory cortex's function is the reception of auditory stimuli. **Wernicke's area**, responsible for the interpretation of language, is located within the superior temporal gyrus, most commonly in the dominant lobe.

Temporal Association Cortex

Situated around the auditory cortex, this area is involved with the recognition and integration of auditory stimuli.

OCCIPITAL LOBE

The occipital lobe lies posterior to the parietal and temporal lobes. There is no anatomical separation of these lobes on the superolateral surface of the hemisphere. However, on the medial surface, the occipital lobe is separated from the parietal lobe by the parieto-occipital sulcus. A further deep sulcus of this surface, the calcarine sulcus, runs anteriorly from the occipital pole (see Fig. 2.2). Areas with known function include the primary visual cortex and the occipital association cortex.

Primary Visual Cortex

This surrounds the calcarine sulcus and receives visual stimuli from the opposite half field of sight.

Occipital Association Cortex

This lies anterior to the visual cortex and is involved with the recognition and integration of visual stimuli.

INSULA (OF REIL)

This is the cortex buried in the floor of the lateral sulcus and is crossed by branches of the middle cerebral artery. Its function is not fully understood; however, it has multiple connections to each of the major lobes as well as the limbic system and basal ganglia. Gustatory and sensorimotor processing are some of its better understood roles, although the area closest to the sensory cortex is probably related to taste. The parts of the frontal, parietal and temporal lobes that overlie the insula are called the operculum. The extreme capsule, claustrum and external capsule lie increasingly medial to the insula (Fig. 2.7).

RADIOLOGICAL FEATURES OF THE CEREBRAL CORTEX

Computed Tomography and Magnetic Resonance Imaging

Identification of lobes on computed tomography (CT) and magnetic resonance imaging (MRI) slices depends on identification of their boundaries. The advent of high-resolution volumetric imaging of the brain with multiplanar reformatting for both CT and MRI have facilitated identification of the major fissures. The sylvian cistern and fissure separating the frontal and temporal lobes are easily identified on axial CT or MR slices (Fig. 2.3). The central sulcus that forms a boundary between the frontal and parietal lobes can be more difficult to identify, however. Because CT images are obtained parallel to the canthomeatal line, on upper images the central sulcus is quite posterior in position. This lies at a transverse level just posterior to the anterior limit of the lateral ventricles.

There are a number of landmarks and signs that have been described to facilitate identification of the central sulcus. For example, on axial images the central sulcus has been described as having an inverted omega-shaped curve that marks the position of the hand motor cortex (see Fig. 2.3D). Also on axial imaging, the L-sign describes the junction of the superior frontal gyrus and precentral gyrus with the central sulcus lying posterior to this. The T-sign is the sulcal equivalent of this, with the superior frontal sulcus and precentral sulcus meeting intersecting as a T-shape (see Fig. 2.3E). The central sulcus is the sulcus posterior to this. Additionally the cortex of the precentral gyrus is thicker than that of the post central gyrus (see Fig. 2.3D).

The parieto-occipital sulcus on the medial surface of the hemisphere can be seen on CT at the level of the lateral ventricles and on midline sagittal MRIs (see later Fig. 2.5). The parieto-occipital junction on the lateral surface has no anatomical landmark but lies at approximately the same transverse level as the sulcus.

Midline sagittal images also show the cingulate gyrus and callosal and cingulate sulci. The insula and the frontal, parietal and temporal opercula can be seen on axial CT and on MRI in all planes.

In adults the white matter is myelinated. In this setting, grey matter is T2 hyperintense and T1 hypointense relative to white matter.

On an unenhanced CT the grey matter is relatively hypodense compared to the white matter.

ULTRASOUND EXAMINATION OF THE NEONATAL BRAIN

The intracranial structures are amenable to ultrasound-guided assessment in neonates and infants while the anterior fontanelle is open. This is the first-line evaluation for most neonates requiring neuroimaging and can be performed at the bedside.

Sulci and gyri can be identified including the interhemispheric fissure, the lateral sulcus, insula and operculum on coronal images, and the corpus callosum and cingulate gyri on midline sagittal views (see later Fig. 2.10).

RADIOLOGY PEARL

The medial wall of the atrium of the lateral ventricle is indented by the white matter over the calcarine sulcus, the calcar avis. In parasagittal views on cranial ultrasound of the newborn, this can be mistaken for thrombus in the ventricle, but imaging in the coronal plane confirms its continuity with normal parenchyma.

White Matter of the Hemispheres

White matter is primarily composed of myelinated axons and supporting glial cells. White matter forms fibre tracts which relay information and help coordinate actions between different parts of the brain and spine.

There are three main types of fibre within the cerebral hemispheres:

■ Commissural fibres, which connect corresponding areas of the two hemispheres.
■ Association (arcuate) fibres, which connect different parts of the cortex of the same hemisphere.
■ Projection fibres, which join the cortex to lower centres.

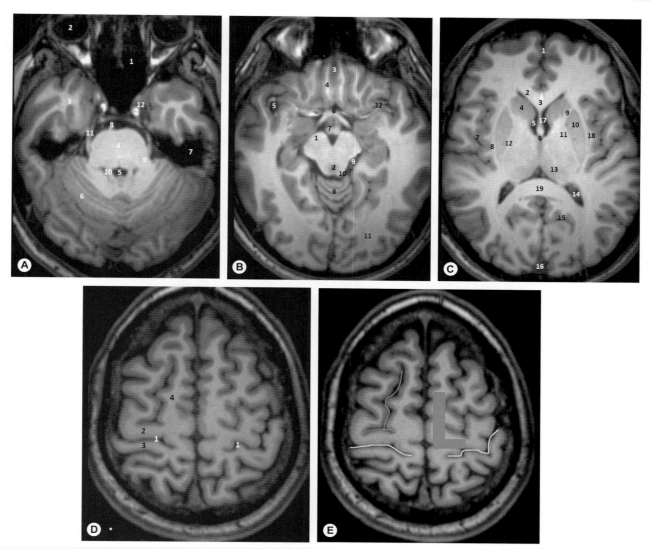

Fig. 2.3 Magnetic resonance image of the brain. (A) Level of the pons. (B) Level of the midbrain. (C) Level of the lateral ventricles. (D) Above the lateral ventricles. (E) Right superior frontal sulcus *(red line)* intersecting with the right precentral sulcus *(green line)* to form the T-sign. The sulcus immediately posterior to this is the central sulcus *(yellow line)*. The right superior frontal gyrus and precentral gyrus intersect to form the L-sign *(in blue)*.

(A)
1. Ethmoid sinus
2. Globe
3. Right temporal lobe
4. Pons
5. Fourth ventricle
6. Right cerebellar hemisphere
7. Petrous part of temporal bone
8. Basilar artery
9. Middle cerebellar peduncle
10. Superior cerebellar peduncle
11. Fifth cranial nerve
12. cavernous sinus

(B)
1. Crus of midbrain
2. Aqueduct of Sylvius
3. Interhemispheric fissure
4. Gyrus rectus
5. Sylvian fissure
6. Optic chiasm
7. Mamillary body
8. Vermis of the cerebellum
9. Ambient cistern
10. Quadrigeminal plate
11. Left occipital lobe
12. Middle cerebral artery

(C)
1. Interhemispheric fissure
2. Tapetum
3. Genu of corpus callosum
4. Head of caudate nucleus
5. Anterior horn of right lateral ventricle
6. Interventricular foramen
7. Sylvian fissure
8. External capsule
9. Anterior limb of internal capsule
10. Putamen of lentiform nucleus
11. Globus pallidus of lentiform nucleus
12. Posterior limb of internal capsule
13. Thalamus
14. Atrium and choroid plexus of lateral ventricle
15. Calcarine sulcus
16. Superior sagittal sinus
17. Septum pellucidum
18. Claustrum
19. Splenium of corpus callosum

(D)
1. Central sulcus – note characteristic inverted omega shape on left side
2. Precentral gyrus
3. Post central gyrus
4. Superior frontal gyrus

COMMISSURAL FIBRES

The Corpus Callosum (Figs. 2.4, 2.5)

The corpus callosum is a large midline mass of commissural fibres, each of which connects corresponding areas of both hemispheres. It is approximately 10 cm long and becomes progressively thicker towards its posterior end. Named parts include the following:

- **Rostrum** – this is the first part, which extends anteriorly from the anterior commissure (see below).

- **Genu** – this is the most anterior part where it bends sharply backwards.
- **Trunk (body)** – this is the main mass of fibres extending from the genu anteriorly to the splenium posteriorly. It lies below the lower free edge of the falx cerebri. Branches of the anterior cerebral vessels run on its superior surface.
- **Splenium** – this is the thickened posterior end.

In cross-section, fibres from the genu that arch forward to the frontal cortex on each side are called **forceps**

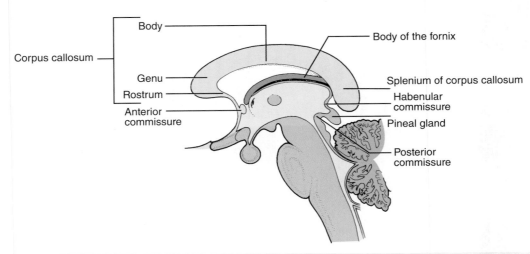

Fig. 2.4 Corpus callosum and other commissures.

minor and fibres from the splenium passing posteriorly to each occipital cortex are called **forceps major**. Fibres extending laterally from the body of the corpus callosum are called the **tapetum**. These form part of the roof and lateral wall of the lateral ventricles.

Anterior Commissure (Figs. 2.4, 2.6)

This is a bundle of fibres in the lamina terminalis in the anterior wall of the third ventricle. The fibres pass laterally in an arc, indenting the inferior surface of the globus pallidus. The anterior commissure runs anterior to the anterior columns of the fornix and caudal to the anterior limb of the internal capsule. The anterior commissure is part of the olfactory system and connects the olfactory bulbs, the cortex of the anterior perforated substance and the piriform areas.

Habenular Commissure

This small commissure is situated above and anterior to the pineal body. It unites the habenular striae, which are fibres from the olfactory centre that pass posteriorly along the upper surface of each thalamus and unite in a 'U' configuration in this commissure.

Posterior Commissure

This is situated anterior and inferior to the pineal body. It lies dorsal to the cerebral aqueduct and forms part of the posterior wall of the third ventricle. It connects the superior colliculi, which are concerned with light reflexes (see brainstem).

Hippocampal Commissure

This is the commissure of the fornix (see below) and connects the two hippocampi. It lies below the body and splenium of the corpus callosum and is in close proximity to the Foramen of Monroe.

PROJECTION FIBRES

These fibres join the cerebral cortex to lower centres in the deep nuclei, cerebellum, brainstem and spinal cord. Some fibres are afferent and some efferent. A number of major projection fibres converge together to form the internal capsule, where they lie lateral to the thalamus and the corona radiata as they fan out between the internal capsule and the cerebral cortex.

Internal Capsule (see Fig. 2.3C)

This contains sensory fibres from the thalamus to the sensory cortex and motor fibres from the motor cortex to motor nuclei in the brainstem, corticobulbar tracts and, in the spinal cord, the corticospinal (pyramidal) tracts. These tracts occupy predictable locations within the internal capsule.

In axial cross-section, the internal capsule has an anterior limb between the caudate and lentiform nuclei and a posterior limb between the lentiform nucleus and the thalamus. Both limbs meet at a right-angle called the genu.

The anterior limb is composed mainly of frontopontine fibres and thalamic radiations. The motor fibres converge at the genu and anterior or thalamolenticular component of

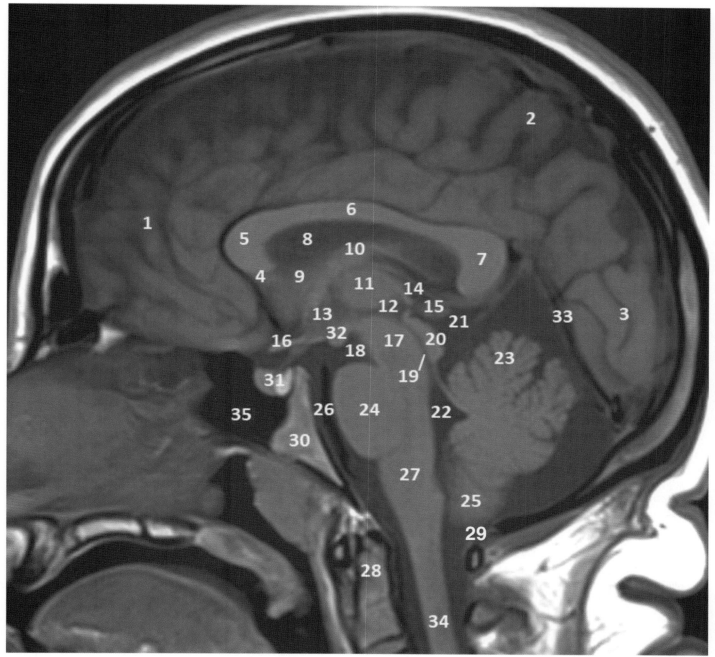

Fig. 2.5 Magnetic resonance image scan of the brain: midline sagittal image.

 1. Frontal lobe
 2. Parietal lobe
 3. Occipital lobe
 4. Rostrum of corpus callosum
 5. Genu of corpus callosum
 6. Body of corpus callosum
 7. Splenium of corpus callosum
 8. Septum pellucidum
 9. Foramen of Monro
10. Fornix
11. Massa intermedia of thalami
12. Third ventricle
13. Supraoptic recess of third ventricle
14. Suprapineal recess of third ventricle
15. Pineal gland
16. Optic chiasm
17. Midbrain
18. Interpeduncular cistern
19. Aqueduct of Sylvius
20. Quadrigeminal plate (superior and inferior colliculi)
21. Quadrigeminal plate cistern
22. Fourth ventricle
23. Vermis of cerebellum
24. Pons
25. Tonsil of cerebellum
26. Prepontine cistern
27. Medulla oblongata
28. Odontoid process
29. Cisterna magna
30. Clivus
31. Pituitary
32. Mamillary body
33. Tentorium cerebelli
34. Spinal cord
35. Sphenoid sinus

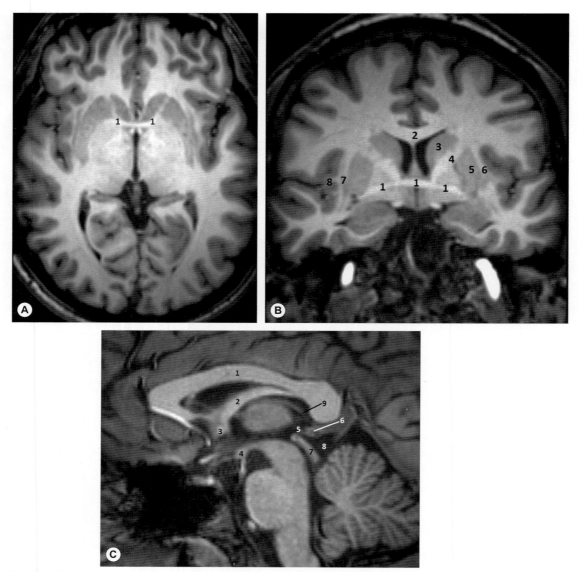

Fig. 2.6 Anterior commissure. (A) Axial T₁ magnetic resonance image. (B) Coronal magnetic resonance image. (C) Midline sagittal magnetic resonance image.

(A)
1. Anterior commissure

(B)
1. Anterior commissure
2. Corpus callosum
3. Head of caudate nucleus
4. Internal capsule
5. Putamen
6. External capsule
7. Claustrum
8. Insula

(C)
1. Corpus callosum
2. Fornix
3. Anterior commissure
4. Mamillary body
5. Posterior commissure
6. Pineal gland
7. Quadrigeminal plate
8. Quadrigeminal plate cistern
9. Habenular commissure

the posterior limb. The corticospinal and corticobulbar tracts are the largest tracts. The most anterior fibres at the genu are those of the head. Fibres to the arm, hand, trunk, leg and perineum lie progressively more posteriorly. Haemorrhage or thrombosis of thalamostriate arteries supplying this area leads to paralysis of these muscles innervated by these fibres.

Behind these fibres on the posterior limb and on the retro-lentiform part of the internal capsule are parietopontine and occipitopontine fibres. More posteriorly are the visual fibres that extend towards the occipital pole as the optic radiation. Most posterior of all are the auditory fibres.

RADIOLOGICAL FEATURES OF THE COMMISSURAL AND PROJECTION FIBRES

Plain Films of the Skull

Calcification of the habenular commissure is a common finding on skull radiographs. It is found anterior and superior to the pineal gland if this is also calcified. Typically, the calcification is C-shaped, with the open part of the letter facing backwards. Some authors suggest that this calcification is in the choroid plexus of the third ventricles – the taenia habenulare – rather than in the commissure.

CT and MRI

The corpus callosum is best assessed on sagittal and coronal imaging. On sagittal imaging the rostrum, genu, body and splenium form a rotated continuous C shape (Fig. 2.5). The anterior and posterior commissures can also be seen on this view. A line joining the anterior and posterior commissures, the AC–PC line, is used as a reference in image-guided procedures.

On coronal MRI scans (Fig. 2.7) the body of the corpus callosum and the tapetum can be seen superior to the lateral ventricles. On this view the anterior commissure may also be visible inferior to the third ventricle, but this commissure is best seen as an arc of fibres on axial MRI (see Fig. 2.6).

On axial imaging the internal capsule is seen as a V-shaped low-attenuation or high T_1 signal structure (see Fig. 2.3C) between the caudate and lentiform nuclei anteriorly and the lentiform and thalamus posteriorly. On coronal imaging it can be seen lateral to the thalami. It is less well visualised on sagittal imaging.

RADIOLOGY PEARL

Superficial subcortical white matter fibres are sometimes called U fibres because of their course on the deep surface of the gyri. These may be specifically involved or spared in different leukodystrophies and white matter disorders. These disorders affect various fibre tracts in different ways, some affecting predominantly deep white matter and some affecting predominantly superficial cerebral white matter and many spare the optic radiation. Optic nerve glioma preferentially affects parts of the optic nerve pathways and its location reflects the anatomical course of these fibres including involving connections to the lateral geniculate body of the thalamus, connections to the temporal lobe (Meyer's loop) and brainstem.

RADIOLOGY PEARL

Unmyelinated immature white matter because of its higher water content is darker on T_1 sequences and brighter on T_2 sequences than mature myelinated white matter. The progression of myelination can therefore be seen on MRI of infants. This progresses in a predictable way from deep to superficial, from posterior to anterior and from inferior to superior (Fig. 2.8)

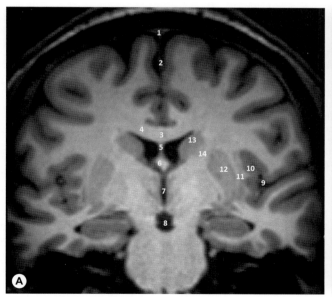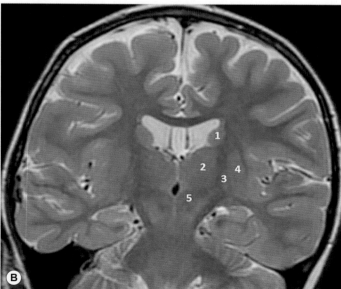

Fig. 2.7 Coronal magnetic resonance image of the brain. (A) Image through the third ventricle. (B) Subthalamic nuclei.

(A)
1. Superior sagittal sinus
2. Interhemispheric fissure
3. Body of corpus callosum
4. Tapetum
5. Septum pellucidum
6. Fornix
7. Third ventricle
8. Interpeduncular cistern
9. Sylvian fissure
10. Insula
11. External capsule, claustrum and extreme capsule

12. Lentiform nucleus
13. Head of caudate nucleus
14. Internal capsule

(B)
1. Head of caudate nucleus
2. Thalamus
3. Globus pallidus
4. Putamen
5. Subthalamic nucleus

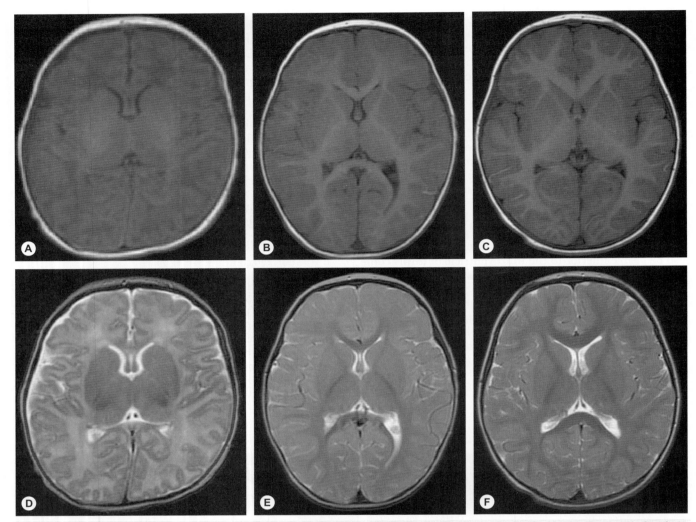

Fig. 2.8 Myelination of an infant brain as seen on T_1 and T_2 magnetic resonance images at level of the internal capsule. (A) T_1 newborn – only the white matter in the posterior limb of internal capsule is bright, indicating that only these fibres are myelinated. (B) T_1 at 1 year old; almost all white matter is bright now. Only the most superficial subcortical fibres have not achieved adult appearance so that grey–white differentiation remains a little blurred. (C) T_1 at 2 years old. All white matter is bright and myelinated now, including the subcortical white matter into the depth of each gyrus. The grey–white differentiation is sharp now. (D) T_2 newborn – only the white matter in the posterior limb of internal capsule is dark, indicating myelination. (E) T_2 at 1 year old. All of the internal capsule, the corpus callosum and the deep white matter (especially posteriorly) are dark. The superficial subcortical fibres have not achieved adult appearance and grey–white differentiation remains blurred. (F) T_2 at 2 years old. All white matter is dark and myelinated now, including the subcortical white matter into the depth of each gyrus.

Magnetic resonance tractography is a technique that uses diffusion tensor imaging to obtain images of fibre tracts within the brain. These scans also give information about fibre direction (Fig. 2.9). Directionality is displayed using different colours with transversely orientated tracts typically presented in red, for example the corpus callosum, craniocaudally orientated tracts typically presented as blue, for example the corticospinal tract, and anteroposteriorly orientated fibres typically presented in green, for example the superior longitudinal fasciculus. Its main clinical application is in preoperative planning in order to preserve critical fibre tract function after surgery.

Ultrasound Examination of the Neonatal Brain (Fig. 2.10)

The corpus callosum can be seen on midline sagittal scans as a thin band of tissue between the pericallosal artery in the pericallosal sulcus superiorly, and the fluid of the cavum septum pellucidum inferiorly. It is seen below the interhemispheric fissure on coronal scans, where both its upper and lower surfaces are perpendicular to the beam. On coronal scans the internal capsule can be seen lateral to the thalamus.

Basal Ganglia (Figs. 2.11, 2.12)

This subcortical grey matter includes:

- The corpus striatum – the caudate and lentiform nuclei
- The amygdaloid body
- The claustrum

The nuclei of the basal ganglia can be divided into input, output and intrinsic nuclei. The regulation of conscious and proprioceptive movements is the primary role of the basal ganglia. This is a complex process with many afferent input pathways including from the cortex,

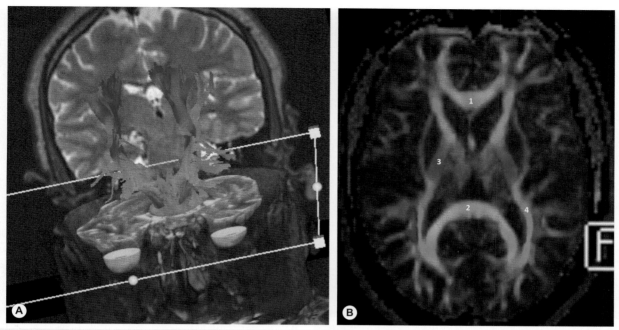

Fig. 2.9 Magnetic resonance tractography. (A) 3D image depicting fibres passing from the brain stem to the cerebral cortex. (B) Reference axial slice shows fibres as they pass through the posterior limb of the internal capsule on both sides. *Red* denotes transversely orientated tracts, *green* denotes anteroposteriorly orientated tracts and *blue* denotes craniocaudally orientated tracts.

(A)
(B)
1. Genu of corpus callosum
2. Splenium of corpus callosum

3. Posterior limb of internal capsule
4. Tapetum and superior longitudinal fasciculus

limbic system and gain-setting nuclei in the brainstem. The basal ganglia interpret these signals and determine which actions will take place through the disinhibition of these signals.

CAUDATE NUCLEUS

This nucleus is described as having a head, body and tail. Its long, thin tail ends in the amygdaloid nucleus. The caudate nucleus is highly curved and lies within the concavity of the lateral ventricle forming a C shape on sagittal imaging. Thus its head projects into the floor of the anterior horn and its body lies along the body of the lateral ventricle. Its tail lies in the roof of the inferior horn of this ventricle.

LENTIFORM NUCLEUS

The lentiform nucleus is shaped like a biconcave lens. It is made up of a larger lateral putamen and a smaller medial globus pallidus. Medially, it is separated from the head of the caudate nucleus anteriorly, and from the thalamus posteriorly by the internal capsule. A thin layer of white matter on its lateral surface is called the external capsule.

Strands of grey matter connect the head of the caudate nucleus with the putamen of the lentiform nucleus across the anterior limb of the internal capsule. The resulting striated appearance gives rise to the term **corpus striatum**.

The function of the corpus striatum is not well understood. It is part of the extrapyramidal system and influences voluntary motor activity. Cortical afferents enter the putamen and caudate nucleus, which send efferents to the globus pallidus. This in turn sends efferents to the hypothalamus, brainstem and spinal cord.

CLAUSTRUM (SEE FIG. 2.12)

This thin sheet of grey matter lies between the putamen and the insula. It is separated medially from the putamen by the external capsule and bounded laterally by a thin sheet of white matter, the extreme capsule, just deep to the insula. The claustrum is cortical in origin. It may have a role in knowledge processing and in the synchronisation of motor and nonmotor processes.

RADIOLOGICAL FEATURES OF THE BASAL GANGLIA

CT and MRI

On axial CT or MRI at the level of the ventricles, the head of the **caudate nucleus** can be seen projecting into the anterior horn of the lateral ventricle (see Fig. 2.3C). The head of the caudate nucleus is usually more radiodense than the lentiform nucleus or the thalamus, especially in older subjects. The body of the caudate nucleus is seen as a thin, dense stripe on the superolateral margin of the lateral ventricle on higher cuts.

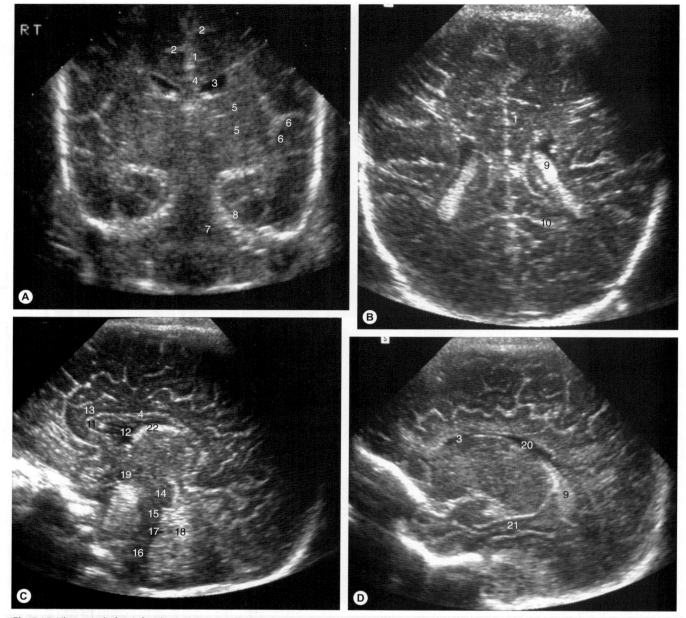

Fig. 2.10 Ultrasound of an infant brain. (A) Coronal image through the frontal horns of the lateral ventricles. (B) Coronal image through the body of the lateral ventricle. (C) Midline sagittal image. (D) Parasagittal image through the lateral ventricle.

1. Interhemispheric fissure
2. Sulci
3. Frontal horn of lateral ventricle
4. Corpus callosum
5. Caudate above, lentiform nucleus below, separated by internal capsule (these three are not distinguished separately)
6. Sylvian fissure
7. Brainstem
8. Parahippocampal gyrus of temporal lobe
9. Choroid plexus in atrium of lateral ventricle
10. Calcarine sulcus
11. Genu of corpus callosum

12. Cavum septum pellucidum
13. Cingulate gyrus
14. Midbrain
15. Pons
16. Medulla
17. Fourth ventricle
18. Vermis of cerebellum
19. Third ventricle
20. Body of lateral ventricle
21. Hippocampus
22. Fornix

The **amygdala** is an ovoid mass of grey matter at the anterior end of the tail of the caudate nucleus and can be seen on MRI anterior to the hippocampus in the medial temporal lobe (see Fig. 2.11 and later Fig. 2.16C).

The connecting fibres between the lentiform and caudate nuclei that cross the anterior limb of the internal capsule and are responsible for the name corpus striatum, may also be seen on MRI.

The **claustrum** can be seen on MRI (see Fig. 2.12) as a stripe isointense with grey matter, separated from the putamen by the external capsule and from the insula by the extreme capsule.

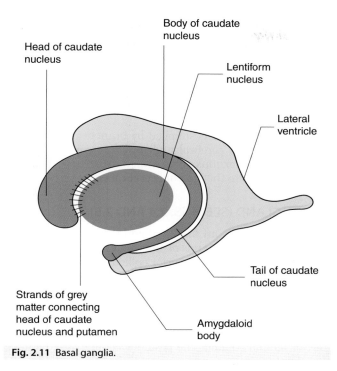

Fig. 2.11 Basal ganglia.

Head of caudate nucleus

Body of caudate nucleus

Lentiform nucleus

Lateral ventricle

Tail of caudate nucleus

Amygdaloid body

Strands of grey matter connecting head of caudate nucleus and putamen

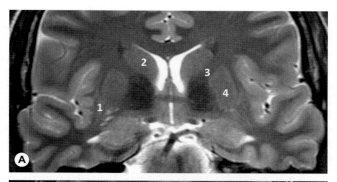

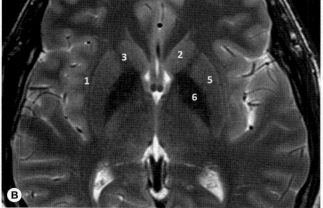

Fig. 2.12 Magnetic resonance image of the basal ganglia. (A) Coronal. (B) Axial.

1. Claustrum
2. Head of caudate nucleus
3. Internal capsule
4. Lentiform nucleus
5. Putamen
6. Globus pallidus

RADIOLOGY PEARL

MRI is sensitive to paramagnetic substances such as iron, which may be deposited in the globus pallidus, giving this a different signal intensity from the lentiform nucleus.

RADIOLOGY PEARL

The tail of the caudate nucleus extends over the roof of the temporal horn of the lateral ventricle, where it should not be confused with heterotopic cortical grey matter.

Ultrasound Examination of the Neonatal Brain (see Fig. 2.10)

The thalami and caudate heads can be seen on coronal images. Parasagittal scans are angled to show most of the lateral ventricle on one image. These show the head of the caudate and the thalamus forming the floor of the lateral ventricle.

RADIOLOGY PEARL

The caudothalamic groove between the head of the caudate and the thalamus on the floor of the lateral ventricle is the commonest site of haemorrhage in preterm infants. The basal ganglia are the most common location for hypertensive haemorrhages in adults.

RADIOLOGY PEARL

A number of neurodegenerative disorders selectively affect different components of the basal ganglia. Huntington's disease results in atrophy of the caudate nucleus.

Thalamus, Hypothalamus and Pineal Gland

The structures around the third ventricle include the thalamus, hypothalamus and pineal gland. Together with the habenula these form the major structures of the diencephalon, a paramedian component of the forebrain.

THALAMUS

These paired, ovoid bodies of predominantly grey matter lie in the lateral walls of the third ventricle, from the interventricular foramen anteriorly to the brainstem posteriorly. Each has its apex anteriorly and a more rounded posterior end called the pulvinar. The thalamus is related laterally to the internal capsule and, beyond that, to the lentiform nucleus. The body and tail of the caudate nucleus are in contact with the lateral margin of the thalamus. The superior part of the thalamus forms part of the floor of the lateral ventricle.

The thalami are connected in the midline by the **massa intermedia** or **interthalamic adhesion** in 60%–90% of humans. Formerly thought to be non-neural connection, however, it does appear to contain some white matter tracts traversing to the contralateral hemisphere, suggesting a role as another commissure.

Most thalamic nuclei are relay nuclei of the main sensory pathways. Each sensory system, with the exception of olfaction, has a thalamic nucleus connected to a cortical area. Medial and lateral swellings on the posteroinferior aspect of the thalamus are called the geniculate nuclei. The medial geniculate nucleus is attached to the inferior colliculus and is involved in the relay of auditory impulses. The lateral geniculate body nucleus is attached to the superior colliculus and is involved with visual impulses. The thalamus receives its blood supply from thalamostriate branches of the posterior cerebral artery.

Separate to and below the thalami are paired nuclei called the **subthalamic nuclei** (see Fig. 2.7B) which make up the majority of the subthalamus. They are connected to the globus pallidus and the substantia nigra. They play an important role in the regulation of movement helping to prevent unwanted movements. Destruction of one of them causes hemiballismus.

RADIOLOGY PEARL

Deep brain stimulation of the subthalamic nuclei has been shown to be effective in the treatment of Parkinson's disease. This technique is dependent on accurate localisation of the subthalamic nuclei in axial and coronal MRIs. MRI also helps to identify anatomic variants or vascular lesions which could impact the approach or ability to perform this procedure.

RADIOLOGY PEARL

Disorders of mitochondrial DNA and respiratory chain disorders may cause abnormalities of the basal ganglia on MRI. Abnormality of the subthalamic nuclei is particularly associated with cytochrome C oxidase deficiency.

HYPOTHALAMUS (FIGS. 2.13, 2.21)

The hypothalamus is a bilateral paramedian group of nuclei surrounding and forming the floor of the third ventricle. It includes the following structures, starting anteriorly:

- Optic chiasm.
- Tuber cinereum – a sheet of grey matter between the optic chiasm and the mamillary bodies.
- Infundibular stalk – leading down to the posterior lobe of the pituitary gland.
- Mamillary bodies – small round masses in front of the posterior perforated substance in which the columns of the fornix (see below) end (Fig. 2.17).
- Posterior perforated substance – the interval between the diverging crura cerebri, which is pierced by central branches of the posterior cerebral artery.

The nuclei of the hypothalamus are connected by white matter, the medial forebrain bundle, to each other, to the frontal lobe anteriorly and to the midbrain posteriorly.

The function of the hypothalamus is maintenance of homeostasis by controlling autonomic, endocrine and somatic activity. As a result, it is widely connected to other structures. These include the cerebral cortex via the medial forebrain bundle, the brainstem via the dorsal longitudinal fasciculus, the hippocampus via the fornix, the amygdala via the stria terminalis, the thalamus via the mammillothalamic tract, the pituitary via the median eminence and the retina via the retinohypothalamic tract.

It has sympathetic and parasympathetic areas and plays a role in the regulation of temperature, appetite and sleep patterns.

The hypothalamus is supplied by branches of the anterior and posterior cerebral and posterior communicating arteries. Intercavernous veins draining the hypothalamus ultimately drain to the internal cerebral veins.

PINEAL GLAND (SEE FIGS. 2.4 AND 2.5)

The pineal gland is an unpaired endocrine gland that lies between the posterior ends of the thalami and between the splenium above and the superior colliculi below. It is closely related to the cerebral aqueduct of Sylvius inferiorly. It is separated from the splenium by the cerebral veins. It lies within 3 mm of the midline.

The pineal stalk has superior and inferior laminae. The superior lamina is formed by the habenular commissure, and the inferior lamina contains the posterior commissure. Between these laminae is the posterior recess of the third ventricle.

The main known function of the pineal gland is in the regulation of the circadian rhythm of sleep through the secretion of melatonin.

Arterial supply is from choroidal branches of the posterior cerebral artery. Venous drainage is to the internal cerebral veins.

RADIOLOGICAL FEATURES OF THE THALAMUS, HYPOTHALAMUS AND PINEAL GLAND

Skull Radiographs

Pineal calcification is visible in approximately 50% of skull radiographs after the age of 10 years and in a greater percentage of CT scans (see section on the skull).

CT and MRI

The structures forming the hypothalamus can best be appreciated on midline sagittal MRI (see Fig. 2.5). The optic chiasm, the tuber cinereum, the infundibular stalk and the interpeduncular cistern, containing the mamillary bodies and in the base of which lies the posterior perforated substance, can be identified. The thalami can be seen on axial or coronal images on each side of the third ventricle (see Fig. 2.3C). Their relationship to the posterior limb of the internal capsule and to the lentiform nucleus can be appreciated on this slice. The pineal gland and its superior and inferior laminae can also be best seen on midline sagittal MRI. Subthalamic nuclei can best be seen on coronal MRI (see Fig. 2.7B).

Ultrasound Examination of the Neonatal Brain (see Fig. 2.10)

In the parasagittal plane the thalamus can be seen in the floor of the lateral ventricle posterior to the head of the caudate nucleus. The relation of the thalami to the internal capsule is best seen on coronal ultrasound scans. On

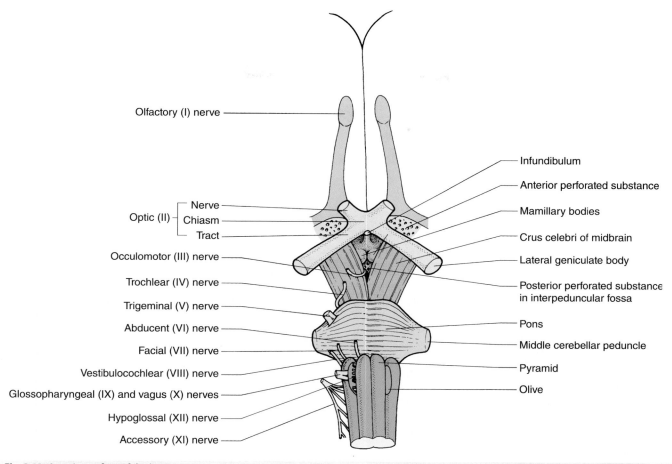

Fig. 2.13 Anterior surface of the brainstem.

coronal views the interthalamic adhesion can be seen within the third ventricle, especially when the ventricle is dilated.

Pituitary Gland (see Fig. 2.14)

The pituitary gland (hypophysis cerebri) lies in the pituitary fossa or sella turcica of the sphenoid bone. On average it measures 12 mm in its transverse diameter, 8 mm in its anteroposterior diameter and 9 mm high. Its size, however, varies with age and gender. It is divided into anatomically and functionally distinct anterior (adenohypophysis) and posterior (neurohypophysis) lobes.

The anterior lobe is five times larger than the posterior lobe. It is developed from Rathke's pouch in the roof of the primitive mouth. (A tumour from remnants of the epithelium of this pouch is called a craniopharyngioma.) The anterior lobe produces hormones in response to release factors carried from the hypothalamus by hypophyseal portal veins, the hypothalamic-hypophyseal portal system.

The pituitary gland has a hollow stalk, the infundibulum, which arises from the tuber cinereum in the floor of the third ventricle. It is directed anteroinferiorly and surrounded by an upward extension of the anterior lobe, the tuberal part. This stalk is composed of nerve fibres whose cell bodies are in the hypothalamus. The posterior lobe is made up of the ending of these nerve fibres and releases hormones in response to impulses from these nerves.

The anterior lobe is adherent to the posterior lobe by a narrow zone called the pars intermedia. This is, in fact, developmentally and functionally part of the anterior lobe.

The relations of the pituitary gland are as follows:
- Above: the diaphragma sellae (dura mater) forming the roof of the sella. Superior to this is the suprasellar cistern which contains a number of structures including the optic chiasm anteriorly (8 mm above dura) and the circle of Willis.
- Below: the body of the sphenoid bone and the sphenoid sinus.
- Laterally: the dura and the cavernous sinus and its contents, the internal carotid artery and abducens nerve with the oculomotor, ophthalmic and trochlear nerves

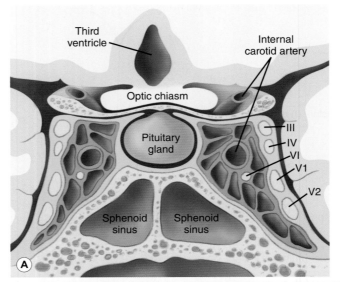

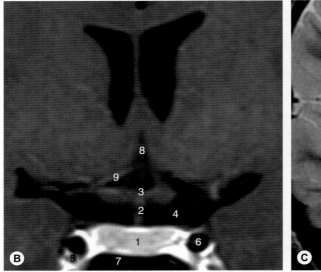

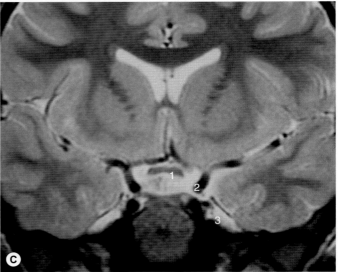

Fig. 2.14 Pituitary gland and cavernous sinus: coronal section. (A) Diagram. (B) Coronal T_1 magnetic resonance image after intravenous contrast. (C) More posterior T_2 view to show Meckel's cave. (A from Winn HR. *Youmans & Winn Neurological Surgery*, 8th ed. Elsevier; 2023.)

(A)– (B)

1. Pituitary gland
2. Pituitary stalk
3. Optic chiasm
4. Suprasellar cistern
5. Cavernous sinus
6. Internal carotid artery in cavernous sinus
7. Sphenoid sinus

8. Third ventricle
9. Right anterior cerebral artery

(C)
1. Optic chiasm
2. Carotid artery
3. Trigeminal ganglion in Meckel's cave

in its walls. Inferior to the ophthalmic division of the fifth nerve is its maxillary division. More posteriorly in the posterolateral wall of the cavernous sinus lies the trigeminal ganglion in its CSF-containing arachnoidal pouch, Meckel's cave (see Fig. 2.14C).

The cavernous sinuses are united by intercavernous sinuses, which surround the pituitary gland anteriorly, posteriorly and inferiorly.

BLOOD SUPPLY

Superior hypophyseal arteries, which arise from each internal carotid artery immediately after it pierces the dura, supply the hypothalamus and the infundibulum. A capillary bed in the infundibulum gives rise to portal vessels to the anterior lobe. The posterior lobe is supplied by inferior hypophyseal arteries which arise from the meningohypophyseal trunk, a branch of the internal carotid arteries in the cavernous sinus.

Venous drainage is to the cavernous and intercavernous sinuses.

RADIOLOGICAL FEATURES OF THE PITUITARY GLAND

Skull Radiographs

The appearance of the bony pituitary fossa is affected by disease processes in the gland. This is dealt with in the section on the skull.

Magnetic Resonance Imaging (see Fig. 2.14)

MRI is the primary modality for evaluation of the pituitary gland. Sagittal and coronal images are most useful. The size and shape of the normal pituitary gland vary. In adult males the gland ranges from 8 to 10 mm craniocaudal dimension in the sagittal plane. The dura above the sella should be horizontal, not convex. In females, the size of the gland varies with the menstrual cycle and pregnancy. In the postpartum period, it may normally exceed 12 mm in height. It is also normal for the gland to have a convex upper border in menstruating or lactating females. During puberty, the gland may also have a convex upper surface in both males and females. With increasing age and in postmenopausal females the gland reduces in volume.

In normal adults the anterior pituitary occupies 70–80% of the total gland volume and is isointense to cerebral white matter on T_1 images. The posterior pituitary usually has high signal intensity on unenhanced T_1 images due to the effect of stored neurosecretory granules on T_1 relaxation time. This so-called **posterior pituitary bright spot** is evident in most babies and children but is less consistently observed with increasing age in adults. The pars intermedia, a vestigial remnant of Rathke's pouch, is not normally visualised on imaging studies. In some cases, a small cyst with variable signal intensity may mark the location of the pars intermedia.

The infundibulum tapers from the floor of the third ventricle to the pituitary gland. The diameter of the infundibulum should be no bigger than 3 mm or the adjacent basilar artery. It is a midline structure and displacement in either direction may signify an underlying pituitary mass. The sella itself is delineated by signal void of the bony cortex and by the high-intensity signal of marrow in the clivus. The optic nerves and chiasm and the intracranial carotid vessels above, and the sphenoid sinus below, are seen clearly on coronal sections.

Computed Tomography

CT has a limited role in the evaluation of the sella and suprasellar structures. The main role of CT is in the assessment of bony anatomy and changes in the sella, in the identification of calcification within lesions which can help narrow the differential diagnosis and in preoperative planning, where an intracranial CT angiogram can help delineate the local vascular anatomy to aid in surgical planning. Fine-cut coronal postcontrast images may be an alternative to MRI in patients who have a contraindication for MRI.

The Limbic Lobe System (see Fig. 2.15)

This is not an anatomical lobe as such, but a large group of functionally related structures which anatomically lie lateral to the thalamus, about the corpus callosum and above the brainstem. The major components include cingulate, splenial and parahippocampal gyri, the hippocampus, amygdala, the dentate gyrus and the fornix, the olfactory bulbs and the hypothalamus.

The cingulate gyrus curves around the genu and body of the corpus callosum and continues around the splenium as the splenial gyrus. This, in turn, is continuous with the dentate gyrus and the hippocampus.

Also included in the limbic lobe are grey matter on the corpus callosum – called the induseum griseum – and white fibres that run along its length – the medial and lateral longitudinal striae.

The limbic lobe contributes to multiple processes including the regulation of emotions and behaviour, especially those needed for survival such as feeding, reproduction and fight or flight responses.

HIPPOCAMPUS (SEE FIG. 2.16)

This is a curved elevation of grey matter within the parahippocampal gyrus of the medial temporal lobe in the floor of the temporal horn of the lateral ventricle. Its enlarged, ridged anterior end has the appearance of a paw – the pes hippocampi. The hippocampus consists of grey matter. A fine covering of white matter overlying this is called the alveus. The hippocampus is divided into an anterior head, a body and a posterior tail. The amygdala lies close to the anterior margin of the head. The internal anatomy of the hippocampus is complex with three distinct zones, different layers and hippocampal subfields all described. Its function is concerned with behaviour patterns, emotion and recent memory.

The uncus is a limbic structure on the anteromedial part of the parahippocampal gyrus of the medial temporal lobe (see Fig. 2.17A).

FORNIX (SEE FIG. 2.15)

This is an efferent pathway from the hippocampus to the mamillary bodies. Fibres of the alveus converge on the medial border of the hippocampus as a band of fibres called the fimbria of the hippocampus. This becomes free of the hippocampus as the crus of the fornix (the posterior pillar of the fornix).

Each crus extends posteriorly to below the splenium of the corpus callosum, where it connects with that of the other side as the commissure of the fornix. Together the two crura form the body of the fornix. The body of the fornix extends anteriorly around the upper surface of the thalami. It is attached posteriorly to the under surface of the corpus callosum and anteriorly to the inferior border of the septum pellucidum.

Above the interventricular foramen, the body divides into two columns, which pass inferiorly between the

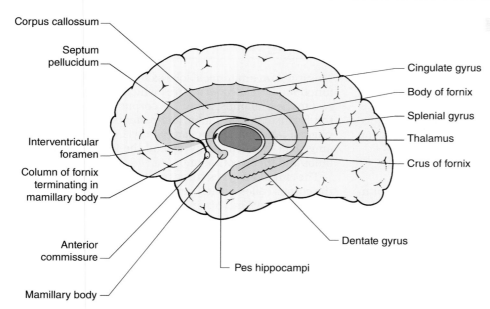

Corpus callossum

Septum pellucidum

Interventricular foramen

Column of fornix terminating in mamillary body

Anterior commissure

Mamillary body

Pes hippocampi

Cingulate gyrus

Body of fornix

Splenial gyrus

Thalamus

Crus of fornix

Dentate gyrus

Fig. 2.15 Components of the limbic lobe.

foramen and the anterior commissure and form the anterior border of the interventricular foramen. The columns then pass to the hypothalamus and the mamillary bodies, in which they terminate. Some fibres from the columns of the fornix, the habenular fibres, turn back over the thalamus to join posteriorly in the habenular commissure.

> **RADIOLOGY PEARL**
>
> The uncus of the parahippocampal gyrus is a common site of temporal lobe seizures.

Herniation of the uncus downward through the tentorial hiatus can be seen on CT or MRI as a marker of increased pressure within cerebral hemispheres, for example in acute cerebral oedema secondary to tumour, stroke or trauma. It can lead to compression of the brainstem and the posterior cerebral arteries in the ambient cistern. Uncal herniation may be unilateral or bilateral.

RADIOLOGICAL FEATURES OF THE LIMBIC LOBE

Magnetic Resonance Imaging

Medial temporal structures and in particular the hippocampus are the most common locus for an identifiable cause of epilepsy with mesial temporal sclerosis, a condition resulting in atrophy and loss of normal internal architecture of the hippocampus, the most common single cause. Dedicated epilepsy protocol imaging includes high-resolution volumetric coronal imaging of the hippocampi with multiplanar reconstructions, ideally with higher field-strength 3 T MRI (see Fig. 2.16).

The body of the fornix is seen in midline sagittal MRI (see Fig. 2.5), extending from the under surface of the corpus callosum posteriorly to the interventricular foramen anteriorly along the under surface of the septum pellucidum.

Fine-cut coronal MRI perpendicular to the axis of the hippocampus and angled axial and sagittal images along its long axis are used to image the hippocampus, especially in the evaluation of epilepsy (see Fig. 2.16).

Ultrasound Examination of the Neonatal Brain (see Fig. 2.10)

The cingulate gyrus can be identified surrounding the corpus callosum. This is absent if the corpus callosum is absent. The body of the fornix can be seen below the septum pellucidum on midline sagittal images. In the coronal plane at the level of the third ventricle the C-shaped echoes of the parahippocampal gyrus are used as a far-field landmark.

The Brainstem (see Fig. 2.13)

The brainstem connects the cerebral hemispheres with the spinal cord and extends from just above the tentorial hiatus to just below the foramen magnum. It is bounded anteriorly by the clivus – the basisphenoid above and the basiocciput below. The pons, the widest part of the brainstem, also grooves the apex of the petrous temporal bone on each side. This bony anterior boundary can cause an artefact in CT scanning of the brainstem, although it does not interfere with MRI studies.

The brainstem has three parts: from superior to inferior, the midbrain, the pons and the medulla.

MIDBRAIN

External Features (see Fig. 2.13)

Anteriorly two cerebral peduncles are seen separated by the interpeduncular fossa. These peduncles, the **crura cerebri**, carry fibres from the internal capsule to the pons. The floor of the interpeduncular fossa is the posterior perforated substance.

The posterior surface of the midbrain presents four rounded prominences – the **corpora quadrigemini** or the superior and inferior colliculi. Each superior colliculus is joined by a **superior brachium** to the lateral geniculate body of the optic tract. Each inferior colliculus is joined by an **inferior brachium** to the medial geniculate body of the auditory system.

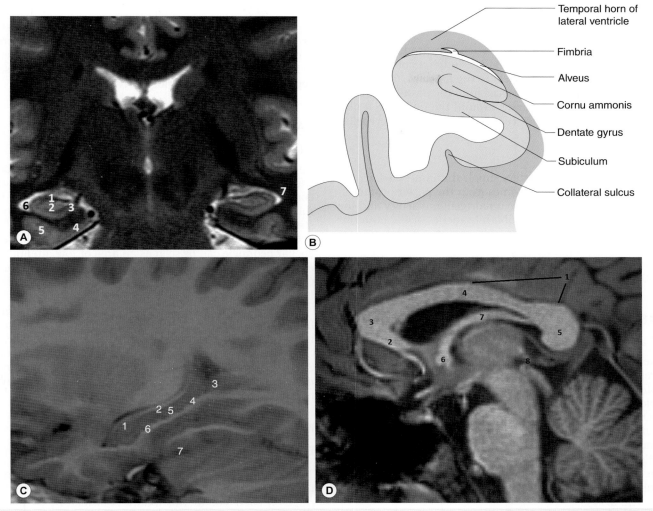

Fig. 2.16 Hippocampus. (A) Coronal T₁ magnetic resonance image (MRI). (B) Diagram of coronal section right hippocampus. (C) Parasagittal MRI showing the hippocampus. (D) Parasagittal MRI showing the indusium griseum.

(A)
1. Alveus
2. Cornu ammonis
3. Subiculum
4. Parahippocampal gyrus
5. Collateral sulcus
6. Temporal horn of lateral ventricle
7. Tail of caudate

(C)
1. Amygdala
2. Temporal horn of lateral ventricle
3. Hippocampal tail
4. Hippocampal body

5. Fimbria of hippocampus
6. Hippocampal head
7. Parahippocampal gyrus

(D)
1. Indusium griseum
2. Rostrum of the corpus callosum
3. Genu of the corpus callosum
4. Body of the corpus callosum
5. Splenium of the corpus callosum
6. Anterior commissure
7. Fornix
8. Posterior commissure

Below the colliculi, the superior cerebellar peduncles converge to form the superior boundary of the fourth ventricle. A thin sheet of white matter between these is the **superior medullary velum**.

Internal Features (see Fig. 2.17)

Cerebral peduncles have a ventral part, the crus cerebri, which contains motor corticospinal tracts, and a dorsal part, the tegmentum. These are separated by the **substantia nigra**. Dorsal to the substantia nigra at the level of the superior colliculi are paired **red nuclei**, which lie close to the median plane. These are part of the extrapyramidal pathway. That part of the midbrain posterior to the aqueduct is called the **tectum** or **quadrigeminal plate**.

Cranial Nerves

The third (III) cranial nerve emerges from between the cerebral peduncles anteriorly. It passes between the posterior cerebral and superior cerebellar arteries and then lies lateral to the posterior communicating artery, where an aneurysm may compress it.

The fourth (IV) cranial nerve emerges from the dorsal surface of the midbrain caudal to the inferior colliculus and winds around its lateral aspect to the ambient cistern. It is the only cranial nerve to emerge from the posterior surface of the midbrain. As it curves around the midbrain it also lies between the posterior cerebral and superior cerebellar arteries.

Blood Supply

Branches of the basilar artery supply the anteromedial midbrain. Additional supply comes from the posterior choroidal arteries laterally and the quadrigeminal artery and the superior cerebellar arteries, both branches of the posterior cerebral artery, posteriorly. Central branches of the superior cerebellar artery supply the midbrain.

Posterior mesencephalic veins curve around each side of the midbrain towards the great cerebral vein.

RADIOLOGICAL FEATURES OF THE MIDBRAIN

CT and MRI

The midbrain is seen on axial CT and MRI at the level of the circle of Willis (see Fig. 2.3B). The crura can be identified anteriorly and the colliculi posteriorly. It is not always possible to identify the cerebral aqueduct.

On contrast-enhanced CT the posterior cerebral arteries or the posterior mesencephalic veins may be seen passing around the midbrain.

Ferritin deposition in the substantia nigra and red nuclei may lead to a lower signal intensity here than in the remainder of the crus cerebri on T_1 and T_2-weighted MRI (see Fig. 2.17).

PONS

External Features (see Fig . 2.13)

The bulbous convex anterior part of the pons consists mainly of cerebellopontine fibres continuous on each side with the middle cerebellar peduncle. This part also transmits corticospinal fibres continuous with the cerebral peduncles of the midbrain. A shallow groove is seen in the midline. The basilar artery may lie in this groove, but often lies lateral to it.

The posterior surface of the pons forms the upper part of the floor of the fourth ventricle.

Cranial nerves

The fifth (V) cranial nerve emerges from the superior anterolateral surface of the pons. There are four trigeminal nuclei, two in the pons, a mesencephalic nucleus in the midbrain, and a spinal nucleus in the medulla and upper cervical cord.

The sixth (VI) cranial nerve emerges at the junction with the medulla, close to the midline anteriorly.

The seventh and eighth (VII and VIII) cranial nerves emerge at the junction with the medulla laterally, that is, at the cerebellopontine angle.

Blood Supply

The pons is supplied by pontine branches of the basilar artery with additional supply by branches of the superior cerebellar artery and posterior inferior cerebellar arteries.

Blood from the pons drains to the anterior pontomesencephalic vein and the inferior petrosal sinus.

RADIOLOGICAL FEATURES OF THE PONS

CT and MRI (see Fig. 2.3A)

The bony anterior relations of the pons – the clivus centrally and the petrous temporal bones laterally – may cause considerable artefact on CT scanning of this area. For this reason, MRI is superior for evaluating posterior fossa structures.

On CT scans, the cerebellopontine fibres of the middle cerebellar peduncle can be seen as an area of low attenuation extending from the pons into each cerebellar hemisphere. On higher cuts the superior cerebellar peduncle forms the lateral border of the fourth ventricle.

The trigeminal nerves can be seen entering and emerging from its anterior surface and the seventh and eighth cranial nerves can be seen exiting at the cerebellopontine angle.

The basilar artery may be seen anterior to the pons. A position to the right or left of the midline is not abnormal. Asymmetry of the cerebellopontine cisterns, however, is usually associated with pathology.

MEDULLA OBLONGATA

External Features (see Fig. 2.13)

The medulla joins the pons to the spinal cord. Anteriorly, the ventral median fissure is deep in its superior part. A ridge on each side of this fissure is formed by pyramidal fibres and is called the pyramid. The pyramids carry motor fibres from the motor cortex. The majority of these fibres decussate in the lower medulla, obliterating the median fissure here and forming the contralateral lateral corticospinal tract in the spinal cord. Lateral to the pyramid on each side in the upper medulla is an oval bulge called the olive, part of the olivocerebellar system. Lateral to the olive lies the inferior cerebellar peduncle – known as the restiform body – joining the medulla to the cerebellum.

Posteriorly, the upper part of the medulla is open as the floor of the fourth ventricle, whereas its lower part is closed around the central canal. Dorsal median and lateral sulci define four columns below the ventricle – gracile columns medially and cuneate columns laterally. A correspondingly named tubercle is found at the upper end of each column. These contain the gracile and cuneate nuclei, respectively, part of the dorsal column-medial lemniscus system.

Cranial Nerves

The ninth and tenth (IX and X) cranial nerves emerge posterior to the olive from the postolivary groove with cranial nerve (CN) IX superior to CN X.

The eleventh (XI) CN has medullary rootlets that arise inferior to those of X, and cervical rootlets that arise from the upper spinal cord and enter the foramen magnum to unite with the medullary roots.

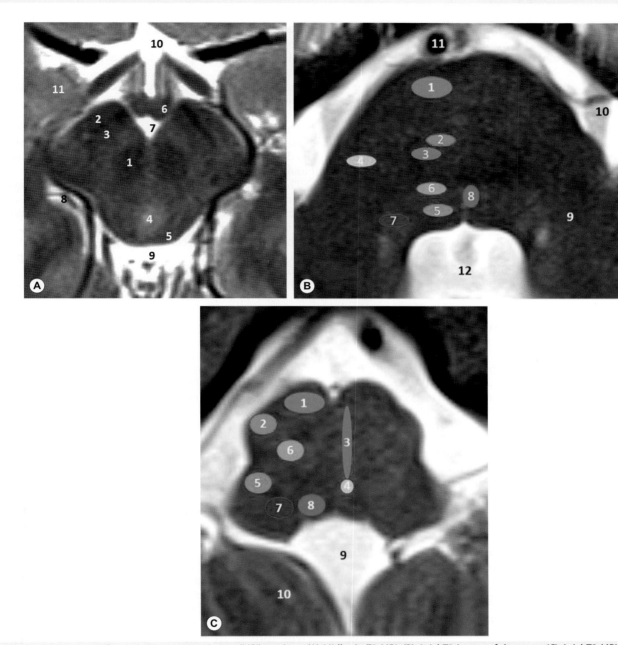

Fig. 2.17 Brainstem axial magnetic resonance image (MRI) sections. (A) Midbrain T2 MRI. (B) Axial T2 image of the pons. (C) Axial T2 MRI of upper medulla.

(A)
1. Red nucleus
2. Crus cerebri
3. Substantia nigra
4. Aqueduct
5. Superior colliculi
6. Mamillary body
7. Interpeduncular cistern
8. Ambient cistern
9. Quadrigeminal cistern
10. Suprasellar cistern
11. Uncus

(B)
1. Corticospinal tract
2. Medial lemniscus
3. Central tegmental tract
4. Cranial nerve V nucleus
5. Cranial nerve VI nucleus

6. Cranial nerve VII nucleus
7. Cranial nerve VIII nucleus
8. Medial longitudinal fasciculus
9. Left middle cerebellar peduncle
10. Cisternal segment of the left cranial nerve V
11. Basilar artery
12. Fourth ventricle

(C)
1. Corticospinal tract
2. Olivary nucleus
3. Medial lemniscus
4. Medial longitudinal fasciculus
5. Cranial nerve V nucleus
6. Cranial nerve IX nucleus
7. Cranial nerve X nucleus
8. Cranial nerve XII nucleus
9. Fourth ventricle
10. Right cerebellar tonsil

The twelfth (XII) CN arises from several rootlets anterior to the olive at the sulcus between the olive and pyramid, in line with ventral spinal roots.

Blood Supply

Cranially the medulla is supplied by the vertebral arteries and branches of the basilar artery laterally and anteriorly, respectively, with the vertebral and basilar arteries suppling the anterior part of the medulla, whereas the posterior inferior cerebellar artery supplies its posterior part. Inferiorly it is supplied by the anterior spinal artery anteriorly and the posterior spinal arteries posteriorly.

Venous drainage is to the occipital sinus posteriorly and the inferior petrosal sinus anteriorly. Inferior medullary veins communicate with spinal veins.

RADIOLOGICAL FEATURES OF THE MEDULLA OBLONGATA

CT and MRI

Sections through the lower medulla are difficult to distinguish from those through the upper cervical cord unless the atlas or foramen magnum can be identified. The upper medulla can be identified easily by the presence of the fourth ventricle and cerebellum posteriorly.

MRI of the medulla gives superior images because of the lack of bony artefact (see Fig. 2.5). The ventral sulcus can be seen anteriorly on axial sections with the pre- and postolivary sulci laterally. The olives give a square configuration to the medulla on this section. The fourth ventricle is seen posteriorly, especially on sagittal sections, with its midline foramen leading to the vallecula. The most inferior part of the fourth ventricle is called the obex. This may be sealed during surgery of a cervical cord syrinx. The fourth ventricle is continuous with the central canal of the spinal cord at the ibex.

In the lowest images, the hypoglossal nerve may be seen entering the hypoglossal canal of the occipital bone.

RADIOLOGY PEARL

There is an array of brainstem syndromes with the clinical features determined by the vascular supply and distribution of nuclei within the brainstem. Foville syndrome or inferior medial pontine syndrome results from infarction of the medial inferior pons which is supplied by paramedian branches of the basilar artery. Infarction results in crossed signs with corticospinal tract and medial lemniscus involvement resulting in contralateral weakness and dorsal column signs and infarction of the middle cerebellar peduncle and CN VI and CN VII, resulting in ipsilateral ataxia and cranial nerve deficits.

Cerebellum (Figs. 2.18, 2.19)

The cerebellum lies in the posterior fossa. It is separated from the occipital lobe by the tentorium and from the pons and midbrain medulla by the fourth ventricle. It is connected to the brainstem by three pairs of cerebellar peduncles:

- Superior cerebellar peduncles (brachium conjunctivum) to the midbrain
- Middle cerebellar peduncles (brachium pontis) to the pons
- Inferior cerebellar peduncles (restiform body) to the medulla

The cerebellum lies on the occipital bone posteriorly and close to the mastoid anteriorly. It closely approximates to the dural venous sinuses, especially the transverse and sigmoid sinuses.

The superior surface of the cerebellum slopes upwards from posterior to anterior. An axial MR or CT image of the upper cerebellum therefore contains cerebellum anteriorly and occipital lobes posterolaterally.

The surface of the cerebellum has numerous shallow sulci that separate tiny parallel folia. Deep fissures separate the hemispheres into lobules.

There are two hemispheres connected by the midline vermis between them.

HEMISPHERES

The two hemispheres extend laterally and posteriorly. These are separated by a shallow median groove superiorly and by a deep groove inferiorly. A midline posterior cerebellar notch lodges the falx cerebelli.

The hemispheres are divided into lobules by fissures, the deepest of which is the horizontal fissure, which extends from the convex posterior border into the depth of the hemispheres. The primary fissure (fissura prima) divides the superior surface and defines a small anterior lobe and a larger posterior lobe.

On each side below the middle cerebellar peduncle is the **flocculus**. This is a small ventral portion of the hemisphere that is almost completely separate from the remainder. It extends laterally from the midline as a slender band with an expanded end. It lies close to the lateral recess and choroid plexus of the fourth ventricle. Together with the nodule, the most inferior part of the vermis, it makes up the flocculonodular lobe, the smallest lobe of the cerebellum. The posterolateral fissure separates the posterior and flocculonodular lobes.

The **tonsils** are the most anterior inferior part of the hemispheres and lie close to the midline.

The cerebellum, like the cerebrum, has a cortex of grey matter and deeper white matter. There are deep nuclei within the hemispheres, the largest of which is the dentate nucleus.

VERMIS

The vermis is the narrow midline portion of the cerebellum. Superiorly this is merely a low median elevation not clearly separated from the hemispheres; however inferiorly the vermis is quite separate and lies in a deep cleft called the vallecula. The vermis is separated into nine named lobules by fissures, each part except the lingula corresponding to an adjoining lobule of the cerebellar hemispheres. The most anterior part of the superior vermis is the lingula, which lies on the superior medullary velum (a thin sheet of white matter between the superior cerebellar peduncles). The most anterior part of the inferior vermis is the nodule.

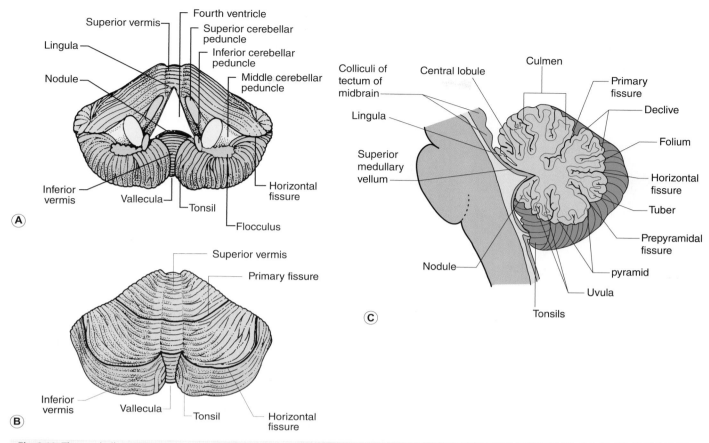

Fig. 2.18 The cerebellum. (A) Anterior view. (B) Posterior view. (C) Midline sagittal section of vermis.

SUBDIVISIONS OF THE CEREBELLUM

- Anterior lobe: lingula, central lobule, culmen
- Posterior lobe: declive, folium, tuber, pyramid, uvula
- Flocculonodular lobe

THE FUNCTION OF THE CEREBELLUM

The cerebellum is best known for its role in the coordination of motor function including voluntary movement, gait and the maintenance of posture. It is important in muscle coordination and in the regulation of muscle tone and posture. Functional MRI studies suggest a broader range of roles of the cerebellum including in learning and memory as well as emotional processing. Unilateral lesions of the cerebellum affect the ipsilateral side of the body.

ARTERIAL SUPPLY

Three pairs of arteries supply the cerebellum, namely:

- Superior cerebellar arteries, also from the basilar artery, supply the superior aspect of the cerebellum.
- Posterior inferior cerebellar arteries (PICAs), most commonly arising from the vertebral arteries, supply the inferior vermis and the inferior part of the hemispheres.
- Anterior inferior cerebellar arteries (AICAs) from the basilar artery supply the anterolateral aspect of the undersurface of the hemisphere and the flocculus.

VENOUS DRAINAGE

(See section on veins of the posterior fossa.)

The precentral cerebellar vein and the superior vermian vein drain to the great cerebral vein. The remainder of the cerebellar veins drain to the nearby dural sinuses as follows:

- The superior and posterior parts to the straight and transverse sinuses.
- The inferior aspect to the inferior petrosal, sigmoid and occipital sinuses.

RADIOLOGICAL FEATURES OF THE CEREBELLUM

CT and MRI

On axial CT and MR sections taken at the level of the pons (see Fig. 2.3A), the cerebellum is seen to be separated from the pons by the fourth ventricle and connected to the pons on each side of this by the middle cerebellar peduncles. At this level the cerebellum is bounded anteriorly by the petrous temporal bones.

More superiorly on axial imaging (see Fig. 2.3B) the cerebellum is separated from the temporal and occipital lobes anterolaterally by the tentorial margins. Close to its bony attachment, the tentorium can be easily seen on contrast-enhanced studies owing to the contained superior petrosal sinus.

The superior vermis can be seen between the occipital lobes on sections through the thalamus.

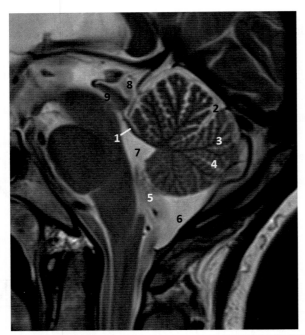

Fig. 2.19 Midline sagittal T$_2$ magnetic resonance image to show vermis of the cerebellum.

1. Lingula on superior medullary velum
2. Primary fissure
3. Horizontal fissure
4. Prepyramidal fissure
5. Foramen of Magendie with some flow artefact
6. Cisterna magna
7. Fourth ventricle
8. Quadrigeminal cistern
9. Aqueduct

The normal flocculus enhances more than the rest of the cerebellum and should not be mistaken for a more anteriorly located acoustic neuroma.

Fissures separating lobes of the cerebellum can be seen on sagittal MRI (see Fig. 2.19).

RADIOLOGY PEARL

The cerebellar tonsils have a variable position. Their position is best evaluated on sagittal CT or MRI. Most commonly they lie above the level of the foramen magnum but can normally extend as far inferiorly as the foramen magnum. Extension through the foramen magnum can represent a benign process called cerebellar tonsillar ectopia without effacement of the CSF spaces at the foramen magnum. A greater degree of inferior extension is associated with Chiari malformations. In Chiari I malformation, one or both cerebellar tonsils project 5 mm or more below the foramen magnum. In Chiari II malformation the cerebellar tonsils and vermis are herniated as well as the brainstem.

Low-lying tonsils may be an acquired phenomenon in the presence of mass effect and increased intracranial pressure causing cerebellar tonsillar herniation. This can have devastating consequences including compression of brain stem structures and obstructive hydrocephalus.

Evaluation of cerebellar tonsillar position is a routine part in the evaluation of a brain CT or MRI, in particular in the setting of trauma, acute cerebral oedema and any intracranial mass.

Ventricles, Cisterns, CSF Production and Flow (Figs. 2.20–2.22)

The ventricles are CSF-filled spaces within the brain related to the development of the nervous system as a tubular structure with a central canal.

Two lateral ventricles represent expansion of the most anterior part of the ventricular system into each cerebral hemisphere. The third ventricle, the aqueduct, and the fourth ventricle are midline in position and are continuous with the central canal of the cord. The ventricular system is also continuous with the subarachnoid space around the brain via foramina in the fourth ventricle. Approximately 25 mL of CSF fills these spaces in an adult.

The ventricles are lined with ependyma, which is invaginated by plexuses of blood vessels called the choroid plexus. These vessels produce the CSF.

THE LATERAL VENTRICLES (FIG. 2.20)

There is a lateral ventricle within each cerebral hemisphere. Each is C-shaped, with the limbs of the C facing anteriorly and a variably developed posterior extension from its midpoint. Each is described as having a frontal (anterior) horn, a body (atrium), a temporal (inferior) horn and an occipital (posterior) horn. The lateral ventricles are separated by a vertically orientated thin membrane called the septum pellucidum which is covered by ependyma on both sides. An interventricular foramen (of Monro) at the junction of the anterior horn and the body of each lateral ventricle connects each lateral ventricle with the third ventricle.

Frontal (Anterior) Horn

This extends into the frontal lobe. Its roof and anterior extremity are formed by the rostrum, genu and anterior body of the corpus callosum and fibres radiating from these, the tapetum. The head of the caudate nucleus makes a prominent impression in the floor and lateral wall of the anterior horn. The medial wall is formed by the septum pellucidum. There is no choroid plexus in the anterior horn.

Body

This is within the parietal lobe and extends from the interventricular foramen anteriorly to the splenium of the corpus callosum posteriorly. As with the anterior horn, the roof and lateral wall of the body of the ventricle are formed by the corpus callosum and its fibres – the tapetum – and the medial wall is formed by the septum pellucidum. The thalamus lies in the floor medially, with the body of the caudate nucleus laterally and the thalamostriate groove and vein between. The body of the fornix lies above the thalamus. The choroid plexus is invaginated into the cavity of the ventricle in a groove – the choroidal fissure – between the fornix and the thalamus.

Temporal (Inferior) Horn

This extends anteriorly into the temporal lobe. It curves down and laterally from the body of the ventricle and then somewhat medially towards the temporal pole. Its lateral wall and lateral roof are formed by the fibres of the tapetum. The tail of the caudate nucleus lies in the medial roof of the temporal horn with the amygdaloid nucleus at its anterior end (see Fig. 2.11). The hippocampus forms the floor of the temporal horn, with the pes hippocampi anteriorly and the crus of the fornix arising from this (see section on the fornix above).

The choroid plexus of the body of the lateral ventricle is continuous with that of the temporal horn.

Occipital Horn

This is the posterior extension of the lateral ventricle that extends into the occipital lobe. The occipital horn may be absent or poorly developed or may extend the full depth of the lobe. The posterior horns of the two lateral ventricles are often asymmetrical.

The roof and lateral wall of the occipital horn are formed by tapetal fibres of the corpus callosum which separate the optic radiation from the ventricle. The floor of the ventricle is formed by white matter that is indented by grey matter at the depth of the calcarine sulcus. This latter indentation forms a bulge called the **calcar avis**. There is no choroid plexus in the occipital horn.

THE CHOROID PLEXUS OF THE LATERAL VENTRICLE

The choroid plexus of the lateral ventricle is responsible for the production of most of the CSF. It also functions as part of the blood–brain barrier. The choroid plexus extends from the roof of the inferior horn to the floor of the body of the lateral ventricle where it is greatest in volume. At the interventricular foramen, the choroid plexus on the floor of the lateral ventricle is continuous with the choroid plexus in the roof of the third ventricle. The choroid plexuses are invaginated into the lateral ventricles medially through the choroidal fissure. The fold of pia containing the plexus is called the tela choroidea. This fold has a narrow, rounded apex anteriorly at the level of the interventricular foramen and is wider posteriorly, where it is continuous with the remainder of the subarachnoid space. If CSF accumulates in this fold, it forms a flat triangular **cavum** (or **cistern of the**) **velum interpositum** that may be visible on axial CT or MRI (see Figs. 2.22 and 2.23).

The vessels supplying the choroid plexus are the anterior and posterior choroidal arteries. The anterior choroidal artery, the most distal branch of the internal carotid artery, enters the choroidal plexus in the anterior part of the temporal horn. It is the major arterial supply for choroid plexus in the lateral ventricles. A smaller contribution comes from the posterior choroidal artery, a branch of the posterior cerebral artery, which also supplies the choroid plexus in the third ventricle. The posterior choroidal arteries are variable in number and pass into the body of lateral ventricle behind and above the thalamus and into the posterior part of the temporal horn below it.

Choroid plexus in the fourth ventricle is supplied by anterior inferior cerebellar arteries and PICAs from the vertebral arteries and basilar arteries, respectively.

The veins draining the plexus unite to form the choroidal vein, which begins in the temporal horn and passes anteriorly to the interventricular foramen, where it joins the thalamostriate vein to form the internal cerebral vein on each side.

The Third Ventricle (see Figs. 2.20–2.22)

This is a slit-like CSF-filled space between the thalami. Its width is between 2 and 10 mm and increases with age. Its lateral walls are formed by the thalami superiorly and part of the hypothalamus inferiorly and are limited inferiorly by the subthalamic (hypothalamic) groove.

- The anterior wall of the third ventricle is a thin sheet of grey matter, the lamina terminalis, which extends from the rostrum of the corpus callosum above to the optic chiasm below. The extension of the cavity inferiorly into the optic chiasm is called the supraoptic recess.
- The floor of the third ventricle is formed by the structures of the hypothalamus, from anterior to posterior.

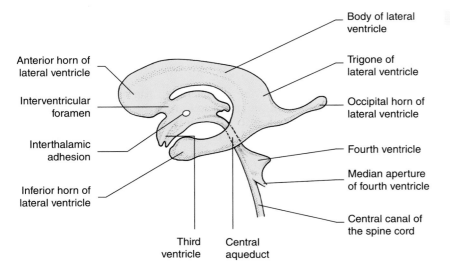

Anterior horn of lateral ventricle

Interventricular foramen

Interthalamic adhesion

Inferior horn of lateral ventricle

Body of lateral ventricle

Trigone of lateral ventricle

Occipital horn of lateral ventricle

Fourth ventricle

Median aperture of fourth ventricle

Central canal of the spine cord

Third ventricle   Central aqueduct

Fig. 2.20 The ventricular system.

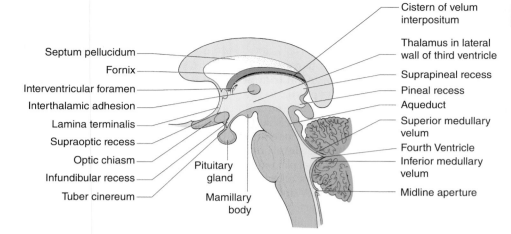

Fig. 2.21 Third and fourth ventricles and related midline sagittal structures.

Cistern of velum interpositum

Thalamus in lateral wall of third ventricle

Suprapineal recess

Pineal recess

Aqueduct

Superior medullary velum

Fourth Ventricle

Inferior medullary velum

Midline aperture

Septum pellucidum

Fornix

Interventricular foramen

Interthalamic adhesion

Lamina terminalis

Supraoptic recess

Optic chiasm

Infundibular recess

Tuber cinereum

Pituitary gland

Mamillary body

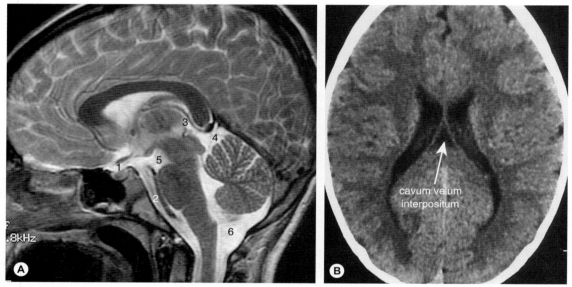

Fig. 2.22 (A) The subarachnoid cisterns. (B) Axial computed tomography scan to show the cavum velum interpositum.

1. Suprasellar cistern
2. Pontine cistern
3. Cavum velum interpositum

4. Quadrigeminal plate cistern
5. Interpeduncular cistern
6. Cisterna magna

These include the optic chiasm, tuber cinereum, mamillary bodies, posterior perforated substance and the tegmentum of the midbrain, including the pituitary gland, whose hollow stalk is the infundibular recess of the ventricle.

■ The posterior wall is formed by the pineal gland superiorly and posterior commissure and cerebral aqueduct inferiorly. The ventricle extends as a small pineal recess into the pineal stalk, and above this into a recess whose size varies from 1 to 3 cm – known as the suprapineal recess.

■ The roof of the third ventricle is formed anteriorly by the anterior commissure, the columns of the fornix and the interventricular foramen. Behind this the roof is formed by the body of the fornix, with the choroid plexus

invaginating below the fornix, in the choroidal fissure, into the upper part of the ventricle.

The thalami are connected in the midline posterior to the interventricular foramina by the **massa intermedia** or **interthalamic adhesion** in 60%–90% of humans. Formerly thought to be a non-neural connection, it does appear to contain some white matter tracts traversing to the contralateral hemisphere, suggesting a role as another commissure.

THE CEREBRAL AQUEDUCT (SEE FIGS. 2.20, 2.21)

This is a narrow channel connecting the posterior end of the third ventricle with the superior end of the fourth ventricle. Measuring 1.5 cm in length and 1–2 mm in diameter, it passes through the brainstem with the tectum (the quadrigeminal plate) posterior to it and the tegmentum and cerebral peduncles anteriorly. The nuclei of the third (III), fourth (IV) and fifth (V) CNs surround the aqueduct and are called the **periaqueductal grey matter**. Given its narrow calibre, it is the most common location for obstruction of the ventricular system.

THE FOURTH VENTRICLE (SEE FIGS. 2.20–2.22)

Posterior to the pons the aqueduct widens as the fourth ventricle and narrows again in the inferior part of the medulla as the central canal of the medulla and of the spinal cord.

The floor of the fourth ventricle lies anteriorly and is formed by the posterior surface of the pons and of the upper part of the medulla. It is diamond-shaped in the coronal plane (the **rhomboid fossa**). The roof appears tent-shaped in the sagittal plane and is formed superiorly by the superior cerebellar peduncles, with the superior medullary velum between, and inferiorly by the inferior cerebellar peduncles and the inferior medullary velum. Over these lies the cerebellum.

In the lower part of the fourth ventricle there are three openings, one median and two lateral. The **median aperture (of Magendie)** is a large opening in the inferior medullary velum beneath the cerebellum, which communicates with the cisterna magna. The cavity of the fourth ventricle is prolonged laterally under the inferior cerebellar peduncle on each side as the lateral recesses of the ventricle. The **lateral apertures (of Luschka)** are at the apex of these recesses and open anteriorly just behind the eighth cranial nerve into the pontine cistern.

Inferiorly, the fourth ventricle is contiguous with the central canal of the spinal cord at the **obex**.

The choroid plexus of the fourth ventricle invaginates the lower part of its roof and is supplied by a branch of the inferior cerebellar artery.

RADIOLOGY PEARL

The fourth ventricle tends to be symmetrical in its anatomy, as do the third ventricle and the aqueduct, and minor asymmetry may be a sign of pathology.

RADIOLOGICAL FEATURES OF THE VENTRICULAR SYSTEM

Skull Radiographs

The ventricular system cannot be seen by plain skull radiography but the position of the lateral ventricles is often indicated in adults by calcification of its choroid plexus. This is seen on a lateral view in the parietal area about 2.5 cm above the pineal gland. On occipito-frontal (OF) or fronto-occipital (FO) views it is seen to be nearly always symmetrical and bilateral.

The normal position of the fourth ventricle is indicated by Twining's line, which runs from the tuberculum sellae to the internal occipital protuberance. The midpoint of this line lies within the fourth ventricle near its floor.

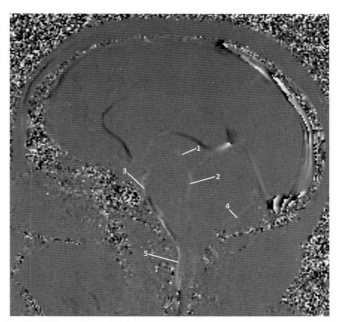

Fig. 2.23 MRI CSF flow study.

1. Cerebral aqueduct
2. Fourth ventricle
3. Interpeduncular and prepontine cisterns
4. Cisterna magna
5. Cervical subarachnoid space

CT and MRI (see Figs. 2.3, 2.7, 2.22)

CT is the primary modality for assessing ventricular size and morphology. Volumetric imaging allows for multiplanar reconstructions and evaluation of the ventricles in all planes. MRI is also frequently performed to evaluate the ventricles. It has better soft tissue resolution and characterisation, allowing for assessment of intraventricular and periventricular pathologies. In particular, high-resolution MRI sequences can identify pathologies obstructing the cerebral aqueduct, for example webs, which cannot be confidently identified on CT.

On axial imaging (see Fig. 2.3A), the fourth ventricle can be seen as a slit-like CSF-filled structure between the brainstem and the cerebellum. At the level of the midbrain (see Fig. 2.3B) it may show the aqueduct as a narrow-calibre CSF-filled structure surrounded by high-attenuation periaqueductal grey matter. The third ventricle is visible more superiorly (see Fig. 2.3C) as a slit-like space between the thalami. At this level, the anterior horns of the lateral ventricles can be seen separated by the septum pellucidum, with the head of the caudate nucleus indenting their lateral walls.

The posterior horns are visible also at this level and calcified choroid plexus is commonly seen in the trigone of the lateral ventricles. The temporal horns are frequently small in younger patients and become more prominent with age related to underlying cerebral volume loss. Superior to this, the bodies of the lateral ventricles are separated by the septum pellucidum. The body and tail of the caudate nucleus can be seen as a high-attenuation structure in its lateral wall.

Sagittal MRIs show the third ventricle, aqueduct and fourth ventricle in continuity with each other and with the central canal of the medulla and of the spinal cord. The communication of the fourth ventricle with the cisterna magna at the foramen of Magendie can also be seen. The recesses of the third ventricle can be seen particularly well on this view (see Fig. 2.22).

RADIOLOGY PEARL

The posterior horns of the two lateral ventricles are often asymmetrical and are bilaterally well developed in only 12% of subjects. If the posterior horn is present on one side only it is usually the left.

RADIOLOGY PEARL

The ventricles may enlarge slightly in old age due to expected cerebral volume loss. Abnormal enlargement disproportionate to any underlying atrophy is termed hydrocephalus. The temporal horns of the lateral ventricles frequently are first to enlarge.

RADIOLOGY PEARL

Raised intraventricular pressure and hydrocephalus due to obstruction at the level of the aqueduct can be treated with external drainage via a ventriculoperitoneal shunt or by bypassing the cerebral aqueduct through the endoscopic creation of a passage through the floor of the third ventricle, an endoscopic third ventriculostomy. In the setting of hydrocephalus, if the floor of the third ventricle is seen to bulge inferiorly on MRI, this indicates that the pressure within the ventricles is greater than the pressure outside the ventricle, and the patient could benefit from a third ventriculostomy.

Ultrasound Examination of the Neonatal Brain (see Figs. 2.10, 2.24)

In anterior coronal views, the frontal horns of the lateral ventricles are seen as triangular in cross-section, with the floor and lateral wall indented by the head of the caudate nucleus. The bodies of the lateral ventricles are also approximately triangular in cross-section, indented inferolaterally by the thalamus medially and the body of the caudate nucleus laterally. Scans through the posterior part of the body of the lateral ventricle show echogenic divergent bands of the choroid plexus. The calcar avis may be seen indenting the medial wall of the ventricle. The mean width of the lateral ventricles is measured at the level of the body and is 9 mm in a 30-week premature infant and 12 mm in the full-term infant.

Parasagittal scans show the full sweep of the lateral ventricle, with the choroid plexus in the floor of the body and in the roof of the inferior horn. The head of the caudate nucleus can be identified anteriorly, the thalamus posterior to this and the thalamocaudate notch between.

The third ventricle may be seen as a slit-like space between the thalami. If not enlarged, this space may not be visible on a normal scan. Superolateral communications with the lateral ventricles at the foramina of Monro can be identified by the presence of the echogenic choroid plexus of the third ventricle in the roof of the third ventricle continuous through the foramen with the choroid plexus in the floor of the lateral ventricles (see Fig. 2.24A). The interthalamic adhesion may be outlined by echo-free CSF.

Midline sagittal scanning identifies the cavum septi pellucidi and vergae above the third ventricle, between the frontal horns and bodies of the two lateral ventricles. These are, in fact, a single structure with that part posterior to the foramen of Monro being named the cavum vergae. They are not normally connected with the remainder of the ventricular system and the term 'fifth ventricle', which is sometimes used, is therefore misleading. The cavum vergae begins to close from posterior to anterior in the sixth gestational month and progresses to complete obliteration of both spaces by 2 months of age in 85% of infants.

The aqueduct is seldom visible on the normal scan, but the echogenic cerebellar vermis helps identify the roof and cavity of the fourth ventricle.

RADIOLOGY PEARL

Germinal matrix is a highly cellular and highly vascularized region in the brain from which cells migrate out during brain development. Residual germinal matrix at the caudothalamic groove in the floor of the lateral ventricle is the location of intraventricular haemorrhage in the preterm infant.

THE SUBARACHNOID CISTERNS (SEE FIG. 2.22)

Because the brain and the internal contours of the skull show marked differences in shape, the subarachnoid space is deep in several places, particularly around the base of the brain. These deep spaces are called cisterns and are named according to nearby brain structures. They contain more CSF than the ventricles. They freely communicate with each other and the remaining CSF space, allowing for normal flow of the CSF.

Cisterna Magna (Cerebellomedullary Cistern)

This is the largest cistern. It lies behind the medulla and below the cerebellar hemispheres and receives CSF from the median aperture of the fourth ventricle. It is continuous through the foramen magnum with the spinal subarachnoid space and continues superiorly for a variable distance behind the cerebellum. On each side its lateral part contains the vertebral artery and its posterior inferior cerebellar branch. Cranial nerves IX–XII pass through this cistern.

Pontine Cistern

This lies between the pons and the clivus, and is continuous below with the cisterna magna and above with the interpeduncular cistern. It receives CSF from the lateral apertures of the fourth ventricle. The pontine cistern contains the basilar artery and its pontine and labyrinthine

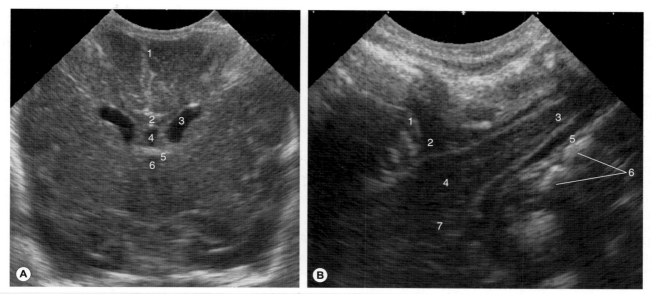

Fig. 2.24 (A) Coronal ultrasound through interventricular foramina. (B) Ultrasound through the foramen magnum.

(A)
1. Interhemispheric fissure
2. Corpus callosum
3. Anterior horn of left lateral ventricle
4. Cavum septum pellucidum
5. Choroid plexus marking position of interventricular foramen
6. Third ventricle

(B)
1. Inferior margin of occipital bone = posterior border of foramen magnum
2. Cisterna magna
3. Cervical cord
4. Medulla oblongata
5. Dura
6. Cervical vertebral bodies
7. Pons

branches, the origins of the AICAs and superior cerebellar arteries. The sixth (VI) CN passes through the pontine cistern.

Interpeduncular Cistern

This cistern lies between the cerebral peduncles of the midbrain and the dorsum sellae. It is continuous below with the pontine cistern, laterally with the ambient cisterns and superiorly with the suprasellar cisterns. It contains the posterior part of the arterial circle of Willis. CN III traverses this cistern.

Quadrigeminal Cistern

This cistern lies posterior to the quadrigeminal plate of the midbrain. It lies between the splenium above and the vermis below and is limited posteriorly by the tentorium. Laterally it communicates with interpeduncular cisterns. Also called the cistern of the great vein, it contains the venous confluence of the internal cerebral veins and the basal veins to form the great cerebral vein (of Galen). This unites with the inferior sagittal sinus to form the straight sinus. It contains portions of the posterior cerebral arteries as well as CN III.

Cistern of the Velum Interpositum (see Figs. 2.21, 2.22)

The space between the layers of the tela choroidea as it passes beneath the splenium of the corpus callosum and the fornix may contain CSF and may be called the cistern (or cavum) of the velum interpositum. It is continuous posteriorly with the quadrigeminal plate cistern through

a narrow slit under the splenium called the transverse fissure. It has a triangular shape on axial sections. The cistern of the velum interpositum contains the internal cerebral veins.

Ambient Cisterns

These extend around both sides of the midbrain between the interpeduncular cistern anteriorly and the quadrigeminal cistern posteriorly. Lateral extensions of the superior part of the ambient cisterns around the posterior part of the thalamus are called the ambient wing cisterns. The posterior cerebral artery and the basal vein lie in the anterior part of each ambient cistern. Each CN IV traverses its ipsilateral ambient cistern.

Suprasellar Cisterns

This cistern is above the pituitary fossa. It lies between the anterior part of the floor of the third ventricle above and the diaphragma sellae below. It is continuous posteriorly with the interpeduncular cistern and extends laterally into the sylvian cistern at the lower end of the sylvian fissure. The optic nerves pass to the chiasm in the anterior part of the suprasellar cistern, and the part of the cistern anterior to this is sometimes referred to as the chiasmatic cistern. The anterior part of the circle of Willis lies in the suprasellar cistern. The infundibulum traverses the cistern, posteriorly extending to the neurohypophysis.

Pericallosal Cistern

The suprasellar and chiasmatic cisterns continue superiorly as the cistern of the lamina terminalis and around the superior surface of the corpus callosum as the pericallosal cistern. This is in turn continuous posteriorly with the quadrigeminal cistern below the splenium. The pericallosal cistern contains branches of the anterior cerebral artery.

RADIOLOGICAL FEATURES OF THE SUBARACHNOID CISTERNS

CT and MRI

The cisterns are visible on axial CT and MR scanning as CSF-filled spaces between parts of the brain and the skull. On axial imaging through the midbrain (see Fig. 2.3B) the interpeduncular, ambient and quadrigeminal cisterns are seen around the midbrain. Anterior to the interpeduncular cistern is the suprasellar cistern and posterior to the quadrigeminal cistern is the superior vermian cistern. At the level of the superior part of the lateral ventricles the pericallosal cistern can be seen between the falx and the genu of the corpus callosum anteriorly, and between the splenium and the falx posteriorly. The marked difference in relaxation constants in MRI between water and brain tissue parenchyma results in particularly good demonstration of small structures in cisterns, where they are surrounded by CSF. This quality can be harnessed using dedicated heavily T2 weighted high-resolution sequences to evaluate cranial nerves, for example CN V, VII and VIII. Additionally, the optic nerve and chiasm in the suprasellar cistern are well evaluated on MRI, for example as part of dedicated orbital or pituitary protocol MRIs. The acoustic nerve in the pontine cistern and vessels in all cisterns are all seen well on T_2-weighted MRI.

The **cavum (or cistern of the) velum interpositum**, if present, is seen as a fluid-filled space inferior to the splenium of the corpus callosum and between the thalamus and the fornix. It is triangular in the axial plane with its apex anteriorly (see Fig. 2.22B).

MRI CSF flow study is a technique using cardiac-gated gradient echo phase contrast MRI to show CSF flow (see Fig. 2.23). It can be used to demonstrate the direction of CSF flow and for distinguishing arachnoid cysts from open CSF spaces. It is also possible to calculate CSF flow velocity in any location and to quantify volumetric flow. MRI CSF flow study demonstrates normal or abnormal CSF flow between ventricles, in the aqueduct, around the fourth ventricular foramina, the basal cisterns and within and around the spinal cord.

CT Cisternography

CT cisternography is a minimally invasive imaging technique used to evaluate the cisterns and subarachnoid spaces. Most commonly the subarachnoid space is accessed via a lumbar puncture with iodinated contrast injected into the thecal sac. The contrast is then encouraged to extend intracranially through manipulation of the patient position, predominantly relying on the Trendelenburg or head down position. CT cisternography can be used to identify skull base CSF leaks and to evaluate suspected arachnoid cysts for communication with the subarachnoid space.

CT cisternography may also be achieved by cisternal puncture into the cisterna magna and the spinal subarachnoid space. A needle is introduced above level C_2 and directed upwards. At a depth of about 3 cm the needle is felt to penetrate the atlanto-occipital membrane and to enter the cisterna magna. Structures at risk of injury by this procedure include the spinal cord and the medulla oblongata anterior to the cistern, and the PICA and its branches within the cistern. A lumbar puncture for cisternography has replaced direct cisternal punctures or cervical myelography in the majority of cases with these approaches reserved for patients with a block to CSF flow in the thoracic or lumbar spine.

Cranial Ultrasound

Images of the cisterna magna and surrounding structures can be obtained in the infant by ultrasound through the foramen magnum by an approach from the posterior aspect of the upper neck (see Fig. 2.24B).

CSF PRODUCTION AND FLOW

The total volume of CSF is about 150 mL, 25 mL of which is within and around the spinal cord, with a further 25 mL within the ventricles. It is produced at 0.4 mL/minute independent of CSF pressure. An adult produces 400–600 mL of CSF every 24 hours, with the entire CSF volume renewed four times a day. The composition of CSF is constant. CSF is produced by the choroid plexuses of all ventricles, but principally by that of the lateral ventricles. It flows through the interventricular foramina into the third ventricle, through the cerebral aqueduct to the fourth ventricle, and from the ventricular system via the midline aperture into the cisterna magna and via the lateral apertures into the pontine cisterns. Some diffusion occurs with fluid from the spinal canal.

From the basal cisterns, some fluid flows down and bathes the spinal cord; the remainder passes upward, over the cerebellum and brain stem and through the tentorial hiatus to diffuse over the surface of the cerebral hemispheres. CSF flow is predominantly secondary to systolic pulsation of arteries within the subarachnoid space. This is aided by respiration, postural changes and pressure within the venous sinuses.

CSF is absorbed through the arachnoid villi. These are herniations of arachnoid through holes in the dura into the venous sinuses. They are most numerous in the superior sagittal sinus and in its laterally projecting blood lakes. In children these villi are discrete; with age they aggregate into visible clumps called arachnoid granulations (Pacchionian granulations). These indent the inner table of the skull beside the dural venous sinuses.

About one-third of the CSF is either absorbed along similar spinal villi or escapes along nerve sheaths into the perineural lymphatics. Hydrostatic pressure differences, lower in the venous sinuses, encourage the reabsorption of CSF. This absorption is passive and dependent on hydrostatic pressure differences.

RADIOLOGICAL FEATURES OF CSF PRODUCTION AND FLOW

RADIOLOGY PEARL

Knowledge of the circulatory pathway of CSF is important in diagnosis, as ventricular dilation proximal to a point of obstruction of its flow indicates the site of the lesion. Thus, a lesion obstructing the cerebral aqueduct causes dilatation of the lateral and third ventricles but not the fourth. Arachnoiditis blocking the exit foramina of the fourth ventricle causes dilatation of all four ventricles.

CT Brain

Arachnoid (Pacchionian) granulations are seen as hypodense foci on noncontrast CT imaging of the brain. They are most prevalent in the superior sagittal sinus, about the torcula and in the transverse sinuses. They can be differentiated from acute thrombus in a venous sinus, which is typically hyperdense on noncontrast imaging. Calcium deposition can occur at the arachnoid granulations and the calcification may be visible on plain films or CT.

Radionuclide Cisternography

MRI is the primary modality for assessing CSF dynamics. [111]Indium-diethylenetriaminepentaacetic acid (DTPA) SPECT/CT cisternography is an alternative technique in patients with contraindications to MRI and provides anatomic and functional imaging. The radionuclide is injected into the CSF via the lumbar route. After 1–3 hours the isotope can be seen in the basal cisterns – the cisterna magna, the pontine and interpeduncular cisterns and the quadrigeminal cistern. After 3–6 hours the radionuclide is seen in the sylvian and interhemispheric fissures. By 24 hours activity surrounds the brain. In children the CSF flow is more rapid, with the basal cisterns being reached at 15–30 minutes and isotope surrounding the brain at 12 hours. At no time is activity normally seen within the ventricles. If indicated, a CT can be performed to further evaluate abnormal findings on SPECT imaging.

Magnetic Resonance CSF Flow Study (see Fig. 2.23)

Dynamic MRI CSF flow sequences can identify the presence of CSF flow through the ventricular system, adjacent cisterns and in and around the spinal cord allowing for estimates of velocity and volume of flow. This is used in the preoperative assessment of patients with Chiari malformations and aqueductal stenosis.

Meninges (Fig. 2.25)

Three layers of meninges cover the brain and spinal cord (spinal meninges). These are, from superficial to deep – the dura mater, the arachnoid mater and the pia mater (see Fig. 2.25).

DURA MATER

The dura mater is also referred to as the pachymeninges. It is a tough membrane described as having two layers.

The outer layer is, in fact, the periosteum of the inner aspect of the skull and is continuous through all the foramina and sutures of the skull with the periosteum on the outside of the skull. The inner layer is the dura mater proper. This is, however, densely adherent to the outer layer in all places except where the layers separate around the dural venous sinuses and where the inner layer projects inwardly as the dural reflections the falx cerebri and cerebelli, and as the tentorium cerebelli and as well as the diaphragma sellae.

The **falx cerebri** is a sickle-shaped dural septum in the median sagittal plane attached to the crista galli in the midline of the floor of the anterior cranial fossa and along the midline of the inner aspect of the vault of the skull to the margins of the superior sagittal sinus. Posteriorly it is wider; here it is attached to the upper surface of the tentorium cerebelli, enclosing the straight sinus. It projects into the interhemispheric fissure and its inferior free edge lies close to the corpus callosum. The inferior sagittal sinus is within this free edge.

The **diaphragma sellae** is a horizontal fold of dura that almost completely covers the pituitary fossa, with a small opening for the pituitary stalk.

The **tentorium cerebelli** is a horizontal septum of dura mater that separates the occipital lobes from the superior surface of the cerebellum. Its outer attached border arises from each posterior clinoid process and is attached along the upper border of the petrous bones, enclosing the superior petrosal sinus on each side. The tentorium is attached to the occipital bone along the margins of the transverse sinuses to the internal occipital protuberance. The anterior free edge of the tentorium, called the tentorial notch, is attached to the anterior clinoid processes and surrounds the midbrain. There is no venous sinus in this free edge. The tentorium is sloped upwards from its attached edge to its free edge and has a midline ridge where the falx cerebri is attached to its superior surface. Close to the posterior clinoid processes an outpouching in the attached edge of the tentorium forms a recess around the trigeminal nerve and ganglion, the trigeminal or Meckel's cave.

The uncus of the temporal lobe and the posterior cerebral artery lie close to the free edge of the tentorium and may be compressed against it if there is increased pressure in the supratentorial part of the brain.

The **falx cerebelli** is a low elevation of dura that projects a small distance into the cerebellar interhemispheric fissure. It is attached from the internal occipital protuberance along the internal occipital crest to the posterior margin of the foramen magnum. The small occipital venous sinus lies in its attached edge.

The **epidural (extradural) space** is a predominantly potential space between the periosteal layer of the dura and the calvarium. This contains arteries and veins but only becomes visible with pathology.

ARACHNOID MATER

This layer of meninges is a delicate avascular membrane which is impermeable to CSF. It lines but is not attached to the overlying the dura mater, separated from it only by a thin layer of lymph in the **subdural (potential) space**. It is separated from the pia mater by the **subarachnoid**

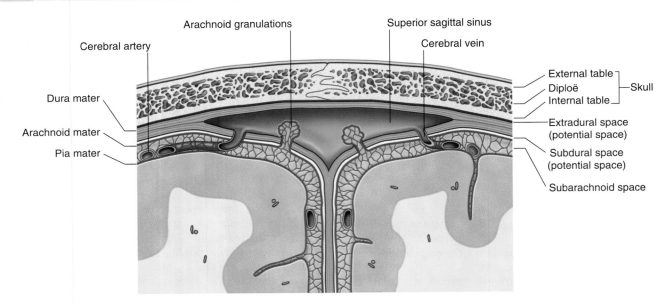

Fig. 2.25 The arrangement of the meninges and spaces between layers of meninges. (Modified from Drake RL, Vogl AW, Mitchell AWM. *Gray's Anatomy for Students*, 5th ed. Elsevier; 2024.)

space, which contains the CSF. The arachnoid mater projects into the interhemispheric fissure and into the root of the sylvian fissure, but otherwise does not dip into the sulci. It surrounds the cranial and spinal nerves in a loose sheath as far as their exit from the skull and vertebral canal.

The arachnoid mater herniates through holes in the dura into the venous sinuses and venous lakes as arachnoid villi or granulations, and only in these villi is the arachnoid pervious to CSF.

PIA MATER

This meningeal layer is closely adherent to the brain surface and dips into all the sulci. It continues along all the cranial and spinal nerves and fuses with their epineurium. It is also invaginated into the surface of the brain by extending along the cerebral arteries and their branches. The perivascular space lies between the vessel walls and pia. The pia invaginates with the choroid vessels into the ventricles, and the layer of pia mater and ependyma together thus formed over these vessels is called the **tela choroidea** of the ventricles.

ARTERIAL SUPPLY OF THE MENINGES

The arterial supply is found mostly between the periosteal and inner layers of the dura mater, the epidural space. Most of the supratentorial dura is supplied by the middle meningeal artery, a branch of the maxillary artery that enters the cranium through the foramen spinosum. It passes laterally in the floor of the middle cranial fossa, then superiorly and anteriorly along the greater wing of sphenoid, where it divides into anterior and posterior branches.

There is additional arterial supply to the meninges in:
- The anterior cranial fossa from meningeal branches of the ophthalmic and anterior and posterior ethmoid arteries.
- Over the cavernous sinus by meningeal branches of the carotid artery and by the accessory meningeal artery from the maxillary artery, which passes through the foramen ovale.

The posterior fossa meninges are supplied by meningeal branches of the vertebral artery, with some additional supply from meningeal branches of the occipital artery through the mastoid and jugular foramina and from meningeal branches of the ascending pharyngeal artery through the jugular foramen and the hypoglossal canal.

Venous drainage is via veins accompanying arteries and the dural venous sinuses.

NERVE SUPPLY OF THE MENINGES

The meninges are supplied supratentorially, mostly by the ophthalmic division of the trigeminal nerve, with some supply in the middle cranial fossa by the maxillary and mandibular divisions of this nerve. In the posterior fossa the meninges are supplied by meningeal branches of the ninth and tenth cranial nerves, with the dura around the foramen magnum being innervated by the C_1–C_3 nerves.

RADIOLOGICAL FEATURES OF THE MENINGES

Extradural (Epidural) Haematoma

This occurs when a vessel in the extradural (potential) space between dura and bone is torn by trauma. In the majority of cases the middle meningeal artery is affected

Calcification of the falx cerebri or of the tentorium can be seen on occipito-frontal (OF) or fronto-occipital (FO) views.

CT and MRI

Above the level of the petrous temporal bones the cerebral hemispheres are separated from the cerebellum by the tentorium. The tentorium is best seen on contrast-enhanced scans because of its contained blood vessels. It is seen as a high-attenuation linear structure extending laterally from the midbrain to the inner table of the skull. Because the tentorium slopes upwards towards the tentorial notch, higher slices (see Fig. 2.3B) show the margins of the tentorium much closer to the midline. A small portion of the upper cerebellum and vermis and the superior vermian cistern are visible between these margins. The occipital lobes may meet the falx in the midline posterior to the tentorium on these slices, giving a Y-shaped configuration to the dural folds here.

The falx cerebri is seen on higher cuts anteriorly and posteriorly extending into the interhemispheric fissure almost to the corpus callosum.

Arterial Supply of the CNS (Figs. 2.26–2.30)

The arterial supply of the CNS is derived from the internal carotid and vertebral arteries. Anastomoses exist between the internal and external carotid arteries but little or no supply to the normal brain is derived from the latter.

All arteries entering the surface of the brain are end arteries, that is, they have no precapillary anastomoses with other arteries and obstruction of them causes infarct of the supplied territory.

INTERNAL CAROTID ARTERY (SEE FIGS. 2.26, 2.27; SEE ALSO THE SECTION ON THE CAROTID ARTERIES IN THE NECK IN CHAPTER 1)

Once the internal carotid artery enters the carotid canal it has a very tortuous course – six bends in all before its terminal division. The reason for this tortuosity is unknown but it may have a role in reducing the pulsating force of the blood supply to the brain.

The internal carotid artery is described as having seven segments, the first or cervical segment, and six intracranial segments, including:

- Petrous or horizontal segment (C2): This component extends anteromedially within the skull base in the carotid canal of the petrous temporal bone. It is separated from the middle and inner ear structures by a thin plate of bone.
- Lacerum segment (C3): Upon exiting the carotid canal it lies superior to the foramen lacerum. Sequential 90-degree turns superiorly and anteriorly lead to the cavernous sinus.
- Cavernous segment (C4): The artery travels anteriorly through the sinus between layers of the dura mater. CN VI lies inferior and lateral to the artery with CN III, CN IV and CN Va lying lateral to the artery from superior to inferior in the lateral wall of the cavernous sinus.
- Clinoid segment (C5): Sequential 90-degree turns superiorly through the proximal dural ring at the anterior margin of the cavernous sinus and posteriorly lead to the clinoid segment of the artery, with the artery lying medial to the anterior clinoid process. The clinoid segment is a short segment extending to the distal dural ring.
- Ophthalmic segment (C6): This segment extends from the distal dural ring to the origin of the posterior communicating artery, with the artery now intradural in location.
- Communicating segment (C7): This segment extends from distal to the posterior communicating artery origin to the carotid terminus and bifurcation.

BRANCHES OF THE INTERNAL CAROTID ARTERY

The cervical portion has no branches. The laceral and clinoid segments usually do not have named branches.
Petrous segment:
- Vidian artery/artery of the pterygoid canal
- Caroticotympanic artery to the tympanic membrane

Cavernous segment:
- **Meningohypophyseal artery:** Supplies the dura of the anterior cranial fossa and sends branches to the pituitary.
- **Inferolateral trunk:** Branches supply part of the dura of the tentorium as well as CN Vb. Additional branches form internal carotid artery–external carotid artery anastomoses.
- **Capsular arteries:** To the wall of the cavernous sinus.

Ophthalmic segment:
- **Ophthalmic artery** (see Fig. 2.28): This is the first intradural branch. It can occasionally arise from the cavernous segment. It passes anteriorly and enters the optic foramen inferior and lateral to the optic nerve. It then crosses the optic nerve superiorly and passes to the medial wall of the orbit. The ophthalmic artery supplies the orbital contents and also has supratrochlear and supraorbital branches to supply the skin over the eyebrow.
- **Superior hypophyseal artery:** Branches supply the optic nerves and chiasm as well as the pituitary gland and infundibulum.

Communicating segment:
- **Posterior communicating artery:** This artery courses posteriorly to join the P1 segment of the posterior cerebral artery. While usually small and the non-dominant contributor to the posterior cerebral artery, the posterior communicating artery may be large and represent the dominant or only supply to the posterior cerebral artery. This a common anatomic variant, a fetal-type or fetal-origin posterior cerebral artery.
- **Anterior choroidal artery:** This vessel is small but is readily identifiable on angiograms. It passes posteriorly, giving branches to the crus cerebri and to the lateral geniculate body before entering the lateral ventricle at the anterior tip of its inferior horn to supply the choroid plexus of this ventricle (along with the posterior choroidal arteries of the posterior cerebral artery). It also supplies branches to the basal ganglia and to the hippocampus. The plexal or choroidal point is an apparent kink in the vessel on anteroposterior

(AP) or lateral angiograms that marks the point where the vessel enters the choroidal fissure.

- The terminal branches of the communicating segment are the anterior cerebral artery and middle cerebral artery.

Anterior Cerebral Artery

This arises from the internal carotid artery at the anterior perforated substance and passes anteriorly, superior to the optic chiasm. It winds around the genu of the corpus callosum and passes posteriorly on its superior surface to supply the medial and superolateral aspect of the cerebral hemisphere posteriorly as far as the parieto-occipital surface (see Fig. 2.26).

It is also divided into segments; the main segments are:

- A1: Extending from the carotid terminus to the origin of the anterior communicating artery.
- A2: Originating at the anterior communicating artery origin and extending along the rostrum of the corpus callosum to its bifurcation into pericallosal and callosomarginal branches.
- A3: The pericallosal artery is the largest terminal branch of the anterior cerebral artery with the callosomarginal artery being variably absent. It extends over the genu of the corpus callosum in the pericallosal sulcus.

Branches of the anterior cerebral artery:

A1 segment:
- **Medial lenticulostriate arteries:** Supplying the anterior limb of the internal capsule and caudate nucleus.
- **Anterior communicating artery:** Anastomosis of the A1 segments of both anterior cerebral arteries.

A2 segment:
- **Recurrent artery of Huebner:** This may arise from the distal A1 or proximal A2 segment. It supplies the anterior limb of the internal capsule, corpus striatum and portions of the hypothalamus.
- **Orbitofrontal artery:** Supplies the inferior part of the frontal lobe including the gyri recti.
- **Frontopolar artery:** This arises before the vessel curves over the superior surface of the corpus callosum. It passes anterosuperiorly towards the anterior pole of the frontal lobe.

A3 segment:
- **Pericallosal artery:** This is the continuation of the anterior cerebral artery on the superior surface of the corpus callosum.
- **Callosomarginal artery:** This arises near the genu and passes up to the superior border of the hemisphere at the frontoparietal region. It is variably absent.

Central branches are small branches arising from A1, the anterior communicating artery and A2. These supply the corpus callosum, the septum pellucidum, the anterior part of the lentiform nucleus and the head of the caudate nucleus.

There are multiple small terminal frontal and parietal branches.

Middle Cerebral Artery

This is the largest and most direct of the branches of the internal carotid artery and is therefore the most prone to embolism. It passes laterally and ends as branches on the insula, the overlying opercula and most of the lateral surface of the cerebral hemisphere. It is also divided into segments; however, the terminology used for these segments varies. The system described is determined by the major branching points of the artery:

- M1 segment: Originates at the carotid terminus and extends laterally adjacent to the sphenoid. It terminates into major branches, most commonly a bifurcation.
- M2 segment: Most commonly originates as a bifurcation of the M1 segment with anterior/superior and posterior/inferior divisions. These course posteriorly in the Sylvian fissure over the insula.
- M3 segment: The main branches arising from the M2 divisions.
- M4 segment: Further smaller branches arising from the M3 branches.

It passes laterally and ends as branches on the insula, the overlying opercula and most of the lateral surface of the cerebral hemisphere.

The middle cerebral artery has an array of branches; some of the major branches by segment include:

M1 segment:
Branches of the middle cerebral artery are:
- **Medial and lateral striate (or lenticulostriate) arteries:** These arise at the anterior perforated substance and are seen on AP angiograms arising from the upper surface of the middle cerebral artery trunk. They have a tortuous course superiorly, running at first medially for a short distance, then laterally and finally medially again. On lateral angiograms they are usually hidden by overlying branches of the middle cerebral vessels. One of these branches tends to be larger than the others and is called the artery of cerebral haemorrhage, as it is the artery of the brain most frequently ruptured. The striate arteries supply the basal ganglia and the anterior part of the internal capsule.
- **Anterior temporal artery and temporopolar arteries:** Both arteries supply the polar and anterolateral temporal lobe.

M2 segment:
Superior division:
- **Lateral orbitofrontal artery:** While variable in origin, it most commonly arises as the first branch of the superior division. It supplies the lateral orbitofrontal cortex.
- **Prefrontal sulcal arteries:** Fan out to supply the middle and inferior frontal gyri. Terminal branches anastomose with branches of the pericallosal artery of the anterior cerebral artery.
- **Prerolandic artery:** Supplies the posterior parts of the middle and inferior frontal gyri as well as the precentral gyrus.
- **Rolandic arteries:** These supply part of the precentral and postcentral gyri.

Inferior division:
- **Temporal arteries:** Middle and posterior temporal arteries supplying portions of the middle temporal gyrus and posterior temporal lobe, respectively.
- **Angular artery:** Divides into two branches supplying the angular gyrus, supramarginal gyrus and posterior superior temporal gyrus.
- **Parietal lobe branches**.

VERTEBROBASILAR SYSTEM (SEE FIGS. 2.27, 2.29)

Vertebral Artery

The vertebral artery arises from the posterosuperior aspect of the first part of the subclavian artery. The left vertebral artery is the dominant artery in 80% of cases. Each artery enters the foramen transversarium of the sixth cervical vertebra (occasionally the seventh, fifth or fourth) and ascends through the foramina of the upper six (or seven, five or four) cervical vertebrae. Within the foramen, the artery passes anterior to the ventral ramus of the spinal nerve and is accompanied by sympathetic nerves from the inferior cervical ganglion and a plexus of veins that unite inferiorly to form the vertebral vein. Having exited from its foramen, the vertebral artery passes posterior to the lateral mass of the atlas and enters the skull through the foramen magnum. It pierces the dura and arachnoid mater and passes anterior to the medulla until it unites with its fellow at the lower border of the pons.

The vertebral artery is also divided into segments:
- V1: From its origin to the transverse foramen of C6 (or another variant vertebra).
- V2: From the transverse foramen of C6 (or other) to the transverse foramen of C2.
- V3: From distal to the C2 transverse foramen to the foramen magnum.
- V4: From the foramen magnum to the formation of the basilar artery. This segment is intradural.

In the neck the branches of the vertebral artery (small branches rarely seen on angiograms) are as follows:
- **Spinal branches:** To the vertebrae and passing into the intervertebral foramina help to supply the spinal cord.
- **Muscular branches:** To the deep muscles of the neck. These anastomose with the branches of the occipital and ascending pharyngeal arteries of the external carotid artery.

V4 segment branches include:
- **Meningeal branch:** To the cerebellar fossa and falx.
- **Posterior spinal artery:** (More frequently arises as a branch of PICA). It descends as two branches anterior and posterior to the dorsal roots.
- **Anterior spinal artery:** Unites with its fellow anterior to the medulla and descends as a single anterior spinal artery.
- **Small branches to the medulla oblongata**.
- **PICA:** The largest branch of the vertebral artery. It is occasionally absent. The PICA normally arises from the intracranial part of the vertebral artery. Occasionally it can arise extradurally or as a common origin with the anterior inferior cerebellar artery from the basilar artery, an AICA-PICA complex. It has a tortuous course, passing posteriorly and ascending at first to the lower border of the pons. It then courses inferolaterally around the fourth ventricle to reach the inferior surface of the cerebellum in the midline. It supplies branches to the lateral part of the medulla and to the choroid plexus of the fourth ventricle. PICA terminates as two branches:
  - **Medial branch (inferior vermian artery)** to the inferior vermis and adjacent inferior surface of the cerebellar hemispheres.
  - **Lateral branch** to the lateral aspect of the inferior surface of the cerebellum.

Basilar Artery

Formed by the union of the two vertebral arteries at the lower border of the pons, the basilar artery lies close to (but seldom exactly in) the midline, anterior to the pons in the pontine cistern. When it deviates away from the midline it does so to the side away from that of a dominant vertebral artery.

The branches of the basilar artery are as follows:
- **Pontine artery:** Comprises several small branches to the adjacent pons.
- **Labyrinthine (internal auditory) artery:** This is a small branch (not visible on angiography) with variable origin, more commonly arising as a branch of the AICA. It extends to the internal acoustic meatus (IAM) with the VII and VIII CNs.
- **AICA:** This runs laterally and posteriorly. It supplies the anterior and lateral aspect of the undersurface of the cerebellum and may form a loop into and out of the IAM with the labyrinthine artery arising from the summit of the loop.
- **Superior cerebellar artery:** This arises very close to the terminal division of the basilar artery and runs laterally around the cerebral peduncle of the midbrain to the superior surface of the cerebellum, which it supplies. This artery also sends branches to the pons and to the pineal gland.
- **Right and left posterior cerebral arteries:** The basilar artery terminates by dividing into these.

POSTERIOR CEREBRAL ARTERIES

The posterior cerebral artery receives the posterior communicating artery of the internal carotid artery to complete the circle of Willis. It runs laterally and posteriorly around the cerebral peduncle parallel and superior to the superior cerebellar artery, and separated from this artery laterally by the tentorium. It reaches the inferior surface of the occipital lobe and supplies this and the inferior part of the posteromedial temporal lobe.

The posterior cerebral artery is divided into segments:
- P1 segment: Is situated within the interpeduncular cistern. Extends from the bifurcation of the basilar artery to the confluence with the posterior communicating artery coursing over CN III.
- P2 segment: From the confluence of P1 and posterior communicating artery this extends around the midbrain within the ambient cistern coursing over the tentorium cerebelli to the quadrigeminal cistern.
- P3 segment: From the quadrigeminal cistern to the sulci of the occipital lobe.
- P4 segment: Branches within the occipital lobe.

The main branches of the posterior cerebral artery are as follows:
- **Central perforating branches:** These include thalamoperforating, thalamogeniculate and peduncular perforating arteries. Supply is to cerebral peduncles, the posterior thalamus, the medial geniculate body, and the quadrigeminal plate and walls of the third ventricle.
- **Thalamostriate arteries:** Branches that enter the posterior perforated substance to supply the thalamus and the lentiform nucleus.

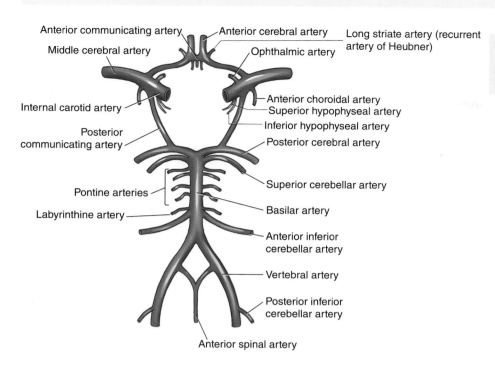

Anterior communicating artery
Middle cerebral artery
Anterior cerebral artery
Long striate artery (recurrent artery of Heubner)
Ophthalmic artery
Internal carotid artery
Anterior choroidal artery
Superior hypophyseal artery
Posterior communicating artery
Inferior hypophyseal artery
Posterior cerebral artery
Pontine arteries
Superior cerebellar artery
Labyrinthine artery
Basilar artery
Anterior inferior cerebellar artery
Vertebral artery
Posterior inferior cerebellar artery
Anterior spinal artery

Fig. 2.27 The arterial circle of Willis and arteries of the brainstem. (Modified from Rollins JH, Long BW, Curtis T. *Merrill's Atlas of Radiographic Positioning & Procedures*, 15th ed. Mosby; 2023.)

- **Medial and lateral posterior choroidal arteries:** One medial and one or two lateral arteries on each side. These pass around the lateral geniculate body supplying branches to this, to reach the posterior part of the inferior horn of the lateral ventricle to supply (with the anterior choroidal artery) the choroid plexus of this ventricle.
- **Multiple cortical branches:** Some of the major branches include:
  - The **posterior temporal branch**, which supplies the inferior aspect of the posterior part of the temporal lobe.
  - The **medial occipital branch**, which passes to the medial aspect of the occipital lobe and divides terminally into **calcarine and parieto-occipital arteries**.

THE ARTERIAL CIRCLE OF WILLIS (SEE FIGS. 2.27, 2.30)

This anastomosis between right and left internal carotid arteries, their branches and the posterior cerebral arteries forms a circle that encloses the optic chiasm and the pituitary stalk in the suprasellar and interpeduncular cisterns. The arteries taking part can be identified in Figs. 2.27 and 2.30.

The circle of Willis is subject to many variations and is complete without absence or hypoplasia of any vessel in approximately 25% of people. The reported incidence of each variant depends on the methods used to identify the vessels of the circle of Willis. The most commonly variant vessel is the posterior communicating artery. The circle of Willis provides a potential route of collateral flow in cases of arterial occlusion or stenosis.

Commonest Variants of the Circle of Willis

The quoted prevalence in different studies vary widely and the provided examples are approximations.

- Hypoplastic posterior communicating artery (approximately 30%).
- Large posterior communicating artery associated with a reduction in size of the proximal part of the ipsilateral posterior cerebral artery so that the posterior cerebral artery effectively receives its supply from the middle cerebral artery (approximately 20%). Such an artery is called a 'fetal' posterior communicating artery.
- Hypoplastic proximal segment of the anterior cerebral artery (the precommunicating horizontal A1 segment) on one side, with both anterior cerebral vessels supplied from that of the other side (approximately 15%).
- Hypoplastic anterior communicating artery (approximately 5%).
- The anterior cerebral artery may be fused as a single trunk, an azygos anterior cerebral artery (approximately 1%).

RADIOLOGICAL FEATURES OF THE ARTERIAL SUPPLY OF THE CNS

Plain Radiographs

The arteries are not visible unless calcified. This occurs most commonly in the carotid siphon near the pituitary fossa as well as in the vertebrobasilar system.

Angiography of the Carotid and Vertebral System (see Figs. 2.28, 2.29)

This can be achieved via the aortic arch by a single femoral or radial artery injection. The internal (or common) carotid arteries are catheterized in turn and views of both vertebral arteries are usually possible via contrast injection into one vertebral artery, with retrograde filling of the other from the basilar artery. The left vertebral artery is catheterized first as the vertebral arteries are often unequal in size and the right vertebral artery is bigger in only 20% of cases. Variation

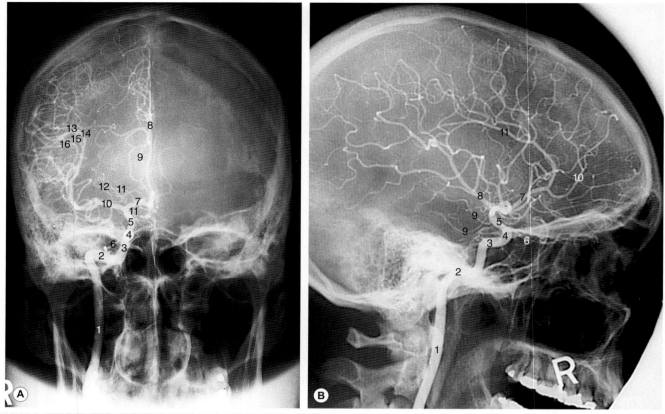

Fig. 2.28 Internal carotid angiogram. (A) Anteroposterior view. (B) Lateral view. The posterior communicating artery does not fill in this case.

(A)
1. Internal carotid artery in the neck
2. Petrous part of the internal carotid artery (carotid canal)
3. Cavernous part of the internal carotid artery
4. Carotid siphon
5. Intracranial part of the internal carotid artery
6. Ophthalmic artery
7. A1 segment of the anterior cerebral artery
8. Pericallosal artery
9. Callosomarginal artery
10. Middle cerebral artery
11. Anterior choroidal artery
12. Lenticulostriate arteries: medial and lateral
13. Sylvian point
14. Posterior parietal artery
15. Angular artery
16. Posterior temporal artery

(B)
1. Internal carotid artery in the neck
2. Internal carotid artery in the petrous bone
3. Internal carotid artery in the cavernous sinus
4. Carotid siphon
5. Intracranial part of the internal carotid artery
6. Ophthalmic artery
7. Anterior cerebral artery
8. Middle cerebral artery
9. Anterior choroidal branches
10. Callosomarginal artery
11. Pericallosal artery

also occurs in the origin of the vertebral artery, with the left vertebral artery arising directly from the arch of the aorta, between the origins of the left common carotid and left subclavian arteries in 5% of cases (see also aortic arch).

On the lateral view of the internal carotid angiogram (see Fig. 2.28B) the sharp angulation of the branches of the middle cerebral artery at the upper and lower borders of the insula approximately form a triangle, which is called the **sylvian triangle**.

The uppermost point of these vessels as seen on AP views is called the **sylvian point**. The sylvian vessels and the sylvian points should appear symmetrical on both sides.

The **arterial supplies of the right and left side of the brain** are connected at the anterior communicating artery and at the union of the vertebral arteries as the basilar artery. Competence of these communications is demonstrated angiographically by selectively injecting contrast into one carotid artery while maintaining steady pressure on that of the other side.

CT and MRI

CT angiography is the usual first modality of choice for evaluation of the intracranial arteries. Rapid volumetric acquisition allows for multiplanar reconstructions and interrogation of the vessels in all planes. This improves detection of aneurysms and other vascular malformations. It is an essential tool in the evaluation of acute stroke patients who may be candidates for endovascular thrombectomy. Reformatted images using maximum-intensity projections can help exaggerate stenoses within arteries.

The major arteries are visible as flow voids on T2 and T2 FLAIR (fluid-attenuated inversion recovery) MRI of the brain. More accurate assessment can be performed using dedicated MR angiographic techniques. Time of

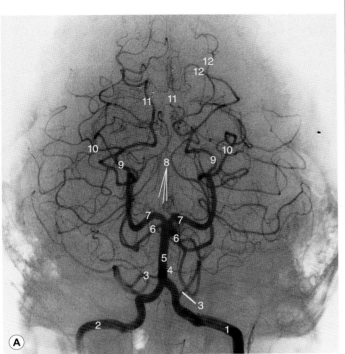

Fig. 2.29 Vertebral angiogram. (A) Anteroposterior view. (B) Lateral view.

(A)
1. Left vertebral artery
2. Right vertebral artery (reflux of contrast)
3. Posterior inferior cerebellar artery
4. Anterior inferior cerebellar artery
5. Basilar artery
6. Superior cerebellar artery
7. Posterior cerebral artery
8. Thalamoperforate branches
9. Internal occipital artery
10. Posterior temporal artery
11. Calcarine branch of the internal occipital artery
12. Parieto-occipital branch of the internal occipital artery

(B)
1. Vertebral artery
2. Posterior inferior cerebellar artery (PICA) – anterior medullary segment
3. Lateral medullary segment of PICA

4. Posterior medullary segment of PICA
5. Inferior tonsillar loop of PICA
6. Supratonsillar loop of PICA
7. Retrotonsillar segment of PICA
8. Vermis branch of PICA
9. Tonsillohemispheric branch of PICA
10. Hemispheric branch
11. Superior cerebellar artery
12. Posterior cerebral artery
13. Posterior communicating artery
14. Thalamoperforate branches of posterior cerebral artery
15. Medial posterior choroidal branches
16. Lateral posterior choroidal branches (arise distal to **15**)
17. Superior vermian branches of **11**
18. Internal occipital branch of **12**
19. Parieto-occipital artery
20. Calcarine artery

flight angiography allows for visualisation of flow within the arteries without the use of a contrast agent (see Fig. 2.30). Contrast-enhanced MR angiography can also be performed and has better spatial resolution and less associated artefact. It is the preferred technique for assessing the patency of intracranial vascular stents.

Ultrasound Examination of the Neonatal Brain (see Fig. 2.10)

On neonatal ultrasound of the brain the collagen sheaths of the vessels give them echogenicity, and on real-time studies pulsation of the middle cerebral vessels can be seen in the insula. The anterior cerebral artery can be seen in the inter-hemispheric fissure on coronal scanning and, on parasagittal scanning, the pericallosal and callosomarginal arteries may be identifiable. Doppler ultrasound can be used to demonstrate patency and flow within vessels.

Venous Drainage of the Brain (Figs. 2.31–2.34)

The veins draining the central nervous system do not follow the same courses as the arteries that supply it. Generally,

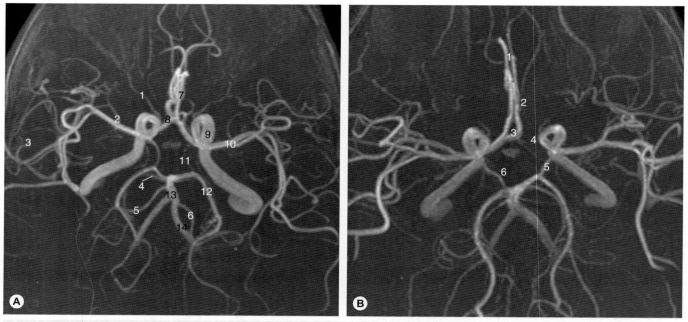

Fig. 2.30 Magnetic resonance angiogram (MRA) of the cerebral circulation. (A) MRA as viewed from above. (B) A variant on the circle of Willis on MRA. Note the absence of the first segment of the left anterior cerebral artery. The remainder of this artery is filled through the anterior communicating artery from the right side.

(A)
1. Ophthalmic artery
2. Anterior temporal artery
3. Opercular branches of MCA
4. Superior cerebellar artery
5. Anterior inferior cerebellar artery (AICA)
6. Posterior inferior cerebellar artery (PICA)
7. Left ACA
8. ACoA
9. Left ICA
10. Left MCA
11. Left PCoA (small)

12. Left PCA
13. BA
14. VA

(B)
1. Right ACA
2. Left ACA
3. ACoA
4. Absent horizontal segment of left ACA
5. Left PCoA
6. Right PCoA

venous blood drains to the nearest venous sinus, except in the case of that draining from the deepest structures, which drains to deep veins. These, in turn, drain to the venous sinuses. The intracerebral veins do not have valves.

Venous Sinuses (see Fig. 2.31)

These are large, low-pressure veins within the folds of dura – between fibrous dura and endosteum, except for the inferior sagittal and the straight sinuses which are between two layers of fibrous dura. The venous sinuses receive blood from the brain and the skull (diploic veins) and communicate with veins of the scalp and face (emissary veins).

The **superior sagittal sinus** starts anteriorly at the foramen caecum and runs posteriorly in the midline to the internal occipital protuberance. It is triangular in cross-section and increases in size from anterior to posterior. Veins enter the sinus obliquely against the flow of blood. Three or four venous lakes or lacunae project laterally from the sinus bilaterally between the dura and the endosteum. Into these the arachnoid (Pacchionian) granulations and villi project to return CSF to the blood. Posteriorly the sinus turns to one side – usually the right – to become the transverse sinus.

The **inferior sagittal sinus** runs in the lower free edge of the falx cerebri superior to the corpus callosum. It receives blood from deep and medial components of both cerebral hemispheres. Posteriorly it joins with the great cerebral veins to become the straight sinus. It is often quite small and poorly developed.

The **straight sinus** runs in the tentorium, where the falx is attached to it, to the internal occipital protuberance – the confluence of the sinuses (torcula Herophili). Here it turns to one side – usually the left – to become the transverse sinus.

The **transverse and sigmoid sinuses** – the transverse sinuses run right and left from the confluence of the sinuses to the mastoid bone, where they turn inferiorly and become the sigmoid sinus (the transverse and sigmoid sinuses are sometimes referred to together as the lateral sinus), which continues at the jugular foramen as the internal jugular vein. A focal dilatation of the vein within the foramen is called the jugular bulb.

The **cavernous sinus** (see Fig. 2.14) – this sinus is on either side of the pituitary gland and the body of the sphenoid bone connected across the midline by intercavernous sinuses. It lies between layers of dura mater. The internal

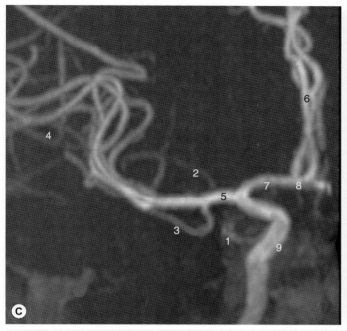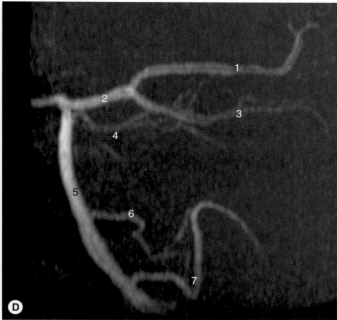

Fig. 2.30, cont'd (C) MRA of the right internal carotid and middle cerebral artery and anterior cerebral artery. (D) MRA of posterior circulation, lateral view. *ACA,* Anterior cerebral artery; *ACoA,* anterior communicating artery; *BA,* basilar artery; *ICA,* internal carotid artery; *MCA,* middle cerebral artery; *PCoA,* posterior communicating artery; *PCA,* posterior cerebral artery; *VA,* vertebral artery.

(C)
1. Ophthalmic artery
2. Lenticulostriate artery
3. Anterior temporal artery
4. Opercular branches of MCA
5. MCA
6. Vertical segment of ACA
7. Horizontal segment of ACA
8. ACoA
9. Right ICA

(D)
1. Parieto-occipital artery
2. Posterior cerebral artery
3. Calcarine artery
4. Superior cerebellar artery
5. Basilar artery
6. Anterior inferior cerebellar artery – AICA confluence of vertebral arteries
7. Posterior inferior cerebellar artery – PICA

carotid artery passes through this sinus with the VI CN lateral and inferior to it. The III and IV CNs and the ophthalmic and maxillary divisions of the fifth cranial nerve pass along the lateral wall of the cavernous sinus. The maxillary division of the fifth cranial nerve lies in or in close proximity to the inferolateral cavernous sinus. After emerging from the sinus, the carotid artery folds back on itself so that it comes to lie on the roof of the sinus. Above the sinus lies the optic tract. The cavernous sinus receives the ophthalmic veins and superficial cortical veins, the sphenoid sinus and the superficial middle cerebral vein, and drains via the petrosal sinuses to the sigmoid sinus and ultimately the internal jugular vein.

The **superior petrosal sinus** runs from the cavernous to the sigmoid sinus in the attached margin of the tentorium on the superior border of the petrous part of the temporal bone.

The **inferior petrosal sinus** runs from the cavernous sinus to the internal jugular vein at the base of the petrous temporal bone. It is usually larger than the superior petrosal sinus and leaves the cavernous sinus under the petroclinoid ligament.

The **sphenoparietal sinus** runs along the free edge of the lesser wing of the sphenoid bone to the cavernous sinus. It may drain the anterior temporal diploic vein, a large vein in the wall of the middle cranial fossa, or the latter may drain separately to the cavernous sinus.

SUPERFICIAL CEREBRAL VEINS (SEE FIG. 2.31)

These veins include superior, middle and inferior cerebral veins and are very variable. They drain to the nearest dural sinus – thus the superolateral surface of the hemisphere drains to the superior sagittal sinus and the posteroinferior aspect drains to the transverse sinus. These named veins are variably seen:
- **The superior anastomotic vein (of Trolard)** overlies the lateral frontoparietal region. It connects the superior sagittal sinus and the superficial middle cerebral vein (of Sylvius). It runs in or adjacent to the postcentral sulcus.
- **The inferior anastomotic vein (of Labbé)** runs from the Sylvian fissure over the temporal lobe to the transverse sinus, connecting the superficial middle cerebral vein to the transverse sinus.
- **The superficial middle cerebral vein (of Sylvius)**, which runs anteriorly along the lateral sulcus to drain to the cavernous sinus or sphenoparietal sinus. It frequently anastomosis to other superficial cerebral veins as described.

DEEP CEREBRAL VEINS (SEE FIG. 2.32)

Several veins unite just behind the interventricular foramen (of Monro) to form the internal cerebral vein. The largest are:

- **The choroidal vein**, which runs from the choroid plexus of the lateral ventricle.
- **The septal vein**, which runs from the region of the septum pellucidum in the anterior horn of the lateral ventricle.
- **The thalamostriate vein**, which runs anteriorly in the floor of the lateral ventricle in the thalamostriate groove between the thalamus and caudate nucleus.

The septal veins of the septum pellucidum usually drain into the thalamostriate vein; however they can join the confluence directly.

The point of union of these veins is called the **venous angle**, which marks the posterior margin of the interventricular foramen.

The **internal cerebral veins** of each side run posteriorly in the roof of the third ventricle and unite with the basal veins of Rosenthal beneath the splenium of the corpus callosum to form the great cerebral vein.

The **great cerebral vein (of Galen)** is a single short (1–2 cm), thick vein that passes posterosuperiorly behind the splenium of the corpus callosum in the quadrigeminal cistern. It receives the basal veins and posterior fossa veins and drains to the anterior end of the straight sinus where this unites with the inferior sagittal sinus.

The **basal vein (of Rosenthal)** begins at the anterior perforated substance by the union of three veins:

- The anterior cerebral vein, which accompanies the anterior cerebral artery
- The deep middle cerebral vein from the insula
- The striate veins from the inferior part of the basal ganglia via the anterior perforated substance

The basal vein of each side passes around the midbrain to unite with the internal cerebral veins forming the great cerebral vein.

VEINS OF THE POSTERIOR FOSSA (SEE FIG. 2.32)

The **anterior pontomesencephalic vein** runs on the anterior surface of the pons and midbrain in relation to the basilar artery. Inferiorly it drains via the petrosal veins to the superior petrosal sinuses. Superiorly this vein is connected to the posterior mesencephalic vein.

The **posterior mesencephalic vein** runs around the upper midbrain to drain into the great cerebral vein.

The **precentral cerebellar vein** arises between the cerebellum and the posterior midbrain in the midline and passes superiorly to drain to the great cerebral vein.

The **superior vermian vein** drains also to the great vein, and the **inferior vermian veins** (paired) drain to the straight sinus.

The **pontine veins** drain laterally to the petrosal sinuses. A midline pontine vein may exist which drains to the basal veins.

Inferior medullary veins drain to the sphenoid or petrosal sinuses.

RADIOLOGICAL FEATURES OF THE CEREBRAL VEINS AND VENOUS SINUSES

Skull Radiographs

The course of the venous sinuses can be seen where they groove the inner plate of bone. The arachnoid granulations may also indent the skull and show as lucencies on each side of the superior sagittal sinus on the skull radiograph (see section on the radiology of the skull, p. 62).

CT Venography

CT venography is the most sensitive noninvasive study for the evaluation of the dural venous sinuses, superficial cerebral veins and deep cerebral veins. The veins demonstrate homogenous enhancement. Filling defects may represent arachnoid granulations or venous sinus thrombosis.

MR Venography (see Fig. 2.33)

MR venography is an additional noninvasive method of evaluating the cerebral veins and the venous sinuses. A nonenhanced time of flight sequence can be performed to demonstrate flow within the veins. This sequence is prone to artefact related to slow flow or flow in a vessel parallel to the scan plane which can become desaturated.

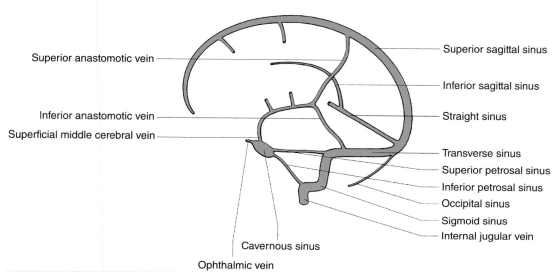

Fig. 2.31 Superficial cerebral veins and venous sinuses.

Superior anastomotic vein

Inferior anastomotic vein

Superficial middle cerebral vein

Cavernous sinus

Ophthalmic vein

Superior sagittal sinus

Inferior sagittal sinus

Straight sinus

Transverse sinus

Superior petrosal sinus

Inferior petrosal sinus

Occipital sinus

Sigmoid sinus

Internal jugular vein

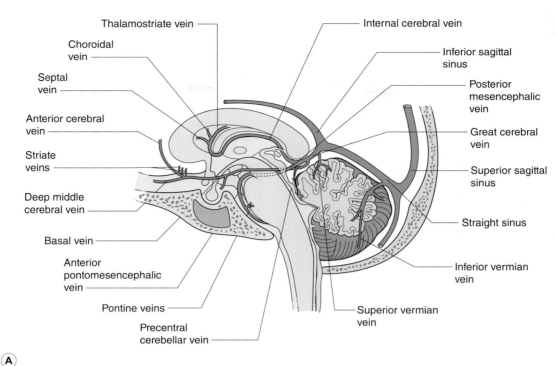

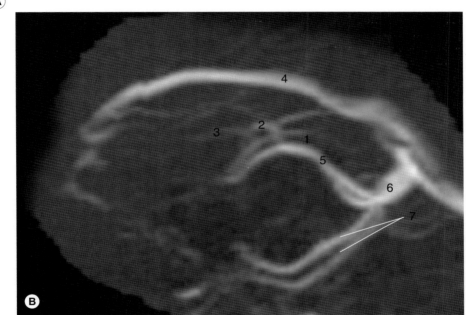

Fig. 2.32 Deep cerebral veins. (A) Diagram. (B) Deep veins on magnetic resonance venogram.

(B)
1. Thalamostriate vein
2. Choroidal vein
3. Septal vein

4. Inferior sagittal sinus
5. Internal cerebral veins
6. Great cerebral vein
7. Basal veins

A two-dimensional time of flight technique is used, which is most sensitive to flow perpendicular to the imaging slice. Coronal scans are thus most useful for evaluation of the sagittal sinuses and the internal cerebral veins but are limited for evaluation of the vertical posterior part of the superior sagittal sinuses and the sigmoid and petrous sinuses. A contrast-enhanced MR venogram can be performed to negate this artefact and has the added benefit of potentially assessing for signs for venous ischaemia with the draining territories.

Angiography During the Venous Phase (see Fig. 2.34)

Superficial veins are seen to fill before deep veins and frontal veins before posterior veins. Of the superficial veins, the superior or inferior anastomotic vein is often visualised, but

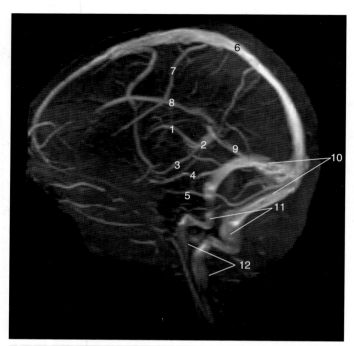

Fig. 2.33 Magnetic resonance venogram.

1. Internal cerebral vein
2. Great cerebral vein
3. Basal vein
4. Superior petrosal sinus
5. Inferior anastomotic vein
6. Superior sagittal sinus
7. Superior anastomotic vein
8. Inferior sagittal sinus
9. Straight sinus
10. Transverse sinus
11. Sigmoid sinus
12. Internal jugular vein

both are seldom seen on one angiogram. The deep veins are more constant than the superficial veins.

CT and MRI (see Fig. 2.3)

The tentorium and falx are seen as relatively hyperdense structures owing to the venous sinuses that they enclose. Venous sinuses may also be seen at the internal occipital protuberance. A high division of the superior sagittal sinus may occur as an unusual normal variant and should not be mistaken for sinus thrombosis. On axial imaging, at the level of the midbrain the posterior mesencephalic vein may be seen winding around the upper midbrain. In higher slices, the posterior end of the internal cerebral veins and the great cerebral vein may be seen in the quadrigeminal cistern.

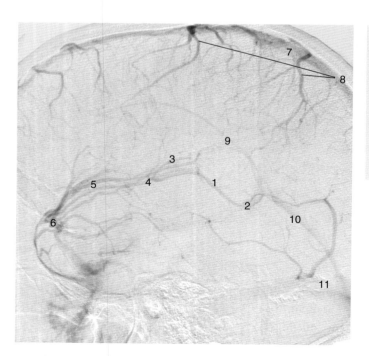

Fig. 2.34 Venous phase of an internal carotid angiogram.

1. Internal cerebral vein
2. Great cerebral vein
3. Thalamostriate vein
4. Venous angle
5. Superficial middle cerebral vein
6. Cavernous sinus
7. Superior sagittal sinus
8. Superficial cortical veins
9. Inferior sagittal sinus
10. Straight sinus transverse sinus
11. Sigmoid sinus

3 The Spinal Column and Its Contents

TERENCE FARRELL and JOHN HYNES
EDITED BY STEPHEN EUSTACE and STEPHANIE RYAN

CHAPTER CONTENTS

The Vertebral Column 101
Joints of the Vertebral Column 109
Ligaments of the Vertebral Column 111
The Intervertebral Discs 113
Blood Supply of the Vertebral Column 114

The Spinal Cord 114
The Spinal Meninges 118
Blood Supply of the Spinal Cord 118

The Vertebral Column

The vertebral column has 33 vertebrae – 7 cervical, 12 thoracic, 5 lumbar, 5 sacral (fused) and 4 coccygeal (fused) vertebrae.

The spine of the fetus is flexed in a smooth C shape. This is referred to as the 'primary curvature' and is retained in the adult in the thoracic and sacrococcygeal areas. Secondary extension results in lordosis – known as the 'secondary curvature' – of the cervical and lumbar spine.

A TYPICAL VERTEBRA

A typical vertebra has a vertebral body anteriorly and a neural arch posteriorly. The neural arch consists of pedicles laterally and laminae posteriorly.

The pedicles are notched superiorly and inferiorly so that adjoining pedicles are separated by an intervertebral foramen, which transmits the segmental nerves. There are 31 segmental spinal nerves – 8 cervical, 12 thoracic, 5 lumbar, 5 sacral and 1 coccygeal. The first seven cervical nerves emerge above the correspondingly named vertebra; the eighth cervical nerve emerges below C7 and the others emerge below the correspondingly named vertebra.

A transverse process arises at the junction of the pedicle and the lamina and extends laterally on each side. The laminae fuse posteriorly as the spinous process.

Articular processes project superiorly and inferiorly from each lamina. Articular facets on these processes face posteriorly on the superior facet and anteriorly on the inferior facet. The part of the lamina between the superior and inferior articular facets on each side is called the pars interarticularis.

THE CERVICAL VERTEBRAE

Typical Cervical Vertebra (Fig. 3.1)

The most distinctive feature is the presence of the foramen transversarium in the transverse process. This transmits the vertebral artery (except C7) and its accompanying veins and sympathetic nerves. The transverse processes have anterior and posterior tubercles. Small lips are seen on the posterolateral side of the superior surface of the C3–C7 vertebral bodies, the **uncinate processes**, with corresponding bevels on the inferior surface. Small joints, called **neurocentral joints (of Luschka)** or uncovertebral joints, are formed between adjacent cervical vertebral bodies at these sites. These are not true synovial joints although they are often called so, but are due to degenerative changes in the disc.

The cervical vertebral canal is triangular in cross-section. The spinous processes are small and bifid, whereas the articular facets are relatively horizontal.

The Atlas – C1 (Fig. 3.2)

The atlas has no body as it is fused with that of the axis to become the odontoid process. A lateral mass on each side has a superior articular facet for articulation, with the occipital condyles in the atlanto-occipital joint, also an inferior articular facet for articulation with the axis in the atlantoaxial joint.

The anterior arch of the atlas has a tubercle on its anterior surface and a facet posteriorly for articulation with the odontoid process.

The posterior arch is grooved behind the lateral mass by the vertebral artery as it ascends into the foramen magnum.

The Axis – C2 (Fig. 3.3)

The odontoid process, which represents the body of the atlas, bears no weight. Like the atlas, the axis has a large lateral mass on each side that transmits the weight of the skull to the vertebral bodies of the remainder of the spinal cord. Sloping articular facets on each side of the dens are for articulation in the atlantoaxial joint.

Vertebra Prominens – C7

This name is derived from its long, easily felt, nonbifid spine. Its foramen transversarium is small or absent and usually transmits only vertebral veins. The anterior tubercle of the transverse process is smaller than other cervical vertebrae.

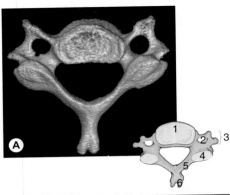

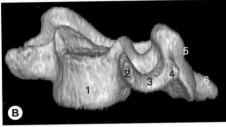

Fig. 3.1 Cervical vertebra. (A) Three-dimensional computed tomography (CT) scan of a cervical vertebra viewed from above. (B) Three-dimensional CT scan of a cervical vertebra anterolateral view.

(A)
1. Body
2. Foramen transversarium
3. Transverse process with anterior and posterior tubercles
4. Superior articular facet
5. Lamina
6. Bifid spinous process

(B)
1. Body
2. Anterior tubercle
3. Transverse process
4. Posterior tubercle
5. Lamina
6. Spinous process

THE THORACIC VERTEBRAE (FIG. 3.4)

These have articular facets on the lateral aspects of the vertebral bodies for articulation with the ribs. A demi-facet is found on the upper and lower aspect on each side on T2–T10 vertebrae. T1 has a complete facet superiorly and a demi-facet inferiorly, whereas a single complete facet is seen at midlevel on T11 and T12. Articular facets are also found on the anterior surface of the transverse processes for the costotransverse articulations.

The spinous processes of the thoracic vertebrae are long and slope downwards. The facets on the articular processes are relatively vertical.

THE LUMBAR VERTEBRAE (FIG. 3.5)

These have larger vertebral bodies and strong, square, horizontal spinous processes. The articular facets face each other in a sagittal plane. A prominence on the posterior aspect of each superior articular process is the mamillary process.

The transverse processes of the upper four lumbar vertebrae are spatulate and increase in size from above downwards. The transverse process of the fifth lumbar vertebra is shorter but strong and pyramidal and, in contrast to those of the other vertebrae, does not arise from the junction of the pedicle and lamina but from the lateral aspect of the pedicle and the vertebral body itself (see Fig. 3.5C).

THE SACRUM (FIG. 3.6)

This is composed of five fused vertebrae. It is triangular in shape and concave anteriorly. A central mass is formed on the pelvic surface by the fused vertebral bodies. The superior border of the central mass is the most anterior part of the sacrum and is called the sacral promontory. Four anterior sacral foramina on each side transmit the sacral anterior primary rami. Lateral to these is the lateral mass of the sacrum, the upper anterior surface of which is called the ala of the sacrum.

On the posterior surface the laminae are also seen to be fused. The fusion of the spinous processes forms a median sacral crest. A sacral hiatus of variable extent inferiorly is caused by nonfusion of the laminae of S5 and often S4 in the midline. The transverse processes are rudimentary. Four posterior sacral foramina transmit the posterior primary rami. The sacral hiatus transmits the fifth sacral nerve.

Laterally there is a large articular facet, called the auricular surface, for articulation with the pelvis in the sacroiliac (SI) joint. Differences in the sacrum between males and females include:
- The width of the body of the first sacral vertebra is less than that of the ala in the female and wider in the male.
- The articular surface of the SI joint occupies two vertebrae in the female and two-and-a-half vertebrae in the male.
- The anterior surface of the female sacrum is flat superiorly and curves forward inferiorly, whereas that of the male is uniformly concave.

THE COCCYX

This comprises four vertebrae that are fused into a triangular bone which forms part of the floor of the pelvis.

RADIOLOGICAL FEATURES OF THE VERTEBRAE

Radiographs of the Vertebral Column (Figs. 3.7–3.9)

The component parts of the vertebrae – the body, pedicles, laminae and the transverse, articular and spinous processes – can be seen. Oblique views, particularly of the lumbar spine, are used for better visualization of the neural foramina and the pars interarticularis.

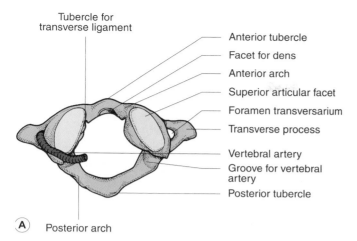

Tubercle for
transverse ligament

Anterior tubercle
Facet for dens
Anterior arch
Superior articular facet
Foramen transversarium
Transverse process
Vertebral artery
Groove for vertebral artery
Posterior tubercle

(A)   Posterior arch

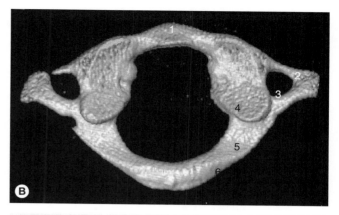

(B)

Fig. 3.2 The atlas. (A) Diagram of superior view. (B) Three-dimensional computed tomography (CT) scan of the atlas viewed from above. (C) T2 magnetic resonance image through lateral masses of the atlas showing the course of the upper part of the vertebral arteries.

(B)
1. Anterior tubercle
2. Transverse process
3. Foramen transversarium
4. Superior articular facet
5. Groove for vertebral artery
6. Posterior arch
7. Posterior tubercle

(C)
1. Dens
2. Lateral mass of atlas
3. Vertebral artery
4. Spinal cord

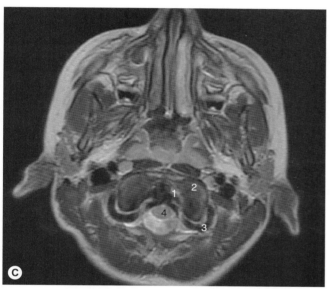

(C)

The point of exit of the basivertebral veins can be seen on lateral views as a defect in the cortex of the posterior surface of the vertebral body.

The anteroposterior (AP) **width of the spinal canal** is measured on a lateral film from the posterior cortex of the vertebral body to the base of the spinous process. The lower limit of normal is taken as 13 mm in the cervical spine at C5 level and 15 mm in the lumbar spine at L2.

The width of the spinal canal is measured as the **interpedicular distance** on AP [CT] (and more easily on coronal computed tomography (CT) reconstruction) and reflects the width of the spinal cord. It is maximum in the cervical spine at C5/C6 and in the thoracic spine at T12, as these are the sites of expansion of the cord for the limb plexuses. The interpedicular distance increases from L1 to L5.

Transitional vertebrae with features intermediate between the two types of typical vertebrae are developmental anomalies. These occur at the atlanto-occipital junction,

where the atlas may be assimilated into the occipital bone or where an extra bone may occur – known as the occipital vertebra. Transitional vertebrae may be found at the cervicothoracic junction at the level of C7; these may have long, pointed transverse processes with or without true rib (cervical rib) formation. Similarly, at the thoracolumbar junction vestigial ribs may be seen on T12 or L1 vertebrae. At the lumbosacral junction, the last lumbar vertebra may be partly or completely fused with the sacrum – known as sacralization – or the first sacral segment may be separated from the remainder of the sacrum – known as lumbarization.

RADIOLOGY PEARL

The possibility of transitional vertebrae must be borne in mind when numbering vertebrae, especially prior to a surgical procedure.

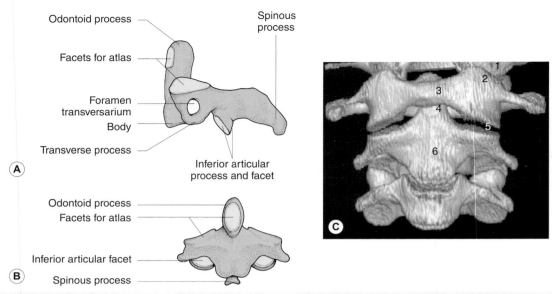

Fig. 3.3 The axis. (A) Lateral view. (B) Anterior view. (C) Anterior view of three-dimensional computed tomography scan of the upper cervical vertebrae.

(C)
1. Occipital condyle
2. Atlas
3. Anterior arch of atlas
4. Dens
5. Atlantoaxial joint
6. Body of axis

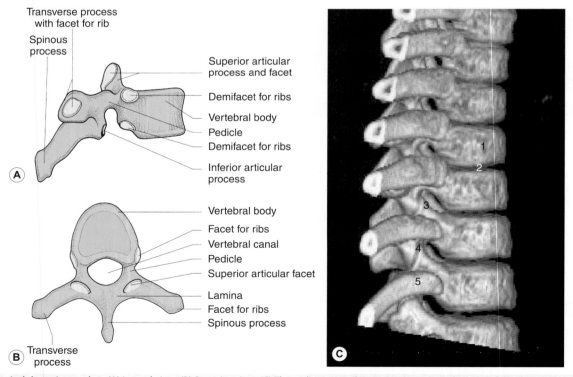

Fig. 3.4 Typical thoracic vertebra. (A) Lateral view. (B) Superior view. (C) Three-dimensional computed tomography scan of the thoracic vertebrae and ribs, lateral view.

(C)
1. Vertebral body
2. Intervertebral disc
3. Pedicle
4. Facet joint
5. Rib

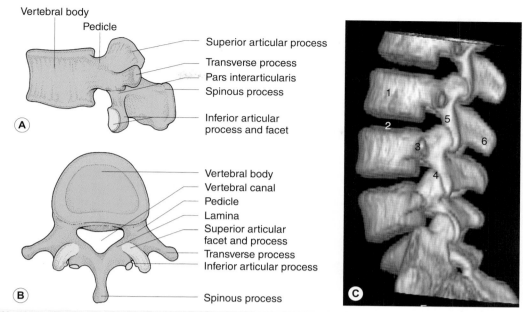

Vertebral body
Pedicle
Superior articular process
Transverse process
Pars interarticularis
Spinous process
Inferior articular process and facet

(A)

Vertebral body
Vertebral canal
Pedicle
Lamina
Superior articular facet and process
Transverse process
Inferior articular process
Spinous process

(B)

(C)

Fig. 3.5 Typical lumbar vertebra. (A) Lateral view. (B) Superior view. (C) Three-dimensional computed tomography scan of the lumbosacral spine.

(C)
1. Vertebral body
2. Intervertebral disc
3. Transverse process
4. Facet joint
5. Pars interarticularis
6. Spinous process

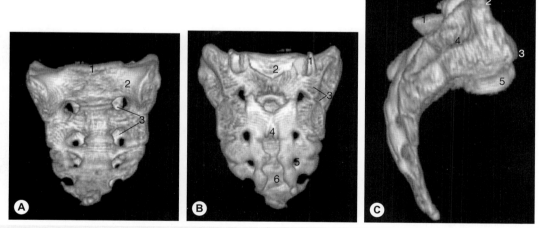

(A)　(B)　(C)

Fig. 3.6 The sacrum, three-dimensional computed tomography scan. (A) Pelvic surface. (B) Dorsal surface. (C) Lateral view of the sacrum showing the sacroiliac joint surface.

(A)
1. Sacral promontory
2. Ala
3. Pelvic sacral foramina
5. Dorsal sacral foramen
6. Lower end of sacral canal

(B)
1. Superior articular process
2. Upper end of sacral canal
3. Depressions for sacroiliac ligament
4. Spinous tubercle

(C)
1. Spinous tubercle
2. Superior articular facet
3. Sacral promontory
4. Depressions for sacroiliac ligament
5. Auricular surface

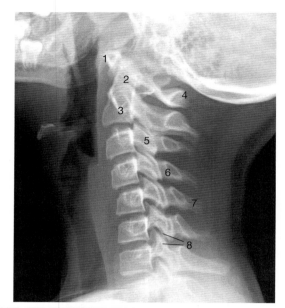

Fig. 3.7 Lateral radiograph of the cervical spine.
1. Anterior arch of atlas
2. Dens
3. Body of axis
4. Posterior arch of atlas
5. Pedicle
6. Lamina
7. Spinous process
8. Articular facets

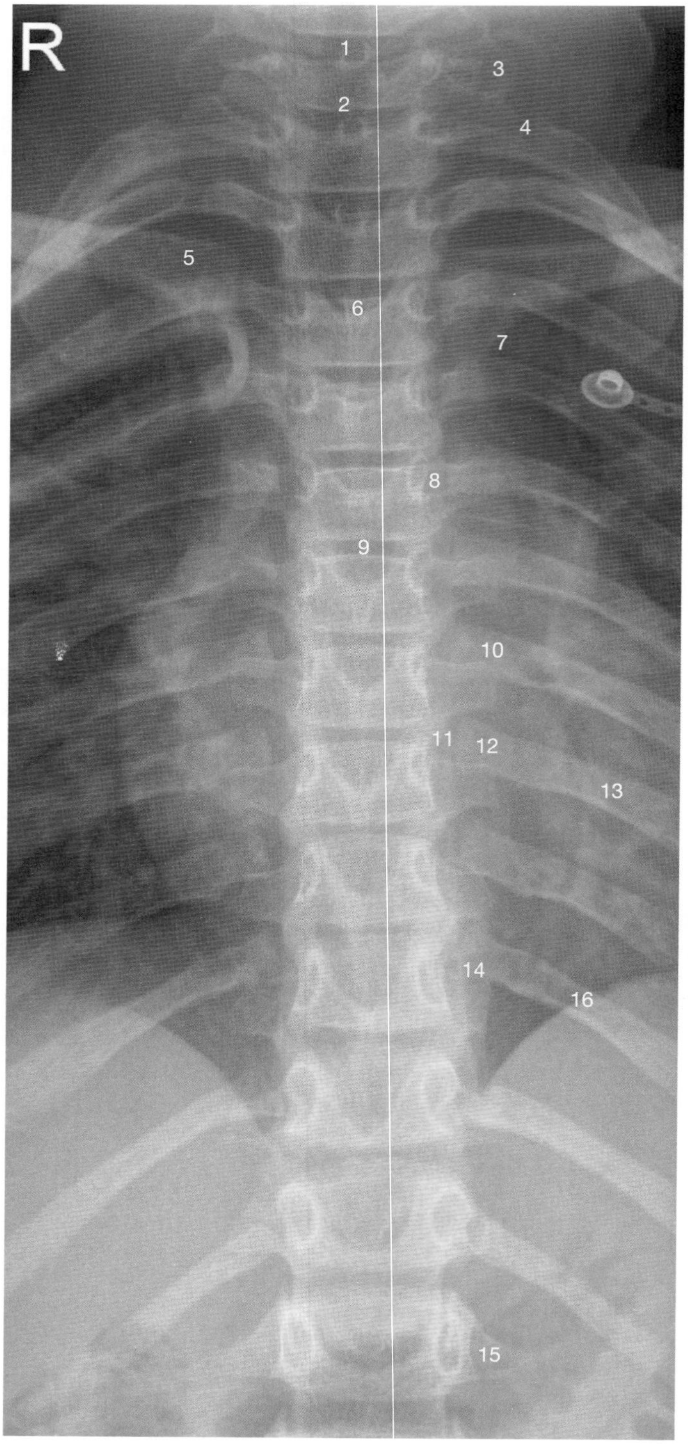

Fig. 3.8 Anteroposterior radiograph of the thoracic spine.
1. Trachea
2. Spinous process of C7
3. Left transverse process of C7
4. Tubercle of first rib, articulating with transverse process of T1
5. Medial end of clavicle
6. Superior margin of manubrium sterni
7. Lateral margin of manubrium sterni
8. Left pedicle of T5
9. T5/T6 intervertebral disc space
10. Tubercle of seventh rib, articulating with transverse process of T7
11. Head of eighth rib
12. Neck of eighth rib
13. Shaft of eighth rib
14. Left paraspinal line
15. Left transverse process of L1
16. Dome of left hemidiaphragm

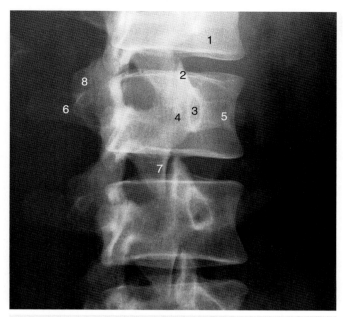

Fig. 3.9 Oblique radiograph of the lumbar spine.
1. Vertebral body of L2
2. Superior articular process of L3
3. Pedicle of L3
4. Pars interarticularis
5. Transverse process of L3
6. Transverse process of L3
7. Inferior articular process of L3
8. Spinous process of L2

Radiographs of the Cervical Spine

The alignment of the cervical spine with respect to the foramen magnum can be assessed radiographically. The following lines have been described:

- **Chamberlain's line** (on a lateral view): from the posterior tip of the hard palate to the posterior lip of the foramen magnum. Less than 2 mm of odontoid is normally above this.
- **McGregor's line** (on a lateral view): from the posterior tip of the hard palate to the base of the occiput (often easier to identify than the lip of the foramen magnum). Less than 5 mm of odontoid should lie above this.
- **Digastric line** (on an occipitofrontal [OF] view of the skull): the atlanto-occipital joints should be below a line between the digastric notches of both mastoid processes.

In basilar invagination (a congenital developmental anomaly where the cervical spine is displaced upward into the foramen magnum) these relationships are abnormal.

RADIOLOGY PEARL

Cervical ribs are distinguished from thoracic ribs by the orientation of the transverse process. Cervical transverse processes are orientated inferiorly, thoracic transverse processes point upwards.

Radiographs of the Thoracic Spine (see Fig. 3.8)

In AP views of the thoracic spine **paraspinal lines** are seen between the paravertebral soft-tissue shadows and the air in the lungs. Only lymph nodes, intercostal vessels, sympathetic nerves and fat normally lie between the vertebrae and pleura, so that displacement of the paraspinal lines on a radiograph is a marker of pathology in these structures or in the vertebrae (see also mediastinal lines).

Radiographs of the Lumbar Spine

Anterior wedging of the L5 vertebra is a normal finding on lateral radiographs, as is narrowing of the L5/S1s disc space, and should not be taken as a sign of disease.

Oblique views of the lumbar spine (see Fig. 3.9) are used to visualize the intervertebral foramina and the pars interarticularis.

Computed Tomography (see Figs. 3.1–3.6, 3.10)

The vertebral body anteriorly and the pedicles, laminae and spinous process posteriorly are seen as a bony ring around the spinal canal. Transverse processes are seen lateral to this, and because they are not truly horizontal they appear separate from the remainder of the vertebra on many images.

Where the CT slice passes through the intervertebral foramen, it is seen as a gap between the body and the posterior vertebral elements. The intervertebral foramen, being oval in shape, appears narrower in cuts through its upper and lower ends.

The dimensions of the spinal canal can be measured directly. Lower limits of normal for the midsagittal distance are taken as 12–15 mm and 20 mm for the interpedicular distance. Other factors in spinal stenosis can also be determined, for example the soft-tissue elements such as the ligamenta flava, the thickness of the lamina (14 mm is the upper limit of normal) and the development of bony spurs at the disc margins and at the facet joints.

Compact bone and cancellous bone components of the vertebrae can easily be distinguished on CT. In order to maintain the axial load imposed by weight bearing, the vertebral body is composed of both a thick outer cortical shell of compact bone and an inner supporting network of vertically orientated trabeculae or cancellous bone. The posterior element of the vertebral body has less of a role in weight bearing and functions primarily to stabilize and prevent subluxation. It is composed of compact cortical bone alone.

RADIOLOGY PEARL

In adulthood up to 50% of the vertebral body is cancellous bone, whereas in the femoral neck the cancellous bone constitutes only 30% by volume. This explains why changes of osteoporosis occur earlier in the vertebral body than in the femoral neck, and explains why screening for osteoporosis is aimed primarily at the vertebral body.

Magnetic Resonance Imaging (Fig. 3.11)

Magnetic resonance imaging (MRI) is widely used to visualize the spinal column and its contents. T1- and T2-weighted

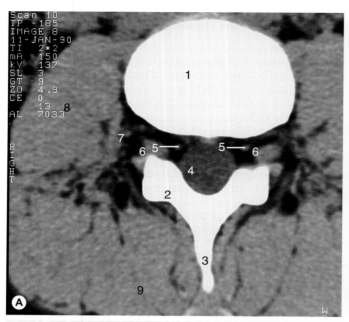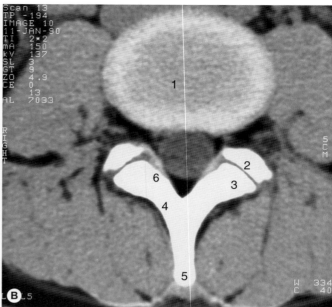

Fig. 3.10 Computed tomography scan through (A) L4 vertebral body and (B) L4/L5 intervertebral disc space.

(A)
1. Body of L4
2. Right lamina of L4
3. Spinous process of L4
4. Thecal sac containing cauda equina
5. Epidural veins
6. Dorsal root ganglia of L4 nerve
7. Intervertebral foramen of L4/L5
8. Psoas muscles
9. Erector spinae muscles

(B)
1. Disc of L4/L5
2. Inferior articular process of L4
3. Superior articular process of L5
4. Right lamina of L5
5. Spinous process of L5
6. Ligamentum flavum

images give information about the morphology and integrity of discs and vertebrae, the intervertebral foramina and facet joints, and an outline of the spinal cord. The vertebrae have a low-signal outer rim surrounding the high-signal cancellous bone. The signal intensity derived from the vertebral body in the spine is dependent on the quantity of yellow marrow relative to haemopoietic red marrow. In adulthood, yellow marrow predominates and results in signal hyperintensity throughout the vertebral body on both T1 and fast-spin echo T2 images. The presence of small quantities of red marrow produces some signal heterogeneity and signal suppression.

Focal fatty deposits frequently appear within the vertebral body during ageing and show signal characteristics of epidural fat. T2 fat-suppressed or STIR sequences can null the signal due to fat in the marrow and help distinguish the high signal due to normal fatty marrow deposits from the high signal due to inflammatory or other pathology.

The basivertebral venous trunk is well seen on MRI in midsagittal sections and can be identified as a horizontal band along the posterior margin of the vertebral body midway between the superior and inferior endplates.

OSSIFICATION OF THE VERTEBRAE (FIG. 3.12)

Typical vertebrae have three primary ossification centres: the body and on each side of the neural arch. These appear in the eighth fetal week. Secondary centres appear for the upper and lower parts of the body, for each transverse process and for the spinous process at 16 years, and fuse by the 25th year. Posterior neural arch fusion starts in the lumbar region at 1–2 years and proceeds cephalad to the cervical region up to 7 years of age. Fusion in the sacral region occurs last. Neural arch to the centrum fusion starts in the cervical region at 3 years and proceeds caudad to the lumbar region by 6 years. Fusion in the sacral region again occurs last.

The **atlas** has only three primary ossification centres, one for the anterior arch and one each for each lateral mass. These unite at 6 years of age. Failure to fuse posteriorly results in a **posterior spina bifida**. Occasionally there are two centres for the anterior arch that fuse at 8 years of age. Failure of fusion of these centres causes an **anterior spina bifida**.

The **axis** has two extra centres – those for the odontoid process, at its base and at its tip.

RADIOLOGY PEARL

The odontoid process in adulthood may remain separated from the axis by a cartilaginous disc and simulate an ununited fracture.

The **seventh cervical vertebra** also has two extra centres, for the attachment of costal processes on each side.

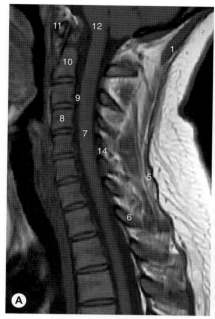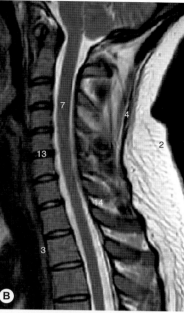

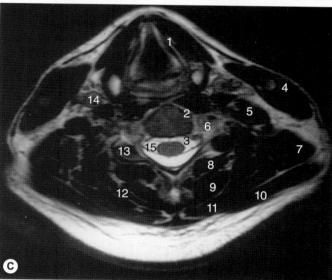

Fig. 3.11 Magnetic resonance image of the cervical spine. (A) Midline sagittal T1-weighted and (B) fat-suppressed inversion recovery images. (C) Axial T2-weighted image in the midcervical spine at the level of the true vocal cords or fourth cervical vertebral body.

1. Obliquus capitis superior
2. Rectus capitis posterior minor
3. Semispinalis capitis muscle
4. Ligamentum nuchae
5. Interspinous ligament
6. Spinous process of C7
7. Spinal cord
8. C4 vertebral body
9. Posterior longitudinal ligament
10. Odontoid peg
11. Anterior arch of C1
12. Medulla oblongata
13. Vertebral body haemangioma
14. Ligamentum flavum
15. Basivertebral vein
16. Anterior longitudinal ligament

(C)
1. Thyroid cartilage and vocal cords
2. Vertebral body and longus colli muscles
3. Ventral nerve root
4. Sternocleidomastoid muscle
5. Scalenus medius
6. Vertebral artery in the foramen transversarium
7. Levator scapulae
8. Semispinalis cervicis
9. Semispinalis capitis
10. Trapezius
11. Splenius capitis
12. Splenius capitis
13. Facet joint
14. Carotid sheath
15. Posterior nerve root

Lumbar vertebrae have extra primary centres for the mamillary processes on each side. In the lumbosacral spine, defects in ossification of the neural arch give rise to a **spina bifida defect** in 5%–10% of the population.

> **RADIOLOGY PEARL**
>
> **Persistent epiphyses in the transverse process** of the lumbar vertebrae are common and should not be mistaken for a fracture line.

Joints of the Vertebral Column

Although the movement between individual vertebrae is small, the additive effect of this is great, allowing significant movement of the vertebral column. Maximum movement is at the atlanto-occipital and atlantoaxial joints, and at the cervicothoracic and thoracolumbar junctions.

The joints between the vertebral bodies at the **intervertebral discs** are secondary cartilaginous joints. The surface of the vertebral bodies in contact with the disc is coated with hyaline cartilage.

Small joints between vertebral bodies, called **neurocentral joints**, occur in the cervical spine as already described.

Facet joints occur between the articular processes of the neural arches of the vertebrae. These are synovial joints with a simple capsule attached just beyond the margins of the articular surface. The capsules are looser in the cervical spine than in the thoracic or lumbar spine.

The **atlanto-occipital joint**, between the occipital condyle on each side of the foramen magnum and the superior articular surface of the atlas, is a synovial joint. A fibrous

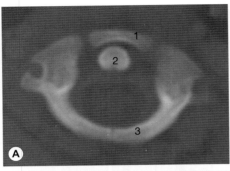

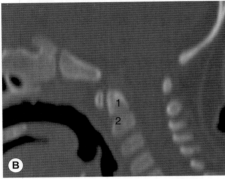

Fig. 3.12 Ossification of the cervical spine, computed tomography (CT) scan of a 2-year-old boy. (A) Axial image through C1 and C2. (B) Midline sagittal CT reconstruction of the cervical spine.

(A)
1. Ossification centre for anterior arch of atlas
2. Dens
3. Ossification for left lateral mass

(B)
1. Ossification centre for odontoid
2. Ossification centre for body of axis

capsule surrounds the synovial membrane and is thickened posteriorly and laterally. In addition, the joint is strengthened by the anterior atlanto-occipital membrane (from the anterior margin of the foramen magnum to the anterior arch of the atlas) and by the posterior atlanto-occipital membrane (from the posterior margin of the foramen magnum to the posterior arch of the atlas). These joints act as a single joint and allow flexion and extension (nodding of the head) and some lateral motion.

Three joints make up the **atlantoaxial joint**:

■ A small synovial joint between the anterior surface of the dens and the posterior aspect of the anterior arch of the atlas.
■ A synovial joint between each of the two lateral masses of the atlas and of the axis.

These joints are strengthened by:

■ The **membrana tectoria**, which is an upward continuation of the posterior longitudinal ligament from the axis to the anterior margin of the foramen magnum.
■ The **cruciform ligament**, which has a transverse band attached to the atlas and a vertical band anterior to the membrana tectoria from the posterior aspect of the body of the axis to the margin of the foramen magnum.
■ The **apical and alar ligament**s, which join the tip of the dens to the margin of the foramen magnum.

The atlantoaxial joint allows rotation about a vertical axis of the head and atlas on the second cervical vertebra.

The **sacroiliac joints** (see Fig. 3.6 and Chapter 6) between the auricular surfaces (so-called because of their ear shape) of the sacrum and ilium on each side are true synovial joints with cartilage-covered articular surfaces and a synovial capsule. The articular surfaces have several elevations and depressions that fit into each other and contribute to the stability of the joint. The fibrous capsule is thickened posteriorly with the dense sacroiliac ligaments, which are the strongest ligaments in the body. Accessory ligaments include the iliolumbar ligament from the transverse process of the fifth lumbar vertebra to the iliac crest, and the sacrotuberous and sacrospinous ligaments from the sacrum to the ischial tuberosity and ischial spine, respectively. Only a small amount of rotatory movement is allowed at this joint, with some increase in the range of movement during pregnancy.

RADIOLOGICAL FEATURES OF THE JOINTS OF THE VERTEBRAL COLUMN

Plain Radiographs (see Figs. 3.7–3.9)

The distance from the anterior border of the odontoid process to the posterior border of the anterior arch of the atlas – the **atlantoaxial distance** – is used as a measure of the integrity of the atlantoaxial joint. Normal measurements are up to 3 mm in the adult and 5 mm in the child – the latter reflects the presence of unossified cartilage in the young spine.

The **sacroiliac joints** lie obliquely at an angle of approximately 25 degrees to the sagittal plane and are best radiographed by oblique views. Alternatively, by placing the patient in the prone position, the diverging beams passing at approximately 25 degrees pass through both joints simultaneously.

The plane of the sacroiliac joints is perpendicular to the plane of the facet joint of the same side and so these support each other structurally. As a result of this relationship, AP oblique views show best the facet joint nearest the film and the sacroiliac joint farthest from the film.

Facet (Apophyseal Joint) Arthrography

This may be performed to visualize these joints or as a prelude to the administration of anaesthetic or steroid or other agents, which are injected by a posterior oblique approach under fluoroscopic control. On AP views the joints are seen as smooth, oval synovial cavities. On a lateral view the joint cavity is S-shaped. In spondylolysis adjacent facet joints may be seen, on arthrography, to communicate via an abnormal tract.

Computed Tomography

The facet joints are well seen on axial CT (see Figs. 3.1, 3.5 and 3.10). The articular process anterior to the joint is that of the vertebra below, and that posterior to the joint is that of the vertebra above.

The sacroiliac joints and the dense sacroiliac ligament are also seen on axial views. Reconstruction in other planes is useful in addition to axial views of the atlanto-occipital and atlantoaxial joints.

Magnetic Resonance Imaging

The C1/C2 Articulation. Sagittal images clearly demonstrate the C1/C2 articulation. Immediately behind the odontoid, an area of decreased signal intensity represents the transverse ligament. The transverse ligament arches across the ring of the atlas and retains the odontoid process in contact with the anterior arch of the atlas. A small fasciculus extends upward and another extends downwards from the transverse ligament as it crosses the odontoid. The upper fasciculus attaches to the basilar portion of the occipital bone and the lower fasciculus is fixed to the posterior surface of C2. This entire ligament is named the cruciate ligament of the atlas. Axial and coronal images through the top of the odontoid show a portion of the alar ligaments. The alar ligaments attach to the top of the odontoid and insert on the medial aspect of the occipital condyles. The transverse ligament is present posterior to the odontoid process, attaching to the ring of C1. Anterior and posterior synovial joints make up the median atlantoaxial joint. The former is between the anterior arch of C1 and the odontoid, and the latter is between the odontoid and the transverse ligament. On either side of the odontoid are the lateral atlantoaxial joints, which are gliding joints. The rotation of the head occurs at the atlantoaxial joints.

Lumbar Facet Joints. The lumbar articular facets are curvilinear, with an anterior component that is orientated toward the coronal plane and a posterior component orientated toward the sagittal plane.

When a lumbar facet joint is viewed on an axial plane, the anterior facet belongs to the caudad vertebra and the posterior facet to the cephalad vertebra. The facet joints are true synovial joints, with articular surfaces covered by hyaline cartilage 2–4 mm thick. The capsule of the facet joint is a continuation of the ligamentum flavum. Chronic joint effusion may lead to the development of a synovial cyst, which may extend to the epidural space.

> **RADIOLOGY PEARL**
>
> Some disease processes, for example, rheumatoid arthritis, affect synovial rather than cartilaginous joints. In the spine this is manifest as involvement of the joints about the atlas and axis (this can lead to erosion of the dens, which is surrounded by synovial joints), the facet joints and the sacroiliac joints.

Ligaments of the Vertebral Column (Figs. 3.13, 3.14)

The **anterior longitudinal ligament** extends from the basilar part of the occipital bone along the anterior surface of the vertebral bodies and intervertebral discs as far as the upper sacrum. It is firmly attached to the discs and less firmly to the anterior surface of the vertebral bodies.

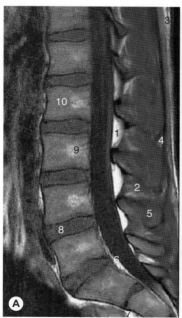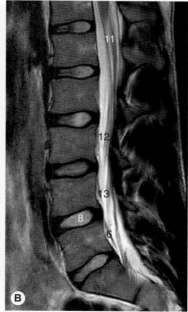

Fig. 3.13 Magnetic resonance image of the lumbar spine. (A) T1-weighted midline sagittal image. (B) T2-weighted midline sagittal image.

1. Posterior epidural space
2. Interspinous ligament
3. Subcutaneous fat
4. Latissimus dorsi muscle attachments
5. Spinous process of L4
6. Anterior epidural fat pad
7. Presacral fat space
8. Intervertebral disc (central nucleus pulposus)
9. Basivertebral vein
10. L2 vertebral body
11. Conus at L1
12. Cauda equina nerve roots
13. Posterior longitudinal ligament

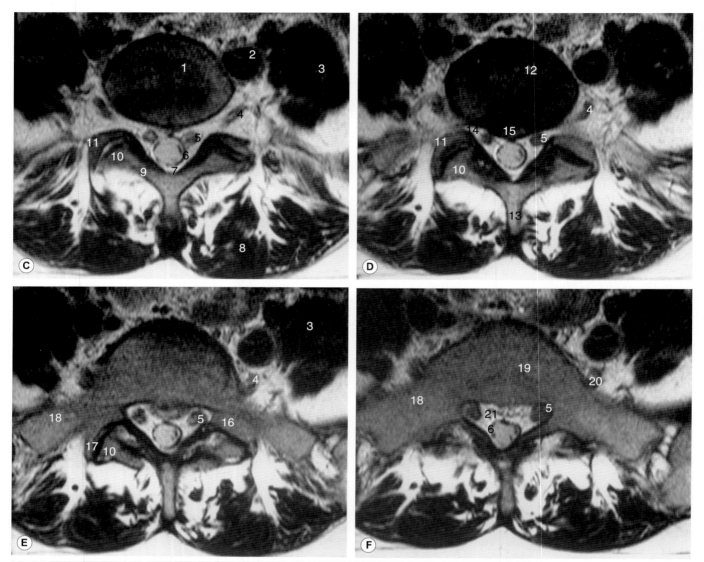

Fig. 3.13, cont'd Sequential axial images through L5 to S1: (C) at the level of the inferior endplate of L5; (D) at the level of the L5/S1 disc; (E) at the level of the superior endplate of S1; (F) at the level of the mid-S1 vertebral body.

(C–F)
1. L5 vertebral body
2. Common iliac veins
3. Psoas muscle
4. L5 nerve root (exited at foramen above the L5/S1 disc space)
5. S1 nerve root in the lateral recess
6. Thecal sac
7. Posterior epidural space
8. Erector spinae muscle
9. Lamina of L5
10. Inferior articular facet of L5

11. Superior articular facet of S1
12. L5/S1 intervertebral disc
13. Spinous process of L5
14. Exit foramen at L5/S1
15. Central disc bulge to anterior epidural fat
16. Pedicle of S1
17. L5/S1 facet joint
18. Transverse process of S1 (sacral ala)
19. S1 vertebral body
20. Presacral plexus
21. Anterior epidural space

The **posterior longitudinal ligament** passes along the posterior surface of the vertebral bodies from the body of the axis to the sacrum. It is firmly attached to the intervertebral discs but separated from the posterior surface of the vertebral bodies by the emerging basivertebral veins. The posterior longitudinal ligament continues superiorly as the membrana tectoria from the posterior aspect of the body of the axis to the anterior margin of the foramen magnum.

The **supraspinous ligament** is attached to the tips of the spinous processes from the seventh cervical vertebra to the sacrum.

Above level C7 it is represented by the **ligamentum nuchae**, which is a fibrous septum lying in the midline sagittal plane that extends from the spines of the cervical vertebrae to the external occipital protuberance and the external occipital crest.

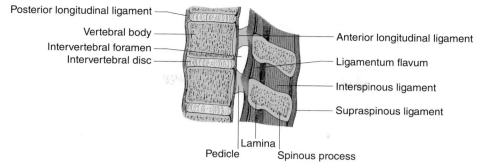

Fig. 3.14 Ligaments of the vertebral column.

Adjoining laminae are connected by **ligamenta flava**, which pass from the anterior surface of one lamina to the posterior surface of the lamina below. There is a right and a left ligament at each level. Anterolaterally, the ligament continues as the capsule of the facet joint. The yellow colour that gives them their name is due to their significant fat content of elastic tissue. They are the only markedly elastic ligament in humans, and can stretch on flexion without forming folds on extension that could impinge on dura.

Relatively weak ligaments connect adjacent transverse processes – the **intertransverse ligaments** – and adjacent spinous processes – the **interspinous ligaments**.

RADIOLOGICAL FEATURES OF THE LIGAMENTS OF THE VERTEBRAL COLUMN

Lumbar Puncture for Myelography

A needle is passed between and parallel to the spinous processes of the lumbar vertebrae (i.e. with slight cranial angulation): (1) through the skin and subcutaneous tissues, (2) through the supraspinous and interspinous ligaments, (3) through the ligamenta flava if these join in the midline (a gap between these to admit midline vessels is variable in size) and (4) through the dura to the subarachnoid space.

Myelogram

The **posterior longitudinal ligament** as it passes posterior to the disc may bulge slightly and impinge upon the thecal sac in myelography. This effect is more marked in extension and disappears in flexion.

CT and MRI (see Figs. 3.10, 3.11)

The ligaments can be viewed directly on both CT and MRI. The anterior and posterior longitudinal ligaments and the ligamentum nuchae and supraspinous ligaments are best seen on sagittal images. The ligamentum flavum lies within the spinal canal arising from the lamina. Because the lamina slopes posteroinferiorly, the ligamentum flavum appears thicker in successively lower axial slices.

The Intervertebral Discs

The vertebral bodies are joined by fibrocartilaginous discs, which are adherent to thin cartilaginous plates on the vertebral bodies above and below them. These joints are amphiarthrodial, with only slightly movable articulations connected by fibrocartilage. Although only a slight amount of motion is possible at each joint, the spine has considerable motion because of the number of joints present. The discs are wedge-shaped in the cervical and lumbar regions and consequently contribute to lordosis in these regions; however in the thoracic region they are flat. The intervertebral discs contribute one-fifth of the total height of the vertebral column.

The major components of the intervertebral disc are the nucleus pulposus, the anulus fibrosus and the cartilaginous endplates. The nucleus pulposus, located centrally in the intervertebral disc, is composed of fibrocartilage that is predominantly type 2 collagen and proteoglycans, which include hyaluronic acid and sulphated glycosaminoglycans. The disc absorbs and retains water because of the negative charge of the proteoglycans. The nucleus pulposus, which is gelatinous in the young subject, becomes more fibrous with age. The nucleus pulposus is surrounded by an anulus fibrosus of tough fibrous tissue. The anulus is stronger anteriorly, being firmly attached to the anterior longitudinal ligament, than posteriorly where the attachment to the posterior longitudinal ligament is loose. The anulus is also relatively thin posteriorly and this is the usual site of rupture in the degenerate disc.

The cartilaginous endplate has a peripheral part which is fibrocartilaginous and covers the apophyseal ring, and a central part which is hyaline cartilage and covers the vertebral endplate.

SOMATIC AND AUTONOMIC NERVE SUPPLY TO THE LUMBAR INTERVERTEBRAL DISC

The anatomic basis for the origin and mediation of clinical signs and symptoms relating to discogenic dysfunction is complex but relates primarily to influences from somatic innervation and from the neural rami arising from the paravertebral autonomic neural plexus.

Discogenic pain arises partly from fibres that arise from the recurrent meningeal nerve of Luschka supplying the posterior longitudinal ligament, the meninges, the blood vessels, the posterior extent of the outermost fibres of the anulus fibrosus, a portion of the periosteum of the vertebral bodies and the underlying bone. In addition, a variable small branch from the ventral ramus of the somatic spinal nerve root may directly innervate the posterolateral aspect of the vertebral body.

Posterior spinal elements, including the facet joints, receive their innervation primarily from the dorsal rami of the spinal nerves.

In addition to somatic innervation, sympathetic fibres arising from the paravertebral autonomic plexus extend posteriorly and form the bulk of the recurrent meningeal nerve to supply the bulk of the disc periphery. Pain referred to the lumbosacral zones of the head is thought to reflect autonomic nerve impulses derived from the segmental embryologic expression of the somatic tissues.

RADIOLOGICAL FEATURES OF THE INTERVERTEBRAL DISCS

Plain Radiographs

The disc space rather than the disc itself is visible. The disc space at L5/S1 level is narrow and this without other degenerative change should not be taken as a sign of disease.

Discography

Discography is performed by injection of contrast medium through the anulus fibrosus into the nucleus pulposus of the intervertebral disc. It may be performed in the lumbar region to establish whether a disc above a proposed fusion is normal. Discography is also performed prior to chemonucleolysis (intentional chemical destruction of the disc). It can be performed by a posterior approach through the dura or by a posterolateral approach without going through the dura.

A normal disc is seen to have a smooth, central, unilocular or bilocular nucleus pulposus, and contrast medium remains within the confines of the anulus fibrosus.

Computed Tomography (see Fig. 3.10)

On CT, the intervertebral discs are seen as low-attenuation structures between the vertebral bodies. It is not possible to distinguish between the nucleus pulposus and the anulus fibrosus.

Magnetic Resonance Imaging

Multiple discs can be examined simultaneously by sagittal MRI (see Figs. 3.11 and 3.13).

In adults, the **nucleus pulposus** is hyperintense on T2-weighted scans and has indistinct boundaries with the anulus fibrosus. The **anulus fibrosus** has a lower water content than the nucleus pulposus, and so they can be distinguished from each other. The anulus fibrosus, which is a highly ordered laminated structure, is divided into an outer and an inner ring. The outer ring inserts onto the ring apophyses of the adjacent vertebrae and the adjacent cartilaginous endplates. The outer ring is made of type 1 collagen and is hypointense on MRI; the inner ring is made of type 2 collagen with more proteoglycan and fluid, and is hyperintense on MRI, indistinguishable from the nucleus pulposus. Hyaline cartilage makes up the cranial and caudal aspects of the disc and attaches to the osseous endplates by numerous collagenous fibres. In the vertebral endplate are numerous pores through which the vascular channels extend. Diffusion of gadolinium into the disc has been shown through these channels.

In youth, the water content of the nucleus pulposus is as high as 80%, although this decreases with age. On MRI the relative signal intensity of the disc varies with water content. In health, a collagen band is often noted to traverse the equator of the disc and is termed the intranuclear cleft.

Intranuclear Cleft

In adults a septum-like structure can be seen to transect the middle of the nucleus pulposus in the horizontal plane. On T2-weighted images of the normal lumbar discs there is often a linear area of reduced signal traversing the centre of the nucleus from anterior to posterior on sagittal views – the so-called intranuclear cleft. This is thought to represent a remnant of the collagenous skeleton of the disc, being a zone of more prominent fibrous tissue than the surrounding nucleus.

Blood Supply of the Vertebral Column

The vertebral bodies and associated structures are supplied by the ascending cervical artery and intercostal and lumbar segmental arteries.

Venous drainage of the vertebral bodies is by a pair of basivertebral veins that emerge from the posterior surface of the body to drain to the internal vertebral venous plexus, which in turn drains to the segmental veins. These large valveless veins allow reflux of blood draining from other viscera into the vertebral bodies and are a potential route of spread of disease – particularly malignancy – into the vertebral bodies.

RADIOLOGICAL FEATURES OF THE BLOOD SUPPLY OF THE VERTEBRAL COLUMN

Spinal Angiography

The blood supply to the vertebral bodies arises from the same arteries that supply the spinal cord. In spinal angiography, therefore, the relevant hemivertebra is opacified when the radicular arteries are opacified.

The Spinal Cord (Fig. 3.15)

The spinal cord is a cylindrical structure extending from the medulla oblongata at the foramen magnum proximally to

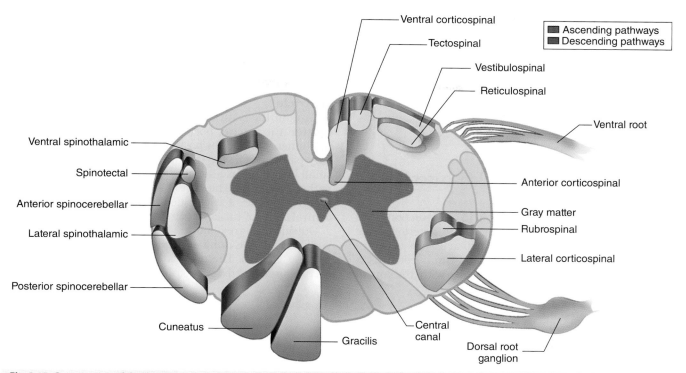

Fig. 3.15 Cross-section of the thoracic spinal cord. (Modified from Williamson P et al. *The Human Body in Health & Disease,* 8th ed. Elsevier; 2024.)

the cone-shaped tapered conus medullaris distally. It extends the entire length of the vertebral canal in a 3-month-old fetus, however, because of greater growth in length of the vertebral column than in the spinal cord, the conus lies at the level of the L2 vertebra at birth and between T12 and L2 at skeletal maturity (most commonly at L1). The conus may lie even higher in the flexed position, which may be used during myelography. The anterior median fissure forms a deep longitudinal midline cleft in the anterior cord with a shallower depression in the midline posterior cord forming the posterior median sulcus. Additional shallow depressions bilaterally are termed the anterolateral and posterolateral sulci. These represent the exit site of the ventral nerve roots and entry point of the dorsal nerve roots, respectively.

Beyond the conus; medullaris, a prolongation of pia mater covered by spinal dura and arachnoid meninges extends as a thin cord – the filum terminale. This is attached to the posterior aspect of the first coccygeal segment.

From the spinal cord, 31 segmental nerves arise on each side – 8 cervical, 12 thoracic, 5 lumbar, 5 sacral and 1 coccygeal.

Although there is no trace of segmentation on the surface of the cord, the part of the spinal cord from which a pair of spinal nerves arises is called a spinal segment. Each spinal nerve arises from a series of rootlets which fuse to form a dorsal root, with a dorsal root ganglion that carries sensory nerves and a ventral root with motor and autonomic nerves. The dorsal and ventral roots unite at the intervertebral foramen to form the spinal nerve.

Spinal nerves C1–C7 exit above the pedicles of the corresponding vertebrae and all other spinal nerves exit below the pedicles of the corresponding vertebrae. Thus the C8 nerve passes under the pedicle of C7 (there is no C8 vertebra) and the L5 nerve passes under the pedicle of the L5 vertebra. Having left the vertebral canal, the spinal nerves divide into dorsal and ventral rami, each of which carry motor and sensory nerves.

Owing to the difference in length between the spinal cord and the vertebral canal, the spinal segment from which a nerve arises is separated from the correspondingly named vertebra and the exit foramen. Thus, cord segments in the lower cervical spine are one level above the exit foramina, those in the lower thorax two levels above, and those in the lumbar spine three levels above their exit foramina.

Similarly, expansions in the diameter of the spinal cord due to the brachial plexus (C5–T1) and the lumbosacral plexus (L2–S3) cause expansion of vertebral interpedicular distances at higher levels C4–T2, maximal at C5 for the brachial plexus and T9–L1/2 (the conus) for the lumbar plexus.

Nerve roots take an increasingly greater downward course from cord to exit foramen in the cervical, thoracic and lumbar spinal cord. The lumbar, sacral and coccygeal roots that exit below the conus at L1/L2 are contained within the dura as far as its lower limit at S2, and are called the cauda equina.

ventricle. It extends inferiorly for 5–6 mm into the filum terminale. While this canal is truly central in the upper lumbar cord, it lies anterior to the midline in the cervical and thoracic cord and is posteriorly placed in the conus. A fusiform dilation of the central canal in the conus about 10 mm long and triangular in cross-section is termed the **terminal ventricle**.

Around the central canal is an H-shaped area of **grey matter**, the anterior horns of which have cell bodies of the motor neurons and the posterior horns have cells in the sensory pathways. In the thoracic and upper lumbar regions, small lateral horns are found that have cell bodies for sympathetic neurons. The grey commissure centrally connects the grey matter of each side of the cord and contains the central canal of the cord.

Outside the grey matter is the **white matter** of the cord, which has long ascending and descending tracts (see Fig. 3.15B). The posterior (dorsal) columns, between the posterior horns, have tracts that convey sensations of

CROSS-SECTION OF THE SPINAL CORD (SEE FIG. 3.15)

The spinal cord is somewhat elliptical in cross-section, with its greater diameter from side to side. The anterior spinal artery courses within the anterior median fissure.

A narrow-calibre **central canal** transmits cerebrospinal fluid (CSF) and is continuous above with the fourth

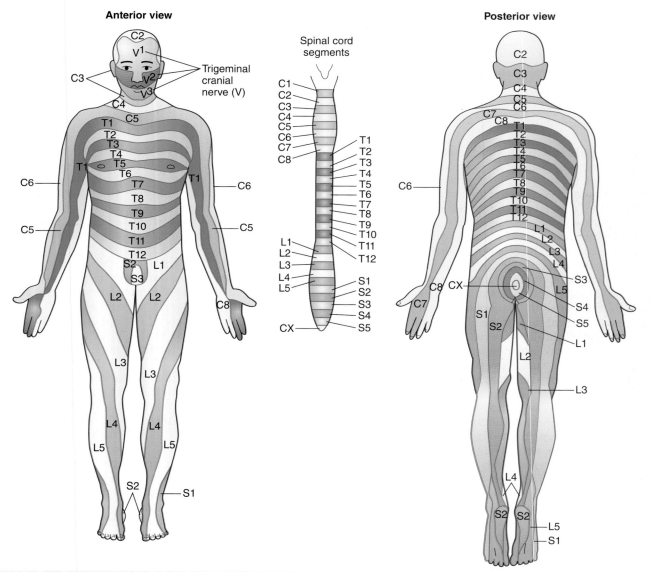

Fig. 3.16 Dermatomes of (A) legs and (B) arms. (From Patton KT et al. *The Human Body in Health & Disease*, 8th ed. Elsevier; 2024.)

pressure, vibration, position, movement and touch. The anterior columns contain descending motor fibres forming multiple different tracts. Other sensations are carried in the lateral columns to the thalamus – the spinothalamic tracts – and to the cerebellum – the spinocerebellar tracts. Additional descending motor tracts are also located within the lateral columns.

The Spinal Canal

The spinal cord lies within the osseous spinal canal surrounded by the anterior and posterior elements of the vertebra and extending from the foramen magnum to the inferior sacrum. The canal is divided anatomically into different regions, or zones (Fig. 3.17). Different pathologies may result in stenosis in one or more of these zones, potentially compressing the neural components within the affected zone/s.

The Subarticular Zone or Recess

The anterolateral portion of the spinal canal is called the subarticular recess or zone. It is bound anteriorly by the posterior surface of the intervertebral disc and vertebral body, laterally by the pedicle and posteriorly by the superior articular process/facet joint. The descending nerve root corresponding to the immediately caudal vertebral body lies in the subarticular recess. The subarticular recess is usually more than 3 mm in AP diameter, narrowing being produced posteriorly by hypertrophic change in the superior facet of the vertebral body below as well as thickening of the ligamentum flavum and anteriorly by posterior bulging of the vertebral body and endplate.

The Neural Foramen

This is a fibro-osseous canal, lateral to and directly continuous with the subarticular recess. It extends superoinferiorly from the pedicle above to the pedicle below, and from the

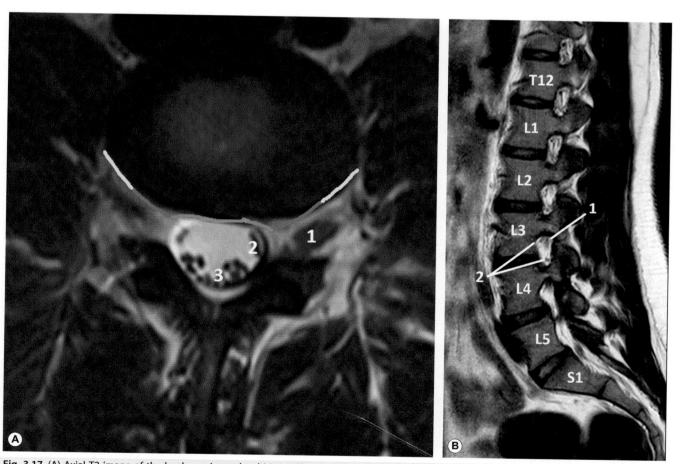

Fig. 3.17 (A) Axial T2 image of the lumbar spine at level L3–L4. The spinal canal zones are depicted: central zone *(red)*, subarticular zones *(green)*, foraminal zones *(blue)* and extraforaminal zones *(yellow)*. (B) Sagittal T2 magnetic resonance image of the lumbar spine at the level of the neural foramen.

(A)
1. Exiting left L3 nerve
2. Descending left L4 nerve
3. Remaining nerves of the cauda equina

(B)
1. Right L3 nerve in the right L3–L4 neural foramen
2. Surrounding vessels within the neural foramen

posterior margin of the vertebral body anteriorly to the superior and inferior facets posteriorly. It has a wider upper portion that contains the exiting nerve roots, the dorsal root ganglion and their accompanying arteries and veins surrounded by fat. The sinuvertebral or recurrent nerve originates partly from the spinal nerve in the neuroforamen and re-enters the spinal canal. It supplies the posterior portion of the annulus, the posterior longitudinal ligament and the periosteum of the vertebral body.

The Spinal Meninges (Fig. 3.18)

Three layers of meninges – the pia, arachnoid and dura mater from deep to superficial – cover the spinal cord as well as the brain. All three layers extend along the nerve roots to the intervertebral foramina.

The **pia mater** is applied closely to the surface of the spinal cord, entering its anterior and posterior sulci just as it does on the brain surface. The pia is thickened laterally between the nerve roots as the **denticulate ligament** up to the level of the twelfth thoracic nerve, attaching to the overlying dura. It is so-called because of teeth-like projections that attach to the dura at intervals. Inferiorly the pia is thickened with glial tissue as the filum terminale. The pia mater helps with stabilization of the cord.

The **arachnoid mater** lines the dura and forms an incomplete posterior median septum. The subarachnoid space, which contains CSF, lies between the arachnoid and the pia mater. The subarachnoid space extends along the nerve roots to the intervertebral foramina, allowing visualization, on myelography, of the nerve roots in their sheaths to this point. The subdural space is a potential space between the arachnoid and the dura, and contains only lubricating serous fluid.

Unlike the cranial dura mater, the spinal dura mater has only one layer, the **meningeal layer**. This is a loose sheath around the spinal cord representing the inner layer of the cerebral dura. The extradural (epidural) space lies external to this between the dura and wall of the vertebral canal and contains loose areolar tissue, fat and a plexus of veins. It extends laterally for a short distance beyond the intervertebral foramina along the spinal nerves, together with the arachnoid mater to form the epineurium.

The dural sac or thecal sac extends interiorly as far as the S2 vertebral level. Below this the arachnoid and dura blend to cover the filum terminale.

Blood Supply of the Spinal Cord (Figs. 3.19 and 3.22)

The spinal cord is supplied by two posterolateral spinal arteries that supply the posterior white columns and part of the grey matter of the dorsal horns, and a single midline anterior spinal artery that supplies the remaining two-thirds of the cross-sectional area of the spinal cord. At the lower end of the cord (i.e. the conus) the anterior artery divides in two and anastomoses with each posterior spinal artery. A small 'twig' continues on the filum terminale. Additionally pial anastomoses between the anterior and posterior spinal arteries encircle the surface of the cord throughout its length, forming the arterial vasocorona and supplying the peripheral lateral aspect of the cord.

The posterolateral spinal arteries arise by one or two branches on each side from the vertebral artery or, more commonly, its posterior inferior cerebellar branch. The anterior spinal artery also arises from the vertebral artery by union, in the midline, of a branch from each side. These arteries receive further supply at intervals along the length of the cord from branches of the deep cervical branch of the subclavian artery, the cervical part of the vertebral artery, and by branches from the intercostal and first lumbar arteries.

These segmental branches pass into the intervertebral foramen and along the nerve roots towards the spinal cord. Branches along the anterior nerve root may arise with or separately from those to the posterior nerve root. The majority of these are **radicular arteries** (i.e. supply mainly the nerve root), but some are **radiculomedullary arteries** and give a significant supply to the cord. The level of origin and number of radiculomedullary arteries is variable, but there are usually four to nine and they arise mainly in the lower cervical, lower thoracic and upper lumbar regions. One of these is often larger than the others and is called the **arteria radicularis magna** or the **artery of Adamkiewicz**. This arises at the lower thoracic level between T9 and T12 (on the left side in two-thirds of cases) and supplies the cord both above and below this level. Radiculomedullary arteries reinforce the supply of both the anterior and posterior spinal arteries, and their supply to the cord is critical to its function.

VENOUS DRAINAGE OF THE SPINAL CORD

The spinal cord drains to a plexus of veins anterior and posterior to the cord which in turn drains into radicular veins and subsequently along the nerve roots to segmental veins. The plexus communicates with:
- The veins of the medulla at the foramen magnum
- The vertebral veins in the neck

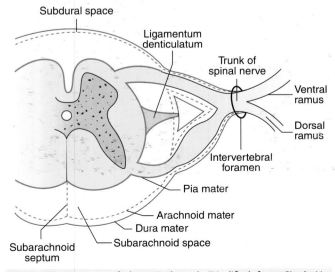

Fig. 3.18 Meninges of the spinal cord. (Modified from Singh V. *Textbook of Clinical Neuroanatomy*, 4th ed. Elsevier; 2021.)

- The azygos veins in the thorax
- The lumbar veins in the lumbar region

RADIOLOGICAL FEATURES OF THE SPINAL CORD, ITS MENINGES AND BLOOD SUPPLY

Myelographic Technique

Lumbar puncture for myelography is performed at a level below the termination of the conus medullaris. The highest point of the iliac crest is at L4, and this is used as a landmark to identify the interspaces above and below it. The procedure is usually performed under fluoroscopic guidance.

Nerve roots leave the cord anterolaterally; they are therefore foreshortened in AP views and are best seen in **oblique views**.

Inadvertent injection of contrast other than into the CSF in the subarachnoid space causes characteristic patterns owing to the anatomy of the spinal meninges. **Extradural (or epidural) injection** between the dura and the vertebral bone causes collection of contrast around the dura and extension of contrast along the nerve roots to beyond the intervertebral foramina. **Subdural injection** between the dura and the arachnoid gives an angular collection of slow-moving contrast on AP views, which extends along the nerve roots only as far as the intervertebral foramen. In both subdural and extradural injection contrast is dense because it is not, with CSF. Injection into an **epidural vein** is recognized by the rapid disappearance of contrast with blood flow.

Myelographic Appearance

Cervical. On the AP view the cervical expansion, maximal at C6, can be seen. The cord occupies 50%–75% of the interpedicular distance. Nerve roots and their sheaths can be seen leaving the cord almost horizontally. The odontoid peg and spinal vessels, vertebral arteries or posterior inferior cerebellar arteries may cause normal filling defects. On lateral views, the transverse ligament of the atlas may cause a filling defect posterior to the odontoid peg.

Thoracic. On the AP view a thin line of contrast on each side outlines the spinal cord, which fills most of the interpedicular distance. The path of the nerve roots is, as a result, short but somewhat more vertical than in the cervical region. On lateral views the cord is seen to be more anterior in position than in the cervical region.

Lumbar (Fig. 3.20). The spinal cord tapers suddenly to end at L1/L2 level as the conus medullaris. The filum terminale can be seen as a long, thin, central filling defect extending from the conus to the end of the thecal sac. It is surrounded by the nerve roots – the cauda equina – which lie laterally until they reach their exit points. The S1 nerve root can be identified passing to the first sacral foramen. The lumbar roots pass beneath the pedicle of the correspondingly numbered vertebra. Roots are compressed by a protrusion of the disc above the exit level (e.g. the L5 root is compressed by a disc at L4/5 level).

The level at which the thecal sac ends are variable and may lie at L5/S1 or extend to S2. The thecal sac fills

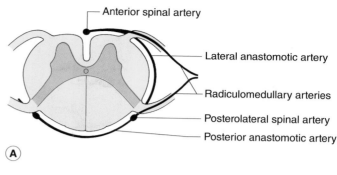

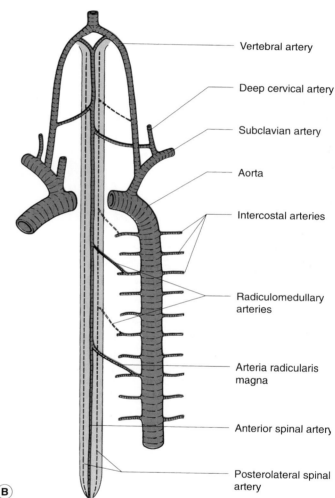

Fig. 3.19 Arterial supply of the spinal cord. (A) Axial section. (B) Coronal view.

30%–80% of the interpedicular distance and is also variable on the lateral view, usually lying close to the vertebral bodies and discs, but occasionally a wide epidural space separates the thecal sac from the L5/S1 disc space and may hide a disc protrusion here.

The Epidural Space

This space contains the epidural veins, fat and nerve roots. The diameter of the anterior epidural space increases progressively towards the sacrum, being a few millimetres

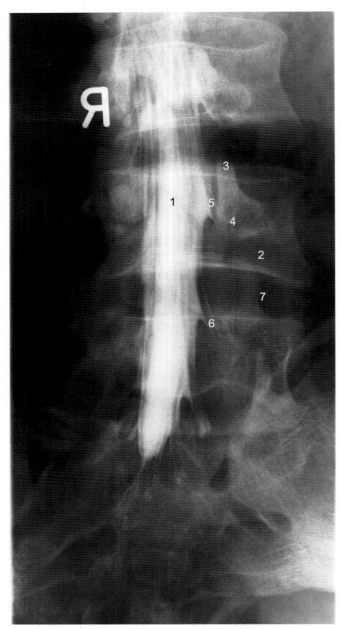

Fig. 3.20 Lumbar myelogram: left posterior oblique view to show nerve roots. Below the level of C7 each nerve root emerges *below* the pedicle of its corresponding vertebral body.

1. Nerves of the cauda equina in the thecal sac, outlined by contrast
2. Body of L4
3. Left superior articular process of L4
4. Left pedicle of L4
5. Left L4 root
6. Left L5 nerve root
7. L4/L5 disc space

the septum does not exist. The posterior epidural space is most extensive at the L3/4 and L4/5 interspaces, and for this reason is most frequently chosen as the site for epidural injections. The caudal extent of the spinal cord is the conus medullaris, from which extends the filum terminale. The filum terminale (also known as the filum terminale internum) extends within the dural sac to its inferior point behind S2. It continues inferiorly below this point as the filum terminale externum to insert on the first coccygeal segment.

Computed Tomography (see Fig. 3.10)

CT of the spinal cord and canal is usually performed following intrathecal injection of contrast, a CT myelogram. This is usually reserved for patients with contraindications to MRI. It can also be performed to identify arachnoid cysts in the spinal canal and in the evaluation of craniospinal hypotension, looking for a spinal source of CSF leak. Intrathecal contrast allows for visualization of the nerve roots as their sheaths fill with contrast. The nerve roots of the cauda equina are also outlined by contrast. The cord is elliptical in cross-section, with its wide axis lying transversely in the cervical region and in the centre of the subarachnoid space. In the thoracic region the cord is circular in cross-section and lies more anteriorly. No cord is visible in cuts taken below the level of L2.

Low-density epidural fat outlines the thecal sac. On non-contrast imaging of the spine CSF is of water density and the higher-density cord can be seen within it.

Magnetic Resonance Imaging (see Figs. 3.11, 3.13, 3.17)

MRI is the modality of choice for evaluation of the spinal cord and its surrounding structures. The spinal cord is well seen against the CSF in either T1- or T2-weighted images. The enlargements of the cord in the cervical and lower thoracic areas are visualized, and the cauda can be seen close to the posterior aspect of the subarachnoid space beyond the lower limit of the cord. Differentiation between grey and white matter within the cord is best seen on axial imaging but often limited in its resolution.

The central, paracentral and subarticular zones are best assessed on axial imaging. The intervertebral foramen is best assessed on axial imaging in the cervical spine and on sagittal imaging in the thoracic and lumbar spine. MRI allows for accurate determination of the extent of stenosis in these zones if present.

Nerve roots are visible, especially where they are outlined by fat in the intervertebral foramen. Epidural fat is invariably present posteriorly and, to a lesser extent, anteriorly. The amount of epidural fat in the nerve roots increases from their cranial to their caudal ends. In contrast-enhanced MRI, bright epidural veins contrast with negligible signal from nerve roots. The spinal nerves of the cauda equina can be seen outlined by the CSF, usually lying posteriorly in the thecal space, except for those passing anteriorly from the exit foramina.

MR angiography of the spine allows for assessment of spinal arterial vasculature and is used in the pretreatment assessment of vascular lesions of the spinal canal, for example dural arteriovenous fistulas.

behind the L5/S1 body. The anterior epidural space is divided by a midline fibrous septum attached to the posterior margin of the vertebral body and the posterior longitudinal ligament. At the level of the disc, the posterior longitudinal ligament attaches directly to the outer annulus and

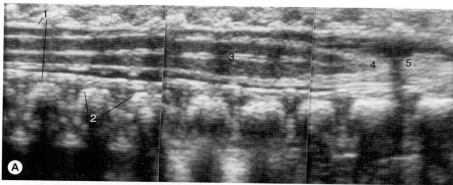

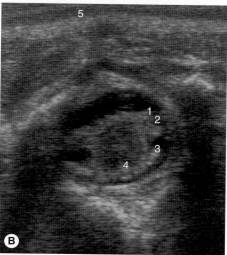

Fig. 3.21 Spinal ultrasound. (A) Composite sagittal view of the lower cord and conus. (B) Transverse section through the spinal cord.

(A)
1. Dura
2. Vertebral bodies
3. Central echo complex
4. Conus
5. Cauda equina

(B)
1. Dorsal nerve root
2. Denticulate ligament
3. Ventral nerve root
4. Anterior median sulcus
5. Unossified spinous process.

Spinal Ultrasound (see Fig. 3.21)

Ultrasound scanning is most useful in the first few weeks of life before the posterior elements of the vertebra ossify.

The spinal cord is seen on ultrasound as a hypoechoic band which is broader at the cervicothoracic junction and in the upper lumbar level, corresponding to the levels of origin of the brachial and lumbar plexi. The central linear echo within the cord has been shown to be due to the interface between the anterior median fissure and the ventral white commissure rather than to the central canal itself. The central canal may be visible, however, especially if this is widened. The denticulate ligament can be seen on either side of the cord on an axial view.

Spinal nerves can be seen to arise from the cord. On axial views the dorsal and ventral nerve roots can be seen. The nerves of the cauda equina almost fill the thecal sac distal to the conus. The normal filum terminale often cannot be distinguished within the cauda equina. If visible, it should not be thicker than 2 mm diameter.

Ultrasound of the spinal cord is more limited in the baby older than 3 months or in the older child. A limited intersegmental view may be achieved by placing the probe lateral to the midline and pointing medially, thus getting an interlaminar view.

Spinal Angiography (Fig. 3.22)

This is a lengthy procedure involving injection of contrast into the vertebral arteries, the deep cervical arteries, several intercostal and lumbar arteries, and the sacral branch of the internal iliac artery to identify the radiculomedullary arteries, which are variable in number and level of origin. No single injection will opacify the entire anterior spinal artery. The main feeding vessel in spinal vascular malformations may arise distant from the lesion and may be missed if a thorough examination is not performed.

The arteria radicularis magna (artery of Adamkiewicz) usually arises on the left side between T_8 and T_{12}. When opacified it is seen to turn cranially from its origin towards the midline of the spinal cord and to bifurcate into a small ascending and a large descending contribution to the anterior spinal artery. This angiographic feature is called the 'hairpin appearance'.

MR angiography is often performed prior to a formal interventional spinal angiogram and may help guide the vessels of interrogation, limiting the number of vessels requiring evaluation.

Spinal angiography is also a therapeutic option for the treatment of some spinal vascular malformations with a range of embolization materials utilized.

RADIOLOGY PEARL

In the catheterization of intercostal arteries and their branches, such as for **bronchial angiography** and in particular for bronchial embolization, there is a risk of damage to the blood supply of the cord by inadvertent embolization to the radiculomedullary branches.

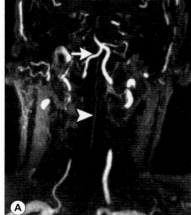

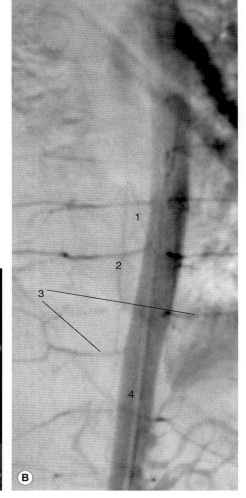

Fig. 3.22 (A) Coronal magnetic resonance angiogram. The anterior spinal artery *(arrowhead)* is seen within the cervical region anterior to the cord. In this patient the artery arises from the right vertebral artery *(arrow)*. No radiculomedullary feeders are visualized. (B) Angiogram. (A, from Sheehy, N., Boyle, G., Meaney, J. F. M. (2005). High-resolution 3D contrast enhanced MRA of the normal anterior spinal arteries within the cervical region. *Radiology 236*(2), 637-641, with permission from the authors.) (B)
1. Arteria radicularis magna
2. Anterior spinal artery
3. Intercostal arteries
4. Aorta

THERAPEUTIC INTERVENTIONS

- **Epidural injection:** Image-guided injection into the posterior epidural space following contrast epidurography. This can be used to perform epidural steroid injections of one or more spinal nerves.

- **Transforaminal nerve root block:** Image-guided selective injection of a spinal nerve root at its extra-foraminal or foraminal component. This can be used for selective nerve root steroid injection.
- **Facet joint block:** Image-guided injection of the facet joint, usually with steroid and local anaesthetic.

CHAPTER CONTENTS

The Thoracic Cage 123
The Diaphragm 129
The Pleura 135
The Extrapleural Space 138
The Trachea and Bronchi 138
The Lungs 143
The Mediastinum 152
The Heart 153
The Great Vessels 167

The Oesophagus 170
The Thoracic Duct and Mediastinal Lymphatics 172
The Thymus 173
The Azygos System 174
Important Nerves of the Mediastinum 175
The Mediastinum on the Chest Radiograph 177
Cross-Sectional Anatomy 179

The thorax is the portion of the trunk that lies between the lower neck and the upper abdomen. It is made up of the chest wall (the thoracic cage and associated soft tissues) and the visceral contents of the thoracic cavity. The diaphragm separates the thorax from the abdomen. The boundary between the lower neck and the thorax is less clearly demarcated.

The Thoracic Cage

The thoracic cage or bony thorax is bounded superiorly by the suprapleural membrane, a layer of fascia attached to the C7 transverse process, the inner margins of the first rib and first costal cartilage and the mediastinal pleura. The thoracic cage is made up of: (1) 12 thoracic vertebrae (see Chapter 3); (2) 12 ribs and their costal cartilages and (3) the sternum.

THE RIBS

There are usually 12 pairs of ribs (i.e., the ribs that articulate with the 12 thoracic vertebrae from T1 to T12); however, there is a variation in rib number (see variant anatomy in the ribs). The ribs can be classified into true ribs, false ribs and floating ribs based on their costal cartilages and articulations with the sternum (see costal cartilages paragraph). The posterior portions of the ribs have a relatively horizontal orientation, while the mid and anterior portions of the ribs course inferiorly. This manifests on chest radiograph as horizontal posterior ribs and more vertical/oblique anterior ribs. On cross-sectional imaging, portions of several adjacent ribs can be seen on a single axial image. The ribs also provide attachment for some of the muscles that make up the chest wall. The primary ossification centre for the body of the ribs appears at the eighth fetal week. Secondary ossification centres for the rib epiphyses (head and costal tubercle) become visible around puberty and only fully fuse around 20 years of age.

THE TYPICAL RIB (FIG. 4.1)

The third to ninth ribs are considered typical ribs. A typical rib has a head, neck and body with a costal tubercle posteriorly, separating the neck and the body of the rib (see Fig. 4.1). The anterior portion of a typical rib is cartilaginous while the posterior portion is bony and forms two separate articulations: the costovertebral and the costotransverse joints, both of which are synovial joints. The head of the typical rib has two facets for articulation with two adjacent vertebral bodies (the costovertebral joint); for example the head of the sixth rib articulates with the inferior portion of T5 and the superior portion of T6, spanning the T5/T6 intervertebral disc. The costal tubercle has a facet medially for articulation with its own transverse process; for example, the tubercle of the sixth rib articulates with the T6 transverse process. The costal tubercle also has a nonarticular part laterally for ligament attachment. The neck of the rib is attached by a ligament to the transverse process of the vertebra above without forming a joint. A typical rib possesses a costal groove anteroinferiorly to accommodate the intercostal neurovascular bundle. The first rib is relatively immobile. The second to twelfth ribs move like bucket handles up and down. In inspiration, accessory muscles of inspiration draw the ribs upwards, which serves to increase the anteroposterior (AP) diameter of the thorax. Increasing the volume of the thoracic cavity decreases the internal pressure and draws gas into it.

> **RADIOLOGY PEARL**
>
> The costal groove can project as a fine line inferior to the rib, which can be confused with a pneumothorax.

RADIOLOGY PEARL

As the heads of the typical ribs articulate with two adjacent vertebrae, it can be difficult to match the rib with its numerically corresponding vertebra. The costotransverse joint can be an easier way to determine with which vertebra a particular rib is matched, on both chest radiograph and on computed tomography (CT).

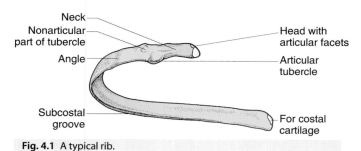

Neck
Nonarticular part of tubercle
Angle
Head with articular facets
Articular tubercle
Subcostal groove
For costal cartilage

Fig. 4.1 A typical rib.

ATYPICAL RIBS

First Rib (Fig. 4.2)

This is the shortest, flattest and most curved rib, and it plays a vital role in protecting vital organs. It articulates with T1 only. Along with its costal tubercle posteriorly, the first rib possesses a scalene tubercle along its inner margin, which serves as the site of insertion of the scalenus anterior muscle; this may be visible on chest radiograph as a superior protuberance. The superior aspect of the first rib has a groove for the subclavian vein anteriorly and a groove for the lowest trunk of the brachial plexus posteriorly. The subclavian artery directly abuts the nerve trunk and not the rib. These two grooves are separated by the scalene tubercle along with the distal scalenus anterior muscle itself (see Fig. 4.2B and C).

Second Rib

This is less curved and twice as long as the first rib. Like the first rib, it has additional tubercles for the attachments of serratus anterior and scalenus posterior.

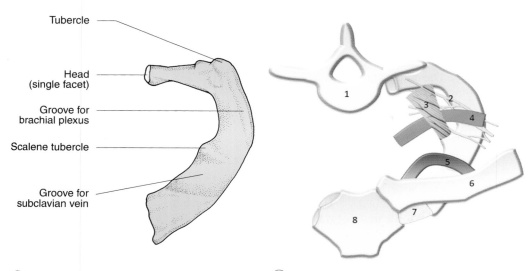

Tubercle
Head (single facet)
Groove for brachial plexus
Scalene tubercle
Groove for subclavian vein

Fig. 4.2 (A) The first rib. (B) Structures crossing the first rib. (C) T1-weighted sagittal MRI of the neck demonstrating the anatomy of the structures crossing the first rib

(B)
1. First thoracic vertebra
2. Brachial plexus (yellow)
3. Scalenus anterior muscle
4. Subclavian artery
5. Subclavian vein
6. Clavicle
7. First costal cartilage
8. Manubrium of the sternum

(C)
1. Subclavian vein
2. Scalenus anterior
3. Subclavian artery
4. Brachial plexus

(A)   (B)

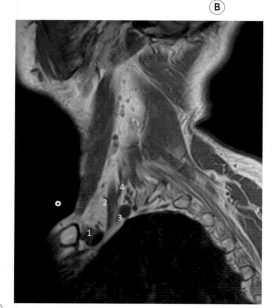

(C)

Tenth Rib

This differs from the typical ribs by having only one articular facet on its head.

Eleventh Rib

This also has only one articular facet on its head. It has no costal tubercle for articulation with the transverse process.

Twelfth Rib

This has only one articular facet on its head; it has no costal tubercle and no costal groove.

VARIANT ANATOMY IN THE RIBS

Cervical Rib (Fig. 4.3)

A supernumerary bony or fibrous rib articulates with C7 posteriorly and fuses with the first rib anteriorly. This occurs in approximately 0.5% of people and when present, is bilateral in up to 50% of these cases. Cervical ribs can predispose

to thoracic outlet compression. It can be difficult to distinguish a cervical rib from an abnormally elongated C7 transverse process.

Short Rib

A short rib or hypoplastic rib occurs when one or more of ribs 1–10 is abnormally short and does not extend anteriorly to the sternum. This is likely due to premature closure of the physis. The rib often fuses with a rib above or below, simulating a partial rib resection. Short rib occurs in up to 16%.

Bifid Rib (Fig. 4.4)

Bifid or forked rib occurs when the anterior portion of a rib divides into two separate processes. This most commonly affects the fourth ribs. Its incidence is unknown.

Absent Ribs

Absence of at least one rib is common, with up to 8% only having 11 ribs. While it can be associated with congenital

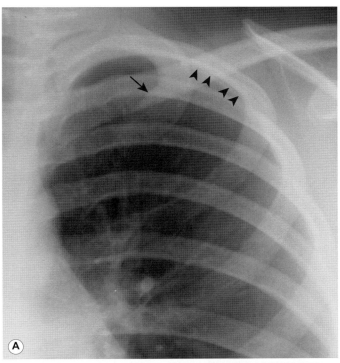

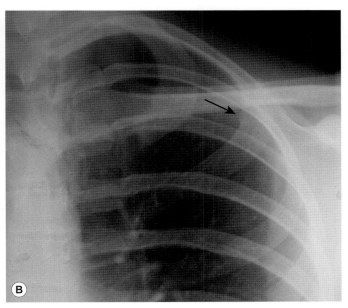

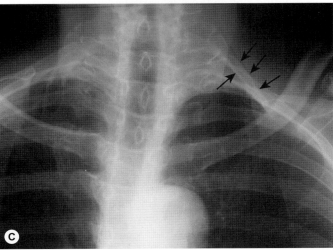

Fig. 4.3 The ribs. (A) Costal groove clearly visible below the second left rib (*arrowheads*). Note also the scalene tubercle on the first rib (*arrow*). (B) Prominence on the upper surface of the second rib due to the insertion of part of scalenus anterior muscle. (C) Cervical rib – a well-developed bony cervical rib on the left side (*arrows*).

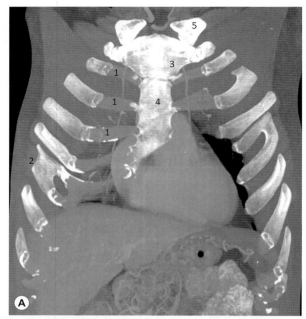

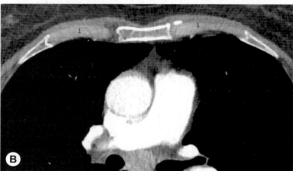

Fig. 4.4 Costal cartilages. Coronal maximum-intensity projection (MIP) computed tomography (CT) thorax. (B) Axial CT thorax with contrast.

(A)
1. Costal cartilages
2. Bifid rib
3. Manubrium of the sternum
4. Body of the sternum
5. Medial end of the left clavicle

(B)
1. Costal cartilages

RADIOLOGY PEARL

Due to the large variation in the number of ribs, the upper-most and lower-most ribs cannot be assumed to be arising from T1 and T12, respectively, when trying to determine vertebral level.

RADIOLOGY PEARL

Cervical ribs may be distinguished from the first rib by the orientation of the transverse process – that of C7 points downward, whereas that of T1 is horizontal or points upward.

RADIOLOGY PEARL

As the first rib is closely associated with the subclavian vessels and is protected anteriorly by the overlying clavicle, a fracture of the first rib in trauma has a significant association with neurovascular injury and should not be considered a typical rib fracture.

disease, it is much more commonly a normal anatomic variation.

Lumbar Rib

This may represent a true accessory rib arising from L1, a nonfused transverse process or an elongated transverse process. This is seen in approximately 1% of the population. The presence of a lumbar rib is commonly associated with transitional spinal anatomy.

COSTAL CARTILAGES (SEE FIG. 4.4)

The costal cartilages are the cartilaginous anterior ends of the ribs which slope obliquely upwards to join with the sternum. The junctions between the bony and cartilaginous portions of a rib, the costochondral junctions, are primary cartilaginous joints/synchondroses for all 12 ribs. The costochondral junctions permit little or no movement. The unions between the medial ends of the costal cartilages and the sternum vary in nature. The first costal cartilage forms a synchondrosis with the manubrium which, along with its primary cartilaginous costochondral junction, explains the relative immobility of the first rib. The second to seventh sternocostal joints form synovial joints which permit mobility. The second costal cartilage articulates with the manubriosternal joint and the third to seventh costal cartilages articulate directly with the body of the sternum. The eighth to tenth costal cartilages attach to each other in series and then with the seventh costal cartilage to join the body of the sternum. This combination of the eighth to tenth costal cartilages creates the costal arches which form the upper boundaries of the anterior abdomen. The eleventh and twelfth costal cartilages are small in size with pointed ends that terminate in the muscles of the abdominal wall. The first to seventh ribs are considered true ribs as they articulate directly with the sternum; the eighth to tenth are considered false ribs as they articulate indirectly, and the eleventh and twelfth ribs floating ribs as there is no articulation with the sternum. Calcification of the costal cartilages is normal with advancing age, seen in 6% in the third decade of life and in 45% in the ninth decade of life. It affects the first costal cartilage earliest and most prominently.

RADIOLOGY PEARL

Prominent calcification of the first costal cartilages, along with first sternocostal joint osteophytes, often simulates apical lung nodules on chest radiograph.

The Intercostal Space and Vessels

The spaces between consecutive ribs are known as the intercostal spaces and are designated by the rib above, for example, the first intercostal space lies between the first and second ribs and the eleventh intercostal space lies between the eleventh and twelfth ribs. Hence, there are 11 intercostal spaces bilaterally; the regions below the twelfth ribs are known as the subcostal regions. The intercostal spaces are filled by the intercostal muscles, described below. The neurovascular bundle lies between the internal and innermost muscle layers.

Intercostal Arteries. The first to ninth intercostal spaces receive dual arterial blood supply from anterior and posterior intercostal arteries which arise from different parent vessels. The tenth and eleventh intercostal spaces are supplied solely by posterior intercostal arteries. The intercostal arteries also help to supply the skin of the chest wall and the parietal pleura.

POSTERIOR INTERCOSTAL ARTERIES
- The first and second intercostal spaces receive posterior supply from branches of a single superior or supreme intercostal artery, which in turn arises from the costocervical branch of the subclavian artery.
- The third to eleventh posterior intercostal arteries arise individually from the descending thoracic aorta and supply their corresponding intercostal space.
- As the descending thoracic aorta lies to the left of the thoracic spine, the right posterior intercostal arteries are longer than the left and they must course anterior to the vertebra before entering the posterior portion of the intercostal space.
- The posterior intercostal arteries can often be identified on CT.

ANTERIOR INTERCOSTAL ARTERIES
- The first to sixth anterior intercostal arteries arise directly from the internal thoracic artery (a branch of the subclavian artery).
- The seventh to ninth anterior intercostal arteries arise from the musculophrenic artery, the continuation of the internal thoracic artery.
- The tenth and eleventh intercostal spaces have no anterior intercostal artery.
- The anterior intercostal arteries are generally not visible on CT, in contrast to the posterior intercostals.

Intercostal Veins. Most of the intercostal spaces are drained by paired anterior and posterior intercostal veins, similar to the intercostal arterial supply; however, the posterior intercostal venous drainage is anatomically unique.

POSTERIOR
- The first posterior intercostal veins arch over the pleura to drain into the brachiocephalic veins as the supreme intercostal veins.
- The second to fourth intercostal veins unite to form the right and left superior intercostal veins. The right superior intercostal vein drains to the azygos vein. The left superior intercostal vein courses laterally and then posteriorly around the aortic arch to drain into the left brachiocephalic vein or the accessory hemiazygos vein. As it travels along the lateral aspect of the aortic arch from anterior to posterior, it can create a small, rounded opacity adjacent to the aortic knuckle on chest radiograph known as the aortic nipple. This normal variant

is reportedly seen in 10% of posteroanterior (PA) chest radiographs and can be confused with pathology.
- The right fifth to eleventh posterior intercostal veins drain into the azygos vein.
- The left fifth to eighth posterior intercostal veins drain into the accessory hemiazygos vein and the ninth to eleventh into the hemiazygos vein.

ANTERIOR
- The anterior intercostal veins mirror the anterior intercostal arteries draining to the internal thoracic and musculophrenic veins.

RADIOLOGY PEARL

Reflecting the position of neurovascular structures in the subcostal groove immediately inferior to the rib, needle puncture into the pleural space should be through soft tissues immediately above the upper margin of the rib.

RADIOLOGY PEARL

Notching of the inferior margins of the posterior ribs is most frequently seen in postductal coarctation of the aorta (congenital focal stenosis of the thoracic aorta just distal to the left subclavian artery). This rib notching reflects abnormally high pressures in the posterior intercostal arteries as blood flows retrogradely through these vessels in order to bypass the stenotic segment of aorta and drain into the descending thoracic aorta distal to the site of coarctation. The first and second posterior intercostal arteries cannot bypass a postductal coarctation in the aortic arch as they arise proximal to the coarct from the thyrocervical trunk (from the subclavian arteries), so rib notching is seen in the third to eleventh ribs, but not the first and second.

MUSCLES OF THE THORACIC CAGE

The intercostal muscles are made up of the external, internal and innermost intercostal muscles but they cannot be reliably distinguished from each other on imaging and appear as a single muscle group. The intercostal neurovascular bundle runs between the internal and innermost intercostal muscles. Their order from superior to inferior is vein, artery and then nerve (VAN). The transverse thoracic muscle arises on the deep surface of the sternum and adjacent lower costal cartilages and passes superolaterally to the deep surface of the anterior ribs.

Other thoracic cage muscles that can be seen on cross-sectional imaging include the pectoral major and minor muscles anteriorly, the serratus anterior and the teres major laterally, the rhomboids, the erector spinae and trapezius posteriorly and the subclavius and levator scapulae superiorly. The rotator cuff muscles are also well delineated on CT and magnetic resonance imaging (MRI) but not considered part of the thoracic cage. Sternalis is a rare accessory muscle that can be identified on CT and occasionally confused with pathology. It runs craniocaudally along the superficial surface of the sternum just medially to the pectoralis major.

'Companion shadow' is a radiographic term used to denote the smooth, homogeneous, well-defined radiodense stripes that can parallel bones on radiographs. Companion shadows are created by the soft tissues that accompany bones. They are often seen along the superior borders of the clavicles, the medial borders of the scapulae and the inferior margins of the ribs. Rib companion shadows are created by the intercostal fat and soft tissues, primarily the intercostal muscles. Companion shadows can simulate pleural pathology.

THE STERNUM (FIG. 4.5)

The sternum measures up to 17 cm in length and is composed of three components: the manubrium, the body and the xiphoid process.

- The manubrium is a broad polygonal bone making up the upper sternum directly opposite the T3 and T4 vertebral bodies. Its superior notch is known as the suprasternal notch and is usually visible as a surface depression in the skin of the lower neck. Superolateral notches form the sternoclavicular joints, the most superior articulation of the sternum. A pair of notches immediately inferior to

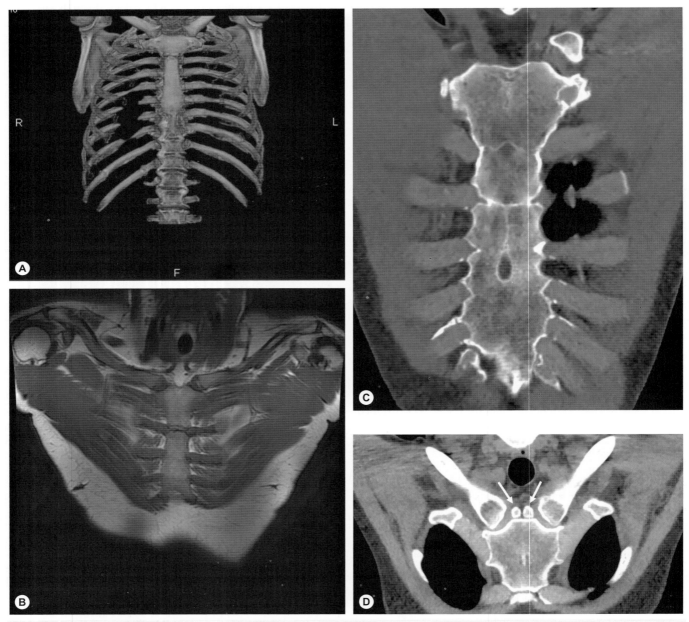

Fig. 4.5 The sternum. (A) Coronal reformatted computed tomography (CT) image of the sternum. (B) Magnetic resonance image of the sternum. (C) Reformatted coronal CT thorax, bone windows. This image demonstrates an unfused sternal body and a sternal foramen, both of which are normal variant anatomy. (D) Coronal CT thorax demonstrating episternal ossicles at the superior aspect of the manubrium of the sternum *(arrows)*.

this are for articulation with the costal cartilage of the first ribs. The manubriosternal joint (also known as the sternal angle or the angle of Louis) is a secondary cartilaginous joint and lies opposite the T4/T5 intervertebral disc space. The second costal cartilage articulates with both the manubrium and the sternal body, centred at the manubriosternal joint. This joint permits little movement and is completely fused in 5%.

- The body of the sternum is a large flat bone opposite T5–T9. The sternal body articulates directly with the third to sixth costal cartilages. It has demifacets superiorly and inferiorly for partial articulation with the second costal cartilage (shared with the manubrium) and the seventh costal cartilage (shared with the xiphoid).
- The xiphoid process (also known as the xiphisternum) usually remains cartilaginous well into adult life but eventually ossifies. The xiphoid usually points inferiorly but can be angled anteriorly (where it can be palpated) or posteriorly.

RADIOLOGY PEARL

The manubriosternal joint, being a secondary cartilaginous joint between the manubrium and body of the sternum, may become inflamed as part of axial seronegative arthropathies such as ankylosing spondylitis.

Ossification of the Sternum

The sternum is made up of six primary ossification centres (one for the manubrium, four for the sternal body and one for the xiphoid), also known as sternebrae. The sternebrae ossify from superior to inferior from 6 months of fetal life onwards with some not yet ossified at birth. Between 15 and 25 years of age, sternebrae fuse from inferior to superior. Incomplete fusion of these ossification centres can result in large sternal foramina (see Fig. 4.5C) which are seen in 5% of the population. These are most commonly seen in the second to fourth sternebrae in the body of the sternum. The xiphoid process fuses with the body at 40 years of age and the body and manubrium fuse in old age, if at all. Accessory ossification centres above the manubrium; episternal ossicles (see Fig. 4.5D), another common variant, are seen in 4%.

RADIOLOGICAL FEATURES OF THE STERNUM

Plain Films

On a frontal chest radiograph, the manubrial borders may simulate mediastinal widening. The remainder of the sternum is not seen. The sternum can be evaluated on lateral and oblique radiographs.

The Diaphragm (Fig. 4.7)

The diaphragm is an anatomically complex, dome-shaped skeletal muscle separating the thorax from the abdomen. In radiology, it is frequently subdivided into the left and right hemidiaphragms but these are descriptive terms for imaging studies and anatomically the diaphragm is a single structure. Unlike typical skeletal muscles, the diaphragm

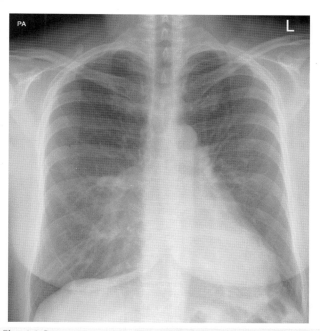

Fig. 4.6 Pectus excavatum. Posteroanterior chest radiograph demonstrating the typical appearance of the pectus excavatum. The right heart border is indistinct and the ribs display a '7' configuration with horizontal posterior ribs and more acute downsloping of the anterior portions of the ribs.

RADIOLOGY PEARL

Variation in sternal configuration includes: (1) depression of the lower end, known as pectus excavatum and (2) prominence of the mid-portion, known as pectus carinatum. Pectus excavatum can be objectively assessed on CT using the Haller index (maximum transverse diameter/narrowest AP length of chest), usually <2. Pectus excavatum causes characteristic findings on chest radiograph including exaggeration of the vertical course of the anterior ribs (7-shaped ribs) and loss of the normal right heart border due to displacement of the heart to the left (Fig. 4.6).

RADIOLOGY PEARL

Reflecting the presence of vascular red marrow within the sternum through adulthood, it is commonly seeded by bloodborne infection or bony metastatic disease, and is a common site for myelomatous deposits.

has a large number of tendinous origins from bones and ligaments around the internal circumference of the lower chest. Rather than having a tendinous insertion into a bone, its numerous muscle fibres converge to insert centrally as a large central tendon within the substance of the muscle itself such that the periphery of the diaphragm is composed of muscle fibres and the centre is composed of tendon. This unique design allows it to pull its centre downwards in inspiration. As previously described, increasing the volume of the thoracic cavity decreases its internal pressure and results in air being drawn into the lungs. The central tendon is, in fact, not central but closer to the sternum.

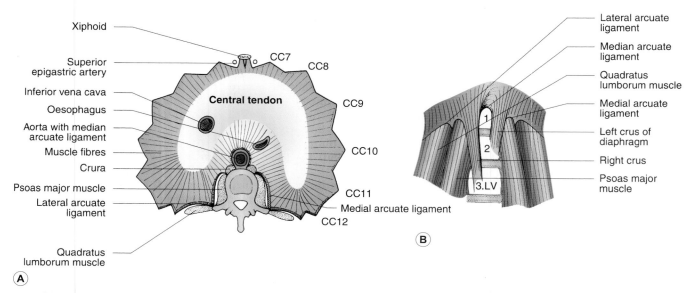

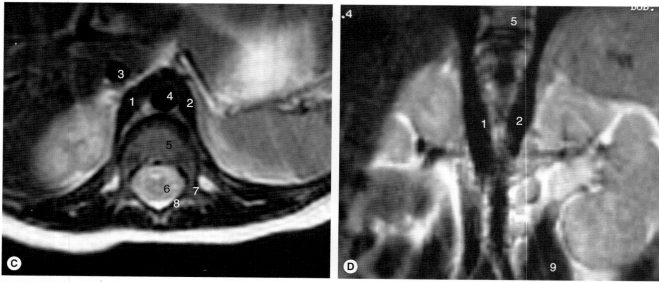

Fig. 4.7 Diaphragm. (A) View from below showing origin and openings; (B) Crura and arcuate ligaments. (C and D) Crura of the diaphragm as seen on axial (C) and coronal (D) magnetic resonance image. *CC*, Costal cartilage; *LV*, lumbar vertebra.

1. Right crus of diaphragm
2. Left crus of diaphragm
3. IVC
4. Aorta
5. Vertebral body

6. Spinal cord
7. Pedicle
8. Lamina
9. Psoas muscle

The multiple peripheral origins of the diaphragm can be grouped into:

Anterior

- Sternal origin: Two small slips from the posterior surface of the xiphisternum make up the sternal origins of the diaphragm.

Lateral

- Costal origin: The costal part of the diaphragm arises in multiple slips from the lower six costal cartilages.

Posterior

- Vertebral origin: Two large tendons called the diaphragmatic crura (singular crus) arise from the left and right sides of the upper lumbar vertebrae. The right crus is longer than the left arising from the lateral aspects of the L1–L3 vertebral bodies. Superior fibres of the right crus encircle the oesophagus as it traverses the diaphragm. The smaller left crus arises from the vertebral body and disc of the L1 and L2 vertebrae. The crura blend with the anterior longitudinal ligament of the spine. Both crura form muscular fibres superiorly which course anteriorly towards the central tendon. These fibres make up a significant portion of the overall diaphragm (the crural portion of the diaphragm).

- Ligamentous origin: Medial and lateral arcuate ligaments also serve as posterior origins for the diaphragm.

They are actually focal fascial thickenings rather than true ligaments. The medial arcuate ligaments are thickenings of the psoas major fascia that extend from the L1/L2 intervertebral discs to the transverse processes of the L1 lumbar vertebra. Medially, they are continuous with the adjacent diaphragmatic crura. The lateral arcuate ligaments extend from the transverse processes of the L1 vertebra to the twelfth ribs and are thickenings of the quadratus lumborum fascia. The median arcuate ligament, also a misnomer, is a single thickened fibrous arch connecting the anterior aspects of the right and left crura in the midline. No portion of the diaphragm arises from the median arcuate ligament.

OPENINGS IN THE DIAPHRAGM

These are as follows:
- Aortic – at level T12: The aorta passes posterior to the diaphragm, between the right and left crura, immediately posterior to the median arcuate ligament rather than through a true opening in the diaphragm. The thoracic duct and the azygos vein pass with the aorta.
- Oesophageal hiatus – at level T10: this is to the left of the midline but is surrounded by fibres of the right crus. With the oesophagus it transmits the right and left vagus nerves, branches of the left gastric artery, veins and lymphatics. Hiatus hernia is a common finding and refers to upward herniation of abdominal contents through the oesophageal hiatus.
- Caval opening – at level T8: transmits the inferior vena cava (IVC), whose adventitial wall is fused with the central tendon, and the right phrenic nerve.
- Behind the medial arcuate ligament – the sympathetic trunk.
- Behind the lateral arcuate ligament – the subcostal nerves and vessels.
- Between sternal and costal origins – the superior epigastric vessels.

RADIOLOGY PEARL

The median arcuate ligament lies immediately anterior to the aorta as it passes from the thorax into the abdomen and the inferior margin of the ligament often abuts the superior margin of the coeliac trunk. When low-lying or thickened, the median arcuate ligament can cause varying levels of stenosis of the proximal coeliac trunk. Median arcuate ligament syndrome is the occurrence of postprandial pain or other symptoms suggestive of coeliac ischaemia in the setting of coeliac stenosis due to compression by the median arcuate ligament. However, asymptomatic stenosis of the coeliac trunk due to the median arcuate ligament is common and this syndrome should not be diagnosed on imaging alone.

STRUCTURES THAT PIERCE THE DIAPHRAGM

The structures that pierce the diaphragm are as follows:

- Terminal branches of the left phrenic nerve pierce the central tendon.
- The greater, lesser and least splanchnic nerves pierce each crus.
- The lymph vessels between the abdomen and thorax pierce the diaphragm throughout, especially posteriorly.

EMBRYOLOGY OF THE DIAPHRAGM

The anterior half of the diaphragm arises from the continuous septum transversum, which ultimately forms the central tendon. The posterior half of the diaphragm forms from left and right pleuroparietal membranes which give rise to the majority of the muscular diaphragm. These membranes are separated by the dorsal oesophageal mesentery which gives rise to the openings in the diaphragm. The pleuroparietal membranes eventually fuse with the septum transversum anteriorly as well as contributions from the thoracic mesoderm posteriorly and posterolaterally, forming a continuous diaphragm. Failure of fusion of the pleuroparietal membranes results in Bochdalek hernias. A congenital fusion defect between the sternum and the septum transversum gives rise to Morgagni hernias. Small anterior and posterior diaphragmatic defects are a common finding at cross-sectional imaging.

BLOOD SUPPLY TO THE DIAPHRAGM

The diaphragm is supplied from its abdominal surface by the inferior phrenic arteries from the abdominal aorta. The costal margins are supplied by the intercostal arteries.

NERVE SUPPLY TO THE DIAPHRAGM

Right and left phrenic nerves from C3 to C5 roots provide the motor supply of the diaphragm. The phrenic nerves descend from the neck along the lateral aspects of the mediastinum and then course from medial to lateral along the central domes of the left and right hemidiaphragms. The phrenic nerves can be visualized on CT coursing along the diaphragms. Sensory impulses from the central part of the diaphragm pass with the phrenic nerves, and those from the peripheral part with the intercostal nerves.

RADIOLOGY PEARL

While the diaphragm is one single structure, the left and right sides are innervated separately by the left and right phrenic nerves, respectively. Hence unilateral diaphragmatic paralysis can occur, and so use of the terms left and right hemidiaphragm is appropriate in the context of imaging interpretation. The highest central portion of a hemidiaphragm is often referred to as the dome of the hemidiaphragm.

RADIOLOGICAL FEATURES OF THE DIAPHRAGM (SEE FIG. 4.7)

Frontal Chest Radiograph (Fig. 4.8)

The central tendon represents the highest portion of the diaphragm; therefore on frontal chest radiographs, the

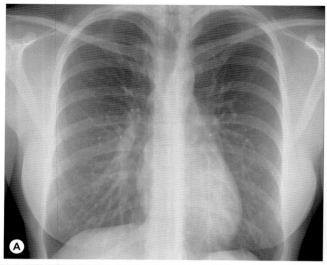

Fig. 4.8 Posteroanterior chest radiograph. (A) Clear. (B) Annotated.

1. Right brachiocephalic vessels *(dark blue dotted line)*
2. Right paratracheal stripe *(purple dotted line)*
3. Azygos vein *(purple circle)*
4. Superior vena cava draining into right atrium *(blue dotted line)*
5. Right hilar point *(red)*
6. Interlobar artery *(green dotted line)*
7. Confluence of the right pulmonary veins with the left atrium *(orange dotted line right side of mediastinum)*
8. Right heart border *(right atrium, red dotted line)*
9. Left paratracheal interface *(commonly made up of the left subclavian artery, dark orange dotted line)*
10. Aortic knuckle *(green dotted line)*
11. Aortopulmonary window *(dark blue dotted line)*
12. Pulmonary trunk *(yellow dotted line)*
13. Left atrial appendage *(light orange dotted line left side of mediastinum)*
14. Left lower lobe pulmonary artery *(turquoise dotted lines)*
15. Left heart border *(left ventricle, purple dotted line left side of mediastinum)*
16. Trachea
17. Left main bronchus
18. Right main bronchus
19. Lateral wall of the descending thoracic aorta
20. Right hemidiaphragm
21. Left hemidiaphragm
22. Right clavicle
23. Companion shadow of the right clavicle
24. Coracoid process of the right scapula

medial portion of the diaphragm is higher than the lateral portions, and the anterior portions are higher than the posterior. The dome of the hemidiaphragm should be at least 1.5 cm above a straight line from the medial cardiophrenic angle to the lateral costophrenic angle. The right hemidiaphragm is typically higher than the left by approximately 2 cm. The left hemidiaphragm can be higher than the right in the normal subject, especially with gas in the colon, but causes of abnormal diaphragmatic elevation should be considered in this case. Position of the diaphragm relative to the ribs on PA chest radiographs is often used to evaluate for hyperinflation of the lungs. Due to the inferior angulation of the anterior ribs, more of the posterior ribs will project above the diaphragm than anterior ribs. True position of the anterior ribs relative to the diaphragm may be more accurate than the posterior ribs, as the apex of the diaphragm is nearer to the anterior ribs and to the detector (on PA chest radiographs), and is therefore less subject to distortion by magnification or beam angulation. Typically, up to 10 posterior ribs and 6 anterior ribs project above the hemidiaphragms and an increase in this number can indicate hyperinflation. However, this should be interpreted with caution given the natural asymmetry of the left and right hemidiaphragm position. Additionally, the diaphragm can be significantly depressed in maximal inspiration in normal health, particularly in young athletic individuals. Loss of the normal convexity is a more accurate marker of hyperinflation; this is easier to judge on lateral chest radiographs.

Lateral Chest Radiograph (Fig. 4.9)

On lateral chest radiographs, the right and left hemidiaphragms appear as smooth interfaces between the inferior lungs and the upper abdomen. They are highest anteriorly and course inferiorly towards the posterior costophrenic recesses. It can be surprisingly difficult to distinguish the left from the right hemidiaphragm, but the following anatomical details can help to identify them:

- A portion of the left ventricle sits on the medial left hemidiaphragm. This will obscure the anterior 20%–30% of the left hemidiaphragm silhouette, whereas the dome of the right hemidiaphragm does not abut the heart and can usually be traced anteriorly to the anterior chest wall. This is typically the most reliable differentiator. As lateral chest radiographs are conventionally acquired with the left chest wall adjacent to the detector, the right hemithorax will be magnified by up to 10% due to its distance from the detector by the diverging X-ray beam. This causes the right posterior costophrenic angle to project more inferiorly and posteriorly than the left. The hemidiaphragm, which can be traced to the more posteroinferior costophrenic angle, is usually the right.
- The IVC may be seen piercing the right dome.
- Air within the gastric fundus lies under the left diaphragm. It is often more anterior than you might think.

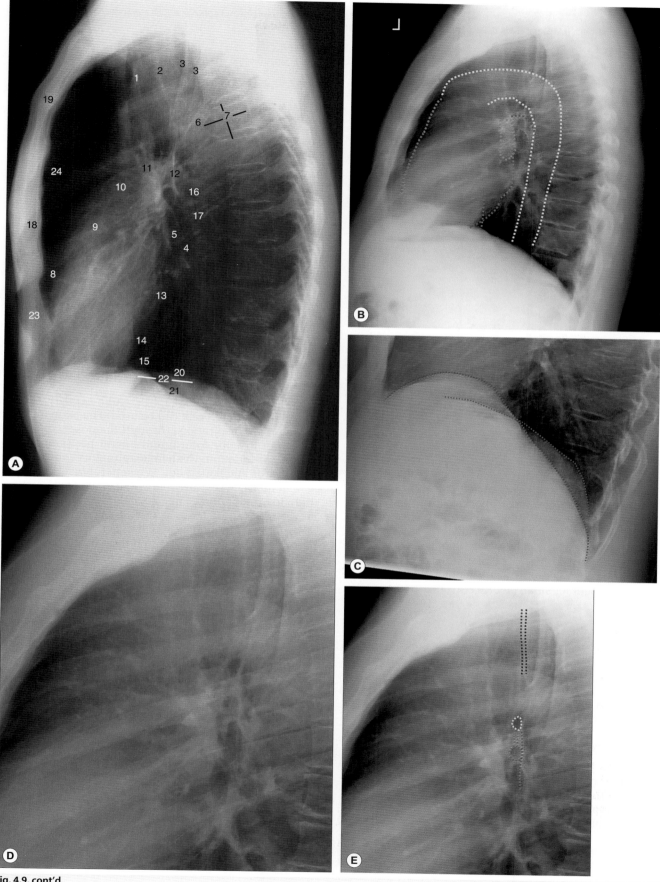

Fig. 4.9, cont'd

Fig. 4.9 (A) Lateral chest radiograph. (B) Lateral chest radiograph. (C) Lateral chest radiograph: Hemidiaphragms. (D) Lateral chest radiograph, zoomed in on superior aspect. (E) Lateral chest radiograph, zoomed in on superior aspect, annotated.

(A)
1. Anterior wall of the trachea
2. Posterior tracheal stripe
3. Scapulae
4. Left lower lobe bronchus
5. Right lower lobe bronchus
6. Aorta (not well seen)
7. Vertebral body of T4
8. Anterior aspect of the right ventricle
9. Pulmonary outflow tract
10. Main pulmonary artery
11. Right pulmonary artery
12. Left pulmonary artery
13. Left atrium
14. Left ventricle
15. Inferior vena cava
16. Horizontal (minor) fissure
17. Oblique (major) fissure
18. Sternum
19. Manubriosternal joint
20. Left hemidiaphragm
21. Right hemidiaphragm
22. Stomach bubble
23. Lung projected anterior to sternum in intercostal space
24. Retrosternal airspace

(B)
Red line: Anterior wall of right ventricle
Light blue line: Right ventricular outflow tract
Yellow lines: Thoracic aorta
Purple lines: Left pulmonary artery
Orange circle: Right Pulmonary artery
Green line: Left atrium
Pink line: Left ventricle
Dark blue line: Inferior vena cava

(C)
Blue line: Left hemidiaphragm
Red line: Right hemidiaphragm

(E)
Blue lines: Posterior tracheal stripe
Yellow circle: Right upper lobe bronchus
Green circle: Left upper lobe bronchus
Purple line: Posterior wall of the bronchus intermedius

There is apparent thickness of the diaphragm on radiographs:
- With the pleura and peritoneum when there is air in the peritoneum: 2–3 mm thick.
- With the pleura and fundal wall of stomach: 5–8 mm thick.

> **RADIOLOGY PEARL**
>
> The posterior costophrenic angle (visible on a lateral chest radiograph) lies more inferiorly than the lateral costophrenic angle (visible on frontal chest radiograph), making it the most dependent portion of the pleural space and the point where fluid will collect first in the standing position. Therefore lateral chest radiographs are considerably more sensitive than frontal in the assessment for small pleural effusions.

Curvature of the Dome

Similar to the frontal radiograph, the perpendicular height of the dome of the diaphragm from a line between the posterior costophrenic and the anterior cardiophrenic angles should be at least 1.5 cm. Flattening of the hemidiaphragm is typically the most sensitive assessment for hyperinflation.

Fluoroscopy

Continuous fluoroscopy can be used to assess normal diaphragmatic movement. The range of movement of the diaphragm with respiration is as follows:
- Quiet respiration: 1 cm
- Deep inspiration/expiration: 4 cm (wide range of normal)

In each case the left hemidiaphragm moves more than the right. The variation of the diaphragm with posture is as follows:
- Supine: higher
- Lateral decubitus: dome on the dependent side is higher

In cases of suspected diaphragmatic paralysis (phrenic nerve palsy), a sniff test can be used. The patient is asked to take rapid inspirations through the nose (sniffs) while screening in both frontal and lateral positions. In normal motor function, the hemidiaphragms contract/move downwards and flatten out. When paralyzed, the affected hemidiaphragm can remain stable or move upwards (paradoxical motion). The reason for paradoxical upward movement is the accessory muscles of inspiration, which are still functional. These will still contract with sniffing, increasing the volume and decreasing the pressure within the hemithorax. As the affected hemidiaphragm is paralyzed, it can no longer resist the pressure drop and is drawn upwards.

> **RADIOLOGY PEARL**
>
> Eventration is focal thinning of a portion of the diaphragm resulting in upward ballooning of a portion of the diaphragm. This is a common finding, most commonly seen in the anteromedial right hemidiaphragm. This can be confused with diaphragmatic paralysis as well as other pathologies.

Ultrasound

The diaphragm is readily imaged by ultrasound, using the liver or spleen as an acoustic window. It is seen as an echogenic line outlining the upper surface of these organs. The diaphragmatic interdigitations may occasionally be pronounced to give the spurious impression of an echogenic mass on the surface of the liver.

Computed Tomography

Portions of the diaphragm, in particular the dome of the right hemidiaphragm adjacent to the liver, are frequently indistinguishable from the adjacent viscera. The costal and posterior origins of the diaphragm are usually well delineated. The costal origins frequently form well-defined slips rather than a continuous structure. When these slips are large, they can indent the lateral aspect of the liver, simulating a nodular liver contour. The right and left crura are usually visible on the anterior surface of the upper lumbar vertebrae and can be confused with lymph nodes. Defects in the posterior (ligamentous) portions of the diaphragms are common, seen in at least 1% of cases.

> **RADIOLOGY PEARL**
>
> On axial CT scans of the upper abdomen in healthy subjects, the abdominal viscera, particularly the gastric fundus and liver, are separated from the posterior abdominal wall by intact posterior diaphragm. Following diaphragmatic rupture, the gastric fundus or liver fall to lie immediately against the posterior abdominal wall, the so called 'dependent viscera sign'.

Magnetic Resonance Imaging (see Fig. 4.7)

This technique yields excellent sagittal and coronal images of the diaphragm as a thin muscular septum of intermediate signal intensity. The crura are elegantly displayed on coronal images.

The Pleura (Fig. 4.10)

The pleura is a serous membranous closed sac that has two components:
- The visceral pleura, the inner layer covering the lung and extending between the lobes of the lungs into the major, minor and accessory fissures.
- The parietal pleura, the outer layer adherent to the inner thoracic wall and mediastinum. Parts of the pleura and pleural space are named according to site, for example costal, diaphragmatic, mediastinal and apical.

The visceral pleura conforms to the contour of the lung and changes dynamically with inspiration/expiration. The position of the parietal pleura is fixed and extends deeper into the costophrenic and costomediastinal recesses than do the lungs and visceral pleura (see Table 4.1 for lower limits of lungs and pleura). The parietal pleura is supplied by the systemic vessels. The visceral pleura receives arterial supply from both the bronchial and the pulmonary circulation.

INFERIOR PULMONARY LIGAMENTS

The lung roots/hila are surrounded by pleura, which is the continuation of the visceral pleura lining the medial surface of the lung and the parietal pleura lining the lateral aspect of the mediastinum. This pleura is closely adherent to the superior, anterior and lateral surfaces of the hilar structures but inferiorly the double layer of pleura continues caudally to the diaphragm as the inferior pulmonary ligaments. The

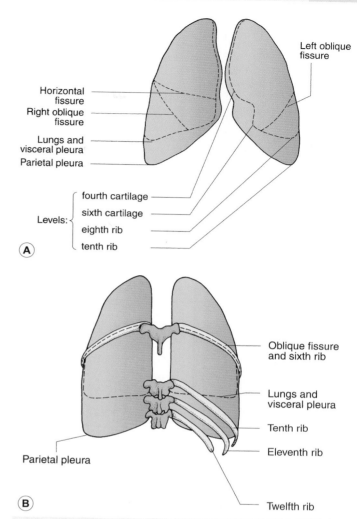

Fig. 4.10 Pleura. (A) Anterior view. (B) Posterior view.

inferior pulmonary ligaments contain lymphatic tissue including lymph nodes as well as connective tissue and the diaphragmatic courses of the phrenic nerves. They allow the lung root to move with respiration and also for distension of the pulmonary veins, which lie inferiorly in the lung root. The inferior pulmonary ligaments therefore divide the medial portion of the pleura space, below the level of the hila, into anterior and posterior compartments. The inferior pulmonary ligaments can usually be identified on CT.

> **RADIOLOGY PEARL**
>
> The lower limits of the parietal pleura are more inferior than is intuitive, particularly when there is a shallow depth of inspiration and there is a large distance (up to 5 cm) between the inferior-most parietal pleural reflection and the lung. This is an important consideration when planning intercostal approaches to upper abdominal interventions as the parietal pleura will commonly be traversed. As long as the visceral pleura (lung) is not traversed, pneumothorax would not be expected but traversing the pleural space with a needle or catheter creates a temporary communication between the abdominal and pleural cavities, potentially contaminating the pleural space with infection/tumour.

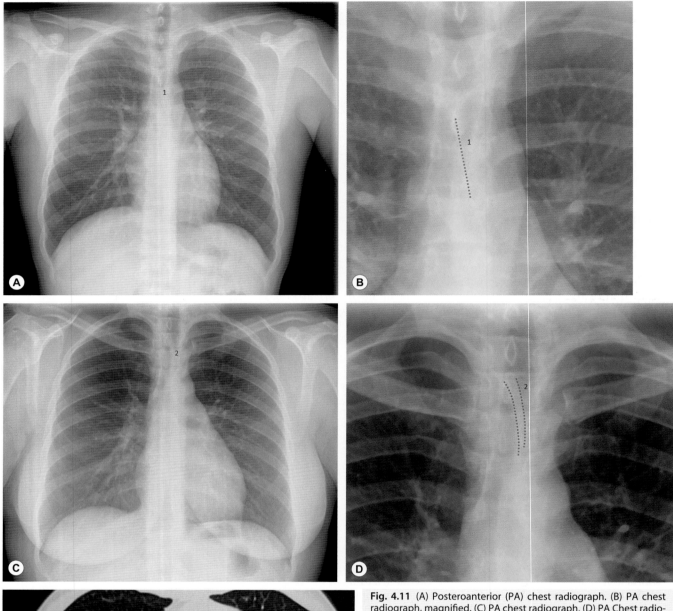

Fig. 4.11 (A) Posteroanterior (PA) chest radiograph. (B) PA chest radiograph, magnified. (C) PA chest radiograph. (D) PA Chest radiograph, magnified. (E) Axial high-resolution CT scan of lungs which shows fissures as fine white lines *(arrows)*.

(A)
1. Anterior Junction Line

(B)
1. Anterior junction line (blue), four layers of pleura, 24.5%–57% of frontal chest radiographs.

(C)
2. Posterior junction line, four layers of pleura, more fat – more of a stripe, 32% of posteroanterior chest radiographs.

(D)
2. Posterior Junction Line (purple)

Table 4.1   Lower Limits of Lung and Pleura at Rest

	Visceral Pleura and Lung	Parietal Pleura
Anterior	6th costal cartilage	7th costal cartilage
Midaxillary line	8th rib	10th rib
Posterior T10	T10	T12

The healthy pleural space is continuous throughout the hemithorax and so the position of air or fluid in the pleural space is related to patient position and gravity. In supine position, pleural air will collect along the anterior chest wall, predominantly at the anterior costophrenic recess. In standing position, pleural air will collect at the apex of the pleural space and laterally in the lateral decubitus position.

RADIOLOGICAL FEATURES OF THE PLEURA

Radiography

As with all structures, the pleura is only visible on a chest radiograph if a sufficient amount of it is tangential to the X-ray beam to attenuate the beam and if there are structures of a different density (non-soft tissue) adjacent to it. As the pleura is a very thin structure, it is often not visible on chest radiography and its position has to be inferred.

The pleura may be visible in a normal subject at:

- Fissures that are tangential to the X-ray beam, which varies with frontal and lateral views (see interlobar fissures section).
- Sites where the parietal pleura lies on prominent extrapleural fat.
- Junction lines (or junctional lines): Formed by the apposition of the pleural layers ± intervening mediastinal fat where both lungs meet, these lines will not necessarily be visible on all normal chest X-rays (CXRs; see Figs. 4.8 and 4.11):
  - Anterior junction line: Formed by the lungs meeting anteromedially anterior to the arch of the aorta. This line courses obliquely across the upper two thirds of the sternum on a PA chest radiograph and should not extend above the manubriosternal joint.
  - Posterior junction line: Formed by the lungs meeting posteromedially, which is more superiorly located compared to the anterior junction line. This line may be seen above the clavicles, projected over the trachea to the level of the aortic arch.

The anterior junction line, when visible, can serve as an important marker of midline shift in a tension pneumothorax as it puts up much less resistance to free air than the mediastinum.

While the pleura usually abuts the ribs on one side and the lung on the other side (both structures are of a different density to the soft tissue-density pleura), it cannot usually be discerned from the high-density bones. Prominent low-density fat in the extrapleural space, when abundant enough, can provide enough contrast to resolve the pleura. Similarly, when a pneumothorax is present, the air in the pleural space provides contrast, so the radiodense line that you can see is the visceral pleura rather than just the edge of the lung parenchyma. Identifying this thin white line is essential in distinguishing a pneumothorax from a skin fold.

Radiology parlance with regard to the pleura can be confusing. The use of the "pleural" to describe a lesion should be reserved for lesions that directly arise from or involve the pleura. The term 'subpleural' is a localizing term to describe something that is in close proximity to the pleura but without arising from it. "Peripheral" is the preferred term for such lesions however subpleural is commonly used. A lesion that does not arise from the pleura, but has contact with it, should be described as "pleura-based".

A glossary of terminology for thoracic imaging has been published by the Fleischner Society, and can be a helpful reference when interpreting thoracic imaging. If you think something is arising from the either the lung parenchyma or the pleura, say so! If you are unsure, say that you are unsure and just describe the location.

CT of the Pleura

As with radiographs, the pleura can also be very difficult to identify on CT and the pleura cannot usually be distinguished from the thoracic wall or mediastinum unless it is thickened. It will be reliably seen in the same locations as on radiographs (fissures, junction lines and adjacent to extrapleural fat). Due to CT's ability to be reconstructed in any plane, all fissures will be visible on CT, regardless of orientation. The inferior pulmonary ligaments are also usually visible on CT extending below the inferior pulmonary vein caudally and posteriorly to the diaphragm. The right inferior pulmonary ligament lies close to the IVC, whereas the left lies close to the oesophagus.

The pleura usually enhances most vividly with contrast after a delay of 70 seconds (not the typical scanning delay of a routine CT thorax). A delayed protocol could be employed to try and highlight pleural pathology.

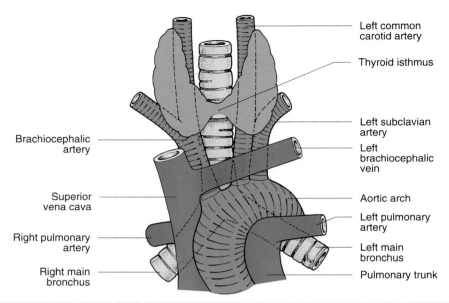

Fig. 4.12 Trachea and main bronchi: anterior relations.

The Extrapleural Space

The extrapleural space is the space external to the pleura, located between the parietal pleura and the inner margin of the ribs. It usually contains, fat, lymphatic tissue including lymph nodes, blood vessels and the innermost intercostal muscles. Typically, it is difficult to visualize the extrapleural space at radiography and cross-sectional imaging unless distended with fat (common in obesity and corticosteroid treatment). It is not a common site of primary pathology and often overlooked, but is commonly involved by pathological process arising from the chest wall or pleura.

RADIOLOGY PEARL

Prominent extrapleural fat simulates pleural thickening/pathology on chest radiographs; however it will be of a lower (fat) density.

The Trachea and Bronchi (Figs. 4.12 and 4.13)

THE TRACHEA

The trachea is the inferior continuation of the respiratory tract beyond the larynx. It begins at the lower border of the cricoid cartilage at the level of the C6 vertebra. It extends to the **carina**, the point where it divides into the left and right main bronchi, at the level of the sternal angle (T5 level, T4 on inspiration and T6 on expiration). The trachea is 15 cm long and 2 cm in diameter. Its inner layer consists of ciliated columnar epithelium which circumferentially lines its anterior, lateral and posterior walls. Fifteen to twenty thick, but incomplete rings of cartilage are present in the walls of the trachea outside the mucosa. These cartilage rings protect

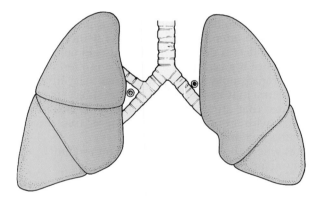

Fig. 4.13 Diagrammatic representation of normal anatomy: situs solitus.

the anterior and lateral walls of the trachea (the cartilaginous trachea). The posterior wall of the trachea is devoid of cartilage and is lined by a longitudinal muscle called the trachealis instead. The posterior wall of the trachea is also known as the membranous trachea and can freely collapse inwards into the lumen of the trachea whereas the cartilaginous trachea is a solid fixed structure.

Relations of the Trachea

Cervical (see Figs 1.34, 1.35). The anterior relations are as follows:

- Anterior:
  - Isthmus of thyroid anterior to the second, third and fourth rings
  - Inferior thyroid veins
  - Strap muscles: sternohyoid and sternothyroid
- Posterior:
  - Oesophagus (often left posterolateral at the 4 or 5 o'clock position)

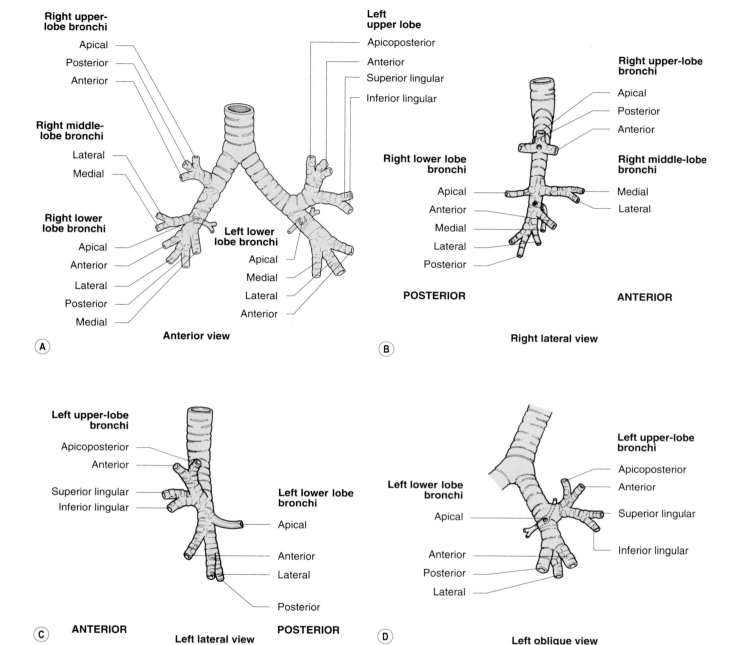

Fig. 4.14 Bronchial tree – main and segmental anatomy as seen on bronchography. (A) Anterior view. (B) Right lateral view. (C) Left lateral view. (D) Left oblique view.

- Lateral:
  - Left and right lobes of the thyroid gland
  - Common carotid artery
  - Recurrent laryngeal nerves
  - Inferior thyroid arteries

Thoracic (see Fig. 4.9). The thoracic relations are as follows:

- Anterior:
  - Brachiocephalic trunk and left common carotid arteries
  - Anterior jugular veins
  - Left brachiocephalic vein
  - Arch of the aorta
- Posterior:
  - Oesophagus (again, usually left posterolateral)
  - Left recurrent laryngeal nerve
- Left lateral:
  - Left common carotid and left subclavian arteries
  - Left recurrent laryngeal nerve
- Right lateral:
  - Right innominate vein/superior vena cava (SVC)
  - Right vagus nerve
  - Arch of the azygos vein
  - Pleura (in direct contact unlike the other side)

Blood Supply of the Trachea

The upper trachea is supplied by the inferior thyroid artery and the lower part is supplied by branches of the bronchial arteries. Venous drainage is to the inferior thyroid venous plexus.

RADIOLOGY PEARL

Tracheal deviation on a chest radiograph occurs with asymmetrical changes in volume between the hemithoraces. For example, in the case of volume loss (e.g. **pulmonary fibrosis) the trachea may deviate towards the abnormality, whereas in pathologies with volume expansion** (e.g. **pneumothorax) the trachea will deviate away from the abnormality**.

RADIOLOGY PEARL

The dynamic nature of the carina is an important consideration in positioning of the tip of an endotracheal tube. A tube tip that projects close to the carina in inspiration may enter into one of the main bronchi in expiration. Some radiologists use 3 cm above the carina as the minimum safe distance for endotracheal tube tip position.

AIRWAYS (FIG. 4.14)

'Airways' is a collective term for the bronchi and bronchioles (the trachea can be included in this term but is often considered separately). Like the anatomy of the lung parenchyma, there is significant asymmetry between the airway anatomy of the left and right lungs. The airway of a right or a left lung follows a general blueprint but there is a large amount of variation from one person to the next. Airways undergo successive divisions into two or more smaller calibre airways with 23 divisions between the trachea and the alveoli. The airways branch in tandem with the pulmonary artery branches which lie immediately adjacent to them. Successive airway divisions can be referred to as successive 'generations' with the first, second and third generations representing the main bronchi, the lobar and the segmental bronchi based on the unit of lung they supply. All generations distal to the segmental bronchi can be termed the subsegmental airways. An airway is designated a bronchus (plural = bronchi) based on the presence of cartilage in its submucosa (this cartilage is C-shaped like in the trachea and serves to keep the airway patent). An airway lacking cartilage is referred to as a bronchiole (plural – bronchioles or bronchioli) and they maintain their patency through the elastic recoil of the surrounding parenchyma. Bronchioles begin around the sixth-generation airways. The diameter of an airway depends on its generation and the wall thickness depends on its diameter. CT can only resolve airways with a diameter of 2 mm and a wall thickness of 0.2–0.3 mm, so the vast majority of bronchioles cannot be seen on CT. These bronchioles are referred to as 'small airways'.

RADIOLOGY PEARL

Airways in the peripheral lungs, within 1 cm of the pleura, have undergone numerous divisions and should have a diameter and wall thickness that cannot be resolved with current CT resolution. Visualization of the lumen of an airway within 1 cm of the pleura is abnormal and can be termed bronchiolectasis.

Carina

The carina is the bifurcation of the trachea into the left and right main bronchi and typically lies at the level of the T4/T5 intervertebral disc (also the level of the manubriosternal joint) but moves significantly with breathing (T4 on inspiration and as low as T6 on expiration). The carinal angle measures approximately 65 degrees – that is, 20 degrees to the right of the midline and 40 degrees to the left. This asymmetry gives the right main bronchus a more vertical downward course and the left main bronchus a more horizontal course. This angle is slightly larger in children. The carinal angle increases by 10 degrees to 15 degrees in recumbency.

RADIOLOGY PEARL

Widening of the carinal angle on a PA chest radiograph above 65 degrees can be a marker of enlargement of the left atrium and the carinal angle should be considered before calling a heart enlarged on chest radiograph.

RIGHT MAIN BRONCHUS

The right main bronchus courses from the mediastinum into the lung along with the pulmonary vessels and lymphatics but has already divided by the time it reaches the root of the lung (rounded opening in the medial aspect of the lung devoid of pleura/interstitium that transmits major structures). As the trachea and carina lie slightly to the right of midline, the right main bronchus is shorter and more vertically orientated than the left main bronchus, measuring 2.5 cm in length and forming an angle of about 25 degrees to the vertical median (left main bronchus: 5 cm long and 40-degree angle). It is also a wider bronchus measuring 1.5 cm in diameter versus 1.2 cm on the left. The course of the right main bronchus lies posteriorly and parallel to the right main pulmonary artery. This fact helps identify it on both lateral chest radiographs and sagittal CTs.

Relations of the Right Main Bronchus

The relations of the right main bronchus are as follows:
- Anterior:
  - SVC
  - Right main pulmonary artery
- Posterior:
  - Azygos vein
- Superior:
  - Azygos arch

The right main bronchus gives rise to three lobar bronchi supplying the upper, middle and lower lobes of the right lung. The bronchus to the upper lobe is also known as the eparterial bronchus (epi – above). This arises from the superior aspect of the right main bronchus and it is the only one of the lobar bronchi on either side to branch above the level of a main pulmonary artery. This is important as it is a consistent marker of right-sided pulmonary anatomy. Determining whether a lung has the correct anatomy for the side of the body that it is on can be important in congenital anomalies. The right upper lobe bronchus arises almost immediately after the tracheal bifurcation and enters the hilum of the lung separately to the bronchus intermedius. The right upper lobe bronchus then trifurcates into the apical, anterior and posterior segmental branches. The short segment of combined bronchus distal to the branching of the right upper lobe bronchus and before the division into the right middle and lower lobar bronchi is called the bronchus intermedius. This airway courses almost directly inferiorly so it is identifiable on a lateral radiograph as it is tangential to the beam.

The lobar bronchi divide into segmental bronchi supplying the bronchopulmonary segments of each lobe along with a corresponding pulmonary arterial branch. There are 10 bronchopulmonary segments in total in the right lung.

Right upper lobe bronchus segmental divisions:
- Apical
- Posterior
- Anterior

Right middle lobe bronchus segmental divisions:
- Lateral
- Medial

Right lower lobe bronchus segmental divisions:
- Superior (this comes off opposite to the right middle lobe bronchus)
- Medial
- Anterior
- Lateral
- Posterior

LEFT MAIN BRONCHUS

The left main bronchus is twice as long as the right main bronchus (5 cm vs 2.5 cm), having to travel to the left lung from the right side of the mediastinum. It courses more horizontally than the left (40 degrees from vertical vs 25 degrees) and it is narrower (1.2 cm vs 1.5 cm). The left main bronchus also courses more posteriorly than the right main bronchus, which is more or less parallel to the horizontal in the axial plane. This explains its more posterior position than the right on a lateral chest radiograph. In contrast to the right main bronchus, the left main bronchus travels inferior to the left main pulmonary artery rather than posterior to it. The left main pulmonary artery runs from posterior to anterior, almost perpendicular to the left main bronchus. This pattern of the left main pulmonary artery running over the top of the left main bronchus distinguishes the left hilum from the right where the bronchus and artery run in parallel with the vessel anteriorly and the airway posteriorly.

Relations of the Left Main Bronchus

The relations of the left main bronchus are as follows:
Anterior:
- Pulmonary trunk
Posterior:
- Oesophagus
- Descending aorta
Superior:
- Aortic arch
- Left main pulmonary artery

The left main bronchus divides into the left upper and lower lobar bronchi within the lung (distal to the root of the left lung). The hyparterial bronchus (hyp – below) describes a segmental bronchus branching below the level of the main pulmonary artery. 'Hyparterial' could technically describe all segmental bronchi except the eparterial right upper lobe bronchus, but the term hyparterial bronchus conventionally refers to the left upper lobe bronchus to highlight the difference between left- and right-sided airway anatomy. Again, this can be helpful in cases of congenital anomalies. There are 8 left bronchopulmonary segments and corresponding bronchi in comparison to the right lung's 10.

Left upper lobe bronchus segmental divisions:
- Apicoposterior: The posterior and apical segmental bronchi usually have a common apicoposterior bronchus, which then subdivides into separate apical and posterior segmental branches.
- Anterior.
- Lingular bronchus comes off the upper lobe bronchus. This divides into:
  - Superior lingular segment
  - Inferior lingular segment.
Left lower lobe bronchus segmental divisions:
- Superior
- Anteromedial
- Lateral
- Posterior

The anatomy of the bronchial tree is shown diagrammatically in Fig. 4.14. Naming basal bronchi laterally to medially is easier if the constant relationship of anterior, lateral and posterior (ALP) is remembered, with only the medial bronchus in the right lung changing its relative position.

RADIOLOGY PEARL

Mnemonics for memorizing the bronchial divisions and their associated bronchopulmonary segments:
- Right lung: **A PALM Seed Makes A Little Palm**
- Left lung: **ASIA ALPS**

BRONCHIAL VARIANT ANATOMY (FIG. 4.15)

- A cardiac bronchus is an anatomical variant bronchus projecting medially (towards the heart) arising from the bronchus intermedius. In 50% of cases, the cardiac bronchus is a short rudimentary blind-ending bronchus.
- A tracheal bronchus is a bronchus arising from the trachea before it bifurcates at the carina. This typically

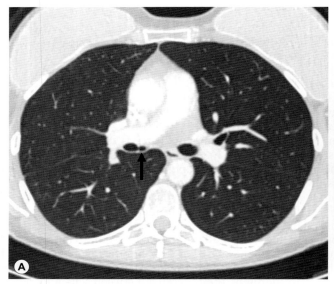

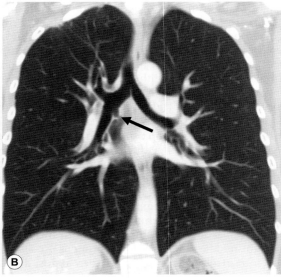

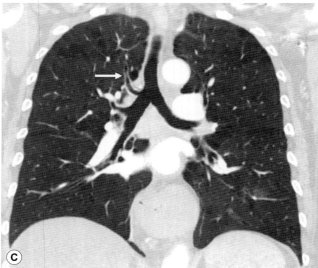

Fig. 4.15 Bronchial variant anatomy. (A) Axial computed tomography (CT) thorax. B) Coronal CT thorax, lung windows. Cardiac bronchus arising medially from the bronchus intermedius *(black arrow)*. (C) Coronal CT thorax with contrast demonstrating a normal variant accessory tracheal bronchus *(white arrow)* supplying the apical segment of the right.

supplies at least a portion of the right upper lobe (usually the apical segment). The tracheal bronchus is usually a displaced rather than accessory bronchus. If the tracheal bronchus supplies the right upper lobe it is termed a 'pig bronchus' or 'bronchus suis', as this is the typical anatomy for the airways of the pig.

RADIOLOGY PEARL

When blind ending, a cardiac bronchus can easily opacify with mucus and simulate a necrotic subcarinal lymph node.

RADIOLOGY PEARL

As the tracheal bronchus arises above the carina, an endotracheal tube can occlude its orifice causing seemingly unexplained right upper lobe collapse. This fact, along with its fun association with swine, make it an absolute favourite of examiners.

BLOOD SUPPLY

The lungs receive dual blood supply. Ninety-nine percent of the blood to the lungs is deoxygenated blood from the pulmonary arteries for gas exchange. The bronchial arteries (which derive their name from the fact that they follow the course of the bronchi) deliver 1% of blood flow to the lungs in the form of oxygenated blood from the left heart and provide nutritive supply to multiple structures including the pulmonary interstitium, pleura, larger vessel walls, a portion of the oesophagus as well as the bronchi and bronchioles.

Bronchial artery anatomy is highly variable in both number of vessels and the origin of those vessels.

The typical (orthotopic) bronchial artery arises from the descending thoracic aorta between T5 and T6 (just below the level of the carina). A typical bronchial artery may arise directly from the descending thoracic aorta as an individual vessel or share a short common stem with a posterior intercostal artery (an intercostobronchial trunk) and then branch into separate intercostal and bronchial arteries.

Bronchial arteries are considered atypical or ectopic if they branch outside of this location, most commonly arising from the more proximal aortic arch or the right third intercostal artery. Bronchial arteries may also arise from the subclavian artery or from its internal thoracic branch. Seventy percent of people have one right and two left bronchial arteries, with the most common configuration being the right bronchial artery arising from an intercostobronchial trunk from the right lateral aspect of the descending thoracic aorta and the two left arteries arising directly from the anterior and left lateral aspect of the descending thoracic aorta between T5 and T6.

Normal bronchial arteries are small-calibre vessels measuring between 0.5 and 1.5 mm and so can be difficult to see on CT but they usually can be identified on a CT angiogram with modern scanners.

The bronchial arteries can be visualized with greater accuracy using digital subtraction angiography, usually performing a descending aortogram close to the level of T5/T6.

The bronchial arteries are responsible for 90% of cases of massive haemoptysis, and catheter angiography has the benefit of allowing therapeutic embolization.

BRONCHIAL VEINS

Tissues supplied by the bronchial arteries drain via the bronchial veins. Bronchial veins form two distinct systems. The deep veins form a network of veins around the pulmonary interstitium and communicate freely with the pulmonary veins. They also form a bronchial vein trunk that drains to the pulmonary system. The superficial bronchial veins drain to the azygos vein on the right side and to the accessory hemiazygos vein on the left side.

RADIOLOGY PEARL

The bronchial arteries hypertrophy (diameter >2 mm) and become more tortuous in response to increased requirements by their target organs. Bronchiectasis is a particularly common cause of bronchial artery hypertrophy. They can also deliver blood for gas exchange when blood flow to the lung is reduced, for example in chronic thromboembolism. This phenomenon is called parasitization of the bronchial arteries.

RADIOLOGY PEARL

A major complication of bronchial artery embolization is transverse myelitis as embolic particles can occlude spinal arteries arising from the posterior intercostal arteries (considering many bronchials arise from intercostobrachial trunks). The artery of Adamkiewicz, the largest anterior medullary branch of the anterior spinal artery, has a variable origin. Embolization of this vessel can have devastating consequences and must be avoided at all costs. This artery usually arises from a left posterior intercostal artery between T8 and T12 and rarely from the typical location of the bronchial arteries (T5–T6 region).

RADIOLOGICAL FEATURES

The radiological features of the trachea and bronchi are discussed in the following section on the lungs.

The Lungs (Fig. 4.16)

The lungs are described as having costal, mediastinal, apical and diaphragmatic surfaces with the lung roots/hila on the mediastinal surfaces. The lungs are subdivided into lobes by the branching pattern of the lobar bronchi. The lobes are partially encased in their own visceral pleura covering, creating the interlobar fissures that separate them. The right lung has three lobes: the right upper, middle and lower lobes. The left lung has two lobes: the left upper and

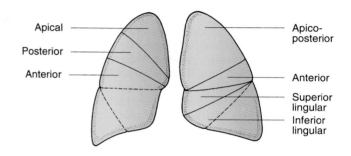

(A)   **Upper lobes**

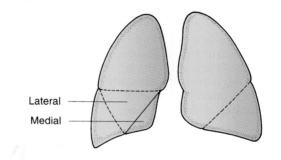

(B)   **Middle lobe**

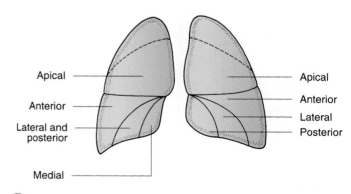

(C)   **Lower lobes**

Fig. 4.16 Bronchopulmonary segments as seen on posteroanterior chest radiograph. (A) Upper lobes. (B) Middle lobes. (C) Lower lobes.

lower lobes, with the lingula of the left upper lobe analogous to the right middle lobe but typically not separated by its own pleural covering.

INTERLOBAR FISSURES (SEE FIG. 4.10)

The depth of fissures varies from a superficial slit to complete separation of lobes. The major and minor fissures are made up of two separate but adjacent layers of visceral pleura.

The Oblique (Major) Fissure

On the left, the major fissure separates the left upper lobe from the left lower lobe. On the right, the major fissure separates the right upper and middle lobes from the right lower lobe (with the posterosuperior right major fissure separating right upper and lower lobes and the anteroinferior portion separating the right middle and lower lobes). The major fissures are not straight flat membranes as they are often depicted. They have undulating, sine wave-like shapes in both the coronal and sagittal plane. The highest point of the left major fissure is more superior than the right beginning at T3/T4 on the left and T4 (just above the carina) on the right. This gives the left major fissure a slightly more vertical course when viewed side-on. Above the level of the hilum, the medial aspects of the major fissures are higher than the lateral, whereas below the hilum the medial portion lies more inferior than the lateral. The anterior portion of the major fissures parallel the anterior arcs of the sixth ribs bilaterally. The medial aspects of the major fissures course to the roots of the lungs bilaterally.

The Transverse (Transverse/Minor) Fissure

The minor fissure is understood to refer to the right-sided horizontal/transverse fissure, without having to specify laterality. It separates the upper and middle lobes of the right lung. It runs horizontally from the hilum to the anterior and lateral surfaces of the right lung at the level of the fourth costal cartilage. Its posterior limit is the right oblique fissure, which it meets at the level of the sixth rib in the midaxillary line if viewed from the side. It is anatomically complete in only one-third of subjects and is absent in 10%.

ACCESSORY FISSURES

The Azygos Fissure (Fig. 4.17)

This is in fact a downward invagination of the azygos vein through the apical portion of the right upper lobe due to embryological descent of the azygos arch through the lung rather than through the mediastinum. It therefore drags with it four pleural layers – two visceral and two parietal – folded in on themselves. The term 'azygos lobe' describes the portion of the right upper lobe medial to the azygos fissure, but the term is inappropriate as there is no corresponding change in lobar architecture. An accessory azygos fissure is reported to be present in up to 1% of the population.

The Superior Accessory Fissure

The superior accessory fissure can occur on either side but is more common in the right lower lobe. When present, the superior accessory fissure separates the superior segment of the lower lobe from other basal segments. It lies parallel and inferior to the transverse fissure and passes posteriorly from the major fissure to the posterior surface of the lung.

The Inferior Accessory Fissure

The inferior accessory fissure separates the medial basal segment from other lower lobe segments. This accessory fissure (also called Twining's line) is equally common in the left and right lower lobes and is an extremely common normal variant, seen in up to 20% of CTs and 8% of PA chest radiographs. It extends from the major fissure posteriorly to the pulmonary ligament, with a convex margin that parallels the right lateral chest wall and inferiorly inserts into the diaphragm. When present on the left side it forms a left medial basal segment (not usually present).

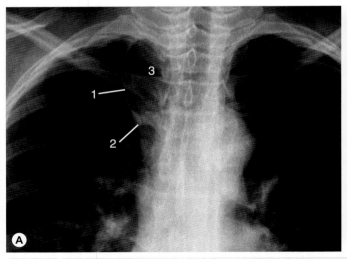 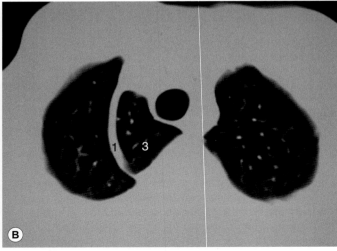

Fig. 4.17 Azygos fissure. (A) Posteroanterior chest radiograph. (B) Computed tomography thorax.

1. Azygos fissure
2. Azygos vein
3. Azygos 'lobe'

Left Transverse Fissure

This is visible in up to 8% of subjects and mirrors the right minor fissure separating the lingula from the remainder of the left upper lobe.

BRONCHOPULMONARY SEGMENTS (SEE FIGS. 4.14, 4.16)

The largest subunit of a lobe of the lung is a bronchopulmonary segment. Each bronchopulmonary segment is supplied by a segmental bronchus, artery and vein making them functionally separate, but they can be connected by collateral air drift. While they are not separated by their own pleural covering like the pulmonary lobes, they are anatomically distinct, separated by interstitium and each bronchopulmonary segment can be individually resected. Each segment takes its title from that of its supplying bronchus, as outlined in the previous section on bronchial anatomy.

Secondary Pulmonary Lobule and the Pulmonary Interstitium

The secondary pulmonary lobule is just one more of many ways to subdivide the lungs, but it is a very important concept in radiological anatomy as it forms the basis of a structured approach to diagnosing lung diseases on CT. The pulmonary interstitium is the connective tissue that supports the lung. It can be subdivided into:

1. The peribronchovascular interstitium, which extends from the hila, insinuating along the airways and arteries to the level of the smallest airways/vessels.
2. The subpleural interstitium, extending along the inner surface of the visceral pleura sending fibrous septae penetrating into the lungs.

The secondary pulmonary lobule is a subsegmental lung unit and is the smallest subunit separated by fibrous septae. Secondary pulmonary lobules:

- Are irregular polyhedral in shape.
- Vary in size, measuring between 1 cm and 2.5 cm, and visible on CT as normal indistinct air-filled lung.
- The outer walls or interlobular septae contain the lymphatics and draining pulmonary veins. The normal septae are too thin to be resolved on CT but become visible when abnormally thickened.
- The centre of the secondary pulmonary lobule contains the feeding pulmonary artery and small bronchiolar branch, which is also too small to be resolved unless abnormally thickened in disease.
- The parenchyma between the central structures and interlobular septae are made up of about eight acini (a subunit smaller than the secondary lobule comprising respiratory bronchioles and alveoli).

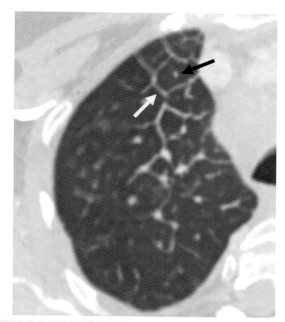

Fig. 4.18 Secondary pulmonary lobule. Axial computed tomography (CT) thorax zoomed in on the right upper lobe. This image demonstrates the anatomy of the secondary pulmonary lobule on CT. The *white arrow* points to the interlobular septa forming the irregular polyhedral shape; the *black arrow* denotes the central arteriole. The secondary pulmonary lobule is visible in this case due to thickening of the interlobular septae from lymphangitis carcinomatosis.

- The secondary lobules also contain fibrous septae, INTRAlobular septae, which weave between alveoli but do not form clear anatomic boundaries in the way that INTERlobular septae do.

THE PULMONARY ARTERY (FIG. 4.19)

The pulmonary trunk leaves the fibrous pericardium and bifurcates almost at once in the concavity of the aortic arch anterior to the left main bronchus. This vessel is usually supplied by the conus branch of the right coronary artery (RCA).

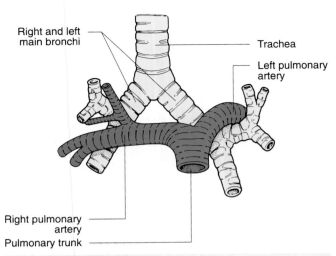

Fig. 4.19 Pulmonary arteries.

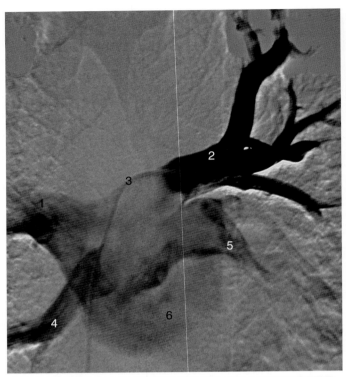

Fig. 4.20 Pulmonary veins: digital subtraction angiography of the pulmonary veins draining into the left atrium. This angiogram was achieved by passing a venous catheter from the right atrium through a 'probe-patent' foramen ovale into the left atrium.

1. Right upper pulmonary vein
2. Left upper pulmonary vein
3. Catheter
4. Right inferior pulmonary vein
5. Left inferior pulmonary vein
6. Left atrium

In contrast to the main bronchi, the right pulmonary artery is longer than the left. It passes across the midline below the carina and comes to lie anterior to the right main bronchus. It bifurcates while still in the hilum of the right lung. An artery to the right upper lobe passes anterior to the right upper lobe bronchus. The interlobar artery (analogous to the bronchus intermedius) supplies the right middle and lower lobes.

The left pulmonary artery passes posteriorly from the pulmonary trunk, arching over the superior aspect of the left main bronchus to reach its posterior surface. It is attached to the concavity of the aortic arch by the ligamentum arteriosum.

The pulmonary arteries further subdivide into segmental arteries that travel with the segmental bronchi, for the most part on their posterolateral surface. The pulmonary arteries supply only the alveoli.

RADIOLOGY PEARL

Pulmonary artery branches lie directly adjacent to an airway whereas pulmonary veins do not. This can be invaluable when a filling defect is seen in a vessel when only a portion of the thorax has been imaged and the vessels cannot be traced back to the hilum, for example the first few slices of a CT abdomen.

RADIOLOGY PEARL

The ligamentum arteriosum, the fibrous remnant of the fetal ductus arteriosus, can routinely be seen on CT as a thin, linear soft tissue–density structure connecting the left main pulmonary artery and the isthmus of the aortic arch. In adults, it usually contains a small portion of calcification. It is important to recognize as it represents the anatomical boundary between lymph node stations (separating 4L from 5) and also designates the location of the left recurrent laryngeal nerve.

RADIOLOGY PEARL

Normal lung parenchyma receives its blood supply from the pulmonary arteries; rarely, segments of lung receive arterial supply from the bronchial arteries and are termed bronchopulmonary sequestrations, defined as being intralobar when venous drainage is to the pulmonary veins or extralobar when drainage is to the systemic or portal venous systems. Such sequestrations fail to ventilate and remain collapsed and often chronically infected, presenting as a pulmonary mass.

THE PULMONARY VEINS (FIG. 4.20)

The pulmonary veins return oxygenated blood from the lungs to the left atrium. These do not follow the bronchial pattern but tend to run in interlobular and intersegmental septae. Typically, small pulmonary veins join to form two large pulmonary veins (the superior and inferior pulmonary veins) which drain each lung. The left upper and lower lobes are drained by the left superior and inferior pulmonary vein, respectively. The right superior pulmonary vein drains the right upper and middle lobes while the right inferior pulmonary vein drains the right lower lobe. The superior pulmonary veins have a relatively vertical course towards the hila whereas the inferior pulmonary veins have a much more horizontal course. The superior pulmonary vein lies lateral to the apical branch of the right upper lobe pulmonary artery as it travels towards the hilum. Within the hila of the lungs, the pulmonary veins lie below the pulmonary arteries and below or at the same level as the main bronchi. The number and configuration of pulmonary vein ostia are highly variable. The most common configuration is a separate ostium in the left atrium for each of the four pulmonary veins; the right superior and pulmonary vein ostia are usually separated by a portion of intervening left atrial wall on the right side of the left atrium; the left superior and inferior pulmonary vein ostia are usually immediately adjacent to each other on the left side of the left atrium with no intervening left atrium. Common variations include conjoined ostia on the left and right as well as supernumerary pulmonary veins.

> **RADIOLOGY PEARL**
>
> Variant pulmonary vein anatomy is not usually of clinical significance (excluding anomalous pulmonary venous drainage into the right circulation) but can be an important consideration prior to some cardiac ablation procedures and some cardiopulmonary surgeries.

> **RADIOLOGY PEARL**
>
> The right superior and inferior pulmonary veins can form an elongated bulbous vestibule gradually entering into the left atrium, particularly if conjoined; this projects as a mediastinal convexity behind the left atrium on chest radiograph and can be confused with a mediastinal mass.

LYMPHATICS (FIG. 4.21)

Mediastinal lymph nodes that drain the lung are named according to their position:
- Pulmonary nodes within the lung substance
- Bronchopulmonary nodes at the hilum
- Carinal nodes below the hilum
- Tracheobronchial nodes above the tracheobronchial junction
- Right and left paratracheal nodes on either side of the trachea

The lymph vessels of the lung are in superficial and deep plexuses. The superficial plexus beneath the pleura drains around the surface of the lungs and the margins of the fissures to converge at the hila and the bronchopulmonary nodes. The deep channels drain with the pulmonary vessels towards the hila. There are few connections between the superficial and deep plexuses except at the hila. The bronchopulmonary nodes drain to the tracheobronchial nodes and the paratracheal nodes, and thence to the bronchomediastinal trunks. Several hilar and mediastinal lymph nodes are visible on CT and measure up to or just above 1 cm in

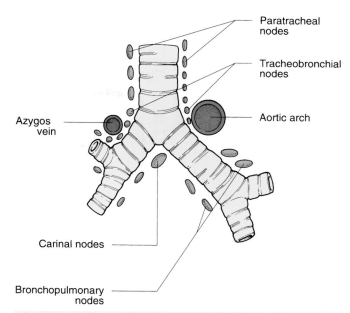

Fig. 4.21 Lymph nodes related to the trachea and main bronchi.

normal health, in particular at the right hilar, right lower paratracheal and subcarinal lymph node stations.

LUNG ROOTS (FIG. 4.22)

The roots and the hila of the lungs are terms that are often used interchangeably. Anatomically, the root of the lung refers to the rounded area on the medial aspect of the lung not covered by visceral pleura that allows structures to exit and enter the lungs to and from the mediastinum. This includes the major pulmonary arteries, major bronchi, bronchial arteries and veins, nerves and lymphatics. In radiography, the hila refer to the composite opacity of these structures encompassing a larger transverse diameter. The roots of the left and right lung are asymmetrical. At the point of the root of the right lung, the right main bronchus has already divided into the right upper lobe bronchus and the bronchus intermedius. The airways lie posteriorly and the right upper lobe bronchus (eparterial bronchus) is the most superior structure. Similarly, the right main pulmonary artery has divided into the right upper lobe pulmonary artery and interlobar artery, both lying anterior in the root. The right superior and inferior pulmonary veins are the most inferior structures. In contrast, the left lung root contains the unbranched left main pulmonary artery anteriorly, the unbranched left main bronchus posteriorly and the left superior and inferior pulmonary veins inferiorly. The roots of the lungs can be somewhat appreciated as 2D structures on lateral chest radiographs, with the right projecting anterior to the left due to the asymmetrical nature of the main pulmonary arteries. The roots of the lungs are surrounded by pleura and form the inferior pulmonary ligaments inferiorly. On frontal chest radiographs, the hila lie at vertebral levels T5–T7. The left hilum is typically higher than right owing to the looping course of the left main pulmonary artery over the left main bronchus. The right lung root lies below the arch of the azygos vein and posterior to

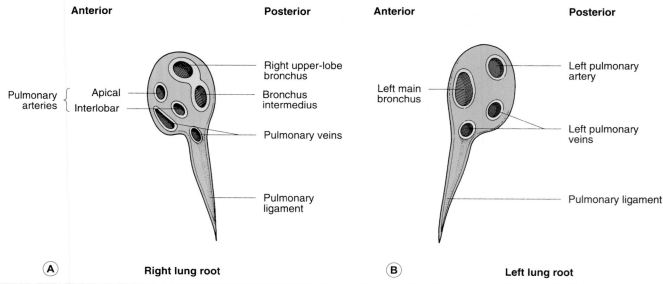

Fig. 4.22 Lung roots. (A) Right lung root. (B) Left lung root.

the SVC and the right atrium. The left lung root lies below the arch of the aorta and anterior to the descending aorta.

RADIOLOGICAL FEATURES OF THE LUNG AND BRONCHIAL TREE

Frontal Chest Radiograph (see Fig. 4.8)

Fissures. Fissures are only seen if tangential to the beam, and because of curvatures in three dimensions they are seldom seen in their entire length. The transverse fissure of the right lung is seen in 80% of dissection specimens but only 50% of chest radiographs. The azygos fissure, although found in 1% of postmortem subjects, is seen in 0.4% of radiographs with the 'teardrop' shadow of the azygos vein in its lower end. The superior accessory fissure is seen in 5% of chest radiographs and, when present, is at a lower level than the transverse fissure. The inferior accessory fissure is seen in 8% of CXRs, 20% of CT scans and 30%–50% of anatomical specimens. The left transverse fissure is seen in less than 2% of CXRs, 8% of CT scans and 18% of anatomical specimens. The major fissures are not usually seen on frontal chest radiograph.

Trachea. The trachea is seen as a midline translucency with a slight inclination to the right in its lower half. Its lumen is 1.5–2 cm in diameter. The right paratracheal stripe (normally <3 mm) is formed by the right wall of the trachea and the pleura, outlined on both sides by air. The left side of the trachea is not seen separately from the mediastinal shadows. A smooth indentation on the trachea is commonly seen just above the bifurcation on the left side. This is caused by the arch of the aorta. The carina lies at T4/T5 at rest. Gross AP or side-to-side (usually to the right side, owing to the aortic arch) displacement may be normal in a child, especially on an expiratory radiograph.

> **RADIOLOGY PEARL**
>
> The adult trachea usually lies to the right of midline on chest radiograph, projecting over the right half of the vertebrae that it overlies. A right-sided aortic arch and unilateral goitre should be considered if it is to the left of midline. The trachea in children is very pliable. It may be deviated to the right at almost 90-degree angulation in a normal expiratory film. It only deviates to the left if the aortic arch is on the right side.

Bronchi. The lumens of the right and left main bronchi are typically visible on frontal chest radiographs, but the visualization of their walls depends on the presence of gas on either side. The right main bronchus is orientated more vertically than the left. The bronchus intermedius can be identified to the right of the cardiac shadow and medial to the density of the interlobar artery. The lower lobe bronchus on the left is not normally seen, as it lies behind the heart shadow. The majority of the rest of the airways of the lungs are not discernible on chest radiographs because they are thin-walled structures filled with air. Exceptions to this are airways that are tangential to the X-ray beam and large enough to attenuate it. These will most likely be seen in the central lungs, close to the mediastinum. The bronchi that are most likely to meet these criteria are the anterior segmental bronchi of the right and left upper lobes, which often run in a directly AP direction. These airways can be seen in up to 50% of chest radiographs and can be a marker of airway disease. Other airways that can sometimes be seen include the posterior segmental bronchus of the left upper lobe and the superior segmental bronchi of the lower lobes bilaterally. Their corresponding pulmonary arteries may be seen accompanying the bronchi as circular densities of about the same size.

The term 'peribronchial cuffing' encompasses bronchial wall thickening usually due to airway inflammation as well as thickening of the periobronchovascular interstitium, most commonly due to pulmonary interstitial oedema. Generalized peribronchial cuffing can manifest as a nondescript increase in pulmonary markings on a chest radiograph. Prior to describing the presence of generalized peribronchial cuffing, it is important to try and identify individual central airways that are tangential to the beam, in particular the right and left upper lobe anterior segmental bronchi as they are often visible, to determine whether they are thickened. If these airways appear normal (pencil-thin walls), the overall appearances may be related to other causes including technical factors.

Bronchopulmonary segments. These are depicted in Fig. 4.16.

The spine should appear progressively more lucent as you move down the thoracic vertebrae until you reach the first hemidiaphragm. This is due to being overlapped by normal lucent lung parenchyma, along with reducing density of the soft tissues of the chest wall below the latissimus dorsi. Increased density over the lower thoracic spine, 'the spine sign' can indicate lower lobe consolidation, collapse, pleura effusion and other abnormalities.

Pulmonary vasculature. The pulmonary arteries and veins account for the large majority of the lung markings on a chest radiograph. The pulmonary trunk forms part of the left border of the heart. The interlobar artery is seen lateral to the bronchus intermedius on the right. This should not measure more than 16 mm midway down its visible length and should have a smooth, nonbumpy contour which gradually tapers.

Bronchi and arteries are seen together radiating out from the hila. Pulmonary veins enter the mediastinum lower than the arteries as they converge toward the posterior aspect of the left atrium. This means that:

■ In the upper zone the veins are inferolateral to the arteries.
■ In the lower zone the veins are almost horizontal and the arteries almost vertical.

The inferior pulmonary veins drain anteriorly and superiorly from the lung bases to the left atrium. Owing to their more horizontal course, if seen end-on on the chest film they may simulate a pulmonary mass.

The left and right hilar points are radiographic terms describing the exact points in the lateral left and right hilum where the superior pulmonary vein crosses the descending pulmonary artery (interlobar on the right and left lower lobar on the left). The upper lobe vein is used and not the upper lobe artery, as the upper lobe vein is a more lateral structure which crosses the descending artery. The right hilar point is projected over the sixth posterior interspace and is usually 1 cm lower than the left. The hilar angle is the angle between the vessels at the hilar point – normally 120 degrees.

The hilar points are an extremely important concept in chest radiography and need to be known well. The right hilar point may be as high as the left hilar point but never higher (again due to the looping of the left main pulmonary artery over the left main bronchus). A right hilar point that is higher than the left could mean volume loss in the right upper lobe dragging it upwards, or volume loss in the left lower lobe dragging the left hilar point down.

The hila contain similar structures and should have a similar density on chest radiograph. Significant density difference between the hila should always prompt scrutiny of the denser hilum as this may be caused by a pathological process adjacent to the normal structures in that hilum or a pathological process in the lung anterior or posterior to that hilum adding to its overall radiographic density.

The combination of the normal vertically orientated interlobar artery/right lower lobe arteries and the horizontally orientated right inferior pulmonary vein can create considerable density in the lower zone of the right lung on chest radiograph. This often appears asymmetric to the contralateral side due to the absence of the overlapping heart on the right. This should be considered when calling pathology in the right base.

Situs inversus. Situs inversus (see Fig. 4.13) can be identified by the position of the heart on chest radiograph. The morphological right lung, whether on the right or the left side of the thorax, is trilobed, has a short main bronchus, and has its bronchus above its pulmonary artery. These features can aid with determining sidedness, for example in heterotaxy syndromes.

Lymphatics. Normal lymph nodes do not form discernible densities on plain radiographs.

Lateral Chest Radiograph (see Fig. 4.9)

Fissures. The major (oblique) fissures may not be visible on lateral chest radiographs at all times. Even when they are visible, it can be challenging to distinguish between the right fissure and the left, just as it is difficult to differentiate between the left and right hemidiaphragms. The left major fissure begins more superiorly than the right (T3/T4 on the left and T4 on the right) and consequently has a more vertical course and reaches the diaphragm more posteriorly than that on the right. The most reliable way to distinguish the major fissures is first to identify the hemidiaphragm from which the fissure appears to be arising. The anterior ends of the major fissures reach the diaphragm 2–3 cm behind the anterior chest wall. As the fissures are undulating, they may appear to be doubled in parts and are often not seen in entirety. For the same reason the posterior part of the transverse fissure may occasionally seem to cross the right oblique fissure and so should not be used as an indicator of laterality of the fissure. Where there is a superior accessory fissure, this extends posteriorly from the major fissure.

Trachea. The trachea is visible on all lateral radiographs, measuring between 1.5 and 2.5 cm in diameter. It enters the thorax midway between the sternum and the vertebrae. Owing to some posterior inclination it ends closer to the vertebrae. The position of the carina is very difficult to identify on lateral chest radiographs because the left and right main bronchi overlap. The position can be estimated from the vertebral level, lying at T4/T5, or at the level of the manubriosternal joint. The posterior tracheal stripe (a stripe of soft tissue density between air in the tracheal lumen and air in the lung posterior to the trachea) is delineated in 50% of lateral chest radiographs and measures between 1 and 6 mm. The reason for this variability in visibility and width is explained by the variation in anatomy. In some patients, the posterior aspect of the trachea is abutted by a portion of the right upper lobe (with the oesophagus lateral to the trachea) creating a reproducible thin posterior tracheal stripe. Alternatively, the oesophagus can lie immediately posterior to the trachea with normal mediastinum and spine posterior to the oesophagus. In this case, the posterior aspect of the trachea will not be clearly defined when the oesophagus is collapsed, but when a column of air is present in the oesophagus, this will outline a thick posterior tracheal stripe, more accurately termed the tracheo-oesophageal stripe. The retrotracheal space, also known as Raider's (pronounced Rider's) triangle is a triangle bounded by the trachea anteriorly, the aortic arch inferiorly and the spine posteriorly.

Bronchi. On the lateral chest radiograph, the trachea terminates as two rounded lucencies, one superior and one inferior. These represent two large bronchi tangential to the X-ray beam and they are the key to recognizing the anatomy of the hilar structures. The more superior lucency is the right upper lobe bronchus (the eparterial bronchus). The more inferior bronchus usually represents the left upper lobe bronchus (the hyparterial bronchus) but can represent the left main bronchus or both airways superimposed, depending on the branching angle of the airways. This left upper lobe bronchus lies at the centre of the chest and is usually well delineated on all lateral chest radiographs. Once this has been identified, the left main pulmonary artery can be identified coursing over the left main bronchus as a comma-shape and the hilar positions can then be determined.

The posterior wall of the bronchus intermedius is usually visible as a thin stripe as it is in contact with the lung. This should not measure more than 3 mm. On the left side, the left main pulmonary artery posterior to the bronchus obscures the view of its posterior wall of the left main bronchus. The left upper lobe apicoposterior segmental bronchus can often be seen arising from the superior aspect of the left upper lobe bronchus as a tubular lucency. The lower lobe bronchi may be seen running in a posteroinferior course in many cases. The left lower lobe bronchus is the more posterior and has a curved configuration in its anterior aspect, merging with the orifice of the upper lobe bronchus.

Vasculature. The right and left main pulmonary arteries are usually clearly delineated on lateral chest radiograph. The right main pulmonary artery is a large oval structure lying anterior to the rounded left and right bronchi. It is larger than might be expected, measuring up to 3 cm. The left main pulmonary artery is again a comma-shaped opacity arching over the left main bronchus. The confluence of the pulmonary veins is seen below the oval density of the right pulmonary artery on the lateral film. The superior veins are more anterior than the inferior pulmonary veins.

RADIOLOGY PEARL

It may be difficult to determine whether or not prominence of hilar structures is real or projectional on a frontal radiograph. On review of a lateral radiograph, lobular enlargement of right hilar structures due to adenopathy produces enlargement of soft tissue structures anterior to the bronchus. In contrast, on review of a lateral radiograph, enlargement due to left hilar adenopathy produces enlargement of soft tissue structures posterior to the bronchus.

RADIOLOGY PEARL

The mnemonic RALPh (Right Anterior Left Posterior) is useful in chest radiology. On lateral chest radiographs: the right main pulmonary artery (and therefore hilum) is anterior to the left; the right hemidiaphragm extends anterior to the chest wall whereas the left stops at the posterior aspect of the heart; and the right major fissure joins its hemidiaphragm more anterior than the left. Also, the RCA arises from the anterior aspect of the aorta, with the left mainstem (LMS) arising more posteriorly.

Pulmonary Angiography

A catheter is inserted via the femoral vein to the IVC, right heart and pulmonary trunk. The pulmonary trunk inclines posteriorly as it leaves the heart and is best seen when the beam is angled at 45 degrees to the anterior chest wall. The pulmonary arteries and branches are seen as described above. Pulmonary veins are seen in the venous phase. Catheter angiography can be used in the investigation of cases of pulmonary hypertension but it is an otherwise uncommonly performed test in a radiology department relative to CT pulmonary angiography (CTPA).

Computed Tomography

High-resolution CT thorax (HRCT) is a historical term coined prior to the widespread use of multidetector CT scanners. The HRCT protocol involved additional acquisition of widely spaced 'step and shoot' slices to obtain 1–1.5-mm slices (high resolution) used for detailed assessment of lung parenchyma, particularly in cases of suspected interstitial lung disease. Images can be reconstructed in any plane.

RADIOLOGY PEARL

All modern-day CT scanners can reconstruct imaging in high resolution, but the term HRCT remains in use, usually referring to a CT protocol geared towards evaluating for interstitial lung disease including 1–1.5-mm axial reconstructions using a hard, high-contrast reconstruction kernel. This is a CT software reconstruction algorithm which accentuates or sharpens the interfaces between tissues of a different density. It can be useful to emphasize the contrast between normal lung and fibrosis. A full HRCT protocol includes the expiratory phase to assess for air trapping and tracheobronchomalacia, and sometimes prone images to better evaluate the lung bases.

Trachea. The normal tracheal wall thickness is between 1 and 3 mm. The cartilaginous rings can be delineated by irregularity of the anterior and lateral walls of the trachea. Like costal cartilages, the tracheal cartilages can undergo senescent calcification with age and become more prominent. The trachea is circular in inspiration/breath hold with a normal diameter range quoted as 13–25 mm. The membranous posterior membrane naturally folds inwards into the lumen in dynamic expiration. This fact can be used to judge the quality of an expiratory CT thorax.

Fissures. On high-resolution CT fissures are seen as sharp lines. On thicker reconstructions, fissures may be seen as areas of relative avascularity where tapering vessels are less visible.

Bronchi. The bronchi may be seen as tubular or circular air-filled structures depending on slice orientation relative to the orientation of the bronchus. The right main bronchus, right upper lobar bronchus and right upper lobe anterior and posterior segmental bronchi can usually be seen on a single axial CT slice, creating an image that is often likened to a whale with the segmental bronchi forming the 'whale tail' (Fig. 4.23). Like the posterior wall of the trachea, the posterior wall of the bronchus intermedius is membranous and visibly bows inwards in dynamic expiration. As a rule of thumb, an airway should have a diameter the same or less than the adjacent pulmonary artery/arteriole. Bronchial walls should become thinner and thinner with successive

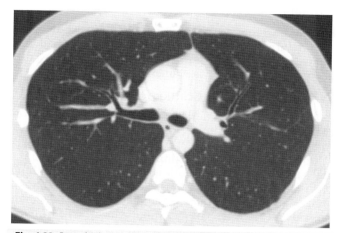

Fig. 4.23 Bronchial anatomy on computed tomography (CT). Axial CT thorax, lung windows. 'Whale tail' appearance of the right main bronchus, right upper lobe and anterior segmental bronchi.

RADIOLOGY PEARL

The posterior wall of the bronchus intermedius should always be a thin structure measuring less than 2 mm. Thickening of this structure to >3 mm can be a sign of pulmonary oedema, lymphadenopathy or even an early primary lung cancer.

RADIOLOGY PEARL

Normal airway diameter increases greatly with age with up to 50% of individuals over 65 having one or more airways greater than the diameter of the adjacent arteriole. Therefore, age should be considered before diagnosing bronchiectasis. Airways should always taper with successive generations and an airway that dilates after branching is always abnormal.

generations and measure 1.5 mm or less. Rather than measuring them, they should appear as 'pencil thin'.

Vasculature. The vessels account for most of the lung markings seen on CT. The relationships of the pulmonary arteries and veins to the bronchi are best seen at hilar level. The right pulmonary artery is anterior to the right bronchus, and the right superior pulmonary vein may be seen anterior to this. The left pulmonary artery is seen anterior to the left main bronchus, and above it on a higher section. The lower lobe artery is seen posterolateral to the lower lobe bronchus. The left superior pulmonary vein is separated from the lower lobe artery at hilar level by the left bronchus.

CTPA has largely superseded conventional pulmonary angiography except in select cases, for example preoperative assessment for surgical thrombectomy in cases of chronic thromboembolic pulmonary hypertension. CTPA is commonly used in the emergency setting to assess for pulmonary embolism (PE).

Magnetic Resonance Imaging

Because the lungs are of very low proton density and move with respiration, they are poorly seen by this method. MRI thorax is mainly used for the characterization of mediastinal masses rather than assessment of the lungs.

Ventilation–Perfusion Scintigraphy

A ventilation (V) scan outlines the trachea and main bronchi in addition to the lungs. In this technique, isotope, most commonly an aerosol of ^{99m}DTPA (technetium-labelled diethylenetriaminepentaacetic acid), is placed in a nebulizer and administered via a mouthpiece during tidal breathing. The isotope is deposited in the airways and aerated alveoli. Images are acquired in multiple planar or single-photon emission CT (SPECT; cross-sectional) views. SPECT images are acquired in a similar fashion to CT, except a gamma camera is used. A gap is seen owing to the mediastinum and a cardiac notch is seen in the anterior border of the left lung on frontal and SPECT images.

Perfusion scanning (Q) is acquired after intravenous injection of 99m MAA (technetium-labelled macroaggregated albumin). Images may show differential isotope distribution from apex to diaphragm owing to variations in blood flow associated with posture. The subject is normally injected with the isotope in a supine position to minimize vertical perfusion gradient and decrease diaphragmatic motion.

RADIOLOGY PEARLS

- Also known as lung scintigraphy or V/Q scan, this is the oldest noninvasive method of detecting PE. With PE, there are regions of hypoperfusion mismatched to areas of ventilation (V/Q mismatch). In the case of parenchymal lung pathology, defects may occur in both ventilation and perfusion components (matched defects).
- CTPA has replaced ventilation/perfusion scanning in the diagnosis of acute PE, but it still plays an important role in the diagnosis of chronic PE as well as quantification of relative lung/lobar perfusion prior to resections.

The Mediastinum (Fig. 4.24)

The mediastinum is the parietal pleura-lined space separating the left and right lungs. It does not include the bones of the sternum or the thoracic spine, which serve as the anterior and posterior boundaries of the mediastinum. Numerous different systems have been devised to divide the mediastinum into separate compartments. These divisions are arbitrary, nonanatomical divisions used to describe the location of pathological processes and narrow the differential diagnosis based on the location. Most of these systems are based on the lateral chest radiograph. One of the most popular systems, the Shields' model, divides the mediastinum into superior and inferior compartments, with the inferior compartment further subdivided into anterior, middle and posterior compartments. The superior mediastinum is above a line drawn from the lower border of the T4 vertebral body to the manubriosternal joint. Below this line are anterior, middle and posterior compartments. The middle mediastinum is occupied by the heart and its vessels. The anterior mediastinum is between the anterior part of the heart and the sternum. The posterior mediastinum is between the posterior part of the heart and the thoracic spine, extending down behind the posterior part of the diaphragm as it slopes inferiorly.

The superior mediastinum contains the:
- Aortic arch and branches
- Brachiocephalic veins and SVC
- Trachea
- Oesophagus
- Thoracic duct
- Lymph nodes
- Nerves

The anterior mediastinum contains the:
- Thymus
- Mammary vessels
- Lymph nodes

The posterior mediastinum contains the:
- Descending aorta
- Oesophagus

Fig. 4.24 Mediastinal divisions.

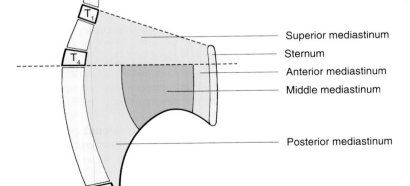

Superior mediastinum

Sternum

Anterior mediastinum

Middle mediastinum

Posterior mediastinum

- Azygos venous system
- Thoracic duct
- Para-aortic, oesophageal and paraspinal nodes

The middle mediastinum contains the:
- Heart and pericardium
- Nerves
- Lymph nodes
- Great vessels

A more recent system of mediastinal divisions that is in widespread use is the International Thymic Malignancy Interest Group system, which is more heavily based on cross-sectional imaging rather than radiographs and divides the mediastinum into previsceral (anterior), visceral (middle) and paravertebral (posterior) compartments.

Ultimately, it is important to recognize that the mediastinum is a single compartment and there are no correct boundaries as different systems are based on nonanatomical boundaries, which vary. However, the process of subdividing the mediastinum into compartments, generally into anterior, middle and posterior compartments, is extremely useful for the generation of differential diagnoses and in widespread use in radiology.

The Heart

GROSS ANATOMY AND ORIENTATION (FIGS. 4.25–4.27; SEE ALSO FIGS. 4.8, 4.9)

The heart is an anatomically complex structure and the descriptive terms for its various surfaces can be confusing. The simplified basic science model of two atria on top and two ventricles on the bottom is more or less accurate but much of the complexity arises from its complex orientation. Taking the simplified model, the heart is shaped like an inverted pyramid with a broader base at the top and a narrower apex at the bottom, much like the prostate. The base represents the portions of the atria where the major systemic and pulmonary veins attach and the apex represents the narrowest most inferior portions of the right and left ventricle. Unlike the prostate, this model is then rotated in all three planes: along the atrioventricular plane so that the apex points towards the sternum and its base towards the spine (causing the ventricles to lie anterior and inferior to the atria); then rotated to the left in space so that its apex points towards the left nipple and its base towards the right lateral chest wall; and lastly along its interventricular axis so that the left atrium and ventricle lie slightly higher than the right. These rotations make the heart a unique organ in the body, whereby structures face in nonintuitive directions relative to axes of the human body, for example, the left atrium faces posteriorly rather than to the left. Much of cardiac imaging is concerned with undoing these rotations to make it more anatomically intuitive.

Relative to the anatomical axes of the body:
- The left atrium with the superior and inferior pulmonary veins draining into its four corners forms the majority of the posterior aspect of the heart.

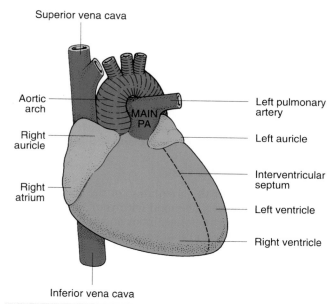

Fig. 4.25 Heart: anterior view. *PA*, Pulmonary artery.

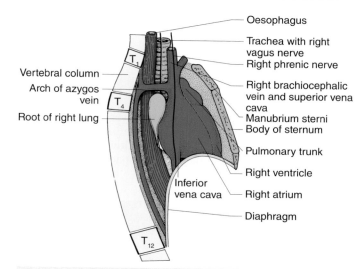

Fig. 4.26 Heart and mediastinum viewed from the right.

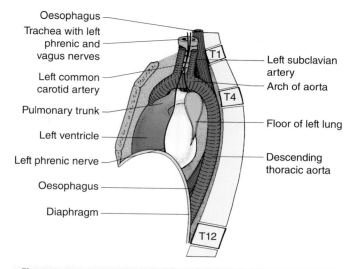

Fig. 4.27 Heart and mediastinum viewed from the left.

- The right atrium forms the right border, with superior and inferior venae cavae draining into its upper and lower parts.
- The apex and left border are formed by the left ventricle.
- The right ventricle forms the anterior part.
- The inferior (diaphragmatic) part of the heart is formed mainly by the inferior walls of the left and right ventricles (confusingly, the inferior walls of the ventricles lie opposite to the anterior walls) and a small part of the right atrium posteriorly where the IVC enters this chamber.

RADIOLOGY PEARL (FIG. 4.28)

A way to remember the orientation of the chambers of the heart is to form a diamond with your index fingers and thumbs, with your longer index fingers representing the larger ventricles and your shorter thumbs representing the smaller atria. Your right digits represent the right chambers and the left digits the left chambers. Now follow the rotations of the cardiac axes pointing the apex (the tips of your forefingers) anteriorly, inferiorly and to the left. Then rotate the left fingers slightly clockwise so that they lie slightly superior to the right fingers. Now your 'chambers' will be correctly aligned relative to the body surfaces with your left thumb (the left atrium) facing posteriorly.

PERICARDIUM (FIG. 4.29)

The pericardium is composed of two layers, the serous and fibrous layers of the pericardium. The inner serous layer is a double layer of mesothelium forming a closed sac just like the peritoneum and pleura. The space within the sac,

the pericardial space, contains 20–25 mL of serous fluid in normal health. The heart is pushed into this double layer apex first (similar to the abdominal viscera being invested into the peritoneum). This creates an inner layer lining the surface of the heart, the visceral layer, and the more superficial outer layer, the parietal layer. The serous pericardium along with its pericardial fluid serve to permit frictionless motion during contraction and relaxation. As the heart is pushed into this double layer, it is not completely encased in visceral pericardium; rather, it reflects back on itself at the origin of the major arteries (aorta and pulmonary trunk) and veins (SVC, IVC and pulmonary veins) at the base of the heart. Parts of the visceral pericardium also encircle the great vessels. These points of reflection and encircling of the pericardium are conceptually difficult but are important in radiology as they create two major pericardial sinuses (pericardial fluid-containing tunnels) and several pericardial recesses (abrupt angulations from visceral to parietal pericardium where pericardial fluid can collect). Many of these are visible on imaging and can be confused with pathological structures. An exhaustive list of these spaces is beyond the scope of this text but the most important are the transverse sinus, the oblique sinus and the superior aortic recess.

- Transverse pericardial sinus: A visceral pericardium-lined tunnel separating the aortic root and pulmonary trunk anteriorly from the superior aspect of the left atrium including the SVC, posteriorly. Surgeons can insert a finger into the transverse sinus posterior to the great arteries and can clamp the ascending aorta through this passage.
- Oblique pericardial sinus: A posterior blind-ending tunnel along the posterior aspect of the left atrium between the left and right pulmonary veins. This projects

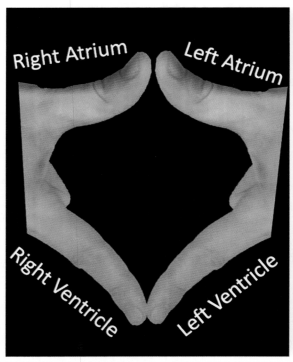
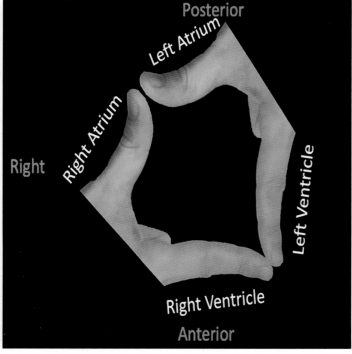

Fig. 4.28 Orientation of the cardiac chambers.

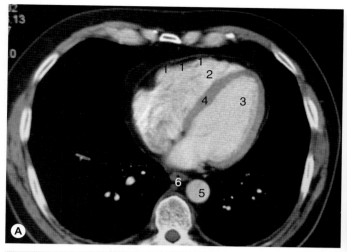

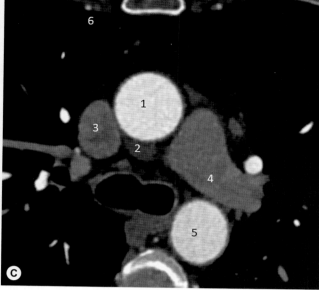

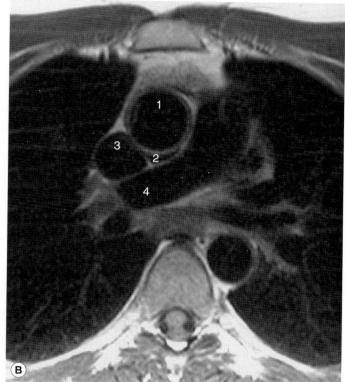

Fig. 4.29 Pericardium. (A) Computed tomography (CT) scan showing the pericardium. (B) Magnetic resonance image showing the pericardial recesses. (C) CT coronary angiogram.

(A)
1. Pericardium
2. Right ventricle
3. Left ventricle
4. Interventricular septum
5. Aorta
6. Oesophagus

(B)
1. Aorta
2. Superior aortic recess of the transverse sinus
3. Superior vena cava
4. Right pulmonary artery

(C)
1. Ascending thoracic aorta
2. Superior aortic recess of the transverse sinus
3. Superior vena cava
4. Left main pulmonary artery
5. Descending thoracic aorta
6. Right internal thoracic (mammary) artery (lateral) and vein (medial)

superiorly from the pericardial space lining the inferior surface of the heart.
- Superior aortic recess. This is a blind-ending pericardial recess projecting superiorly from the transverse sinus to partially surround the ascending thoracic aorta. This can be subdivided into anterior (aortopulmonary), right (right lateral aspect of the ascending aorta) and posterior (tear drop-shaped recess posterior to the ascending aorta).

The visceral pericardium is not directly adherent to the epicardium (the outermost cells of the heart) and is often separated from the epicardium by the fat in which the coronary arteries course. This layer of fat is called the epicardial fat. The fibrous pericardium is the outer layer of the pericardium. This is inseparable from the parietal pericardium that lines it such that there is no potential space between the parietal pericardium and the fibrous pericardium. As its name suggests, the fibrous pericardium is a tough fibrous layer which unlike the serous layer gives some rigidity to the heart. The fibrous pericardium is strongly adherent to the central tendon of the diaphragm inferiorly and the great vessels superiorly and is the structure that keeps the heart in its position in the chest, stopping it from falling to one side or the other when lying on one's side. The other function of the fibrous pericardium is to stop the heart from expanding too much in diastole. Like the serous pericardium, the fibrous pericardium is deficient at the base where the vessels arise. Fat external to the fibrous pericardium is most commonly referred to as pericardial fat (pericardial fat pads when abundant). However, unlike epicardial fat, it is continuous with the fat in the upper mediastinum and can also be referred to as simply mediastinal fat.

RADIOLOGICAL FEATURES OF THE PERICARDIUM

CT and MRI (see Fig. 4.29)

On CT, the serous and fibrous layers of the pericardium cannot be distinguished from each other and the whole structure appears as a single, very thin, soft tissue–density line. It can be difficult to identify on CT when not containing fluid but at least a portion of it is usually visible anterior to the right ventricle where epicardial fat is most abundant. It is difficult to see along the free wall of the lateral ventricle where there is little epicardial fat. When not containing fluid, it is a thin structure with an upper limit thickness of 2 or 3 mm. Accumulation of a small amount of fluid in the pericardial sac is a normal physiological finding and it often accumulates posteriorly along the right lateral ventricle or along the inferior walls of the ventricles at the diaphragm. It does not demonstrate appreciable enhancement with contrast, and marked pericardial enhancement should always be considered abnormal. The same is true for pericardial calcification. On MRI the pericardium appears as a low-signal, thin structure on all sequences and follows the same pattern to the CT appearances.

The transverse and oblique pericardial sinuses and the superior aortic recess are usually visible on CT and MRI as fluid-filled, smoothly marginated structures surrounding the heart. The superior aortic recess is often fluid filled even when there is no appreciable fluid in the pericardial sac proper. The posterior portion of the superior aortic recess appears as a tear drop–shaped structure posterior to the aortic root and the oblique sinus as an ovoid structure in the subcarinal region. Both can be confused with lymph nodes but can be distinguished by their position immediately

adjacent to the walls of the heart and great vessels, smooth margins and fluid density.

CARDIAC CHAMBERS AND VALVES (SEE FIGS. 4.25–4.27, 4.30)

Cardiac Valves

There are four major valves in the heart: two atrioventricular valves (the mitral and tricuspid valves) separating the atria from the ventricles; and two semilunar valves (the aortic and pulmonary/pulmonic valves) separating the left and right ventricular outflow tracts (LVOTs and RVOTs, respectively) from the aorta and pulmonary trunk, respectively. The valves are made of up of cusps or leaflets (these terms are used interchangeably) which are anchored to the heart by a round or oval fibrous annulus. The mitral valve has two cusps, while the tricuspid, aortic and pulmonary valves all normally have three cusps (trileaflet or tricuspid). The commissures represent the fissures between the valve leaflets when they are coapted (closed). The mitral and tricuspid valves are attached to papillary muscles by chordae tendineae to stop them prolapsing into the atria during systole. Sinuses of Valsalva are dilated pouches of the walls of the aorta located just above the aortic valve leaflets that help prevent backflow of blood into the left ventricle during diastole. The pulmonary trunk/valve also technically has sinuses of Valsalva but these are rarely described in anatomy and the term almost exclusively refers to the aortic sinuses. The atrioventricular valves do not possess sinuses of Valsalva.

Right Atrium

This has a smooth posterior wall into which three large systemic veins drain: the SVC drains into the superior aspect of the right atrium; the IVC into its inferior aspect and the coronary sinus (the final confluence of the majority of the cardiac venous drainage) into its posteromedial aspect between the orifice of the IVC and the tricuspid valve. The crista terminalis is a thin muscular ridge that extends along the lateral wall of the right atrium from the orifice of the SVC to the orifice of the IVC. This represents an embryological divide between the smooth-walled posterior right atrium which receives the major vessels and the anterior right

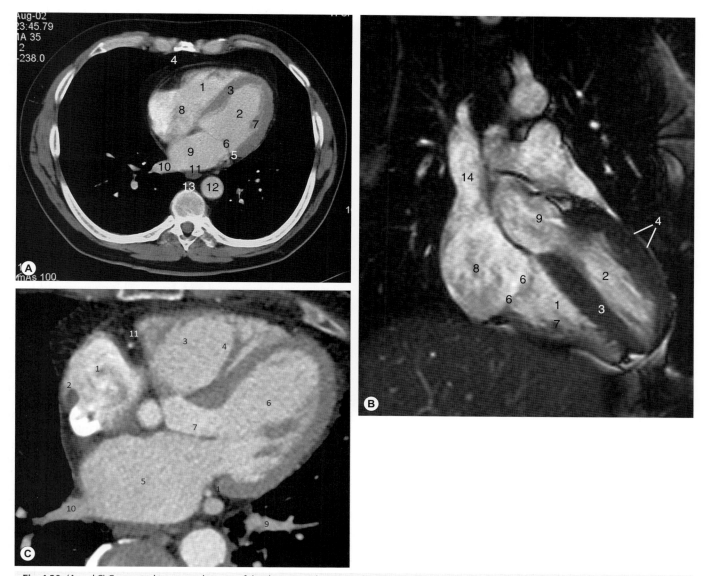

Fig. 4.30 (A and C) Computed tomography scan of the thorax: axial sections through the heart. (B) Oblique sagittal magnetic resonance image through the long axis of the heart.

(A and B)
1. Right ventricle
2. Left ventricle
3. Interventricular septum
4. Pericardium
5. Atrioventricular groove
6. Mitral valve
7. Papillary muscle
8. Right atrium
9. Left atrium
10. Right pulmonary vein
11. Oesophagus
12. Descending aorta
13. Azygos vein
14. Superior vena cava

(C)
1. Right atrium
2. Crista terminalis
3. Right ventricle
4. Moderator band
5. Left atrium
6. Left ventricle
7. Anterior leaflet of the mitral valve
8. Left circumflex coronary artery
9. Inferior left pulmonary vein
10. Inferior right pulmonary vein
11. Right coronary artery

atrium which is ridged by pectinate muscles. The right atrial appendage arises from the anterior aspect of the superior portion of the right atrium and also possesses these muscular ridges which appear as trabeculations. Along with the crista terminalis, the right atrial eustachian valve is

a linear projection into the right atrium that can be seen on CT when there is little motion artefact. The eustachian valve separates the orifices of the IVC and the coronary sinus. The interatrial septum makes up the shared wall of the left and right atria. The interatrial septum is a naturally thin structure measuring 3–4 mm but fat can accumulate within the septum causing it to appear thickened. In its inferior portion, the interatrial septum bears an oval depression named the fossa ovalis which represents the closed foramen ovale through which oxygenated blood from the maternal circulation reaches the left side of the heart in the fetus. The fossa ovalis is a thin structure composed of the fused leaflets of the septum primum and secundum, and usually measures 1 mm. Lipomatous hypertrophy of the interatrial septum spares the fossa ovalis.

> **RADIOLOGY PEARL**
>
> The crista terminalis is often visible on CT and sometimes appears thick and nodular. This should not be confused with a right atrial thrombus or tumour.

> **RADIOLOGY PEARL**
>
> When lipomatous hypertrophy of the interatrial septum is present and sparing the fossa ovalis, it can give the impression of an absent fossa ovalis (secundum atrial septal defect). Caution should be taken when diagnosing atrial septal defects on nondynamic studies such as CT thorax. A dynamic study such as an echocardiogram or cardiac MRI is needed to confirm flow across the apparent defect.

Right Ventricle

The right ventricle (RV) is anatomically different to the left ventricle and recognition of the differences is important when evaluating congenital cardiac diseases. It is roughly triangular when viewed from the side and in short axis (down its barrel) with anterior, septal and inferior/posterior walls (there is some overlap between the posterior and inferior walls but both are opposite the anterior wall with the inferior wall facing the diaphragm and the posterior wall more basally facing the spine). There is no lateral wall. Blood flows into the RV from the right atrium through the tricuspid valve. The three leaflets of the tricuspid valve are named based on their position in the heart: anterior, posterior and septal leaflets. The leaflets attach via the chordae tendineae to the anterior, septal and posterior papillary muscles. The RV papillary muscles are smaller and less well defined than the left ventricle (LV), and are made up of multiple small disparate slips. This pattern makes the internal walls of the RV (including the septum) highly trabeculated, which is a defining feature of the RV. A band of tissue called the moderator band traverses the RV and is part of the conduction system of the heart and is often recognizable on CT and MRI. The shared interventricular septum is as thick as the other walls of the LV. In contrast, the anterior and inferior walls of the RV are much thinner, reflecting its low-pressure system. In the normal heart, the interventricular septum always bulges convex into the RV. Lastly, the RV has an elongated muscular outflow tract called the RVOT, also known as the conus or the infundibulum, which is another distinguishing feature. The pulmonary valve has three semilunar cusps – right and left anterior and a posterior cusp. It faces to the left and slightly posteriorly. It is the most anterior and superior of all the cardiac valves.

Left Atrium

This is square-shaped and smooth-walled, and forms the most superior and posterior part of the heart on the lateral view. It receives the four pulmonary veins in its upper part (see Fig. 4.20). The fossa ovalis can also be seen on the left atrial side of the interatrial side, often with incompletely fused leaflets. The left atrium has a long, narrow, trabeculated appendage that projects anteriorly on the left side of the pulmonary trunk, overlapping its origin. The left atrial appendage also commonly overlies a portion of the left coronary arteries (usually the proximal/mid-left anterior descending [LAD] artery).

Left Ventricle

The LV is by far the most important chamber in the heart in terms of cardiac function, and much of cardiac imaging is centred around imaging it. When viewed in short axis it forms a circle (unlike the triangular RV). This creates anterior, lateral, inferior and septal walls. This plane can be further subdivided into three segments: basal, mid and apical. This model illustrates the coronary vascular territories and serves as the basis for cardiac scintigraphy as well as gadolinium-enhanced cardiac MRI sequences. The anterior, lateral, inferior and septal walls should be equal in thickness (again, best evaluated in short axis). Wall thickness depends on whether the myocardium is imaged in diastole or systole. As a rule of thumb, an end-diastolic (relaxed) LV wall thickness of 15 mm or more is abnormal but it is often <10 mm. The ventricles are separated by the interventricular septum, which is mostly thick and muscular with a short membranous part at the top and again bulges convex into the RV due to the higher pressures in the normal left heart. The mitral valve separates the LV from the left atrium. This valve has two cusps – anterior and posterior – whose free margins are attached to the ventricular wall by chordae tendineae. The LV papillary muscles are thick, well-defined muscles that are easily visualized at cross-sectional imaging. They arise from the anterior and posteroinferior walls and not the septum, which is smooth. Instead of a muscular conus as on the right, the larger anterior cusp of the mitral valve separates inflow and outflow tracts, and blood flows over both its surfaces. The mitral and aortic valves are in fibrous continuity. The aortic valve has three cusps which, like the aortic sinuses, are named after the coronary arteries (see later): right coronary cusp, left coronary cusp and noncoronary cusp.

> **RADIOLOGY PEARL**
>
> As LV thickness varies greatly throughout the cardiac cycle, caution should be taken when diagnosing LV hypertrophy on nongated scans such as a CT thorax.

THE CORONARY ARTERIES AND VEINS

Sinuses of Valsalva (FIG 4.31)

The aorta dilates just above the aortic valve into three saccular aortic sinuses, the sinuses of Valsalva, bounded inferiorly and medially by one of the three aortic valve cusps.

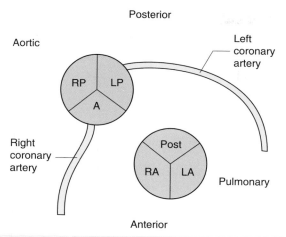

Fig. 4.31 Relationship of aortic and pulmonary valves and origin of the right and left pulmonary arteries. *A*, Anterior; *LA*, left anterior; *LP*, left posterior; *RA*, right anterior; *RP*, right posterior; *Post*, posterior.

The aortic sinuses, like the corresponding valve cusp, derive their name from the coronary artery that arises (or does not arise) from them

- The right coronary sinus of Valsalva (also known as the anterior sinus) points anteriorly and gives rise to the right coronary artery (RCA).
- The left coronary sinus of Valsalva (also known as the left posterior sinus) is orientated posterolaterally to the left and gives off the left coronary artery (LCA) at the 4 o'clock position of the aortic root
- The noncoronary sinus of Valsalva (also known as the right posterior sinus) is orientated posterolaterally to the right and does not give rise to a coronary artery. The noncoronary sinus is always orientated towards the interatrial septum regardless of the plane of reconstruction.

Coronary Artery Dominance

The posterior descending artery (PDA) runs in the posterior interventricular groove and supplies the inferior third of the interventricular septum. The posterolateral branch, also known as the posterolateral artery (PLB or PLA) runs along the inferior wall of the LV supplying this territory. The PDA and PLB have variable origin. The coronary artery/arteries that supply the PDA and PLB determines the coronary dominance.

- If the RCA supplies both of these arteries, typically with a small-calibre distal left circumflex artery, the circulation can be classified as 'right dominant'.
- If the left circumflex coronary artery (LCx), a branch of the left main stem (LMS) coronary artery, supplies both of these arteries, typically with a small-calibre distal RCA, the circulation can be classified as 'left dominant'.
- If the RCA supplies the PDA and the LCx supplies the PLB, the circulation is known as 'co-dominant'.
- Rarely, the LAD supplies the PDA by wrapping around the apex of the LV, along with a small-calibre RCA. This pattern is known as LAD superdominance.

There is variation in the reported relative frequencies of coronary artery dominance. A commonly quoted breakdown is: 70% of subjects are right dominant, 20% are co-dominant and 10% are left dominant.

RIGHT CORONARY ARTERY (FIG. 4.32)

The RCA arises from the right coronary sinus on the anterior (12 o'clock) position of the aortic root and travels through the right atrioventricular groove from the anterior to the posterior aspect of the heart. The RCA measures up to 4 mm proximally and 2 mm distally, but size will depend on dominance. Excluding the PDA and PLB territories, the RCA supplies the conus (RVOT), the sinoatrial node, the atrioventricular nodes, the walls of the right atrium including the interatrial septum, and the anterior and inferior walls of the RV. When reconstructed in a plane along the right atrioventricular groove and put into a thick maximum-intensity projection (MIP) the RCA forms a C-shape. The upper part of the 'C' is the proximal segment, the middle portion the middle segment and the lower part of the 'C' is the distal segment. The junction of the middle and lateral segments is the acute margin of the heart (i.e. where the coronary wraps around on to the inferior/diaphragmatic surface).

Branches

The branches of the RCA are as follows:
Proximal:
- Conus artery to the pulmonary outflow tract.
- Branch to the sinoatrial node, which curves anticlockwise around the SVC to reach the sinoatrial node.
- Atrial branches.

Mid-portion:
- Acute marginal branches which run anteriorly from the RCA to supply the RV (these can be remembered by the acute angle at the bottom of the capital letter **R** in RCA).
Distal:
- Branch to the atrioventricular node.
- PDA and PLB when dominant.

LEFT CORONARY ARTERY (FIGS. 4.33 AND 4.34)

The LCA arises from the left coronary sinus of Valsalva and supplies the remainder of the LV. The initial portion of the LCA, prior to dividing into the LAD and LCx, is the LMS. This is the most significant location in the coronary circulation to have stenoses (often informally called widowmaker lesions). The LMS is a short vessel extending 5–10 mm to the left of the aorta, posterior to the pulmonary trunk before dividing. Sometimes the LMS trifurcates, giving off a supernumerary branch centrally between the LAD and LCx, known as a ramus intermedius branch.

LEFT ANTERIOR DESCENDING ARTERY

The LAD arises and courses anteriorly from the LMS and descends the anterior aspect of the heart in the anterior interventricular groove.

The LAD is divided into segments as follows:
- Proximal: Origin to the first diagonal branch
- Middle: From the first diagonal branch to halfway to the ventricular apex
- Distal: From the end of the mid-segment to the ventricular apex

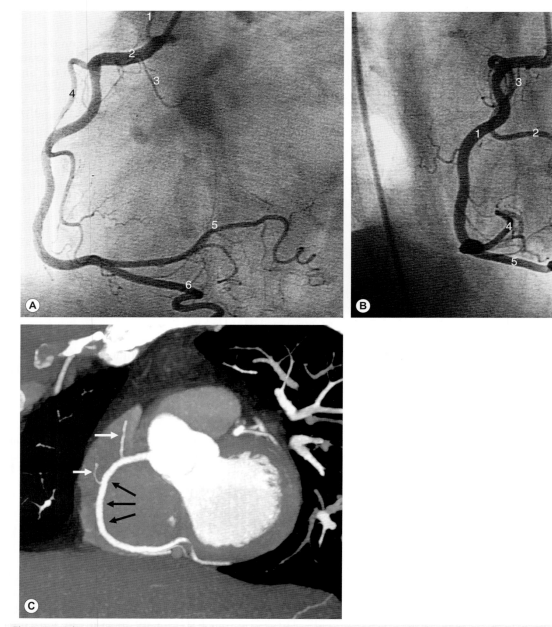

Fig. 4.32 Right coronary angiogram. (A) Left anterior oblique projection. (B) Right anterior oblique projection. The AV nodal branch is not seen. (C) Reformated maximum-intensity projection image of a computed tomography coronary angiogram demonstrating the typical 'C' configuration of the right coronary artery *(black arrows)*. *White arrows* highlight the conal and sinoatrial branches.

(A)
1. Sinus artery
2. Right coronary artery
3. Conus branch
4. Right ventricular branch
5. Posterolateral branch
6. Posterior descending artery

(B)
1. Right coronary artery
2. Right ventricular branch
3. Conus branch
4. Posterolateral branch
5. Posterior descending artery

Branches of the Anterior Descending Artery

These are as follows:
- Septal branches: Short branches coursing from the right side of the LAD, supplying the anterior two-thirds of the interventricular septum.

- Diagonal branches: Larger vessels that run to the left of the LAD over the anterolateral wall of the LV supplying it (remembered by **D** for **d**iagonal and **D** for LA**D**). The diagonal branches are numbered in order of their branching (i.e. D1, D2, D3. D1 and sometimes D2), are

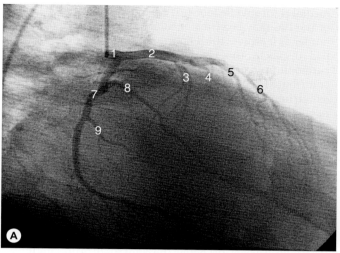
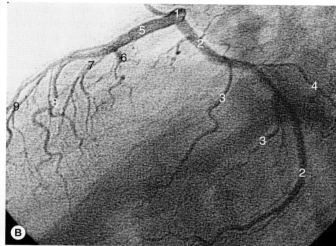

Fig. 4.33 Left coronary angiogram. (A) Right anterior oblique projection. (B) Left lateral projection.

(A)
1. Left main coronary artery
2. Left anterior descending artery (LAD)
3. Septal branch
4. First diagonal branch
5. Second diagonal branch
6. Continuation of the LAD
7. Circumflex artery
8. First obtuse marginal branch
9. Second obtuse marginal branch

(B)
1. Left main coronary artery seen end-on
2. Circumflex artery
3. Obtuse marginals
4. Posterolateral branch
5. Left anterior descending artery (LAD)
6. Septal branch
7. First diagonal branch
8. Second diagonal branch
9. Continuation of the LAD

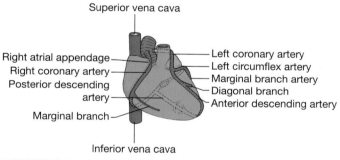

Fig. 4.34 The coronary arteries.

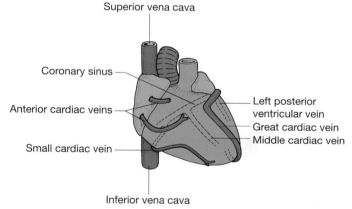

Fig. 4.35 The coronary veins.

usually large branches similar in size to the main coronary arteries. When a ramus intermedius branch is present, it usually replaces one of the diagonal branches and supplies the anterolateral LV wall.
■ A branch to the RV (occasionally).

LEFT CIRCUMFLEX ARTERY

The LCx arises and courses posteriorly from the LMS and descends in the left anterior interventricular groove.

Branches of the Left Circumflex Artery

These are as follows:
■ Obtuse marginal branches, which supply the inferolateral wall of the LV
■ Atrial branches

In general, the RCA (usually dominant) supplies the RV and the inferior part of the LV. The left coronary supplies the remainder of the LV. The interventricular septum is supplied by the LAD anteriorly and the PDA posteriorly. The atria have a variable supply. In more than 50% of cases the sinoatrial node is supplied by the RCA, and in 90% of cases the RCA supplies the atrioventricular node.

THE VEINS OF THE HEART (FIG. 4.35)

Sixty percent of venous drainage of the heart is via veins that accompany the coronary arteries. The vast majority of cardiac veins drain via the coronary sinus into the right atrium. The coronary sinus (not to be confused with the pericardial sinuses and the aortic sinuses of Valsalva) is the largest cardiac venous structure. It is a short (3–5 cm), large-calibre (1 cm) vein which forms on the posterior aspect of the heart between the left atrium and the LV and travels in the posterior/inferior portion of the left atrioventricular groove and drains into the posterior wall of the right atrium to the left of the orifice of the IVC. Its tributaries are:

- The great cardiac vein: This vein begins at the LV apex as the anterior interventricular vein (a part of the great cardiac vein) in the anterior interventricular groove with the LAD. It then runs into the left atrioventricular groove with the LCx before draining into the coronary sinus in the posterior portion of the left AV groove.
- The middle cardiac vein, which ascends in the posterior interventricular groove.
- The small cardiac vein, which accompanies the marginal branches of the RCA on the inferior surface of the heart and then runs posteriorly in the right atrioventricular groove to enter the right side of the coronary sinus.
- The left posterior ventricular vein, which accompanies the obtuse marginals of the LCA, running up the posterior aspect of the LV to drain into the coronary sinus.

The anterior cardiac veins drain much of the anterior surface of the heart and drain into the anterior wall of the right atrium directly. Several small veins, the venae cordis minimae, drain directly into the cardiac chambers.

RADIOLOGY OF THE HEART

Radiography

Frontal Chest Radiograph. The heart is asymmetrically distributed to the left of the spine, reflecting the normal left cardiac orientation. The right heart border is made up primarily by the right atrium which is outlined by air in the medial right middle lobe but a portion of the lateral aspect of the IVC may be visible medial to the right cardiophrenic border as it crosses the diaphragm. Occasionally a fibrofatty pad displaces the right pleura laterally, obscuring the cardiophrenic angle. The right atrial appendage does not contribute to the contour as it is an anterior structure. The left atrium is abutted by lung on its right side but does not usually contribute to the cardiac silhouette as it projects over the spine. When enlarged, it extends further laterally and can be seen as a second contour posterior to the right atrium (double density or double right heart sign). Again, left atrial enlargement should also cause splaying of the carina. As previously described, the confluence of the right superior and inferior pulmonary veins may also be seen behind the right heart. The cavoatrial junction (between the SVC and right heart) can be seen as an abrupt change in contour from the rounded right atrium to the straight SVC. It usually projects just below the right main bronchus which can be very useful for central line placement. The left heart border is entirely made up by the LV. Pericardial fat pads are also often seen on the left. The region of the left atrial appendage is just below the pulmonary trunk contour at the level of the left main bronchus. As previously described, this should never be convex. The density of the left and right heart should be equal with vessels visible through them. On a PA chest radiograph the normal cardiothoracic ratio (ratio of maximal cardiac diameter to maximal horizontal thoracic measurement) is less than 0.50 and up to 0.60 in infants. On an AP chest radiograph, the normal ratio is approximately 0.66. These measurements are crude and significantly influenced by technical factors such as depth of inspiration (Fig. 4.36). Valve position may be deduced on PA and lateral films in relation to the cardiac outline or the sternum and ribs (Fig. 4.37). The aortic and mitral valves are the most important to recognize, as they are most often affected by disease. The lowest part of the aortic valve is very close to the anterior part of the mitral valve, where they are anatomically in fibrous continuity.

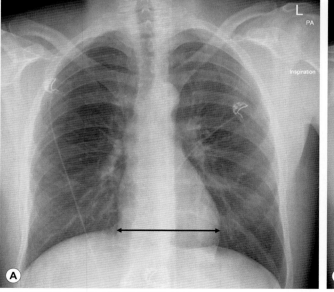
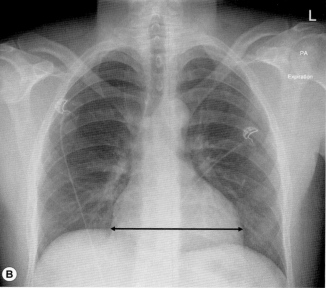

Fig. 4.36 (A) Posteroanterior chest radiograph in (A) inspiration and (B) expiration demonstrating the change in the size of the cardiac silhouette *(black arrow)* depending on the phase of respiration.

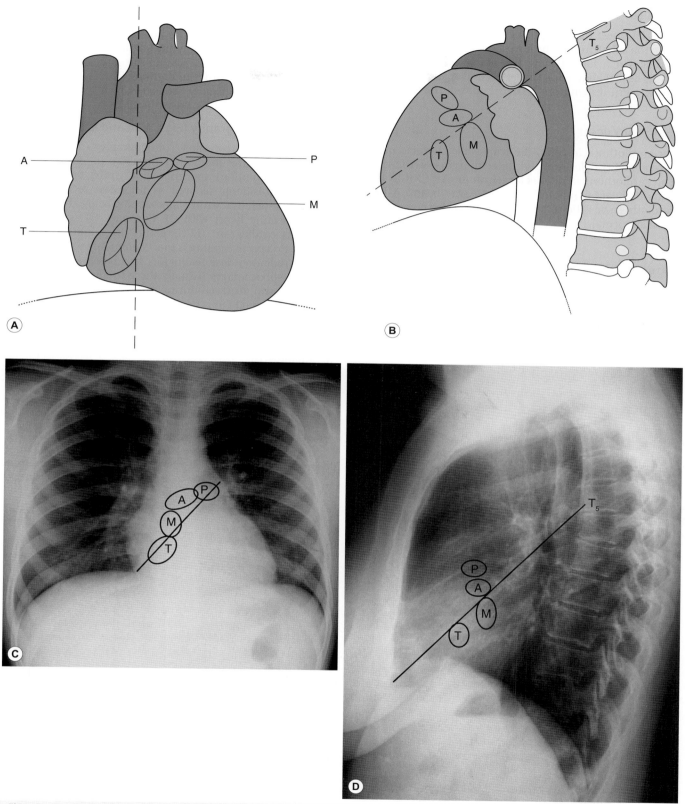

Fig. 4.37 Position of cardiac valves. (A) As seen on anteroposterior (AP) chest radiograph. (B) As seen on lateral chest X-ray (CXR). (C) AP CXR. (D) Lateral CXR. *A,* Aortic; *M,* mitral; *P,* pulmonary; *T,* tricuspid.

RADIOLOGY PEARL

On a PA chest radiograph the valves lie close to a line from the left atrium to the lowest point of the right heart border. On a lateral view the pulmonary and aortic valves lie just above, and the mitral and aortic valves just below, a line drawn from T5 to the apex of the heart.

RADIOLOGY PEARL

For cardiothoracic ratio, the transverse thoracic measurement is made from the inner margins of the ribs. The cardiothoracic ratio is larger on an AP CXR as the anterior heart is magnified by the X-ray beam. A low cardiothoracic ratio of less than 0.40 is also considered to be abnormal.

RADIOLOGY PEARL

The cardiac contour should also be considered, as a rounded or prominent LV may be misdiagnosed as cardiomegaly.

Lateral Chest Radiograph

The anterior aspect of the cardiac shadow is made up entirely by the RV on lateral radiograph. The anterior aspect of the RV usually abuts the sternum so does not form a crisp silhouette. The RV shadow should not occupy more

than one-third of the craniocaudal length of the retrosternal space or it is enlarged. The RV silhouette flows upwards into the RVOT silhouette. The posterior aspect of the cardiac silhouette is made up by the left atrium superiorly and the LV inferiorly. The IVC crossing the diaphragm also contributes to the more inferior contour. The posterior aspect of the LV contour usually projects <3 cm beyond the IVC contour. If it exceeds this, it is enlarged.

Computed Tomography (Figs. 4.38 and 4.39)

Technique. CT coronary angiography has greatly improved with the increasing numbers of detector rows (improved resolution) and improving gantry speeds (faster shorter acquisitions) as well as improved reconstruction algorithms such that we are approaching being able to image the nonbeating heart with CT. Coronary CT is dependent on electrocardiogram (ECG) gating to minimize cardiac motion. Prospective gating is most commonly used as it uses a lower radiation dose technique. It is based on sequential step and shoot images (usually three to four depending on detector rows) acquired during sequential RR intervals on the ECG and modulates dose. Retrospective ECG gating can be used, particularly when heart rate is high or irregular. This technique images continuously throughout several RR intervals until the heart has been entirely imaged without modulating the dose. The images can retrospectively be matched to their point in the RR interval. This allows dynamic assessment (beating heart) but has a much higher dose due to absence of dose modulation as well as using a lower pitch (slower table movement which increases beam overlap, giving more temporal data at the expense of a higher dose).

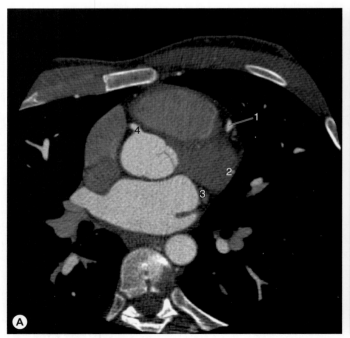
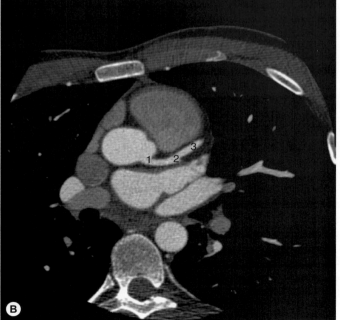

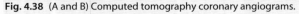

Fig. 4.38 (A and B) Computed tomography coronary angiograms.

(A)
1. Left anterior descending coronary artery
2. Diagonal coronary artery
3. Circumflex coronary artery
4. Origin of the right coronary artery

(B)
1. Origin of the left main stem coronary artery
2. Origin of the circumflex coronary artery
3. Left anterior descending coronary artery

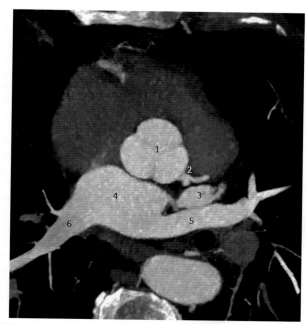

Fig. 4.39 Maximum-intensity projection image of a computed tomography coronary angiogram at the level of the aortic valve.
1. Trileaflet aortic valve
2. Left main stem arising from the left coronary cusp before bifurcating into the left circumflex and left anterior descending coronary arteries
3. Left atrial appendage
4. Left atrium
5. Left superior pulmonary vein draining into the left atrium
6. Right superior pulmonary vein draining into the left atrium

Beta blockers are usually administered to try and reduce the heart rate, ideally to less than 60–65 bpm. Glyceryl trinitrate is also commonly administered to dilate the coronary arteries to facilitate evaluation. Contrast bolus tracking is aimed around optimal contrast in the left heart so the right heart chambers are frequently not opacified. If information on the right heart is pertinent, a different contrast protocol should be used. A prospectively gated noncontrast cardiac CT (CT calcium score) is usually performed prior to contrast phases to allow assessment of the degree of coronary calcification using the Agatston score. Imaging in coronary CT is acquired transaxially and can be reconstructed into any plane in postprocessing as distinct from coronary MRI. The cardiac planes described below are sometimes used. In curved planar reformats of the coronary arteries the vessels are traced and with the aid of postprocessing software are 'laid out' in a linear fashion on two-dimensional images to show their whole length.

As with chest radiographs, cardiomegaly is frequently overcalled on CT. Cardiothoracic ratio is not used on CT and assessment depends on chamber size. These vary from patient to patient and greatly vary with body surface area and sex. On axial slices, a left atrial AP diameter of >5 cm for a male and 4.5 cm for a female is enlarged. LV diameters perpendicular to the interventricular septum of >5.7 cm for a male and 5.3 cm for a female are considered cardiomegaly. As above, the crista terminalis in the right atrium can be misleading. The increased trabeculation of the RV can be appreciated and usually the moderator band

is identified. The tricuspid valve is usually indistinct on CT and leaflets can rarely be delineated. The fossa ovalis is usually visible. Contrast can often be seen to extend between the septum primum and secundum which are often incompletely fused. This is a normal finding. If contrast extends through from the left atrium to the right atrium (which can be recognized if the right heart is not opacified with contrast), a patent foramen ovale can be suspected. This is reportedly present in 25% of all people but not seen at this frequency on CT. The left papillary muscles are well delineated in the LV as large filling defects and should not be confused with pathology. The left ventricular apex is often very thin in normal health. The leaflets of the aortic valve can be clearly delineated on good-quality studies (Fig. 4.39) and valve opening can be assessed on retrospective studies. The pulmonary valve can usually be seen but is less well defined.

The coronary arteries can be assessed throughout their course on a good-quality CT coronary angiogram. When there are multiple branches, the correct vessels can be determined based on their location, for example if there are large diagonal branches, the LAD is the vessel running in the anterior interventricular groove whereas the diagonal runs over the LV anterior wall. Points at which coronary veins cross the coronary arteries can simulate atherosclerotic plaque/stenoses.

RADIOLOGY PEARL

The posterior papillary muscle of the LV is usually supplied only by the PDA. This makes the posteromedial papillary muscle significantly more susceptible to ischaemia, and therefore myocardial infarction involving the PDA is more likely to cause mitral regurgitation.

RADIOLOGY PEARL

There are a wide variety of coronary artery anomalies including anomalous origins and anomalous courses, the list of which is beyond the scope of this text. Eighty percent are not of clinical significance but some are associated with a significant risk of ischaemia. Previously, the course of the anomalous artery was felt to be the most important factor, with an interarterial course between the aorta and pulmonary trunk considered malignant. More recently, there has been increased focus on the angle of take-off of the coronary from the aorta and whether that causes stenosis. The course of the vessel is still relevant but the term 'malignant course' has been phased out.

RADIOLOGY PEARL

Occasionally coronary arteries traverse segments of myocardial muscle, a finding termed myocardial bridging. During muscle contraction in systole, blood flow through such segments is limited and may produce acute ischaemia. This may be one of many causes of sudden cardiac death in athletes.

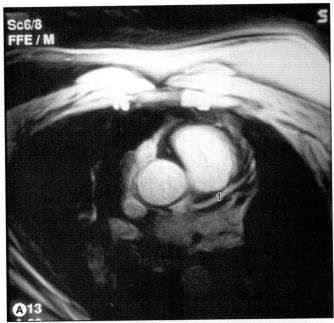

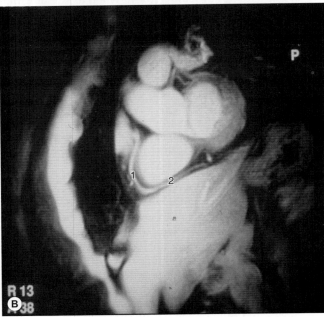

Fig. 4.40 (A and B) Coronary magnetic resonance angiograms.

(A)
1. Proximal left anterior descending coronary artery

(B)
1. Right coronary artery
2. Posterior descending coronary artery

Cardiac MRI

Cardiac MRI combines excellent imaging of the structure of the heart with unmatched functional assessment. Dynamic cine imaging shows cardiac morphology and motion, and also allows measurement of volumes and ejection fraction. Phase contrast imaging (a complex MRI technique in which moving blood is bright) allows flow quantification of flow and velocity measurement. Gadolinium contrast-enhanced imaging assesses late contrast uptake (indicating myocardial scar tissue). Acquisition of images is gated to the ECG to overcome motion artefact, and faster scan times have improved image quality. The cardiac chambers, valves and major vessels may be imaged in any plane. Unlike coronary CT, the plane of imaging is determined in advance and can be well reconstructed in postprocessing. Cardiac MRI uses cardiac imaging planes, many of which are based on ECG planes. The basic planes are essentially axial, sagittal and coronal but with respect to the cardiac axis rather than the body's axis as seen in most other areas of radiology. The horizontal long axis is equivalent to an axial of the heart as well as the echo four-chamber view. The vertical long axis is akin to a sagittal or two-chamber view of the heart and the short axis is like a coronal along the plane of the LV from base to apex or the parasternal short axis. Several other well-established imaging planes exist. The pericardium is shown as a dark line 1–2 mm thick. Cardiac MRI can be useful in pericardial assessment as it can show typical signs of pericardial constriction which would not be perceptible on CT or other nondynamic studies. Cardiac MRI does not image the coronary arteries as well as CT due to its inferior spatial resolution (Fig. 4.40), but it can assess for ischaemia in coronary territories by detecting delayed gadolinium enhancement.

Echocardiography

Two-dimensional echocardiography uses ultrasound to image the heart. A subcostal or intracostal window may be used and images may be obtained in any plane. Longitudinal images through the outflow tracts are usually obtained, as well as cross-sectional images through the valves and chambers. Ultrasound is probably the best modality for imaging the internal anatomy of the heart, the walls, chambers and valves. The movement of the walls and valves may also be assessed dynamically throughout the cardiac cycle. Transoesophageal echocardiography allows much closer inspection of the heart because of the close apposition of the left atrium to the anterior wall of the distal oesophagus, without intervening air or lung.

Coronary Catheter Angiography

Coronary angiography involves selective catheterization of the coronary arteries. A small volume of contrast is injected and images may be obtained in lateral, anterior oblique and AP projections. There is individual variation in the branches of the coronary arteries, which are demonstrated from case to case. This is due to both anatomical variation and technical factors. The major arteries are demonstrated in Figs. 4.32 and 4.33. This is generally performed by interventional cardiologists rather than radiologists.

Myocardial Viability and Perfusion Scintigraphy

Nuclear medicine studies are used mainly for functional assessment of the heart, which in clinical practice is often more important than the demonstration of the anatomy. **Thallium-201 (^{201}Th) and technetium-99m (^{99m}Tc)-labelled MIBI** (2-methoxy isobutyl isonitrile) are taken up by normally perfused myocardium, and images obtained by gamma camera show the heart. The use of SPECT allows images to be constructed in any plane – usually with three sets of images – along the short cardiac axis (at right angles to the long axis of the heart), and along the vertical and horizontal long axes. It also improves the target:background ratio, as neither radiopharmaceutical agent is taken up exclusively by the myocardium. Other functional information on ventricular filling, ejection fraction and so on may be obtained by blood-pool imaging using ^{99m}Tc-labelled red blood cells and ECG-gated acquisition of data.

Positron Emission Tomography CT (Fig. 4.41)

Normal cardiac muscle concentrates or consumes injected 18-fluorodeoxyglucose (essentially uses glucose), reflecting normal pulsatility and cardiac muscular contractions. Targeted cardiac positron emission tomography (PET) CT scanning allows detection of metabolically inactive sites of infarcted muscle. When combined with CT coronary angiography, it may show areas of salvageable 'hibernating' myocardium – which shows persistent metabolic activity despite loss of vascular supply demonstrated at CT angiography.

The Great Vessels (see Figs. 4.12, 4.25 and 4.27)

THE THORACIC AORTA (SEE FIGS. 4.12 AND 4.42)

The thoracic aorta is divided into three components – ascending, arch and descending.

The Ascending Aorta

The ascending aorta begins at the aortic valve at the level of the lower border of the third costal cartilage to the left of the midline. The first few centimetres of the ascending aorta and the pulmonary trunk are enclosed in a common sheath of pericardium. At its origin it lies behind the outflow tract of the RV and the pulmonary trunk, and the right atrial appendage overlaps it. It ascends to the right, arching over the pulmonary trunk to lie behind the upper border of the second right costal cartilage. It continues anteriorly to the right pulmonary artery. The right lung and sternum are anterior. The coronary arteries arise from aortic sinuses of Valsalva – three localized dilatations above the cusps of the aortic valve. The point at which the sinuses meet the normal aortic vessel is called the sinotubular junction.

The Aortic Arch

The arch of the aorta is the continuation of the ascending aorta. A horizontal line drawn from the manubriosternal angle to the T4 vertebral body defines the transthoracic plane of Ludwig. This can be used to determine the starting point of the aortic arch anteriorly and the level at which it becomes the descending aorta posteriorly. The arch passes posteriorly and from right to left, anterior to the trachea and arches over the left main bronchus and pulmonary artery to come to lie to the left of the body of T4.

Anatomical relations of the aortic arch:

- Anterior and to the left of the arch are the pleura and left lung.
- On its right side, from front to back, are the trachea, oesophagus, thoracic duct and body of T4.
- Its inferior aspect is connected to the ligamentum arteriosum, the fibrous remnant of the ductus arteriosus.
- Superiorly are the three branches of the arch that are crossed anteriorly by the left brachiocephalic vein. The

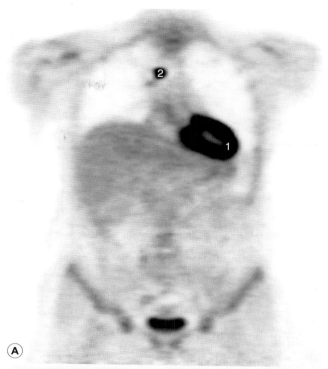

(A)

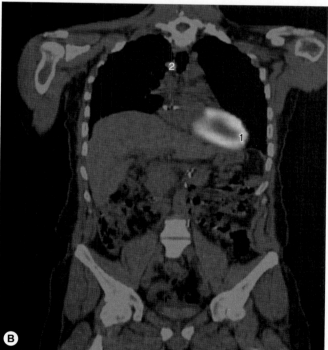

(B)

Fig. 4.41 (A) Positron emission tomography (PET) scan and (B) PET computed tomography scan acquired following injection of 18-fluorodeoxyglucose radiotracer showing avid uptake by healthy contracting cardiac muscle.

1. Left ventricle
2. 18-fluorodeoxyglucose uptake by pathological paratracheal node

left superior intercostal vein runs down to the brachiocephalic vein, passing anterior to the aorta and occasionally causing a small bulge on the arch, which is visible on the chest radiograph. This is a normal variant on CXR known as an 'aortic nipple'.

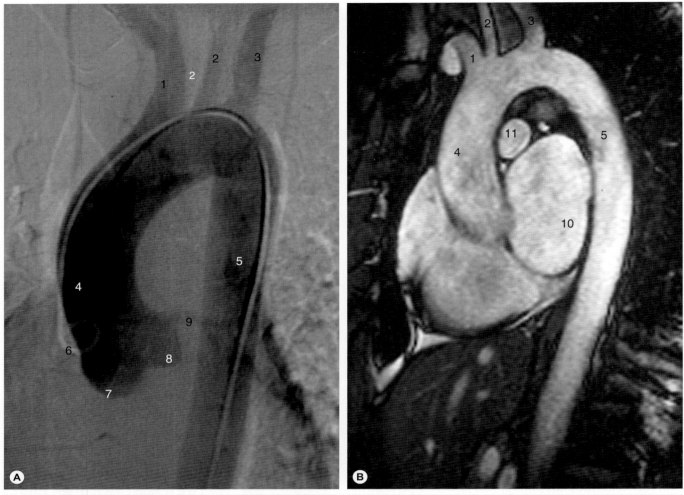

Fig. 4.42 Aortograms. (A) Digital subtraction angiography. (B) Magnetic resonance angiogram.

1. Brachiocephalic artery
2. Left common carotid
3. Left subclavian artery
4. Ascending aorta
5. Descending aorta
6. Angiography catheter

7. Anterior cusp of aortic valve
8. Left posterior cusp of aortic valve
9. Left coronary artery
10. Left atrium
11. Left pulmonary artery

Branches. The branches of the arch of the aorta in order from proximal to distal are the brachiocephalic trunk, the left common carotid and the left subclavian arteries. The brachiocephalic and left common carotid arteries ascend on either side of the trachea in a 'V' shape to come to lie behind the sternoclavicular joints, at which point the brachiocephalic bifurcates into the right common carotid and subclavian arteries. From this point the common carotids ascend symmetrically into the neck.

Variation is common in the branches of the aortic arch, such that the 'normal' pattern as described above is only seen in 65% of subjects. The reported frequency of these variations differs between studies, the figures provided are approximations:

- 14%: Left common carotid arises from the brachiocephalic artery, a 'bovine' arch configuration.

- 3%: Left vertebral artery arises directly from the arch of the aorta, between the origins of the left common carotid and left subclavian arteries.

- 2.7%: Common origin of the left common carotid and subclavian as a left brachiocephalic artery.

- 0.5%: Aberrant right subclavian artery arises distal to the left subclavian artery and passes to the right, posterior to the oesophagus.

- Rare: Right common carotid and subclavian arteries arising separately.

- Very rare: Common carotid is absent so that the internal and external carotid arteries arise separately from the aortic arch on one or both sides.

- The following other arteries may also arise from the aortic arch:
  - One or both bronchial arteries
  - Thyroidea ima artery

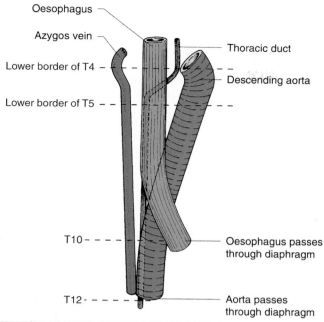

Oesophagus
Azygos vein
Lower border of T4
Lower border of T5
Thoracic duct
Descending aorta
T10
T12
Oesophagus passes through diaphragm
Aorta passes through diaphragm

Fig. 4.43 Posterior mediastinum.

- Inferior thyroid artery
- Internal thoracic artery
- The origins of the brachiocephalic and the left common carotid arteries may also vary. If the vessels arise earlier than normal the left common carotid has to pass anterior to the trachea to assume its position left of the aorta. If the vessels arise more distally the brachiocephalic artery passes anterior to the trachea to get to its right side. Either arrangement may lead to anterior compression of the trachea, which may cause symptoms especially in the infant, whose anterior mediastinum is crowded by the thymus.

RADIOLOGY PEARL

The **aortic isthmus** is the junction of the arch of the aorta and the descending aorta. This area is relatively fixed and is thus prone to injury with the shearing forces of blunt trauma; this is the most frequent site of aortic mural tear and transection.

The isthmus may also be the site of a ductus diverticulum, a focal smooth outpouching of the thoracic aorta. This is a normal variant and should not be confused for a pseudoaneurysm.

The Descending Aorta

The descending aorta passes inferiorly through the posterior mediastinum to the left of the spinal column. It passes through the aortic hiatus in the diaphragm at the level of T12 and continues as the abdominal aorta. As the aorta descends it passes posterior to the left main bronchus and pulmonary artery, the left atrium, the oesophagus and the posterior part of the diaphragm.

Anatomical relations of the descending aorta (Fig. 4.43):
- Left: Left lung and pleura.
- Right: Right lung and pleura. Inferiorly the thoracic duct and azygous vein.
- Posteriorly: Vertebral column and the hemiazygos veins.
- At its highest point the oesophagus lies to the right. The descending aorta then continues behind the oesophagus.

Branches of the descending aorta:
- Nine pairs of posterior intercostal arteries and a pair of subcostal arteries arise from the posterior aspect of the descending aorta to run in the neurovascular grooves of the third to twelfth ribs. These anastomose with the anterior intercostal arteries, which are branches of the internal thoracic aorta. The intercostal arteries give rise to radicular and radiculomedullary arteries to the spinal cord and its nerve roots.
- Two to three bronchial arteries, the origins of which are variable. The right bronchial artery usually arises from the third posterior intercostal artery and the two left bronchial arteries from the aorta itself. The upper left usually arises opposite T5 and the lower left bronchial artery below the left main bronchus.
- Four to five oesophageal branches arise from the front of the aorta. These ramify on the oesophagus, forming a network with oesophageal branches of the inferior thyroid artery and ascending branches of the left phrenic and left gastric arteries.
- Mediastinal branches.
- Phrenic branches to the upper part of the posterior diaphragm (which receives most of its blood supply by inferior phrenic arteries that arise from the abdominal artery).
- Pericardial branches to the posterior pericardium.

SUBCLAVIAN ARTERY (SEE FIG. 1.47)

The right subclavian artery arises from the bifurcation of the brachiocephalic trunk behind the right sternoclavicular joint. The left subclavian artery arises from the arch of the aorta in front of the trachea at the level of the T3/T4 disc space. It ascends on the left of the trachea to behind the left sternoclavicular joint. From this point, both arteries have a similar course.

The subclavian artery has three parts:
- The first part arches over the apex of the lung from the origin of the artery to medial border of the scalenus anterior muscle (which passes from the transverse processes of the upper cervical vertebrae to the inner border of the first rib).
- The second part is posterior to the scalenus anterior muscle, which separates it from the subclavian vein.
- The third part passes from the lateral border of scalenus anterior to the lateral border of the first rib, at which point it becomes the axillary artery (see Chapter 1 for branches).

PULMONARY ARTERIES (SEE FIGS. 4.19, 4.25; SEE ALSO SECTION ON THE PULMONARY ARTERY IN THE LUNGS, P. 126)

The pulmonary trunk carries deoxygenated blood from the RV to the lungs via the left and right pulmonary arteries. It begins at the pulmonary valve and is approximately 5 cm long. At first it lies anterior to the left main bronchus. The entire pulmonary trunk is covered by the pericardium in a common sheath with the ascending aorta. The normal diameter of the pulmonary trunk is less than 2.9 cm.

The right and left atrial appendages and the right and left coronary arteries surround the base of the pulmonary trunk. Anterior and to the left it is in contact with the left lung and pleura.

The right pulmonary artery runs horizontally and to the right, passing behind the ascending aorta and SVC in front of the right main bronchus. It is crossed anteriorly by the right superior pulmonary vein as it drains to the left atrium.

The left pulmonary artery runs to the left, arching over the left main bronchus as it gives off the upper lobe bronchus. It has a slightly higher position in the chest and is slightly shorter and smaller than the right pulmonary artery. It is crossed anteriorly by the left superior pulmonary vein. It is attached to the concavity of the aortic arch by the ligamentum arteriosum, the fibrous remnant of the ductus arteriosus.

GREAT VEINS (SEE FIG. 4.12)

The brachiocephalic veins are formed by the union of the internal jugular and subclavian veins at either side, behind the medial end of the clavicles. On the right, the brachiocephalic vein runs inferiorly behind the right border of the manubrium, anterolateral to the brachiocephalic artery. The left brachiocephalic vein is longer. It descends obliquely behind the manubrium, crossing the origins of the left common carotid and subclavian arteries. It joins with the right brachiocephalic vein to form the SVC behind the junction of the first right costal cartilage with the manubrium.

The **superior vena cava** runs inferiorly behind the right border of the manubrium to enter the right atrium at the level of the third costal cartilage. Its only tributary is the azygos vein, which enters its posterior aspect just above the upper limit of its covering sheath of pericardium.

Tributaries of the Brachiocephalic Veins

These are as follows:

- Internal thoracic (mammary) veins, which drain into the inferior aspect of the brachiocephalic veins.
- Inferior thyroid veins, which arise in the thyroid gland and form a plexus anterior to the trachea. From here, left and right veins drain into the corresponding brachiocephalic vein, close to their confluence.
- Left superior intercostal vein, which drains the left second and third posterior intercostal veins and passes obliquely down anterior to the aortic arch to drain into the left brachiocephalic vein.

RADIOLOGY OF THE GREAT VESSELS

The great vessels may be imaged by two-dimensional echocardiography, angiography, CT or MRI.

In suspected acute thoracic aortic pathology CT angiography is generally the first line of investigation. An ECG-gated acquisition can be performed to reduce the effects of cardiac motion and provide better visualization of the aortic root. This is especially important when imaging type A thoracic aortic dissection to provide accurate assessment of the coronary ostia.

Using MRI, images can be acquired following intravenous gadolinium infusion in coronal, axial or the favoured sagittal oblique plane.

With two-dimensional echocardiography the aortic root and sinuses, and ascending and descending aorta may be visualized using an anterior approach. The arch of the aorta and its branches are occasionally well visualized from a suprasternal approach.

The Oesophagus (Figs. 4.43, 4.44)

This begins at the level of C5/C6 or the lower border of the cricoid cartilage as the continuation of the oropharynx (see also Chapter 1). Its upper limit is defined by the cricopharyngeus muscle, which encircles it from front to back. It descends behind the trachea and thyroid, lying in front of the lower cervical vertebrae. It then inclines slightly to the left in the neck and upper mediastinum before returning to the midline at the level of T5, from where it passes to the left again before sweeping forward to pass through the diaphragm. From superior to inferior in the chest it passes behind the trachea, left main bronchus, left atrium and upper part of the LV; it then passes behind the posterior sloping part of the diaphragm before traversing this at the level of T10. The oesophageal hiatus in the diaphragm is surrounded by a sling of fibres from the right crus of the diaphragm. In its terminal part in the abdomen the oesophagus is retroperitoneal and grooves the posterior aspect of the liver. It enters the stomach at the oesophagogastric junction.

Relations of the thoracic oesophagus:

Left side (superior to inferior):

- Left subclavian artery
- Aortic arch (forms an indentation on the oesophagus)
- Thoracic duct (lies to the posteriorly inferiorly before moving to the left of the midline at T4, continuing to the left of the oesophagus as it ascends)
- Descending thoracic aorta (left initially then posterior as it descends)
- Right side: right lung and pleura
- Crossed by the termination of the azygous vein as it drains into the SVC at the T4 level

Posterior:

- Thoracic vertebrae
- Azygous vein
- Thoracic duct superiorly

Anterior:

- Trachea
- Left recurrent laryngeal nerve
- Left main bronchus
- Left atrium

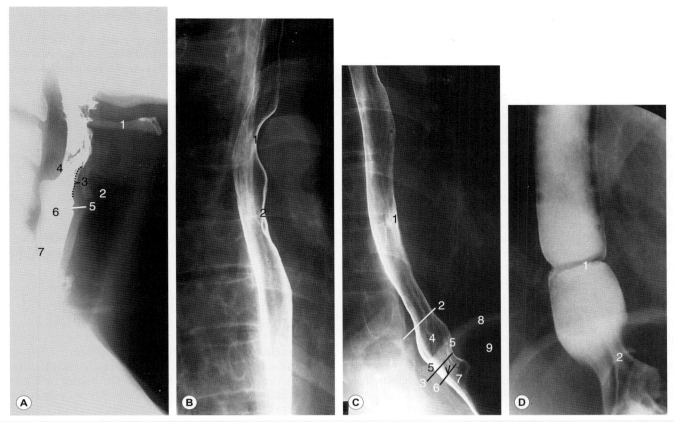

Fig. 4.44 Barium-swallow technique showing the oesophagus. (A) Upper oesophagus and oropharynx, lateral view. (B) Mid-oesophagus, right anterior oblique view. (C) Distal oesophagus. (D) Distal oesophagus in another patient with prominent Schatzki ring.

(A)
1. Hyoid bone
2. Cricoid cartilage
3. Cricoid impression
4. Cricopharyngeus muscle impression
5. Postcricoid venous plexus
6. Oesophagus
7. Impression caused by osteophytes

(B)
1. Impression of aortic arch
2. Impression of left main bronchus

(C)
1. Cardiac impression (mainly left atrium)
2. A ring: upper limit of ampulla (vestibule)
3. B ring (Schatzki ring): lower limit of ampulla
4. Ampulla (oesophageal vestibule)
5. Diaphragmatic hiatus
6. Oesophageal mucosal folds
7. Oesophagogastric junction (Z-line)
8. Diaphragm
9. Air in fundus of stomach

(D)
1. Schatzki ring
2. Gastro-oesophageal junction

BLOOD SUPPLY

The blood supply is organized in thirds (with free anastomosis between each third) as follows:

- Branches of the inferior thyroid artery supply the upper third.
- Branches from the descending aorta supply the middle third.
- Branches from the left gastric artery supply the lower third.

Venous drainage is also found in thirds: to the inferior thyroid veins, the azygos system and to the portal system via the left gastric vein. Thus there is communication of the systemic and portal venous systems in the oesophagus.

RADIOLOGY PEARL

Reflecting vascular supply, tumours of the lower oesophagus tend to metastasize below the diaphragm while tumours of the mid- and upper oesophagus metastasize above the diaphragm.

LYMPH DRAINAGE

This is via a rich paraoesophageal plexus to posterior mediastinal nodes, draining from here to supraclavicular nodes. The lower part drains to left gastric and coeliac nodes.

RADIOLOGY OF THE OESOPHAGUS (FIG. 4.44)

Plain Films

The right wall of the oesophagus and the azygos vein are outlined by the lung, which may be seen on the frontal film as the azygo-oesophageal line. Above the level of the arch of the azygos (at T4 level) the right wall is sometimes seen as the pleuro-oesophageal line. If the oesophagus contains air, the posterior aspect of the anterior oesophageal wall may be seen on the lateral film, behind the trachea. This is known as the 'posterior tracheal stripe'.

Barium Studies

The main radiological method of assessing the oesophagus is the barium-swallow technique, where the oesophagus is outlined by barium. Gas is usually swallowed in addition to give a double-contrast examination and to distend the oesophagus. The use of a paralyzing agent such as intravenous hyoscine butylbromide (Buscopan) stops intrinsic oesophageal contraction, allowing a better appreciation of oesophageal anatomy.

On the frontal view, the oropharynx may be examined. The piriform fossae are outlined by barium and the epiglottis and base of the tongue show as filling defects in the midline. The cervical oesophagus is seen to curve slightly to the left.

On the lateral view the tongue base and epiglottis are seen from the side, with the vallecula between. A posterior indentation caused by the contraction of cricopharyngeus muscle to initiate deglutition indicates the commencement of the oesophagus proper. Just below this, on the anterior wall of the oesophagus, a small impression may be made by a submucosal plexus of veins. The cervical oesophagus is seen to lie on the anterior surface of the vertebral bodies of the cervical spine.

In the chest, the oesophagus is best demonstrated with the subject rotated slightly off lateral – usually in the right anterior oblique position. Three major impressions are seen anteriorly. These are made by the aortic arch, the left main bronchus and the left heart chambers (mainly left atrium) from above down. In this position the oesophagus can be seen to curve anteriorly in its distal part to enter the stomach.

On the frontal view, the oesophagus has a left-sided indentation from the aortic arch. The left main bronchus also makes an impression on its left side and may make a linear impression as it indents the anterior wall. The lower oesophagus curves to the left to enter the stomach. In elderly people the course of the oesophagus may be altered by unfolding of the aorta.

The lower end of the oesophagus has a fusiform dilatation just above the oesophagogastric junction. This is called the oesophageal vestibule. On barium examination, the upper part of the vestibule is defined by a transiently contractile ring known as the 'A ring'. The lower limit of the vestibule is defined by another transiently contractile ring known as the 'B ring', 'Schatzki ring' or 'transverse mucosal fold'. The vestibule corresponds to the manometrically measurable zone of increased pressure that is felt to represent the lower oesophageal sphincter. The upper oesophageal sphincter is formed by cricopharyngeus. In young people the vestibule may span the diaphragm. In this case only the upper ring may be identified radiologically. As the oesophagus passes through the diaphragm the latter makes an indentation on it.

The oesophageal mucosa is arranged in longitudinal folds that are best seen when the oesophagus is not distended. These measure approximately 3 mm in width. The thicker folds of the stomach are seen distally, indicating the oesophagogastric junction. In normal people this may rise into the thorax on swallowing.

Cross-Sectional Imaging

The oesophagus may also be imaged by CT and MRI. On cross-section its relationship to the other structures of the thorax is appreciated. Its visualization is improved if it contains air. When collapsed it is seen as a narrow, thin-walled structure in the posterior mediastinum. Appreciation of the areas in which air-containing lung is adjacent to the oesophagus provides an understanding of the mediastinal lines seen on the frontal chest radiograph.

The Thoracic Duct and Mediastinal Lymphatics (Figs 4.21 and 4.43)

The **thoracic duct** arises from a saccular lymphatic reservoir called the 'cisterna chyli', which lies behind the right crus of the diaphragm, anterior to the bodies of L1 and L2. Lymph from the abdomen and lower limbs passes from here into the thoracic duct, which runs superiorly into the posterior mediastinum, passing through the aortic opening in the diaphragm. The thoracic duct ascends anterior to the vertebral column, with the descending aorta to its left and the azygos vein to its right. The right posterior intercostal arteries run across the vertebral column behind the duct, and the terminal parts of the hemiazygos and accessory azygos veins cross behind it to enter the azygos vein. It ascends behind the oesophagus, coming to lie to the left of this at T5 and then running superiorly on its left side into the neck. It then passes laterally behind the carotid vessels, and at the level of C7 the duct arches anteriorly over the left lung, rising 3–4 cm above the clavicle. It then descends to drain into the left subclavian vein at the jugulosubclavian junction. The thoracic duct has many valves in its last 5 cm.

The thoracic duct typically receives:
- Lymph from the abdomen and legs through the cisterna chyli.
- The left jugular lymph trunk draining the left side of the head and neck.
- The left subclavian lymph trunk draining left axilla and arm.
- The left bronchomediastinal trunk draining left lung and heart.
- The right lymphatic duct at the jugulosubclavian junction.

The **right lymphatic duct** is about 1 cm long with two semilunar valves at its entry to the vein to prevent reflux of blood into the lymphatic channel. It has three converging trunks:
- The right jugular trunk drains the right side of the head and neck.

- The right subclavian trunk drains the right arm, the right half of the thoracoabdominal wall as far inferiorly as the umbilicus anteriorly and the iliac crest posteriorly, and much of the right breast.
- The right bronchomediastinal trunk drains the hemithorax, including the right heart, the right lung and part of the liver.

Variations in thoracic lymph ducts are seen in 40%:
- The right lymphatic trunks may enter into the jugulo-subclavian junction separately, without the formation of a single right lymphatic duct.
- Multiple thoracic ducts may be seen in 20%.
- Multiple terminal channels from any single duct.
- The thoracic duct may terminate in the right jugular vein.

RADIOLOGY PEARL

The Virchow node or enlarged lymph node in the left supraclavicular fossa is often the first site of metastatic lymph nodal spread in patients with stomach and upper gastrointestinal tract tumours, reflecting lymphatic drainage from the cisterna chyli through the thoracic duct to the jugulosubclavian junction.

The **mediastinal lymph nodes** contain numerous lymph node groups which may enlarge in disease states. The anterior mediastinal nodes comprise the internal mammary chain, accompanying the internal mammary vessels, and a preaortic group lying anterior to the ascending aorta. The tracheobronchial nodes lie centrally around the trachea and its bifurcation. They comprise:
- Hilar nodes at the hilum of the lungs
- Carinal nodes below the hilum
- Tracheobronchial nodes above the tracheobronchial junction
- Right and left paratracheal nodes on either side of the trachea
- The azygos node in the right tracheobronchial angle
- Pretracheal nodes anterior to the trachea
- An aortopulmonary node between the concavity of the aortic arch and the pulmonary artery

The posterior mediastinal lymph nodes are found along the aorta and oesophagus and also anterior to and on either side of the spinal column. They take their name from their location, for example paraspinal, para-aortic and so on. Normal nodes are not appreciated on plain chest radiographs. Nodes may be seen on CT; if they measure more than 1 cm in diameter they are likely to be pathologically enlarged.

PET/CT

Pathological lymphadenopathy is best assessed at PET/CT scanning. Tumour-infiltrated nodes typically concentrate 18-fluorodeoxyglucose following intravenous injection and show increased metabolic activity. The associated positron emission is recorded at PET/CT scanning as an elevated specific uptake value (SUV); >2 in malignant nodes or <2 in benign conditions (it should be noted that SUV values are used as a guideline; very rarely malignant infiltrated nodes record SUV values <2; in contrast not uncommonly benign inflammatory enlargement of lymph nodes can lead to increased metabolic activity, with SUV values >2 simulating malignancy.) (See Fig. 4.41.) PET/CT is commonly used to stage lung cancer and lymphoma. It is important to be aware of areas that can accumulate radiotracers normally as this can mimic disease. For example, extensive brown fat in the neck can mimic cervical lymphadenopathy.

Lymphography

Lymphography may be performed by direct injection of groin nodes with contrast and imaging using X-ray or MRI.
See section in Chapter 5.

The Thymus

This organ is part of the lymphatic system and lies in the anterior mediastinum. It has two lobes, the left larger and higher than the right, which extend down as far as the fourth costal cartilage in infancy. It is a soft structure and is moulded into the sternum and ribs anteriorly, and the pericardium, great vessels and trachea posteriorly. It is extremely variable in size and shape, even in the same subject at different times. It may extend into the posterior mediastinum or be entirely below the level of the aortic arch. It is visible on the chest radiograph within 24 hours of birth, gradually involuting after 2 years of age. It is rarely seen on chest radiographs after 8 years of age but may be identified into early adulthood on CT as a small triangular structure in the anterior mediastinum, rarely measuring greater than 1 cm in diameter. The thymus gradually undergoes fatty replacement and is rarely identified beyond the age of 60 years. The rate of involution varies and is affected by factors such as BMI and cigarette smoking. Persistence of thymic tissue into late adulthood is more common in females and should not be mistaken for an anterior mediastinal mass.

RADIOLOGY OF THE THYMUS

Chest Radiograph (Fig. 4.45)

The thymus is visible on the chest radiograph as a mediastinal structure of soft tissue density. It may be focally or diffusely quite large and mass-like. Typically, lung markings can be seen through it; the edges are not sharp, but gradually fade or are wavy because of overlying ribs. Its lower well-defined horizontal border may protrude from the mediastinal contour on the right or the left as a 'sail sign'. It typically has clear lung lateral to it, or clear lung can be seen lateral to it if the patient is oblique enough. A normal thymus does not deviate a normal structure. It should never, for example, cause deviation of the trachea. The thymus appears larger on expiration than on inspiration radiographs. Its anterior location can be seen on a lateral radiograph.

CT and MRI (Fig. 4.46)

The normal thymus can be seen on CT or MRI long after it is no longer visible on a radiograph. In children the thymus can have convex borders; however, as it starts to involute

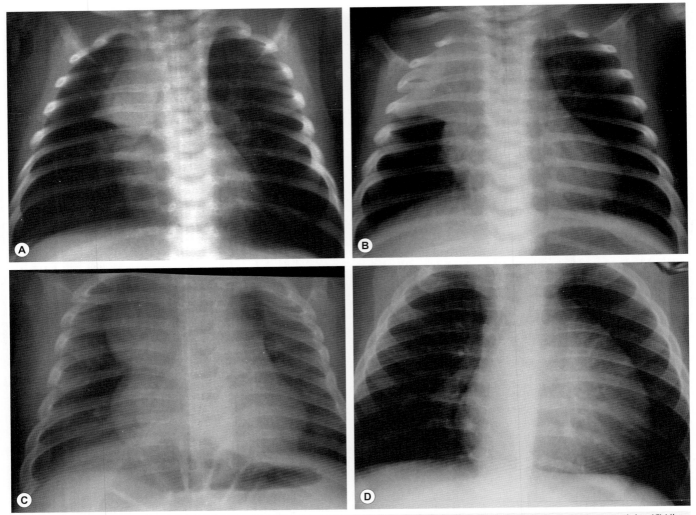

Fig. 4.45 Variable appearance of normal thymus on chest radiographs of young children. (A) Sail-like. (B) Like consolidation of right upper lobe. (C) Like mediastinal mass. (D) Like cardiomegaly.

after puberty it demonstrates a triangular morphology, following the contours of the anterior mediastinum in the axial plane (although the shape of the thymus is variable). On CT it is homogeneous, with a density similar to that of muscle. On T1- and T2-weighted MRI the thymus has a signal greater than that of muscle.

Ultrasound

Using high-frequency high-resolution ultrasound the internal architecture of the thymus may be seen. One can see the vascular septa dividing parenchymal lobules, which have an echogenic medulla centrally and a relatively hypoechoic cortex.

The Azygos System (Figs. 4.26, 4.43, 4.47 and 4.48)

The azygos veins are found in the posterior mediastinum. The system consists of the azygos vein on the right and the hemiazygos and accessory hemiazygos azygos veins on the left.

The azygos vein commences variably anterior to the L2 vertebra, either as a branch of the IVC or as a confluence of the right ascending lumbar vein and right subcostal vein. The aorta, thoracic duct, oesophagus and right vagus nerve lie to its left as it ascends in the thorax. The azygous vein lies anteriorly to the bodies of T12–T5 and the right posterior intercostal arteries, which cross behind it. The right lung and pleura are to its right. It usually passes behind the right crus of the diaphragm to enter the thorax (see Fig. 4.7). At the level of T4 the azygos vein arches anteriorly to drain into the SVC, passing over the right main bronchus as it enters the hilum of the right lung. The azygos vein drains into the SVC just above the upper limit of the pericardium, behind the third costal cartilage.

The azygos vein receives all but the first intercostal vein on the right. The second, third and fourth intercostal veins usually drain via a common channel – the right superior intercostal vein. The hemiazygos and accessory azygos veins drain into the azygos vein at midthoracic level. The right bronchial veins drain into the azygos vein near its termination. It also receives tributaries from the oesophagus, pericardium and mediastinum.

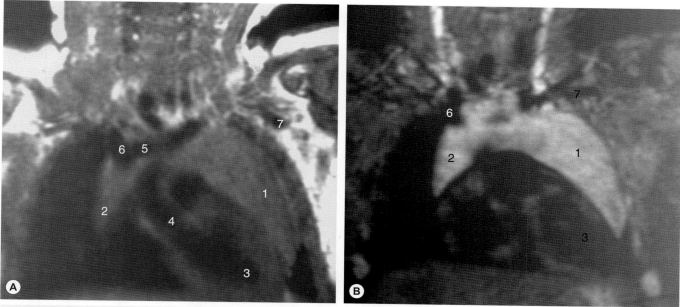

Fig. 4.46 Coronal magnetic resonance image of the thymus. (A) T1 weighted. (B) T2 weighted.

1. Left lobe of thymus
2. Right lobe of thymus
3. Left ventricle
4. Ascending aorta

5. Brachiocephalic vein
6. Right subclavian vein
7. Left subclavian vein

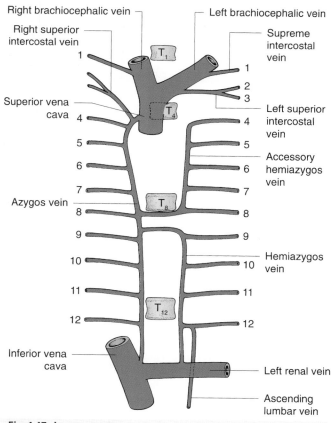

Fig. 4.47 Azygos system.

The hemiazygos vein commences in a similar manner to the azygos vein on the left side of the aorta. Its origin may communicate with the left renal vein, and it ascends anterior to the vertebral column to the midthoracic level (usually T8 or T9), then passes behind the aorta to drain into the azygos vein. It receives the left ascending lumbar and lowest four posterior intercostal veins, as well as mediastinal and oesophageal veins.

The accessory hemiazygos vein receives the fourth to the eighth posterior intercostal veins. (The first to third posterior intercostal veins drain into the left brachiocephalic vein.) It may also receive the left bronchial veins. It descends on the left side of the vertebral column to the midthoracic level, then crosses to the right behind the aorta to drain into the azygos vein. The hemiazygos and accessory hemiazygos veins may drain into the azygos vein separately or via a common trunk.

Important Nerves of the Mediastinum

The **vagus nerves** are the tenth cranial nerves and pass through the neck in the carotid sheath. Composed of parasympathetic, motor and sensory fibres, the vagus nerve enters the superior mediastinum posterior to the internal jugular vein and brachiocephalic veins. It passes behind the main bronchi, forming a posterior pulmonary plexus; branches then pass to the oesophagus, forming anterior

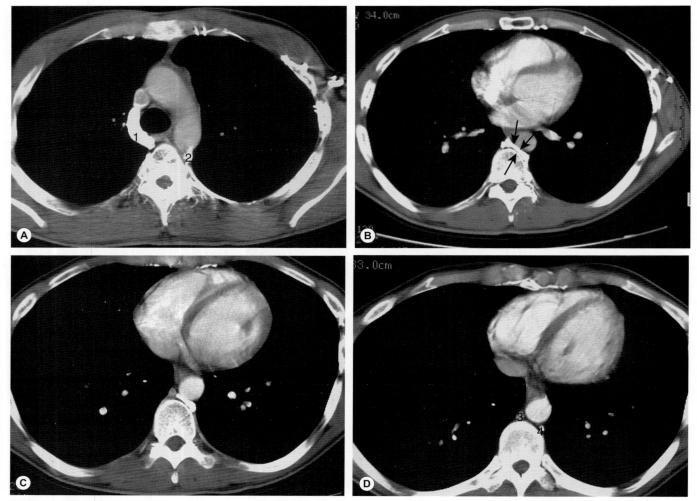

Fig. 4.48 Axial computed tomography (CT) thorax with contrast to show the azygos and hemiazygos system of veins. (A) Contrast densely opacifies the arch of the azygos vein. (B) The accessory hemiazygos vein drains to the azygos system *(arrows)* at T8 level. (C) At a slightly lower level the hemiazygos vein also drains to the azygos vein. (D) Below this both the hemiazygos and azygos veins are visible.

1. Arch of azygos vein
2. Accessory hemiazygos vein
3. Azygos vein
4. Hemiazygos vein

and posterior oesophageal plexuses which continue into the abdomen through the oesophageal hiatus as anterior and posterior vagal trunks. The **recurrent laryngeal nerves** arise from the vagi. On the right the recurrent laryngeal nerve winds around the subclavian artery before ascending through neck between the trachea and oesophagus. On the left it winds around the aortic arch and passes through the aortopulmonary window before ascending between the trachea and oesophagus.

The **phrenic nerves** arise from the third to fifth cervical nerves and are the motor supply to the diaphragm. They enter the chest anterior to the subclavian artery and deep to the vein. The right phrenic nerve runs down in front of the SVC, over the right heart border and IVC to reach the diaphragm. The left phrenic nerve runs down over the aortic arch and left superior intercostal vein, in

front of the left hilum, and runs on the left heart border to reach the diaphragm.

RADIOLOGY PEARL

Phrenic nerve damage resulting in diaphragmatic palsy may be secondary to injury at any point in its course from its origin in the neck through to its path close to the hila.

The **sympathetic trunk** runs inferiorly in the posterior mediastinum in the paraspinal gutters, coming to lie in front of the bodies of T11 and T12 before passing through the diaphragm behind the medial arcuate ligament to continue as the lumbar sympathetic trunk. It is distributed to the thoracic viscera and forms the splanchnic nerves to the abdominal viscera.

The Mediastinum on the Chest Radiograph

UPPER MEDIASTINAL CONTOUR ON THE FRONTAL CHEST RADIOGRAPH (FIG. 4.8)

The heart and great vessels form a characteristic contour on the frontal chest radiograph. The right side of the mediastinal contour is formed from above downward by the right brachiocephalic vein and the SVC. The ascending aorta does not usually contribute to the right upper mediastinal contour as it is anterior but when ectatic or aneurysmal, it will project over the SVC. This can be recognized by its lateral convexity rather than the straight border of the SVC.

The left side of the mediastinal contour is formed by the composite shadow of the subclavian vessels superiorly. The artery is lower and actually forms the contour. This fades out laterally and is usually indistinct. Below this the aortic prominence is termed the 'aortic knuckle'. This is formed by the posterior part of the arch. It may be indistinct in young people and very prominent in older people, especially if there is aortic unfolding. Sometimes a small 'nipple' may be seen projecting from the aortic knuckle. This is caused by the left superior intercostal vein as it crosses the aorta to drain into the left brachiocephalic vein (Fig. 4.49). In older people the left side of the descending aorta may be visible descending from the aortic knuckle. Below the aortic knuckle is an air space called the aortopulmonary window. This may be obscured by lymphadenopathy. Below the aortopulmonary window is the main pulmonary artery, which has a straight upper border, and below this is the LV. The pulmonary arteries and veins form the densities of the hila on the frontal chest radiograph (see radiological features of the lung, p. 128).

RADIOLOGY PEARL

Pathological straightening of the left heart border occurs secondary to left atrial appendage enlargement as part of rheumatic mitral stenosis. In normality, the left atrial appendage does not contribute to the left heart border.

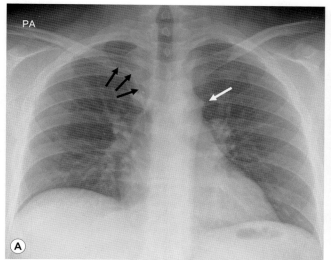

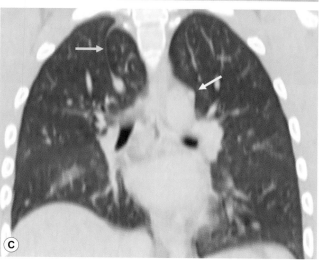

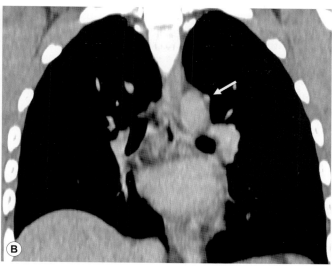

Fig. 4.49 (A) Posteroanterior chest radiograph. Aortic nipple representing the left superior intercostal vein *(white arrow)*. There is a right-sided peripherally inserted central catheter (PICC) in situ *(black arrows)*. (B) Coronal computed tomography (CT) thorax, soft tissue window. Aortic nipple representing the superior intercostal vein *(white arrow)*. (C) Coronal CT thorax, lung windows. Aortic nipple representing the superior intercostal vein *(white arrow)*. Azygous fissure *(yellow arrow)*.

MEDIASTINAL CONTOURS ON THE LATERAL CHEST RADIOGRAPH (SEE FIG. 4.9)

The heart shadow lies behind the lower third of the sternum. The anterior border is formed by the RV and outflow tract. Higher up the lungs are in contact with each other behind the sternum and in front of the ascending aorta, forming the retrosternal air space. The posterior contour of the heart shadow is formed by the left atrium above and the LV below. The IVC may be identified as a triangular structure crossing the diaphragm to enter the right atrium, which lies in a more anterior plane than the left atrium.

The Aorta

The aorta may be invisible in young people but is usually seen, at least in part, in middle-aged subjects. The ascending aorta is indistinct. The arch curves evenly from front to back and the descending aorta is seen anterior to the vertebral column. Its walls should be parallel. In older people, unfolding may cause it to overlie the vertebral bodies.

MEDIASTINAL LINES (SEE FIGS. 4.9, 4.11, 4.8, 4.51 AND 4.50)

Wherever air-filled lung outlines a linear soft tissue structure, the difference in density is detected by the plain radiograph as a **line**. If air outlines two sides of a thin structure the soft tissue density is seen as a **stripe**. This relationship may be appreciated on CT scans.

Right Paratracheal Stripe

The lung is in contact with the trachea from the level of the clavicles to the azygos vein in the right tracheobronchial angle. As the trachea is air filled the right tracheal wall is seen as a stripe, which should not measure more than 3 mm (the left tracheal wall is separated from lung by the aorta and great vessels and is not seen).

Posterior Junction Line (see Fig. 4.11)

This is formed by the apposition of the two lungs posteriorly. It extends from well above the clavicles vertically downwards to the arch of the aorta. The aortic arch separates the lungs and the line disappears. It may reform below the arch. The line represents the four layers of pleura between the posterior parts of the lungs seen from the front.

Anterior Junction Line

This line is formed by the apposition of the lungs anteriorly. It begins below the clavicles and runs inferiorly and to the left. Its oblique course is because of the differing anterior extent of the two lungs. It always ends at the RVOT.

Pleuro-Oesophageal Line

This is formed by the right lung outlining the right wall of the oesophagus above the level of the azygos vein. If the oesophagus happens to be distended with air, the pleuro-oesophageal stripe is seen. The thickness of this represents the thickness of the oesophageal wall and pleura and should not exceed 2 mm.

Azygo-Oesophageal Line (Fig. 4.50)

The azygos vein is closely related to the right posterolateral aspect of the oesophagus in the posterior mediastinum. The

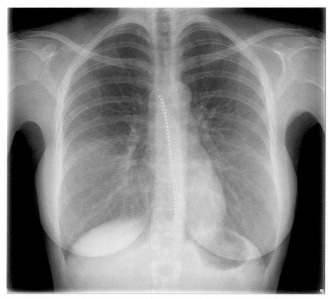

Fig. 4.50 Posteroanterior chest radiograph. Yellow line: azygo-oesophageal recess.

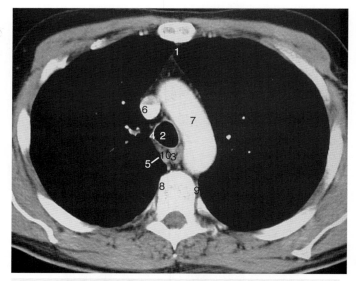

Fig. 4.51 Computed tomography scan of the thorax: upper T4 level showing mediastinal lines.

1. Anterior junction line
2. Air-filled trachea
3. Oesophagus
4. Right paratracheal stripe
5. Azygo-oesophageal stripe
6. Superior vena cava
7. Aortic arch
8. Right paraspinal line
9. Left paraspinal line
10. Azygos vein

right lung abuts the two structures forming the azygo-oesophageal line, tucking in behind them in the azygo-oesophageal **recess**. On the frontal CXRs the line curves to the right as the azygos vein crosses to gain the right tracheobronchial angle before draining into the SVC.

Paraspinal Lines

These are outlined by lung apposing the spinal column. The right line is sharper than the left as the descending aorta tends to reflect the pleura off the thoracic spine on the left, making the line more indistinct. The distance from the lateral border of the spine to the line may vary with body habitus and may be 1 cm on the left in obese people with paraspinal fat deposits. Widening of the paravertebral soft tissue on the right is always abnormal. Widening of the paravertebral soft tissue beyond the transverse process is always abnormal.

Aortopulmonary Mediastinal Stripe

This is the reflected pleura from the aortic arch to the pulmonary trunk and left pulmonary artery. It defines the lateral boundary of the aortopulmonary window.

Posterior Tracheal Stripe

This is seen on the lateral view and represents the posterior wall of the trachea outlined on either side by air. It measures 2–3 mm. If the collapsed oesophagus is apposed to the posterior trachea the stripe may measure 1 cm. If there is air in the oesophagus the stripe represents posterior tracheal and anterior oesophageal walls.

Cross-Sectional Anatomy

(Refer to Figs. 4.52–4.60 for this section.)

LEVEL T3 (FIGS. 4.52 AND 4.53)

This is the superior mediastinal level. The trachea is seen in the midline, with the great vessels anteriorly and the oesophagus behind. The brachiocephalic veins are anterior and lateral to the arteries and unite to form the SVC at

about this level. The left brachiocephalic vein is seen passing anteriorly to the branches of the aortic arch.

LEVEL T4 (FIGS. 4.54 AND 4.56)

This plane passes through the lower border of T4 and the sternal angle. Above this plane is the superior mediastinum. At this level is the lower part of the aortic arch to the left of the trachea, and the arch of the azygos vein to the right, crossing the right hilum to drain into the posterior aspect of the SVC. The oblique fissure, although demonstrated on these figures, is not always seen on CT as a line.

LEVEL T5 (FIGS. 4.55 AND 4.57)

This plane is at, or just below, the tracheal bifurcation. The main pulmonary artery is seen dividing into the right pulmonary artery, which runs anteriorly to its bronchus, and left pulmonary artery, which arches superiorly out of the plane to pass over the left bronchus. The descending lower lobe artery is seen lying posterolateral to the bronchus.

The superior pulmonary veins are seen anteriorly. On the right this is anterior to the interlobar artery. On the left it is separated from the lower lobe artery by the left bronchus.

The ascending aorta is seen in cross-section, lying in a more posterior plane than the origin of the main pulmonary artery.

Anterior to this is the junction of the anterior pleurae of the lungs, which forms the anterior junction line on the frontal chest radiograph.

The oesophagus, azygos veins and descending aorta are seen in the posterior mediastinum. The azygo-oesophageal recess may be seen.

LEVEL T6 (FIG. 4.58)

This section passes through the upper part of the heart. The right atrial appendage may be seen overlapping the origin of the aorta. The coronary arteries come off the aorta at this level. The RVOT is seen anterior to the origin of the aorta. The relationship of the oesophagus to the left atrium is seen.

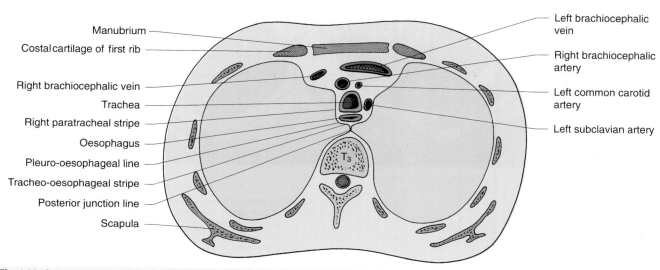

Fig. 4.52 Cross-sectional anatomy: level T3.

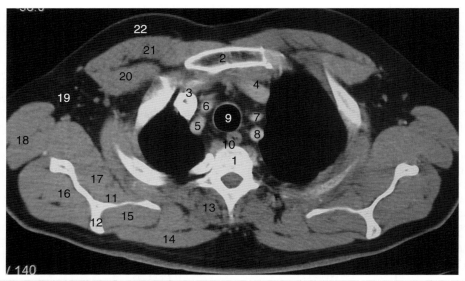

Fig. 4.53 Computed tomography scan of the thorax: level T3.

1. Body of T3
2. Body of manubrium sterni
3. Right brachiocephalic vein
4. Left brachiocephalic vein
5. Right subclavian artery
6. Right common carotid artery
7. Left common carotid artery
8. Left subclavian artery
9. Trachea
10. Oesophagus
11. Right scapula
12. Spine of scapula
13. Erector spinae muscle
14. Trapezius muscle
15. Supraspinatus muscle
16. Infraspinatus muscle
17. Subscapularis muscle
18. Deltoid muscle
19. Fat in axilla
20. Pectoralis minor muscle
21. Pectoralis major muscle
22. Subcutaneous fat

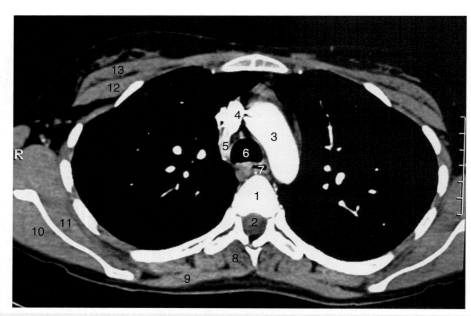

Fig. 4.54 Computed tomography scan of the thorax: level T4.

1. Body of T4
2. Thecal sac and spinal cord
3. Arch of aorta
4. Superior vena cava
5. Azygos vein
6. Trachea
7. Oesophagus
8. Erector spinae muscle
9. Trapezius muscle
10. Infraspinatus muscle
11. Subscapularis muscle
12. Pectoralis minor muscle
13. Pectoralis major muscle

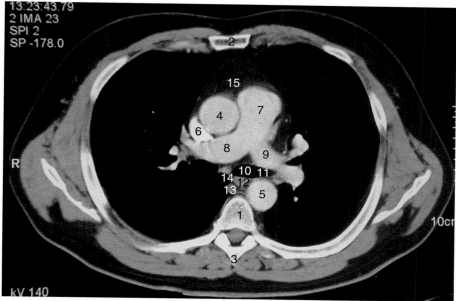

Fig. 4.55 Computed tomography scan of the thorax: lower T5 level.

1. Body of T5
2. Sternum
3. Spinous process of T5
4. Ascending aorta
5. Descending aorta
6. Superior vena cava
7. Main pulmonary trunk
8. Right pulmonary artery

9. Left pulmonary artery
10. Carina
11. Left main bronchus
12. Oesophagus
13. Azygos vein
14. Azygo-oesophageal recess
15. Mediastinal fat

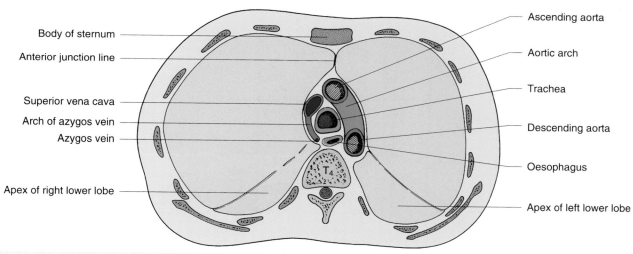

Fig. 4.56 Cross-sectional anatomy: level T4.

Labels (clockwise):
Body of sternum
Anterior junction line
Superior vena cava
Arch of azygos vein
Azygos vein
Apex of right lower lobe

Ascending aorta
Aortic arch
Trachea
Descending aorta
Oesophagus
Apex of left lower lobe

LEVEL T8 (FIG. 4.59)

This section passes through the heart and shows the relationship of the chambers to each other. The left ventricular inflow and outflow tracts are separated from each other by the anterior leaflet of the mitral valve. The aortic sinuses are seen as localized bulges. Note that the right heart border is formed by the right atrium, the anterior border is formed by the RV, the left border by the LV and the posterior border by the left atrium.

LEVEL T10 (FIG. 4.60)

At this level, part of the abdominal cavity is also seen as the dome of the diaphragm reaches the level of

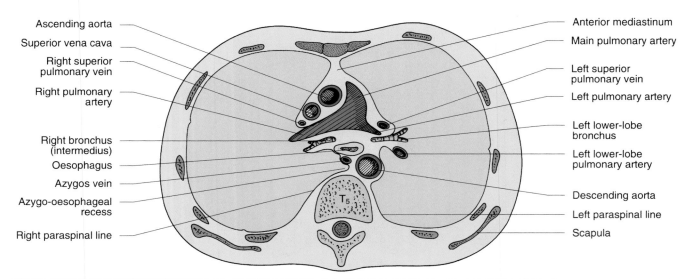

Ascending aorta — Anterior mediastinum
Superior vena cava — Main pulmonary artery
Right superior pulmonary vein — Left superior pulmonary vein
Right pulmonary artery — Left pulmonary artery
— Left lower-lobe bronchus
Right bronchus (intermedius) — Left lower-lobe pulmonary artery
Oesophagus
Azygos vein — Descending aorta
Azygo-oesophageal recess — Left paraspinal line
Right paraspinal line — Scapula

Fig. 4.57 Cross-sectional anatomy: level T5.

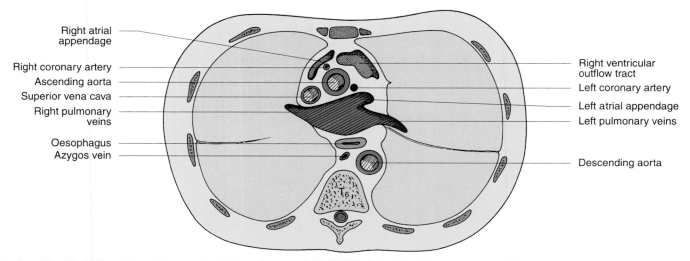

Right atrial appendage
Right coronary artery — Right ventricular outflow tract
Ascending aorta — Left coronary artery
Superior vena cava — Left atrial appendage
Right pulmonary veins — Left pulmonary veins
Oesophagus
Azygos vein — Descending aorta

Fig. 4.58 Cross-sectional anatomy: level T6.

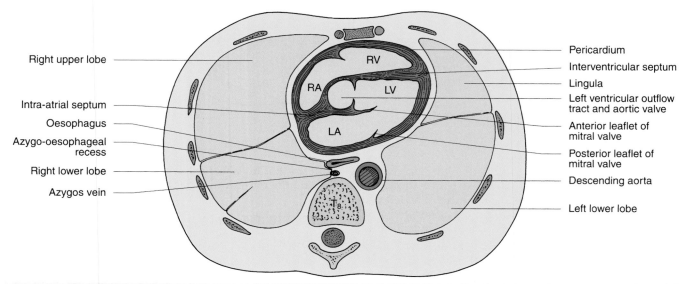

Right upper lobe — Pericardium
— Interventricular septum
— Lingula
Intra-atrial septum — Left ventricular outflow tract and aortic valve
Oesophagus — Anterior leaflet of mitral valve
Azygo-oesophageal recess — Posterior leaflet of mitral valve
Right lower lobe — Descending aorta
Azygos vein — Left lower lobe

Fig. 4.59 Cross-sectional anatomy: level T8.

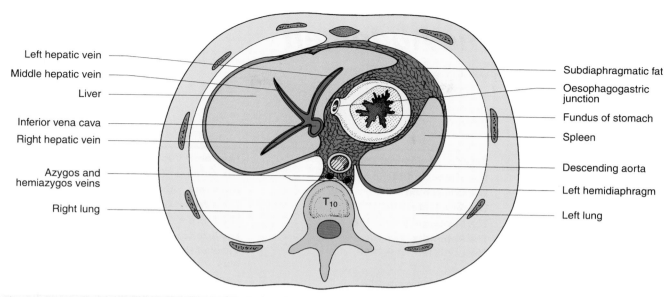

Left hepatic vein
Middle hepatic vein
Liver
Inferior vena cava
Right hepatic vein
Azygos and
hemiazygos veins
Right lung

Subdiaphragmatic fat
Oesophagogastric
junction
Fundus of stomach
Spleen
Descending aorta
Left hemidiaphragm
Left lung

T₁₀

Fig. 4.60 Cross-sectional anatomy: level T10.

approximately T9. The oesophagus traverses the diaphragm at this level, in a relatively anterior position, through the oesophageal hiatus and joins the stomach at the oesophagogastric junction. The fundus of the stomach and part of the spleen and liver are seen. The IVC is situated slightly anteriorly; on higher cuts it enters the right atrium. The descending aorta with azygos and hemiazygos veins on its right and left are posterior.

5 *The Abdomen*

EMMA DUNNE
EDITED BY MICHELLE McNICHOLAS

CHAPTER CONTENTS

Anterior Abdominal Wall 184
The Stomach 185
The Duodenum 189
The Small Intestine 193
The Ileocaecal Valve 196
The Appendix 197
The Large Intestine 198
The Liver 201
The Biliary System 208
The Pancreas 212
The Spleen 218

The Portal Venous System 219
The Kidneys 222
The Ureter 226
The Adrenal Glands 229
The Abdominal Aorta 230
The Inferior Vena Cava 231
Veins of the Posterior Abdominal Wall 232
Peritoneal Spaces of the Abdomen 235
Cross-Sectional Anatomy of the Upper Abdomen 239

Anterior Abdominal Wall

FASCIAL LAYERS

There are two layers of superficial fascia on the abdominal wall; a loose areolar fatty layer named Camper's fascia, and deep to this a fibrous layer named Scarpa's fascia. Camper's fascia extends inferiorly past the inguinal ligament as the subcutaneous fat of the thigh. It extends medially past the pubic symphysis, combining with Scarpa's fascia to form the Dartos fascia of the scrotum in males and the fatty tissue of the mons pubis and labia majora in females. Scarpa's fascia extends deep to the inguinal ligament and posteriorly into the perineum to fuse with Colles' fascia. It does not extend into the thigh but fuses with the fascia lata. A condensation continues onto the dorsum of the penis as a suspensory ligament.

MUSCLE LAYERS (FIG. 5.1)

The wall consists of three principal muscular layers. Each consists of lateral muscular fibres with aponeuroses fibres centrally. The fibrous aponeurotic components ensheath the rectus abdominis around the anterior midline.

The **external oblique** arises on the anterior surface of the lower eight ribs and is inserted into the linea alba, pubic crest, pubic tubercle and anterior half of the iliac crest. Between the anterior superior iliac spine and pubic tubercle the aponeurotic free border of this muscle forms the inguinal ligament. The muscle fibres run inferiorly and medially.

The **internal oblique** arises from the lumbar fascia, the anterior iliac crest and the lateral two-thirds of the inguinal ligament and is inserted into the costal margin, aponeurosis of the rectus sheath and the pubic crest via the conjoint tendon. Muscle fibres run superomedially at right angles to the external oblique.

The **transversus abdominis** arises from the deep aspect of the lower six ribs (interdigitating with the diaphragm), the lumbar fascia, the anterior iliac crest and the lateral inguinal ligament, and is inserted into the linea alba and the pubic crest via the conjoint tendon.

The **rectus abdominis muscle** originates from the fifth, sixth and seventh costal cartilages and inserts into the pubic crest. It has three to four tendinous intersections at intervals along its length, which adhere to the anterior rectus sheath.

The **rectus sheath** is formed by the aponeuroses of the external oblique, internal oblique and transversus abdominus muscles. The aponeurosis of the transversus abdominus runs deep to the rectus sheath. The aponeurosis of transversalis splits to enclose the rectus abdominus muscle. The external oblique aponeurosis is anterior to the rectus muscle. The rectus sheath fuses at the midline to form the linea alba which runs from the xiphisternum to the pubic symphysis.

The posterior lamina of the sheath, formed by the internal oblique aponeurosis (covering the posterior aspect of rectus muscles), terminates inferiorly halfway between the umbilicus and pubis symphysis, whereas the anterior lamina covers the rectus to its insertion into the pubic bone. The free end of the posterior lamina of the sheath is the **arcuate line of Douglas or linea semilunaris**. Superior to the arcuate line, the posterior rectus sheath is made up of the aponeurosis of transverses abdominis and some of the aponeurosis of internal oblique; below the arcuate line there is only transversalis fascia. The arcuate line marks the level at which the inferior epigastric vessels enter the rectus sheath.

A layer of fat separates the muscles of the anterior abdominal wall from the peritoneum and the abdominal contents. This is referred to as extraperitoneal or properitoneal fat.

UMBILICAL LIGAMENTS

The **median umbilical ligament** is an unpaired midline structure. It runs from the bladder fundus, along the deep aspect of the anterior abdominal wall to the umbilicus. It consists of the fibrous remnant of the obliterated fetal urachus. It is covered by a fold of peritoneum called the median umbilical fold.

The **medial umbilical ligaments** are the paired fibrous remnants of the obliterated umbilical arteries and run from the internal iliac artery to the umbilicus on the deep surface of the anterior abdominal wall. These are also covered by folds of peritoneum called the medial umbilical folds.

The **lateral umbilical fold** refers to the fold of parietal peritoneum that covers the inferior epigastric artery as it passes superomedially from the external iliac artery to enter the rectus sheath.

RADIOLOGICAL FEATURES OF THE ANTERIOR ABDOMINAL WALL

Plain Films of the Abdomen (Fig. 5.1)

The muscle layers of the anterior abdominal wall are outlined, especially in obese individuals, between the subcutaneous fat line and the properitoneal fat line. Clearly seen **fat lines** indicate a lack of oedema in these areas; in 18% of normal radiographs the properitoneal line is absent.

Computed Tomography (CT) of the Abdominal Wall (Figs. 5.2-5.5)

The muscle layers of the anterior abdominal wall can be seen in cross-section. Three muscles can be seen antero-laterally: the external oblique is outermost, then the internal oblique, with transversus abdominus deepest. The rectus muscle and its rectus sheath can be seen in the anterior paramedian position superficial to the other muscles.

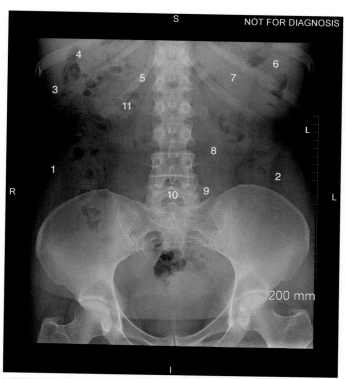

Fig. 5.1 Plain film of the abdomen.

1. Abdominal wall musculature
2. Properitoneal fat line (extraperitoneal fat layer)
3. Inferior border of the right lobe of the liver
4. Gas in the hepatic flexure
5. Right twelfth rib
6. Splenic flexure
7. Left kidney
8. Left psoas muscle
9. Left spinous process of L5
10. Spinous process of L5
11. Small bowel loops

RADIOLOGY PEARLS

- Free intraperitoneal gas may outline the umbilical ligaments and falciform ligament making them visible, thus making a diagnosis of pneumoperitoneum possible on a supine radiograph.
- Rupture of the bulbous urethra results in tracking of urine into the scrotum, perineum and abdominal wall deep to Scarpa's fascia. It cannot track into the thigh due to the attachment of Scarpa's fascia to the deep fascia of the thigh.
- Spigelian hernias emerge lateral to the rectus sheath at the level of the arcuate line, a relative weak point below the lower limit of the internal oblique fascia.
- Skin punctures lateral to the rectus muscles, or in the midline, will avoid the epigastric vessels. Catheter placement that avoids the recti is also better tolerated.

The Stomach (Figs. 5.6, 5.7)

The stomach is J-shaped but varies in size and shape with the volume of its contents, with erect or supine position, and with inspiration and expiration.

The stomach consists of two surfaces (anterior and posterior) and two curvatures (the greater and the lesser). The lesser curve is punctuated by a notch known as the incisura.

The stomach has two **orifices** – the cardia and the pylorus. The cardiac orifice or cardia is so-named because of its proximity to the heart and marks the anatomical junction between the oesophagus and stomach. In clinical practice the junction is known as the gastro-oesophageal junction, oesophagogastric junction and lower oesophageal sphincter.

The dome-like projection of the stomach above the cardia is the **fundus**.

Between the cardia and the incisura is the **body** of the stomach, and distal to the incisura is the **gastric antrum** which leads to the **pylorus**. The lumen of the pylorus is referred to as the **pyloric canal**.

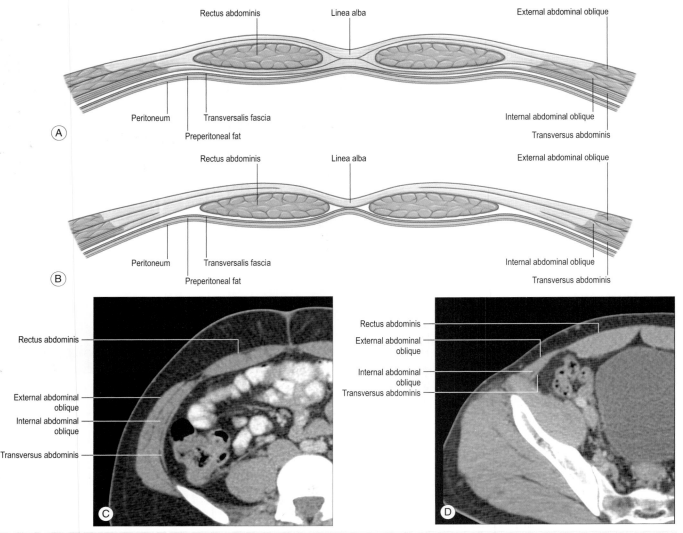

Fig. 5.2 The anterior abdominal wall: Diagrams and axial computed tomography images through the anterior abdominal wall. (A) Diagram immediately proximal to the umbilicus. (B) Distal to the arcuate line. (C) Axial CT images above the arcuate line. (D) Axial CT image below arcuate line. (From Standring S. *Gray's Anatomy: The Anatomical Basis of Clinical Practice*, 42nd ed. Elsevier; 2021.)

The stomach is lined by mucosa, which has tiny nodular elevations called the **areae gastricae** and is thrown into folds called **rugae**. Longitudinal folds parallel to the lesser curve are called the '**magenstrasse**' meaning 'street of the stomach'. Rugae elsewhere in the stomach are random and patternless.

There are three **muscle layers** in the wall of the stomach: (1) an outer longitudinal, (2) an inner circular and (3) an incomplete, innermost oblique layer. The circular layer is thickened at the pylorus as a sphincter, but not at the oesophagogastric junction. Fibres of the oblique layer loop around the notch between the oesophagus and the fundus, and help to prevent reflux.

Peritoneum covers the anterior and posterior surfaces of the stomach and is continued between the lesser curve and the liver as the lesser omentum, and beyond the greater curve as the greater omentum.

ANTERIOR RELATIONS OF THE STOMACH

The upper part of the stomach is covered by the left lobe of the liver on its right and by the left diaphragm on its left.

The fundus occupies the concavity of the left dome of the diaphragm. The remainder of the stomach is covered by the anterior abdominal wall.

RADIOLOGY PEARL

The oblique fibres are responsible for the '**magenstrasse**' and can reduce the volume of the stomach, allowing fluids and food to pass directly and rapidly from the oesophagus along the lesser curve to the duodenum without filling the main lumen of the stomach. This can be seen when liquid contrast is swallowed.

POSTERIOR RELATIONS OF THE STOMACH

Posterior to the stomach lies the lesser sac (refer to section on peritoneal spaces for further detail). The structures that lie behind this are referred to as the stomach bed. The pancreas lies across the midportion of the stomach bed with the splenic artery partly above and partly behind it, and the spleen at its tail. Above the pancreas lie the aorta, coeliac trunk, the coeliac

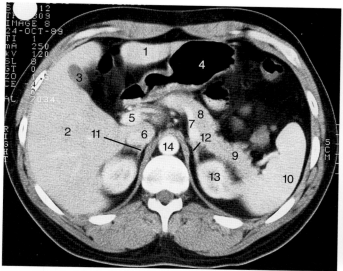
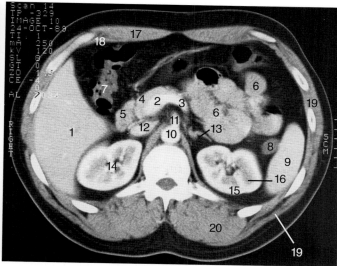

Fig. 5.3 Computed tomography scan: level of body of pancreas (T12).

1. Left lobe of the liver
2. Right lobe of the liver
3. Gallbladder
4. Stomach
5. Portal vein origin
6. Inferior vena cava
7. Splenic vein
8. Body of the pancreas
9. Tail of the pancreas
10. Spleen
11. Right adrenal gland
12. Left adrenal gland
13. Left kidney
14. Aorta

Fig. 5.4 Computed tomography scan: level of pancreatic head (L1).

1. Right lobe of the liver
2. Confluence of the splenic and superior mesenteric veins to form the portal vein
3. Splenic vein
4. Head of the pancreas
5. Second part of the duodenum
6. Loops of the small bowel
7. Hepatic flexure
8. Descending colon
9. Spleen
10. Aorta
11. Superior mesenteric artery
12. Inferior vena cava
13. Left adrenal gland
14. Right kidney
15. Renal cortex
16. Renal pyramid in the renal medulla
17. Rectus abdominis muscle
18. Transversus abdominis muscle
19. Latissimus dorsi muscle
20. Erector spinae muscle

plexus and nodes, the diaphragm, left kidney and left adrenal gland. Attached to the anterior pancreas is the transverse mesocolon which forms the inferior part of the stomach bed.

ARTERIAL SUPPLY OF THE STOMACH (FIG. 5.8, FIGS. 5.9, 5.10)

Branches of the coeliac trunk reach the stomach along its greater and lesser curves as follows:
- The lesser curve is supplied by the left gastric artery (a branch of the coeliac trunk) and the right gastric artery (a branch of the hepatic artery).
- The greater curve is supplied by the right gastroepiploic artery (from the gastroduodenal branch of the hepatic artery) and the left gastroepiploic artery (from the splenic artery).
- The proximal aspect of the greater curve and the fundus are supplied by the short gastric branches of the splenic artery.

The arteries of the stomach anastomose freely within the stomach wall, unlike the arteries of the small and large intestine, which are end arteries.

VENOUS DRAINAGE OF THE STOMACH (FIG. 5.11)

Venous drainage of the stomach follows a similar pattern to arterial supply:
- The right and left gastric veins drain directly into the portal vein

- The short gastric and left gastroepiploic veins drain to the splenic vein
- The right gastroepiploic vein drains to the superior mesenteric vein

LYMPHATIC DRAINAGE OF THE STOMACH

Lymphatic drainage follows the arterial pattern, draining to coeliac nodes which drain into the cisterna chyli:
- The left gastric artery lymphatics drain directly to coeliac nodes
- The right gastric artery lymphatics drain via retroduodenal nodes to coeliac nodes
- The short gastric and left gastroepiploic artery lymphatics drain via nodes in the splenic hilum and behind the pancreas to coeliac nodes
- The right gastroepiploic artery lymphatics drain via retroduodenal nodes to coeliac nodes

Retrograde spread of carcinoma may occur into the nodes at the porta hepatis. The extensive and complex lymphatic drainage of the stomach poses a challenge in the management of gastric cancer.

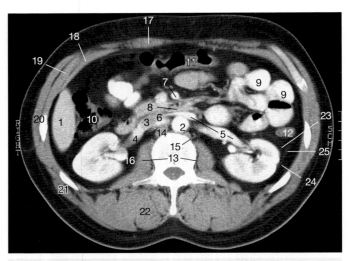

Fig. 5.5 Computed tomography scan: level of renal hila (L2).

1. Right lobe of the liver
2. Aorta
3. Inferior vena cava
4. Right renal vein
5. Left renal vein
6. Left renal artery
7. Superior mesenteric artery
8. Third part of the duodenum passing between the aorta and superior mesenteric artery
9. Loops of small bowel
10. Ascending colon
11. Transverse colon
12. Descending colon
13. Psoas muscle
14. Lower end crus of the right hemidiaphragm
15. Lower end crus of the left hemidiaphragm
16. Right renal pelvis
17. Rectus abdominis muscle
18. Transversus abdominis muscle
19. Internal oblique muscle
20. External oblique muscle
21. Latissimus dorsi muscle
22. Erector spinae muscle
23. Gerota's fascia
24. Fascia of Zuckerkandl
25. Lateral conal fascia (fusion of Gerota's fascia and fascia of Zuckerkandl)

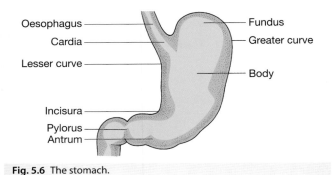

Fig. 5.6 The stomach.

RADIOLOGICAL FEATURES OF THE STOMACH

Plain Film of the Abdomen (see Fig. 5.2)

Erect radiographs demonstrate a wide fluid level at the gastric fundus. This is because the antrum and body contract when empty and a relatively small amount of fluid and gas in the fundus can produce a long fluid level. When the stomach is distended, two fluid levels may be seen, one in the body of the stomach and one in the antrum.

Double-Contrast Barium Meal Examination (Fig. 5.12)

Features of the stomach, such as the greater and lesser curves, the incisura, the cardia, fundus, body, antrum and pylorus, can be seen. The change in position of these with posture and respiration can be appreciated on fluoroscopy.

CT and Magnetic Resonance Imaging (MRI) of the Stomach (Figs. 5.13, 5.14)

The thickness of the stomach wall varies considerably depending on the degree of distension and can appear thickened in the fasting state.

The mucosa of the stomach enhances with intravenous contrast and the stomach layers are best appreciated in the arterial phase of contrast enhancement, This enhancement is best seen when there is no positive contrast in the stomach.

Fig. 5.7 Posterior relations of the stomach (viewed from anterior through the stomach).

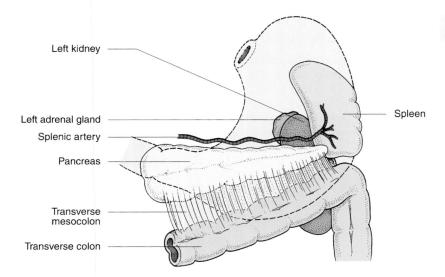

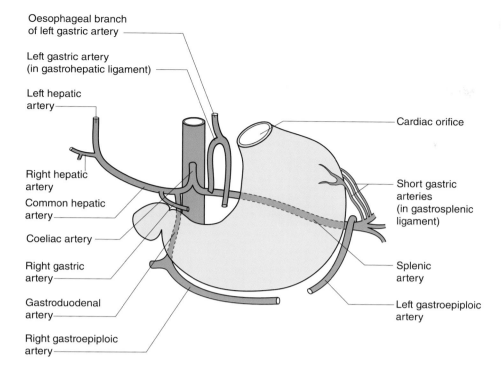

Oesophageal branch
of left gastric artery

Left gastric artery
(in gastrohepatic ligament)

Left hepatic
artery

Right hepatic
artery

Common hepatic
artery

Coeliac artery

Right gastric
artery

Gastroduodenal
artery

Right gastroepiploic
artery

Cardiac orifice

Short gastric
arteries
(in gastrosplenic
ligament)

Splenic
artery

Left gastroepiploic
artery

Fig. 5.8 Arterial supply of the stomach.

Ultrasound Studies of the Stomach

Ultrasound is limited by the presence of intraluminal gas in the stomach. Structures in the stomach bed cannot be seen through the stomach if this is filled with gas. If the stomach is gas free or fluid filled, then the pancreas and the aorta and coeliac trunk can be seen well.

RADIOLOGY PEARLS

- In the infant, ultrasound is used in the study of the pylorus in cases of suspected pyloric stenosis. Pyloric muscle thicknesses greater than 3 mm and muscle lengths greater than 14 mm are considered abnormal.
- The stomach can be filled with gas using effervescent granules to eliminate confusing rugal patterns, and to push other bowel loops out of the field of interest.

RADIOLOGY PEARLS

- The fundus of the stomach may project posteriorly if redundant and may mimic an adrenal mass on CT and MRI.
- Food in the stomach can appear as a pseudomass, especially in the dependent portion.

The Duodenum (Figs. 5.15, 5.16)

The duodenum extends from the pylorus, curving in a C shape around the head of the pancreas to end at the duodenojejunal flexure, where transition to the small bowel proper is marked by the assumption of a longer, more mobile mesentery.

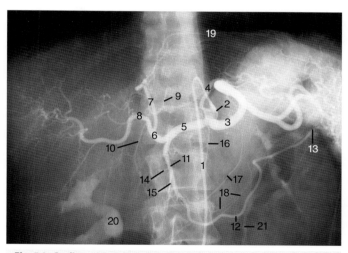

Fig. 5.9 Coeliac axis angiogram.

1. Catheter in the aorta
2. Catheter tip in the coeliac trunk
3. Splenic artery
4. Left gastric artery
5. Common hepatic artery
6. Hepatic artery proper
7. Left hepatic artery
8. Right hepatic artery
9. Right gastric artery
10. Cystic artery
11. Gastroduodenal artery
12. Right gastroepiploic artery
13. Left gastroepiploic artery
14. Posterior superior pancreaticoduodenal artery
15. Anterior superior pancreaticoduodenal artery
16. Dorsal pancreatic artery
17. Transverse pancreatic artery
18. Gastric branches of the gastroepiploic artery
19. Phrenic branch of the left hepatic artery
20. Contrast in right renal pelvis
21. Left ureter

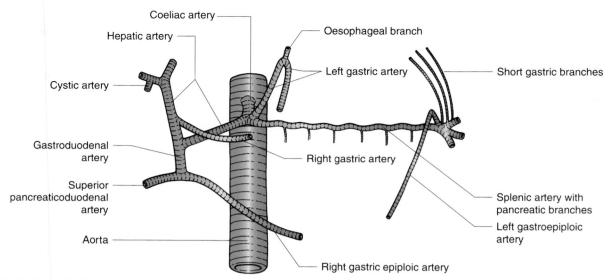

Fig. 5.10 Branches of the coeliac artery.

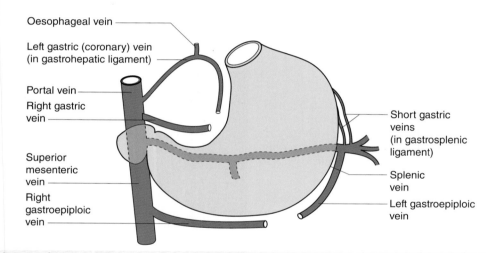

Fig. 5.11 Venous drainage of the stomach.

The first 2.5 cm of duodenum, like the stomach, is attached to the greater and lesser omentum. The remainder of the duodenum is retroperitoneal, with a short mesentery and, as a result, it is less mobile. Its anterior surface is covered by peritoneum, except where the second part is crossed by the transverse mesocolon and where the third part is crossed by the superior mesenteric vessels in the root of the mesentery.

It is described as having four parts: the first (or superior), second (or descending), third (or horizontal) and fourth (or ascending). These measure approximately 2 cm, 8 cm, 8 cm and 4 cm, respectively. The first part is at the level of L1 lumbar vertebra, the second at L2, the third at L3, and the fourth ascends again to L2 level.

■ The **first part (superior)**, called the duodenal bulb/cap, passes posterosuperiorly over a distance of approximately 2 cm on the transpyloric plane at L1. It is covered by the peritoneum, with the lesser omentum

extending from its superior edge and the greater omentum from its inferior. The common bile duct, the portal vein and the gastroduodenal artery pass behind the first part of the duodenum and separate it from the inferior vena cava (IVC). Inferiorly it is in contact with the pancreatic head.

■ The **second part** (descending) of the duodenum is approximately 8 cm long. It runs inferiorly around the head of the pancreas at the level of the L2 and L3 vertebral bodies. The common bile duct (CBD) and the main pancreatic duct open into posteromedial wall of the second part of the duodenum at the ampulla of Vater/dueodenal papilla. This is guarded by the sphincter of Oddi. An accessory pancreatic duct (of Santorini), if present, opens proximal to this.

■ This part of the duodenum is crossed by the transverse mesocolon anteriorly. As a result, its upper half is supracolic and has the liver as an anterior relation. Its lower

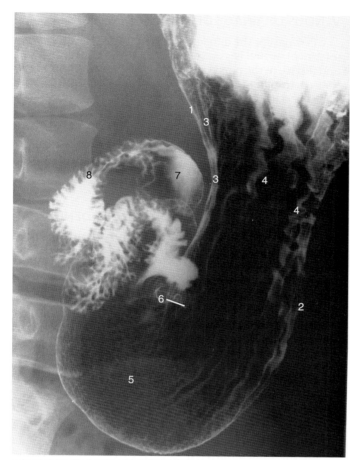

Fig. 5.12 Barium meal technique. This film demonstrates the various rugal and mucosal folds in the stomach and in the nondistended duodenum.

1. Lesser curve of the stomach
2. Greater curve of the stomach
3. Longitudinal mucosal folds ('magenstrasse')
4. Gastric rugae
5. Areae gastricae
6. Incisura
7. Duodenal bulb (partially gas distended)
8. Mucosal pattern of the nondistended duodenum

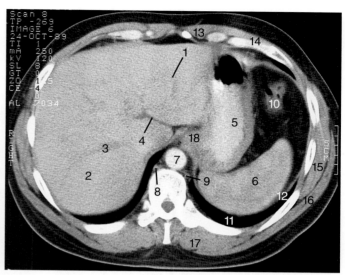

Fig. 5.13 Computed tomography of the upper abdomen: level of the gastro-oesophageal junction (T10).

1. Left lobe of the liver
2. Right lobe of the liver
3. Right hepatic vein
4. Fissure for the ligamentum venosum
5. Contrast medium in the stomach
6. Spleen
7. Descending aorta
8. Azygos vein
9. Hemiazygos vein
10. Splenic flexure
11. Left lung
12. Left diaphragm
13. Rectus abdominis muscle
14. External oblique muscle
15. Serratus anterior muscle
16. Latissimus dorsi muscle
17. Erector spinae muscle
18. Oesophagogastric junction

half is infracolic and has loops of jejunum anteriorly. Its posterior relations are the right kidney and it is in contact with the pancreatic head medially.

- The **third part (horizontal)** of the duodenum runs for approximately 8 cm horizontally across the anterior aspect of the L3 vertebra, the IVC and aorta. Its posterior relations include the right psoas muscle, ureter and gonadal vessels of the posterior abdominal wall. Anteriorly it is crossed by the root of the mesentery and the superior mesenteric vessels. The head of the pancreas is in contact with its superior border.
- The **fourth part** (ascending) of the duodenum passes upwards before turning abruptly anteriorly. Its superior turn is suspended by a peritoneal fold which descends from the right crus of the diaphragm, called the ligament of Treitz. At this ligament the small bowel assumes a longer mesentery, marking the transition to the jejunum. The ligament is not easily identified

radiologically, its lower limit is inferred by the duodenojejunal flexure, normally the highest point of the duodenum. The DJ flexure normally lies on the left side of the aorta, superficial to the left psoas muscle and posterior to the stomach. The inferior mesenteric vessels raise another peritoneal fold lateral to the fourth part of the duodenum.

ARTERIAL SUPPLY (SEE FIG. 5.15)

The first part of the duodenum is supplied by the right gastric and the right gastroepiploic arteries.

The **superior pancreaticoduodenal artery**, a branch of the gastroduodenal artery from the hepatic, supplies the first half of the second part.

The remainder of the duodenum is supplied by the **inferior pancreaticoduodenal artery**, the first branch of the superior mesenteric artery (SMA). At the midpoint of the second part of the duodenum, therefore, there is a transition from supply by the coeliac trunk to supply by the SMA, representing a transition from foregut to midgut.

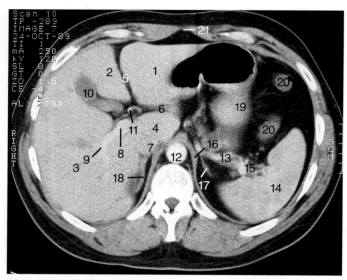

Fig. 5.14 Computed tomography of the abdomen: level of body of the stomach (T11).

1. Left lobe of the liver: lateral segment
2. Left lobe of the liver: medial segment
3. Right lobe of the liver
4. Caudate lobe of the liver
5. Fissure for ligamentum teres
6. Interlobar fissure (for ligamentum venosum)
7. Inferior vena cava
8. Portal vein
9. Right branch of the portal vein
10. Gallbladder
11. Hepatic artery
12. Abdominal aorta
13. Splenic artery
14. Spleen
15. Splenic vein
16. Left crus of the diaphragm
17. Left adrenal gland
18. Right adrenal gland
19. Stomach
20. Splenic flexure
21. Linea alba (aponeurosis of the rectus sheath)

VENOUS DRAINAGE OF THE DUODENUM

The first part of the duodenum drains to the prepyloric vein (of Mayo), which lies on the anterior surface of the pylorus, and thence to the portal vein. The remainder drains to veins that correspond to the arteries. These drain to the portal and superior mesenteric veins.

LYMPHATIC DRAINAGE OF THE DUODENUM

Pancreaticoduodenal nodes drain to pyloric nodes and to coeliac nodes.

RADIOLOGICAL FEATURES OF THE DUODENUM

Barium Studies of the Duodenum (Figs. 5.12, 5.16)

The duodenum is usually examined radiologically as part of a double-contrast barium meal examination (see Fig. 5.12).

The first part of the duodenum passes posteriorly as well as superiorly, therefore it is best evaluated with the right side raised in a right anterior oblique view (it is foreshortened in anteroposterior, [AP] views).

The duodenal bulb may be indented by the normal gallbladder. The bulb has thin mucosal folds that are parallel, or parallel in spiral, from base to apex. Circular valvulae conniventes begin in the second part of the duodenum.

The ampulla is visualized in two-thirds of normal examinations and an opening of an accessory pancreatic duct in less than one-quarter. The accessory duct opens more anteriorly than the main duct.

The third part of the duodenum is indented by the aorta posteriorly and superior mesenteric vessels anteriorly.

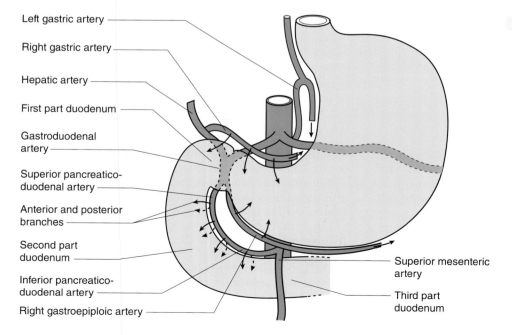

Left gastric artery

Right gastric artery

Hepatic artery

First part duodenum

Gastroduodenal artery

Superior pancreatico-duodenal artery

Anterior and posterior branches

Second part duodenum

Inferior pancreatico-duodenal artery

Right gastroepiploic artery

Superior mesenteric artery

Third part duodenum

Fig. 5.15 Duodenum: arterial supply.

Ultrasound

Gas in the duodenum may hinder visualization of other organs, particularly the common bile duct, which runs behind the first part. The duodenum may be identified adjacent to the head of the pancreas by ultrasound.

The Small Intestine

The small intestine begins at the duodenojejunal flexure and ends at the ileocaecal junction. It has a variable length, averaging 6 m. The mesentery in continuity with the small bowel extends from the left side of L2 to the right sacroiliac (SI) joint (Fig. 5.17). The small intestine is very mobile and

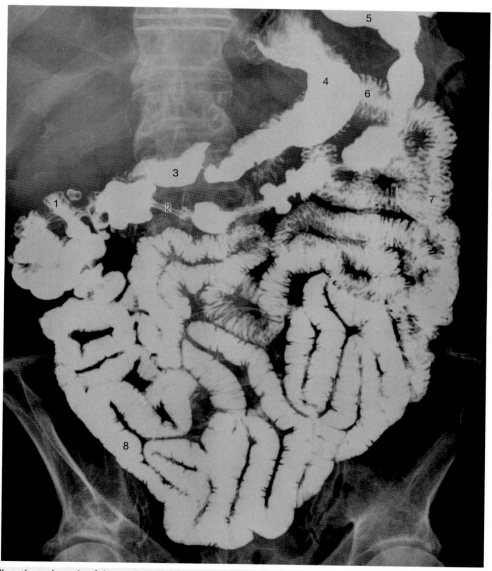

Fig. 5.16 Barium follow-through study of the small bowel. Notice the feathery mucosal pattern of the jejunum compared with the more featureless ileum. The presence of generous mesenteric fat is separating the bowel loops slightly. The valvulae conniventes are thicker and more prominent in the jejunum. The highest part of the duodenum (marking the ligament of Treitz) is hidden by the stomach. Contrast has passed into the colon. Notice the high position of the splenic flexure. Notice the normal linear mucosal pattern of the collapsed colon due to its longitudinal muscle bands (taenia) and its sacculations.

1. Sacculation
2. Collapsed transverse colon
3. Duodenal bulb
4. Stomach

5. Splenic flexure
6. Duodenojejunal junction
7. Jejunum
8. Ileum

lies in mobile coils in the central abdomen. The proximal two-fifths of the small intestine is called the jejunum and the distal three-fifths the ileum, although the boundary between these is not well defined.

Circular mucosal folds – known as **valvulae conniventes** or **plicae semilunaris** – are seen in the duodenum and continued in the small intestine, although they are less prominent distally and may be absent in distended views on barium studies.

Lymphoid follicles found in the mucous membrane throughout the intestinal tract become increasingly more numerous along the length of the small intestine. In the distal ileum they become aggregated together into patches called **Peyer's patches**. They are oval in shape and found on the **antimesenteric border** of the ileum.

Differences between the jejunum and ileum are outlined in Table 5.1.

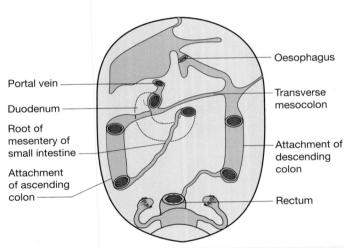

Fig. 5.17 Posterior abdominal wall showing peritoneal attachment of the mesentery.

Table 5.1 Comparison between Jejunum and Ileum

	Jejunum	Ileum
Diameter	Wider (3.0–3.5 cm)	Narrower (2.5 cm)
Wall thickness	Thicker	Thinner
Position	Left upper abdomen	Right lower abdomen
Valvulae conniventes	Thicker and more prominent	Thinner and less prominent
Peyer's patches	Fewer and bigger	More numerous
Arterial arcades	One or two with fewer long branches	Four to five with many short branches

ARTERIAL SUPPLY OF THE SMALL INTESTINE (FIGS. 5.18, 5.19)

The entire small intestine is supplied by the SMA, which arises from the aorta at the L1 vertebral level. Jejunal and ileal branches arise from the left of the main trunk. These branches link with one another in a series of arcades, which are usually single in the jejunum but number up to five in the distal ileum. The arteries that enter the intestinal wall – the vasa recta – are end arteries.

VENOUS DRAINAGE OF THE SMALL INTESTINE

Veins from the small intestine drain to the superior mesenteric vein, which in turn drains to the portal vein (see section on Portal Venous System).

LYMPHATIC DRAINAGE OF THE SMALL INTESTINE

Lymphatic drainage is to the superior mesenteric group of preaortic nodes.

MECKEL'S DIVERTICULUM

This is a true diverticulum that projects from the antimesenteric border of the lower ileum. It represents the persistent intestinal end of the vitellointestinal duct, which

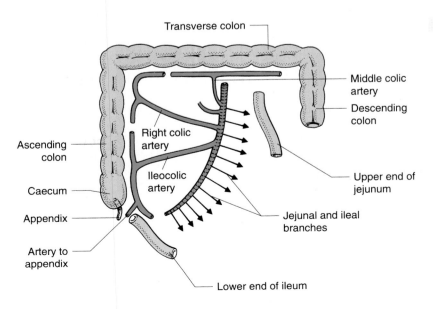

Fig. 5.18 Branches of the superior mesenteric artery.

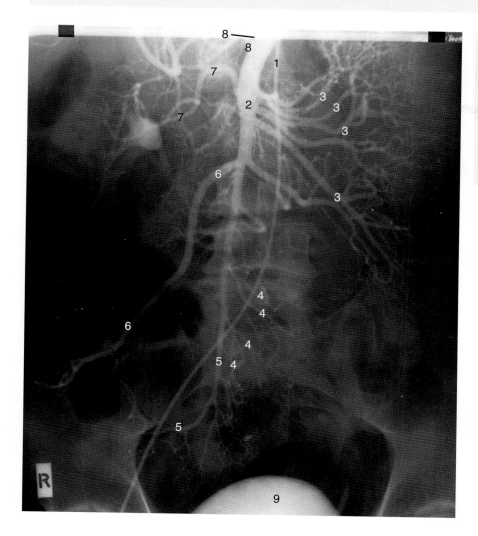

Fig. 5.19 Superior mesenteric angiogram. The inferior pancreaticoduodenal artery (not shown) also arises from the proximal superior mesenteric artery and runs superiorly.
1. Catheter in the aorta
2. Superior mesenteric artery
3. Jejunal branches
4. Ileal branches
5. Terminal superior mesenteric artery
6. Ileocolic artery
7. Right colic artery
8. Middle colic artery running superiorly
9. Contrast-filled bladder

connects the yolk sac to the primitive digestive tube in early fetal life and is found in about 2% of subjects.

Meckel's diverticulum is said to be 5 cm (2 inches) long and situated about 60 cm (2 feet) from the ileocaecal valve. (Old 'rule of 2's': 2%, 2 inches, 2 feet). In fact, its length, position and appearance is very variable.

The apex of the diverticulum may be adherent to the umbilicus or attached to it by a fibrous cord. It may have ectopic gastric, hepatic or pancreatic tissue at its apex.

The vitellointestinal duct may also rarely persist as a **fistula** from the small intestine to the umbilicus; as a **cyst** along the path of the duct; or as a **raspberry tumour** of the umbilicus (the pouting red mucosa of the persistent extremity of the duct).

RADIOLOGICAL FEATURES OF THE SMALL INTESTINE

Plain Films of the Abdomen (see Fig. 5.2)

Gas and fluid levels are often visible in normal loops of small intestine.

Jejunal loops are distinguished from ileal loops by their position, with the former being in the left upper abdomen whereas the ileal loops tend to be in the lower abdomen and the right iliac fossa.

In radiographs of intestinal obstruction the central position of dilated small bowel loops helps distinguish them from loops of dilated colon. Other identifying features of small intestinal loops include the circular valvulae conniventes, as distinct from the incomplete septa formed by colonic haustra (see the section on the colon).

Barium Studies of the Small Intestine (see Fig. 5.16)

The small intestine may be imaged using a variety of contrast techniques. In a **barium follow-through** examination the barium is taken orally and imaged as it passes through to the caecum. In a **small bowel enema** (or **enteroclysis**) a tube is passed to the duodenojejunal flexure and barium is passed directly into the small intestine.

Normal upper limits of diameter are higher for the distended bowel than for the relaxed state. Diameters of up to 4 cm in the jejunum and 3 cm in the ileum are normal in small bowel enemas. Normal valvulae conniventes may be up to 2 mm thick in the jejunum and 1 mm in the ileum. The valvulae conniventes may be absent in the ileum when it is distended, giving it a featureless appearance.

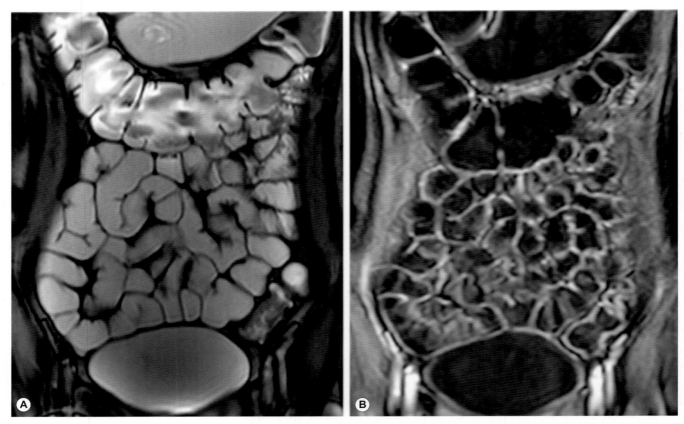

Fig. 5.20 Normal magnetic resonance enterography. (A) Coronal unenhanced image showing good bowel distension with biphasic enteric contrast (mannitol). (B) Coronal postcontrast fat-suppressed T1-weighted gradient echo image showing normal enhancement of bowel wall against a low signal intensity of lumen. (From Amarnath C. *Comprehensive Textbook of Clinical Radiology, Volume IV: Abdomen.* Elsevier; 2023.)

Computed Tomography

Oral contrast may be used to distinguish normal loops of small intestine from abdominal masses. Loops of small intestine fill most of the middle abdomen and the upper pelvis. When adequately filled with oral contrast the thin wall of normal jejunum is almost imperceptible. Fine, transversely thickened areas due to the valvulae conniventes may be seen. These are seldom seen in the ileum. The mesentery along with its vessels, fat and lymph nodes may be easily seen.

Magnetic Resonance Enterography (Fig. 5.20)

MRI of the small bowel is used frequently to assess the primary disease status of patients with inflammatory bowel disease and to assess for complications.

Patients are required to fast for 4–6 hours preprocedure. Over a period of 45 minutes to 1 hour preprocedure, 1–1.5 L of oral contrast solution is administered (this is required to be biphasic, i.e. T1 hypointense and T2 hyperintense; mannitol and polyethylene glycol are frequently used).

Antiperistaltic drugs improve the image quality. Either glucagon or hyoscine butylbromide may be given.

Gadolinium is administered to assess for active inflammation. Other small bowel pathology assessed with MRI includes malabsorption, polyposis syndromes and small bowel malignancy.

Angiography (see Fig. 5.19)

Selective injection of the SMA demonstrates the jejunal and ileal branches and arterial arcades. The mesenteric vessels can also be readily identified on contrast-enhanced and angiographic CT/MR sequences.

The Ileocaecal Valve (Fig. 5.21)

The distal ileum opens into the posteromedial aspect of the large intestine at the junction of the caecum and the ascending colon. Two horizontal crescentic folds of mucosa and circular muscle project into the lumen on the colonic side. These folds are extended laterally as the frenula of the valve. Some thickening of the circular muscle of the ileum at the junction acts as a sphincter.

RADIOLOGICAL FEATURES OF THE ILEOCAECAL VALVE

Plain Films of the Abdomen

Gaseous distension of the colon is seen proximal to a site of colonic obstruction. In some of these cases the ileocaecal valve remains competent, so that marked distension of the caecum can occur without distension of the small intestine.

In other patients the valve is incompetent and there is distension of both large and small intestine without excessive distension of the caecum.

Barium Enema Examinations

The ileocaecal valve may present a filling defect in the posteromedial wall of the caecum. This may be polypoid or bilabial, depending on the state of contraction of the valve. In the contracted valve, barium may fill a narrow slit between the folds like a linear ulcer.

> **RADIOLOGY PEARL**
>
> The ileocaecal valve is at the site of the first completely transverse haustral fold. The thickened posterior ends of this haustra are the frenula of the valve.

Computed Tomography

Fat accumulation around the ileocaecal valve makes it easily visible in many abdominal CT scans. This can be very marked in some individuals, particularly elderly females.

The Appendix (see Figs. 5.21, 5.22)

The appendix arises at the convergence of the taenia coli on the posteromedial wall of the caecum, about 2.5 cm below the ileocaecal valve. It is a thin structure containing lymphoid tissue. Its length is very variable – between 12 and 24 cm long. It has its own mesentery – a triangular fold from the lower border of the ileum – and as a result is mobile. Its position is variable and according to most authors the retrocaecal position is commonest. The possible positions are retrocaecal, pelvic, pre-ileal (anterior to ileum), postileal (behind ileum) or subcaecal (inferior to caecum).

Occasionally it lies beneath the peritoneum of the caecum and may be fused to the caecum or the posterior abdominal wall.

> **RADIOLOGY PEARL**
>
> The lumen of the appendix is wide in the infant and obliterated after mid-adult life. Acute appendicitis, which is usually caused by obstruction of the lumen, is therefore rare in the extremes of life.

> **RADIOLOGY PEARL**
>
> The appendix is supplied by the **appendicular artery**, which reaches it in the mesoappendix from the ileocolic artery. This is its sole supply, and if infection causes thrombosis of this artery, gangrene and perforation of the appendix results (compare with the gallbladder, which receives a rich collateral supply from the liver in the gallbladder bed and in which gangrene and perforation are much less common). Lymph drainage is to the paracolic nodes along the ileocolic artery to the SMA group.

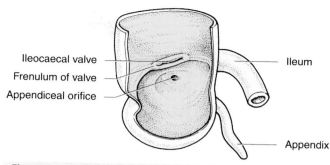
Fig. 5.21 Internal view of the caecum showing the ileocaecal valve and appendix.

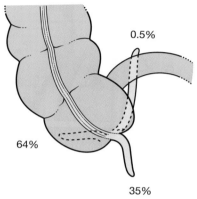
Fig. 5.22 Variation in position of the appendix.

RADIOLOGICAL FEATURES OF THE APPENDIX

Plain Abdominal Film

Faecoliths or fluid levels of the appendix may be visible on plain films of the abdomen in the right iliac fossa in approximately 10% of individuals.

Ultrasound

The appendix is identified as a blind-ended tube arising from the posterior aspect of the caecum. Unlike nearby loops of ileum, it does not display peristalsis. Its position is variable, with the subcaecal appendix being least likely to be obscured by caecal gas. If in a retrocaecal position, visualization of the appendix is aided by compression of the caecum.

The appendix can be found on ultrasound by finding the junction of the terminal ileum with the medial aspect of the colon in the right lower quadrant by sequentially scanning the colon from superior to inferior and then by scanning carefully just below this level. Compression using the ultrasound probe is used to reduce obscuring gas in the overlying bowel and to push overlying bowel loops out of the way.

Barium Enema (Fig. 5.23A)

If the lumen of the appendix is patent, it may fill on barium enema examination. The lumen is often obliterated in patients past mid-adulthood. To fill the appendix the patient should be supine because its orifice is on the posterior aspect of the caecum. Some elevation of the head is also helpful.

CT (Fig. 5.23B) and MRI

The normal appendix can usually be identified arising from the caecum inferior to the insertion of the terminal ileum. It can be followed on sequential images and may have a long and somewhat tortuous course.

RADIOLOGY PEARL

Because the appendix is on a mesentery and mobile, pus from an infected appendix may cause **abscess formation** in a variety of locations. Pus may travel inferiorly to the pelvic peritoneum to the rectovesical (or rectouterine) pouch. Pus may also travel superiorly in the right paracolic gutter to the subhepatic spaces (see section on the peritoneal spaces of the abdomen).

The Large Intestine (See also sections on the rectum and anal canal in Chapter 6)

The length of the large intestine is very variable, with an average length of 1.5 m. It is wider in diameter than the small intestine, with a maximum diameter at the caecum of 9 cm and the transverse colon of 5.5 cm.

Proximal to the rectum, the colon is marked by **taeniae coli**. These are three flattened bands of longitudinal muscle that represent the (incomplete) longitudinal muscle layer of the colon. The taeniae converge on the appendix proximally and the rectum distally, and these two structures have a complete longitudinal muscle layer. The taeniae coli are about 30 cm shorter than the colon and cause the formation

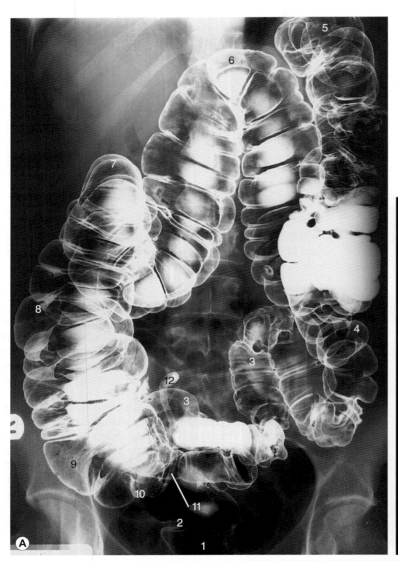
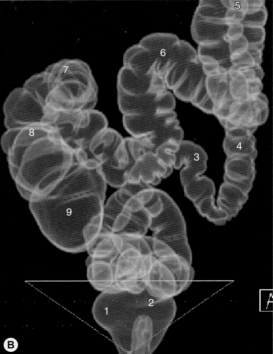

Fig. 5.23 (A) Barium study of the colon. (B) Reformatted computed tomography colonogram (courtesy Siemens Ireland).

1. Rectum
2. Valve of Houston (lateral mucosal fold)
3. Sigmoid colon
4. Descending colon
5. Splenic flexure
6. Transverse colon
7. Hepatic flexure
8. Ascending colon
9. Caecum
10. Caecal pole
11. Base of the appendix
12. Tip of the appendix

of sacculations along its length. On radiographs these give rise to the appearance of incomplete septa, called haustra.

Scattered over the free surface of the large intestine, except for the caecum and rectum, are fat-filled peritoneal tags called **appendices epiploicae**. These are especially numerous in the sigmoid colon. Arteries supplying these perforate the muscle wall. Mucous membrane may herniate through these vascular perforations, giving rise to diverticulosis.

The caecum is a blind pouch of large bowel proximal (inferior) to the ileocaecal valve. It is approximately 6 cm long and usually has its own mesentery, making it mobile and easily distensible.

The ascending colon runs from the ileocaecal valve to the inferior surface of the liver, where it turns medially into the hepatic flexure.

The transverse colon runs from the hepatic flexure across the midline to the splenic flexure.

The descending colon runs from the splenic flexure inferiorly to the sigmoid colon.

RADIOLOGY PEARL

The fatty tags of the colon may twist, leading to ischaemia or infarction and present as acute focal abdominal pain (epiploic appendagitis). This condition often causes diagnostic difficulty with 'negative imaging'. Subtle fat stranding adjacent to the colon at the site of pain may yield the diagnosis.

PERITONEAL RELATIONS OF THE COLON (SEE FIG. 5.17)

The ascending and descending parts of the colon are usually retroperitoneal (covered anteriorly and on both sides by peritoneum). The peritoneal spaces lateral to these are called the paracolic gutters and may act as a route of spread of intraperitoneal infection.

Occasionally the ascending colon has a mobile mesentery. The caecum is usually completely invested in peritoneum and is relatively mobile.

The transverse colon always has a mesentery (mesocolon) on which it hangs in a loop between the hepatic and splenic flexures, which are fixed points. The splenic flexure is attached to the diaphragm by the phrenicocolic ligament. The convexity of the greater curve of the stomach lies in the concavity of the loop of transverse colon. The gastrocolic ligament attaches the stomach and transverse colon. This continues below the transverse colon as the greater omentum (see section on the peritoneal spaces of the abdomen).

The sigmoid colon also has a mesentery. This is attached to the posterior abdominal wall to the left of the midline in an inverted V shape whose limbs diverge from the bifurcation of the common iliac artery over the SI joint at the pelvic brim.

The rectum has peritoneum anteriorly and laterally in its upper third and anteriorly only in its middle third. The lower third of the rectum is below the pelvic peritoneum. (The sigmoid colon, rectum and anus are described fully in Chapter 6.)

RELATIONS OF THE COLON

The parts of the colon that are retroperitoneal have as their **posterior relations** the structures of the posterior abdominal wall; that is the psoas and iliac muscles, the quadratus lumborum muscles and the kidneys. The more mobile transverse and sigmoid colon are related posteriorly to loops of small intestine.

The colon is an anterior structure in the abdomen (see section on development of the colon, below) and has the anterior abdominal wall as an **anterior relation**. The liver, gallbladder and spleen overlap superiorly.

The sigmoid and rectum are related anteriorly to the bladder and retrovesical structures in the male and the uterus in the female.

ARTERIAL SUPPLY OF THE COLON (SEE FIGS. 5.18, 5.19, 5.24, 5.25; SEE ALSO SECTION ON THE RECTUM IN CHAPTER 6)

That part of the colon derived from the midgut (i.e. caecum to the midtransverse colon) is supplied by the **superior mesenteric artery** as follows:

- The ileocolic artery (the lowest right-sided branch of the main trunk of the SMA) supplies the caecum, appendix and the beginning of the ascending colon
- The right colic artery (arising about midway down the right side of the SMA, occasionally from a common trunk with ileocolic artery) supplies the remainder of the ascending colon
- The middle colic artery (arising from the SMA just below the pancreas) supplies the transverse colon to its midpoint
  The **inferior mesenteric artery** supplies the colon as far as the upper rectum as follows:
- The left colic artery to the descending colon
- The sigmoid artery to the sigmoid colon
- The superior rectal (superior haemorrhoidal) artery to the upper rectum

Each of these vessels anastomoses with its neighbour, forming a **marginal artery** (of Drummond) close to the colon. The vessels that enter the bowel are, however, end arteries.

RADIOLOGY PEARL

The region of colon between the supply of the superior and inferior mesenteric arteries (around the splenic flexure) is known as a *watershed* area. This area is more vulnerable to reduced blood flow during hypotensive episodes, leading to ischaemic damage.

VENOUS DRAINAGE OF THE COLON

Veins corresponding with the arteries drain to the superior and inferior mesenteric veins, draining to portal venous system (see below).

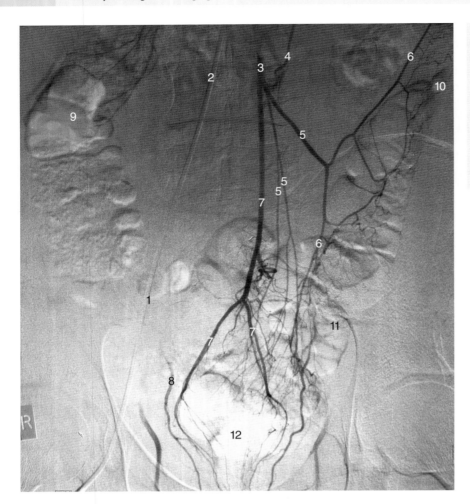

Fig. 5.24 Inferior mesenteric angiogram.
1. Catheter in the right common iliac artery
2. Catheter in the aorta
3. Inferior mesenteric artery
4. Left colic artery
5. Sigmoid arteries
6. Marginal artery of Drummond
7. Superior rectal artery and branches
8. Middle rectal artery (filling by reflux: a branch of the internal iliac artery)
9. Gas in the ascending colon
10. Descending colon
11. Sigmoid colon
12. Rectum

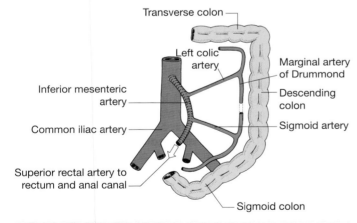

Fig. 5.25 Branches of the inferior mesenteric artery.

LYMPHATIC DRAINAGE OF THE COLON

Lymph drains to nodes near the bowel wall, which drain to nodes in the mesentery and retroperitoneum along with the mesenteric vessels.

- The drainage of the right colon to midtransverse colon is with the superior mesenteric vessels to the peripancreatic nodes and superior mesenteric group of para-aortic nodes.

- The drainage of the left side of the transverse and left colon is along the inferior mesenteric vessels to the inferior mesenteric nodes at the origin of the inferior mesenteric artery at the level of the third lumbar vertebra.

DEVELOPMENT OF THE COLON

In the fifth fetal week the midgut herniates into the umbilical cord, with the vitellointestinal duct at the apex of the hernia. At the tenth week the loops of gut return to the abdominal cavity, proximal bowel before distal and rotating 270 degrees anticlockwise as it does so. This results in the jejunum being to the left and deeper than the colon, and the caecum being to the right and superficial.

In **malrotation** the bowel returns to the abdomen without rotating, leaving the small intestine on the right and the colon on the left. As a result, the small intestinal mesentery is very short and prone to volvulus.

In **exomphalos**, midgut herniation at the umbilicus persists at birth.

RADIOLOGICAL FEATURES OF THE COLON

Plain Films of the Abdomen (see Fig. 5.2)

Gas within the colon outlines the colon or parts of it. The sacculation of the colon by the taeniae coli gives rise to

Table 5.2 Anatomical Features of Small and Large Intestine in Intestinal Obstruction

	Small Intestine	Colon
Position of loops	Central	Peripheral
Septa	Complete (valvulae conniventes)	Incomplete (haustra)
Number of loops	Several	Few
Diameter	<5 cm	>5 cm
Solid faeces	Absent	May be present

septa called haustra. The haustra are fixed anatomical structures in the proximal colon, but in the distal colon require active contraction for their formation. Haustra may be absent distal to the midtransverse colon.

The upper limit of normal diameter of the transverse colon on plain films is taken to be 5.5 cm, and of the caecum 9 cm. Beyond these limits, in the right clinical setting there is a risk of caecal perforation. Numerous gas–fluid levels may be normal and 18% of normal films have fluid levels in the caecum.

In intestinal obstruction, distinguishing dilated loops of small intestine from dilated loops of colon is based on several anatomical features (Table 5.2).

RADIOLOGY PEARL

The transverse colon is mobile and may interpose itself between the liver and the right hemidiaphragm in the normal subject. This is called **Chilaiditi's syndrome** and is commoner in patients with chronic lung disease. It may mimic pneumoperitoneum.

Double-Contrast Barium Enema Examination (see Fig. 5.23A)

The entire colon and appendix may be outlined. The technique for filling the colon with barium and air requires an understanding of anatomy. Because the transverse colon, for example, hangs anteriorly between the relatively posteriorly positioned splenic and hepatic flexures, this is easiest to fill when the patient is prone. Resumption of a supine position allows filling of the hepatic flexure and the ascending colon with barium. The junction of the caecum with both the appendix and the ileum is posterior, and these therefore fill with barium in the supine position.

Visualization of the sigmoid colon may require oblique views and caudally angled views to overcome the problem of overlapping loops. Similarly, views of the ileocaecal area are best obtained with the patient's left side raised because of the posteromedial position of this junction.

The haustra can be seen well on double-contrast views of the colon. Gaseous distension may obliterate these distally as far as the midtransverse colon.

Angiography

For full evaluation of the blood supply of the colon both superior and inferior mesenteric arteries must be shown (see Figs. 5.19 and 5.24).

RADIOLOGY PEARLS

- Small mucous glands in the mucosa of the colon (**crypts of Lieberkühn**) may fill with barium on good double-contrast views. These are up to 1 mm deep and perpendicular to the colonic wall on tangential views, and on 'en-face' views are seen as thin, transverse, parallel lines with short intercommunicating branches called **innominate lines**.
- **Lymphoid follicles** are visible in 13% of adults on double-contrast barium studies. These are low elevations of 1–3 mm in diameter. They are larger in the rectum where a diameter up to 4 mm is considered normal.
- In **malrotation** of the bowel the caecum may be high in partial defects or lie in the left side of the abdomen in complete malrotation.

CT of the Abdomen

The caecum and ascending colon can be seen anterior to the muscles of the posterior abdominal wall on the right side. The right paracolic gutter lies lateral to the ascending colon. The right infracolic space lies medially. The hepatic flexure can be seen lateral to the second part of the duodenum inferior to the right lobe of the liver.

The transverse colon varies in its position because of its variable length and its mobility. Fat, blood vessels and lymph nodes may be seen in the mesocolon. The splenic flexure is seen behind the greater curvature of the stomach and the anterior splenic tip. The descending colon is seen lying on the muscles of the posterior abdominal wall on the left side. The left paracolic gutter lies lateral to the descending colon and the left infracolic space is medial. The sigmoid colon can be distinguished from small intestinal loops by the presence of solid faecal matter and gas, its larger calibre, its relatively featureless smooth wall, and by following its sigmoid course from descending colon to rectum.

CT Colonography

This technique is frequently used to evaluate the colon in patients who are deemed unfit for full colonoscopy and in patients who have failed colonoscopy.

Full-bowel preparation is undertaken, after which a faecal tagging agent such as gastrograffin is administered so that residual stool can be easily differentiated from an underlying lesion. When no contraindication exists, an antispasmodic agent (e.g. hyoscine butylbromide) is administered preprocedure. Optimal colonic distension is critical, and the colon is insufflated with carbon dioxide using a pressure-regulated device, aiming for intracolonic pressures of 15–25 mm Hg. The colon can then be followed from rectum to caecum on sequential CT images to screen the mucosa for polyps or masses.

The Liver (Figs. 5.26–5.28)

The liver, the largest solid organ in the body, is found in the right upper quadrant of the abdomen. Relative to the other

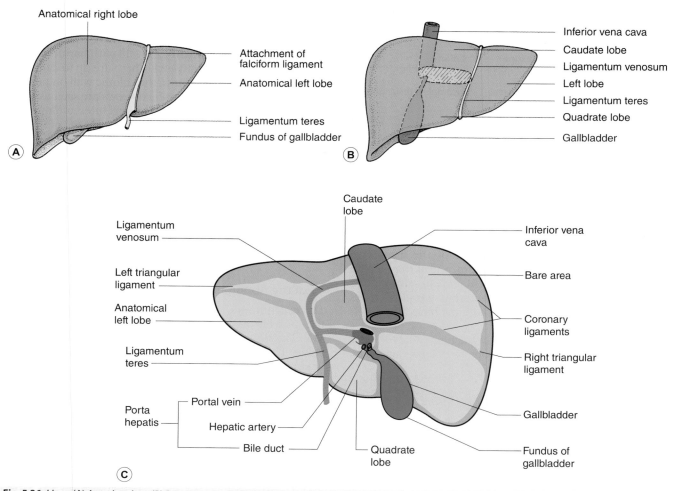

Fig. 5.26 Liver. (A) Anterior view. (B) Posterior view. (C) View through the liver.

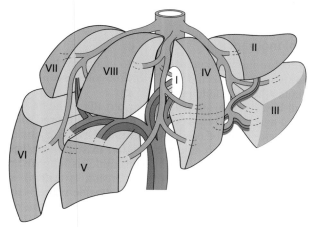

Fig. 5.27 Schematic view of segmental anatomy of the liver. This division is based on the principal divisions of the hepatic artery and portal vein. Hepatic veins run between the segments.

abdominal structures, it is much larger in the fetus and child. The liver assumes the shape of the cavity it occupies. It has two surfaces, the **diaphragmatic surface** and the **visceral surface**.

The diaphragmatic surface is smooth and flat anteriorly and has a smooth, rounded upper surface with a large dome for the right hemidiaphragm and a smaller dome for the left hemidiaphragm. A depression between these marks the site of the **central tendon** and the overlying heart.

The diaphragmatic surface of the liver ends anteriorly at the inferior border of the liver. The inferior border runs along the right costal margin from lateral to a point about 4 cm to the right of the midline, the site of the gallbladder notch. Medial to this, the inferior border ascends less obliquely than the costal margin and lies below the costal margin as it crosses the midline to meet the costal margin of the left side at approximately the eighth costal cartilage. The lateral extent of the left lobe is variable: it may extend only to the midline or may wrap around the stomach or spleen to reach the left lateral abdominal wall.

In addition to the notch for the gallbladder, the inferior border is marked by a notch for the **ligamentum teres**. This ligament is the obliterated remnant of the umbilical vein, which carries blood from the placenta to the fetus. It is also known as the **round ligament of the liver**. It passes, with small **paraumbilical veins**, from the umbilicus to the inferior border of the liver in the free edge of a crescentic fold of peritoneum called the **falciform ligament** (meaning 'sickle-shaped'). This meets the liver just to the right of

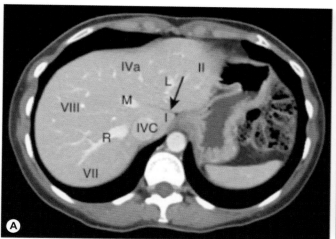 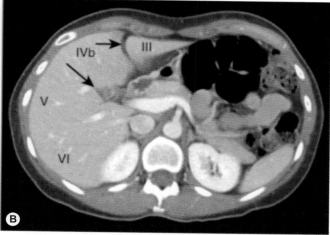

Fig. 5.28 Segmental anatomy of the liver on computed tomography (CT). (A) Axial contrast-enhanced CT image superior to the plane of portal vein shows right *(R)*, middle *(M)* and left *(L)* hepatic veins between hepatic segments that drain to inferior vena cava *(IVC)*. Note fissure for ligamentum venosum *(arrow)* anterior to caudate lobe *(I)*, as well as lateral *(II)*, medial *(IVa)*, anterior *(VIII)* and posterior *(VII)* segments. (B) Axial contrast-enhanced CT image through the liver inferior to the plane of portal vein shows left intersegmental fissure *(short arrow)* and interlobar fissure *(long arrow)*, as well as lateral *(III)*, medial *(IVb)*, anterior *(V)* and posterior *(VI)* segments. (From Ramchandani P, Torigian DA. *Radiology Secrets Plus*, 4th ed. Elsevier; 2017.)

the midline and runs through the liver in a deep fissure to the porta hepatis where it attaches to the left portal vein. The fissure for the ligamentum teres is identified as a deep fissure running from anterior to posterior to the porta of the liver on cross-sectional images. The site of attachment of the falciform ligament marks the sagittal plane of division of the liver into traditional anatomical left and right lobes.

The posteroinferior, or **visceral**, **surface** of the liver is marked by an H-shaped arrangement of structures (see Fig. 5.26C). The crossbar of the H is made by the horizontal hilum of the liver called the **porta hepatis**. This is the entry site of the right and left hepatic arteries and portal veins, and the exit of the right and left hepatic ducts. It also contains autonomic nerves and lymph vessels. It is a deep, short, transverse fissure passing across the medial undersurface of the right lobe of liver. It is seen as a cleft running horizontally in the mediolateral plane from fissure for the ligamentum teres, towards the lesser curve of the stomach on the deep surface of the liver on cross-sectional images.

The gallbladder in its bed (inferior and anterior), and the IVC (superior and posterior), in a deep groove, form the right vertical part of the H. These are separated by the **caudate process of the caudate lobe**.

The left vertical part of the H is formed by the ligamentum teres (inferior and anterior) and the **ligamentum venosum** (superior and posterior). The ligamentum teres runs to its attachment to the left portal vein in the left extremity of the porta hepatis. The fissure for the ligamentum teres is continuous with the **fissure for the ligamentum venosum** (ligamentum venosum = obliterated remnant of **ductus venosum**), a deep fissure lined by peritoneum running in a broad craniocaudal plane between the left lobe of liver and the caudate lobe. It can be seen running superiorly from the transverse fissure on cross-sectional images. The ductus venosum shunts blood from the umbilical vein to the IVC in the fetus, bypassing the liver. At the upper end of the fissure the ligamentum venosum curves laterally to attach to either the left hepatic vein or the IVC.

The visceral surface of the liver lies in contact with, and is slightly moulded by:

- The oesophagus, stomach and lesser omentum on the left
- The pancreas (through the lesser omentum) and the duodenum in the midline
- The right kidney and adrenal and the hepatic flexure of the colon on the right

The peritoneal attachments of the liver determine the distribution of free gas and of fluid in this part of the peritoneal cavity and are discussed in the section on the peritoneal spaces of the abdomen.

SEGMENTAL LIVER ANATOMY (SEE FIGS. 5.27, 5.28)

The **Couinaud** classification divides the liver into eight functionally independent segments. Each segment has its own vascular inflow, outflow and biliary drainage. In the centre of each segment there is the triad of the portal vein, hepatic artery and bile duct. At the periphery of each segment there is venous drainage through the hepatic veins. The hepatic veins are **intersegmental**, draining blood from adjacent segments.

The middle hepatic vein divides the liver into right and left lobes. This is the **principal plane** (also known as **Cantlie's line**) and runs from the IVC to the gallbladder fossa, and a line between these two denotes its position on the visceral surface. There is no external marking of this plane on the anterior surface of the liver, but it lies about 4 cm to the left of the falciform ligament.

The right hepatic vein divides the right lobe into anterior and posterior segments.

The left hepatic vein divides the left lobe into medial and lateral parts.

The portal vein divides the liver into upper and lower segments. The left and right portal veins branch superiorly and inferiorly to run in the centre of each segment.

The subdivision into **segments** is based on branches of the right and left hepatic arteries. Knowledge of these segments is essential in assessment of the location and extent of hepatic pathology prior to liver surgery. Surgery is performed in a segmental fashion; therefore the distribution of disease determines resectability. Segments are numbered in the **Couinaud system**. The caudate lobe is segment I. Segments II and III are the farthest left, divided by the left hepatic vein from segment IV. The left portal vein separates segment II above from segment III below. Segment IV lies between the left hepatic vein and the middle hepatic vein. It is divided into segment IVa above and IVb below by the left portal vein. The right lobe has four segments, divided by the right hepatic vein into anteromedial and posterolateral divisions, and by the plane of the right branch of the portal vein into superior and inferior sections. These four segments are numbered in a clockwise fashion from anterior inferomedial: V, VI, VII and VIII. The segments may also be named descriptively according to their location, for example posterior segment (caudate), **right** posterior lateral, posterior medial, anterior lateral and anterior medial segments, and **left** medial superior, medial inferior and lateral segments.

The functional subunit of the liver is the microscopic **lobule**, which has a central vein and, in spaces between the lobules, portal canals or triads, each with a branch of the hepatic artery, portal vein and bile duct.

The old anatomical description of the liver as having a large right lobe and small left lobe separated by the falciform ligament defines the anatomical left lobe as consisting only of segments II and III.

OLD LOBAR ANATOMY

Traditional anatomic teaching divides the liver into a large right and a small left lobe. These are divided anteriorly by the attachment for the falciform ligament, and on the visceral surface by the grooves for the ligamenta teres and venosum. Two further lobes are described: the caudate lobe posteriorly between the IVC and the fissure for the ligamentum venosum, and the quadrate lobe anteroinferiorly between the gallbladder bed and the fissure for the ligamentum teres. These lobes are part of the conventional right lobe. The caudate lobe is attached to the remainder of the right lobe by the caudate process. This division of the lobes bears no relationship to the functional structure of the liver and has been replaced by new International Anatomical Terminology.

BLOOD SUPPLY OF THE LIVER

The blood supply to the liver is from the portal venous system (75%) and the hepatic artery (25%). The portal venous system supplies nutrient-rich blood from the gastrointestinal tract and spleen, providing approximately half of the liver's oxygen demand and most of its nutrients. The oxygen-rich hepatic arterial system supplies the biliary system.

Arterial Supply

Conventional anatomy (type I) exists in 55%–75% of subjects. Traditionally the common hepatic artery (CHA) originates from the coeliac artery as one of its three branches. It supplies the right gastric and gastroduodenal artery before continuing as the proper hepatic artery, running in the free edge of the lesser omentum. It passes anterior to the portal vein and medial to the CBD. It divides into approximately equal-sized right and left hepatic branches before entering the liver at the porta hepatis.

Variations in Arterial Supply to the Liver

These are common and important to recognize prior to surgery or to hepatic arterial interventional procedures. Tiny anastomoses exist between the vascular territories. Accessory arteries, where they exist, provide a vital arterial contribution to the segments they supply. The hepatic artery normally passes anterior to the portal vein and posterior to the common hepatic duct (CHD). Accessory hepatic arteries originating from the SMA pass posterior to the portal vein and lateral to the CBD. This is an important variation to recognize at surgery as the bile duct could be clamped inadvertently.

Accessory branches may exist *in addition* to the normal origin of the hepatic artery from the coeliac trunk. All or part of either hepatic artery may be *replaced* by a vessel originating in a different manner from the norm. The following variations are some of the more commonly seen variants. Percentages are approximate, various ranges are reported. The prevalence of right or left hepatic artery aberrations approaches 30% (Choi et al., 2021 Radiology; study of 5625 patients); approximately 15% each had aberrant right or left hepatic arteries, in 4.5% cases both vessels were aberrant. The relevance of aberrant arteries is that they have a different course than in conventional anatomy, which should be recognized prior to radiologic or surgical intervention (e.g. hepatic artery embolization or liver resection).

- The entire liver is supplied by a **replaced CHA** arising from aorta or SMA in 2.5%.
- The entire right lobe is supplied by a **replaced right hepatic artery** with separate origin (usually SMA) in 10%.
- Part of the right lobe is supplied by an **accessory right hepatic artery** in 5%.
- The left hepatic artery is replaced by the **left gastric artery** in 10%.
- **Accessory left hepatic arteries** arise from the left gastric in 10%–15%.
- The CHA may **divide early** or trifurcate with the gastroduodenal artery.
- The hepatic artery may **arise separately** from the aorta rather than from the coeliac trunk in 2%.
- The middle hepatic artery usually arises from the left hepatic artery.

When the right hepatic artery arises from the SMA it runs horizontally between the pancreas and vena cava and supplies the cystic artery to the gallbladder.

The left hepatic artery arises from the left gastric artery, it runs medially from the stomach to the porta in fissure for the ligamentum venosum before supplying left and middle hepatic arteries.

PORTAL VEIN (FIG. 5.29, SEE ALSO SECTION ON PORTAL VENOUS SYSTEM BELOW)

The portal system is much less prone to anatomical variation than the hepatic artery. It normally forms posterior to

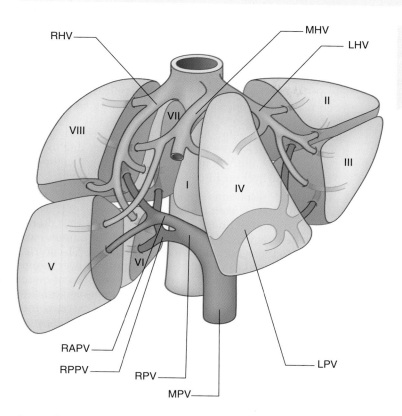

Fig. 5.29 Portal and hepatic veins: segmental anatomy - commonest configuration. *MPV*, main portal vein; *LPV*, left portal vein; *RPV*, right portal vein; *RPPV*, right posterior portal vein; *RHV*, right hepatic vein; *MHV*, middle hepatic vein; *LHV*, left hepatic vein. (Modified from Townsend CM. *Sabiston Textbook of Surgery: The Biological Basis of Modern Surgical Practice*, 21st ed. Elsevier; 2022.).

the neck of the pancreas by the union of the **superior mesenteric vein** (SMV) and the **splenic vein** at the level of the L1/L2 disc space. It ascends anterior to the IVC and passes to the right in the posterior aspect of the free edge of the lesser omentum. It runs posterior to the bile duct and the hepatic artery to the porta hepatis. At the porta, the portal vein branches into right and left portal veins, and the right portal vein divides into right anterior portal vein, supplying segments V and VII, and right posterior portal vein supplying segments VI and VII. This is the usual configuration (see Fig. 5.27). Common variations are trifurcation of the portal vein into right anterior portal vein, right posterior portal vein and left portal vein; and right posterior portal vein arising as the first branch of the portal vein.

In most individuals the inferior mesenteric vein joins the splenic vein close to the confluence of the SMV and splenic vein. In approximately 40% it drains into the SMV. In approximately one-third of individuals the inferior mesenteric vein joins with the SMV and splenic vein in a confluence. Very rarely the portal vein is double, caused by nonunion of the superior mesenteric and splenic veins (see section on the portal venous system).

VENOUS DRAINAGE OF THE LIVER (SEE FIG. 5.27)

The liver is drained by hepatic veins, which drain upwards and posteriorly to the IVC without an extrahepatic course. The hepatic veins assist in the stabilization of the liver. The distribution of the hepatic veins differs from that of the hepatic artery, the portal vein and the bile ducts. Right, middle and left hepatic veins drain corresponding thirds of the liver. The middle hepatic vein lies in the principal plane and may unite with the left hepatic vein and have a common final course to the IVC. A lower group of small veins drain directly to the IVC from the lower parts of the right and caudate lobes. Hepatic veins have no valves.

LYMPHATIC DRAINAGE OF THE LIVER

Lymph from the deep lymphatics of the liver drains in the connective tissues of the portal triads and along hepatic veins. Lymphatics accompany the portal vessels and ducts draining to nodes in the porta hepatis, to hepatic nodes along the hepatic vessels and to ducts in the lesser omentum. From here lymph drains via retropyloric nodes to the coeliac nodes and thence to the cisterna chyli. There is also a superficial network of lymphatics under the capsule of the liver. The anterior parts of the diaphragmatic and visceral surface of the liver drain to the deep lymphatics. The posterior part of the visceral and diaphragmatic surfaces drain toward the bare area of the liver. From here, lymph drains into phrenic lymph nodes, or joins deep lymphatics that run with the hepatic veins towards the IVC. These lymphatics pass through the diaphragm with the IVC and drain into posterior mediastinal lymph nodes.

RADIOLOGICAL FEATURES OF THE LIVER

Plain Films of the Abdomen (see Fig. 5.2)

The margins of the liver are visible where they are outlined by fat; thus the lateral border can be seen where it is flanked by properitoneal fat. Intraperitoneal and omental fat lie near the inferior border. Air in the lungs outlines the pleura and diaphragm over the upper limit of the liver, but gas in the stomach may give a misleading impression of the position of the inferior border of the liver, as the stomach may pass posterior to this border.

CT and MRI (Fig. 5.30)

CT of the Liver. Dedicated CT evaluation of the liver parenchyma is generally conducted using a triple-contrast phase technique. This involves late arterial, portal venous and delayed phase acquisitions.

For diagnosis of and characterization of bleeding, addition of noncontrast imaging should be performed (i.e. four-phase CT). Blood is dense on CT, but its age cannot always be accurately assessed. Subacute hematoma may be dense but if there is active bleeding, additional dense material will be seen accumulating on the arterial-phase CT. Four-phase imaging is also performed if there has been prior chemoembolization as lipiodol contrast (which is mixed with the therapeutic agent) remains in the treated liver lesions. Lipiodol is also dense and might be interpreted as enhancement if not recognized on the noncontrast images.

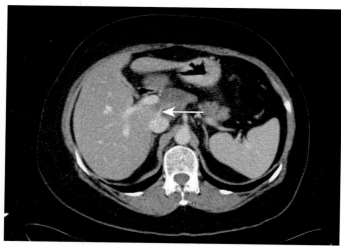

Fig. 5.30 Axial computed tomography of the upper abdomen. The caudate lobe demonstrates focal fatty infiltration resulting in its relatively low density. Note the vein draining directly into the inferior vena cava (arrow).

MRI of the Liver. On MRI the liver is of equal signal intensity to the pancreas and higher on T1 and lower on T2 images than the spleen. Normal hepatic vessels are seen as areas of signal void on standard imaging. The major hepatic veins and the secondary branches of the portal veins are visible. Hepatic arteries are less well seen unless intravenous contrast is given.

The intrahepatic biliary ducts are seen on fluid-sensitive imaging in MR cholangiography (MRCP; see section on the biliary system).

On T2 images the ligamentum venosum and the ligamentum teres are of low intensity but the fat within their fissures is of high intensity.

Many protocol variations exist in the imaging of the liver with MRI; standard protocols will generally include:

- Axial and coronal T2-weighted imaging (T2 half Fourier single-shot turbo spin-echo [HASTE] and T2 fat saturated).
- Axial T1-weighted imaging (in phase, out of phase and fat saturated).
- Axial diffusion-weighted imaging.

- Postcontrast axial imaging using T1 gradient echo sequences in arterial, portal venous, equilibrium and hepatobiliary delayed/excretion.

Contrast for Liver MRI. There are two types of contrast agent used in liver MRI. Extracellular contrast agents have been used for decades and are used in all types of MRI – characterizing lesions based on their vascularity. They are analogous to iodine in CT imaging. Malignant lesions typically enhance more than the normal liver due to their neovascularity and will appear relatively bright compared to the normal liver on T1 contrast-enhanced images.

Gadoxetate disodium (Primovist) is a hepatospecific contrast agent that is taken up by hepatocytes and excreted in the bile on delayed images. Malignant lesions that do not contain hepatocytes (all but hepatocellular carcinoma) will not take up the agent and will appear dark on T1 contrast images compared to the surrounding normal liver parenchyma. It is also used to differentiate between focal nodular hyperplasia (FNH; which contains hepatocytes) and hepatic adenoma (which does not). As it is excreted into the bile, it also allows for the acquisition of an MR contrast cholangiogram which may demonstrate bile leaks and may be useful in hepatojejunostomy evaluation.

- Focal fatty sparing (normal parenchyma in an otherwise fatty liver) tends to occur in segments IV and V, adjacent to the gallbladder fossa.
- A projection of the caudate lobe to the left of the portal vein, called the **papillary process** of the caudate lobe, may mimic a porta hepatis mass on CT if its continuity with the liver is not appreciated.
- Prominent diaphragmatic muscle slips may indent the soft surface of the liver but can be identified by their characteristic location and are usually multiple. Fat covers these diaphragmatic slips, and this also helps to distinguish this variant from a mass.

- Focal fatty infiltration of the liver may be seen in normal subjects and can be confused with pathologic lesions. Typical locations include adjacent to the falciform ligament, portal vein, gallbladder and in the caudate lobe (see Fig. 5.30). Focal fat is seen as a low-density area on CT, has imaging characteristics of fat on MRI (bright on T1 and T2 imaging, with loss of signal on fat-suppression sequences) and is echogenic on ultrasound.
- Fat within fissures, including incomplete accessory fissures on the smooth diaphragmatic surface, may also mimic a mass.

Ultrasound (Fig. 5.31)

As a solid organ, the liver is particularly suitable for ultrasound examination and it is seldom covered by gas-containing bowel. The liver is used as an acoustic window for visualization of other structures, including the right

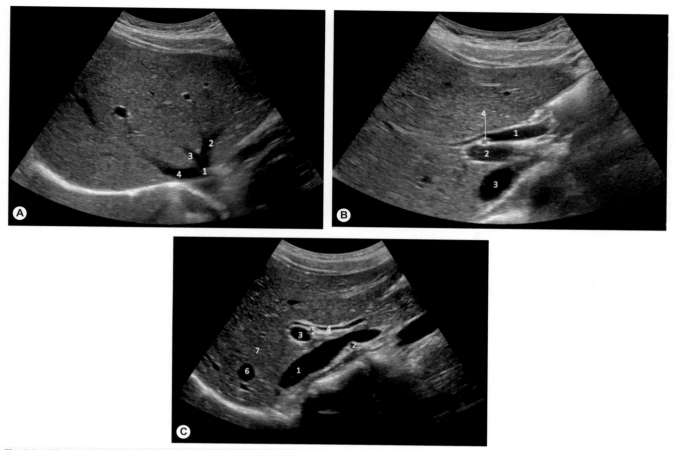

Fig. 5.31 Ultrasound of the liver. (A) Transverse image showing the confluence of hepatic veins. (B) Transverse section through the left lobe of the liver to show the structures at the porta hepatis. (C) Sagittal section of the inferior vena cava in the liver.

(A)
1. Inferior vena cava
2. Left hepatic vein
3. Middle hepatic veins
4. Right hepatic vein

(B)
1. Common bile duct
2. Portal vein
3. Inferior vena cava
4. Hepatic artery

(C)
1. Inferior vena cava
2. Right renal artery
3. Portal vein
4. Common bile duct
5. Hepatic artery
6. Right hepatic vein
7. Right lobe of liver

kidney and adrenal gland, the gallbladder and the pancreas. Vessels and bile ducts of the liver are particularly well seen on ultrasound studies (see section on the biliary system). Blood flow can be studied using colour flow Doppler, and the direction and velocity of flow in the portal vein can be evaluated with pulsed-wave Doppler.

Liver Shear Wave Elastography

In shear wave elastogtaphy (SWE) of the liver, quantification of mechanical and elastic tissue properties of the liver using ultrasound aids evaluation of fibrosis, allowing non-invasive diagnosis and assessment of response to treatment. SWE is more reliable and reproducible than earlier types of elastography. It uses a high-intensity acoustic radiation impulse generated by the ultrasound machine to generate shear waves which propagate perpendicular to the ultrasound beam, causing transient displacements of liver tissue. Shear waves propagate faster through stiff or fibrotic tissue and their velocity can be measured and converted into a liver stiffness measurement measured in kilopascals (kPs) or metres per second.

Scintigraphy

Technetium Sulphur Colloid Scan. Technetium-99m (^{99m}Tc) sulphur colloid is injected intravenously and taken up by the reticulendothelial system of the liver, spleen and bone marrow. Computerized images are acquired using a planar or multiplanar (single-photon emission CT [SPECT]) scintillation gamma camera providing three-dimensional images of the liver and spleen. It gives information on the function of the liver prior to lobectomy.

IR and the Liver. Multiple interventional angiographic procedures are performed in the management of hepatic disease.

For arterial procedures the supply is assessed by performing arteriography of the coeliac and superior mesenteric arteries. Variant hepatic arterial anatomy is present in 30%–50% of the population. Commonly performed procedures requiring access to the hepatic arteries include chemoembolization of hepatic metastases or hepatocellular carcinoma and radioembolization of hepatic malignancy. Embolization of the hepatic artery branches, which are end arteries, or arteries with only tiny anastomoses, does not result in infarction because of the dual supply to the liver, with the portal venous system also bringing blood to the liver.

The hepatic veins are usually accessed via the IVC via a retrograde approach from the right internal jugular vein. Hepatic venous access is utilized in the performance of transjugular liver biopsy and transjugular intrahepatic portosystemic shunt (TIPS).

RADIOLOGY PEARLS

- The ligamentum teres can be identified as an echogenic band running from the left portal vein to the surface
  of the liver in most subjects. It separates segments III and IV.
- The ligamentum venosum can be seen as an echogenic line running posteriorly from the left portal vein separating the lateral part of segment I from the medial part of segment II.
- A benign lesion known as focal nodular hyperplasia (FNH) is occasionally difficult to differentiate on conventional imaging from other lesions, which may require surgery. Because the FNH lesions are caused by hyperplastic growth of normal hepatocytes, they contain hepatocytes as well as biliary canaliculi. FNH behaves as normal liver on ^{99m}Tc hepatobiliary iminodiacetic acid (HIDA) and ^{99m}Tc sulphur colloid scans, taking up the isotope and presenting as an area of normal or increased uptake of isotope, whereas almost all other focal liver lesions appear as photopenic (cold) areas. FNH is treated conservatively as it is benign with a very low risk of bleeding or rupture in contrast to other benign liver lesions, which tend to be removed if large.

The hepatic portal vein is usually accessed using a percutaneous, ultrasound-guided approach. Access to the hepatic portal veins is required prior to portal vein embolization.

Contrast Cholangiography. Access to the intrahepatic bile ducts is achieved using a percutaneous, ultrasound-guided approach. Biliary access is usually required in the setting of obstruction. Confirmation of position within the bile ducts can be achieved by contrast injection. The ducts are usually accessed via a right mid-axillary approach. A 22-gauge needle is inserted under ultrasound or fluoroscopic guidance. Contrast injection is used to confirm the position of the needle. In the portal venous system contrast flows towards the periphery of the liver, filling portal vein branches and sinusoids; in veins contrast clears quickly towards the IVC; contrast in the bile ducts trickles slowly towards the hilum.

Contrast Lymphography (see section on Abdominal Lymphatic System below). There is subspecialized interest in lymphatic imaging and intervention. The liver contributes 40%–50% of lymphatic flow to the thoracic duct. Access to the lymphatics using a 25-gauge needle is possible. The calibre of the normal lymphatics is tiny, with complex and variable anatomy consisting of multiple interconnected networks. Various contrast agents may be injected, although oily agents such as lipiodol may be needed to provide good fluoroscopic or CT fluoroscopic images. Abnormal communications between the liver and duodenum or lymphatic leaks may be detected in this way, and interventional procedures may be performed to embolize abnormal communications or leaks. In addition to communications with the duodenum and proximal small bowel, the liver lymphatics also communicate with the lymphatics in the thoracic cavity through the bare area, as outlined by the hepatic ligaments.

RADIOLOGY PEARLS

- Radiographic demonstration of the patency of the portal system is essential prior to embolization.
- When the right lobe is being embolized the catheter tip should be beyond the origin of the cystic artery. While embolization of the right hepatic artery proximal to the origin of the cystic artery is safe, embolization of the gallbladder should be avoided where possible to decrease the severity of postembolization syndrome.
- The caudate lobe (Fig. 5.30) is drained by small veins that enter the IVC directly and may receive portal supply from both branches of the portal vein. Because of this, the caudate lobe may be spared in cirrhosis or diseases that occlude the main hepatic veins (e.g. Budd–Chiari syndrome). As a result it may undergo compensatory hypertrophy which, if extensive, may itself obstruct the IVC.
- Riedel's lobe is a relatively common variant. It refers to inferior elongation of segment VI. This is an extension of the right lobe anterior to the lower pole of the right kidney and may be accompanied by a smaller left lobe. It is a possible cause of a palpable mass in the right upper quadrant.

The Biliary System

THE GALLBLADDER (FIG. 5.32)

The gallbladder is a pear-shaped sac attached to the extrahepatic bile ducts by the cystic duct. It is very variable in size but normally measures up to 10 cm in length and 3 cm in diameter. It is described as having a fundus, body and neck, and it hangs on its bed on the visceral surface of the liver with its neck lying superiorly and its fundus inferiorly. A pouch called Hartmann's pouch on the ventral surface just proximal to the neck is seen when the gallbladder is dilated in disease; this is not a normal anatomical feature.

The gallbladder is covered by peritoneum on its fundus and inferior surface. It may have a mesentery and hang free from the inferior surface of the liver.

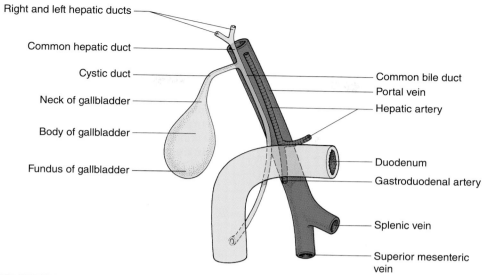

Fig. 5.32 The biliary system and its relations.

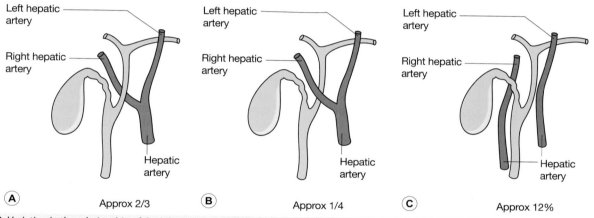

Fig. 5.33 Variation in the relationship of the bile ducts and hepatic artery at the porta hepatis. (A) In two-thirds of individuals the bile duct is anterior to the right hepatic artery. (B) In one-quarter the bile duct passes behind the artery. (C) In 12% the right hepatic artery arises from the superior mesenteric artery and passes behind the bile duct.

The mucosa lining the gallbladder is smooth except at the neck and the cystic duct, where it forms folds that are arranged spirally and called the **valves of Heister**.

Relations of the Gallbladder

These are as follows:
Antero superiorly:
- The gallbladder bed of the liver
- The fundus is related to the anterior abdominal wall at the point where the lateral edge of the right rectus muscle meets the ninth costal cartilage

Posteroinferiorly:
- The neck: lesser omentum
- The body: first part of the duodenum
- The fundus: transverse colon

Normal Variants

These are as follows:
- The lumen may have a septum
- The fundus may be folded back on itself – known as the **phrygian cap**
- Diverticula may occur anywhere, commonest at the fundus

- Location may be retrohepatic or suprahepatic
- Location may be intrahepatic (normal in the fetus up to 2 months)
- Location may be left-sided (if under the left lobe, it has herniated through the epiploic foramen or as part of transposition of the viscera)
- Absent gallbladder – very rare and usually associated with other congenital abnormalities
- Gallbladder duplication – exceedingly rare (reported 1 in 4000); if double they usually share a duct

ARTERIAL SUPPLY

The gallbladder is supplied by the cystic artery, a branch of the right hepatic artery and by branches that supply it directly from the liver in the gallbladder bed.

VENOUS DRAINAGE

Blood from the gallbladder drains via small veins to the liver from the gallbladder bed. Sometimes a cystic vein is formed that drains to the portal vein.

BILE DUCTS (FIGS. 5.32–5.35)

The intrahepatic bile ducts follow the same pattern of distribution as the hepatic arteries. As with the arteries, knowledge of the segmental anatomy is especially important in assessment prior to segmentectomy. The right hepatic duct (RHD) drains the segments of the right lobe (V–VIII) and has two major tributaries – the right posterior duct (RPD) draining the posterior segments (VI and VII), and the right anterior duct (RAD) draining the anterior segments (V and VIII). The RAD has a more horizontal course and usually passes anterior to the RPD, which is orientated more vertically. The RAD usually fuses with the RPD on its medial side to form the RHD. The LHD

is formed by the ducts draining segments II, III and IV. The bile duct draining the caudate lobe (segment I) joins the RHD or LHD. The RHD and LHD have a diameter of up to 3 mm each and these unite outside the liver in the porta hepatis to form the **common hepatic duct (CHD)**. This duct has a variable diameter (7 mm is considered the upper limit of normal; however it may dilate in patients post cholecystectomy and in old age) and lies anterior to the portal vein in the free edge of the lesser omentum, with the hepatic artery on its left side. The CHD is joined after a variable distance (usually 3.5 cm) by the **cystic duct** (usually 3.5 cm long) to form the **common bile duct (CBD)**.

The CBD has a supraduodenal third where it lies in the free edge of the lesser omentum, with the hepatic artery on its left and the portal vein posteriorly. It also has a retroduodenal third where it passes behind the first part of the duodenum with the gastroduodenal artery, and a pancreatic third where it passes behind the pancreas in a tunnel or groove towards the midpoint of the second part of the duodenum. The CBD usually unites with the pancreatic duct in a common dilated terminal **ampulla** (of **Vater**) and empties into the duodenum at the **papilla** 8–10 cm distal to the pylorus. The ampulla is surrounded by a circular layer of involuntary muscle known as the **sphincter of Oddi**. This protrudes slightly into the duodenum, aiding identification at endoscopy.

Variation in the Biliary Ducts

Some variation in the intrahepatic ducts occurs in over 40% of cases. These vary more often than the extrahepatic ducts. The commonest variations are shown in Fig. 5.35A and B.

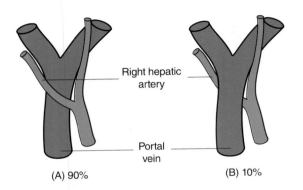

In 90% individuals the right hepatic artery passes anterior to the portal vein

Fig. 5.34 Variation in relationship of the hepatic artery and portal vein.

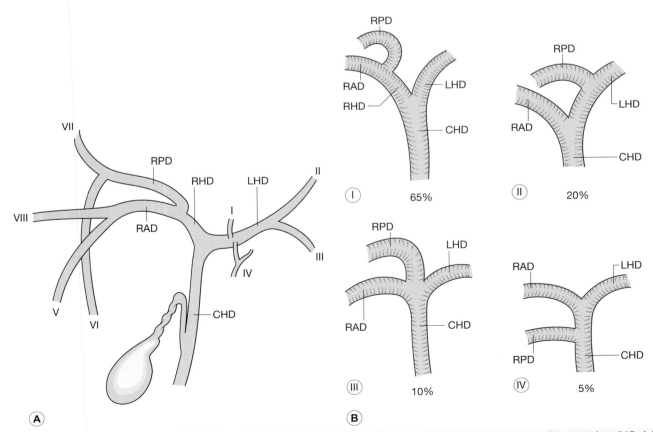

Fig. 5.35 Segmental biliary drainage. (A) Usual configuration. (B) Commonest variations. *CHD*, Common hepatic duct; *LHD*, left hepatic duct; *RAD*, right anterior bile duct; *RHD*, right hepatic duct; *RPD*, right posterior bile duct.

The RPD may drain into the LHD before its confluence with the RAD. This is the commonest variant.

The RAD, RPD and LHD may join in a 'triple confluence' of the ducts.

The RPD may drain into the right side of the RAD and not pass posterior to it.

Accessory hepatic ducts may arise in the liver, particularly in the right lobe, and join the RHD, the main hepatic duct, the common bile duct, the cystic duct or rarely the gallbladder (approximately 2%).

The RHD and LHD may fail to unite, giving rise to a **'double' hepatic duct**.

The **cystic duct** has three common variants:
- A low insertion where it fuses with the distal CHD
- A medial insertion where it passes posterior to the CHD and drains into its left side
- A parallel course where it adheres closely to the CHD for at least 2 cm

RADIOLOGY PEARLS

- Compression of the hepatic duct by calculi in a long cystic duct results in a syndrome known as **Mirizzi's syndrome**.
- The **CBD** and the pancreatic duct may have separate openings close to each other in up to 40% of cases and widely separate from each other in 4% of cases.
- The **papilla** may be positioned as far proximally as the stomach or as far distally as the third part of the duodenum.

RADIOLOGICAL FEATURES OF THE BILIARY SYSTEM

Plain Films of the Abdomen

The normal gallbladder or biliary system is not visible. Gas may be seen in the extrahepatic ducts in the elderly where the ampullary tone is low, after sphincterotomy or after surgical anastomosis of bile ducts to small bowel (choledochojejunostomy). Calcified gallstones may be visualized in the right upper quadrant (only 15%–20% are radiopaque).

Ultrasound Examination of the Biliary System (see Fig 5.31)

Intrahepatic bile ducts are tiny structures that run with portal vein branches. They can often be detected on higher resolution scanning and normally measure less than 2 mm, or less than 40% calibre of the adjacent portal venous branch. Anything larger is abnormal and suggests biliary obstruction. The union of the right and left hepatic ducts can be seen in the porta hepatis. The right hepatic artery can be seen to cross between the main portal vein and the common duct at the porta. The upper limit of normal for diameter of the CBD varies with age. The mean diameter is 3 mm at 20 years of age and 6.5 in asymptomatic subjects over 75 years. However, up to 8 mm is considered normal in older subjects, and up to 10 mm is normal in the postcholecystectomy case.

The gallbladder can be visualized between the liver and the right kidney. Its wall thickness varies with the degree of distension. The size of the gallbladder also varies between fed and fasting states. The position of the fundus can be as low as the pelvis.

The hepatic and common bile ducts can sometimes be visualized throughout their course, but part of the CBD is often obscured by gas as it passes posterior to the first part of the duodenum.

RADIOLOGY PEARLS

- The normal gallbladder wall is seen as a thin echogenic line less than 3 mm thick.
- The upper limit of normal of the CBD is approximately one-tenth of the age of the subject in millimetres – 4 mm at 40 years of age, 7 mm at 70 years of age, etc.

RADIOLOGY PEARL

- The spiral **valves of Heister** in the gallbladder neck and the cystic duct may cast acoustic shadows that must not be confused with calculi.

Contrast and Cross-Sectional Examinations (Fig. 5.36)

A variety of contrast examinations of the gallbladder and biliary tree are possible, depending on the clinical circumstances. Some, such as intravenous cholangiography and oral cholecystography, have been replaced by ultrasound. Others such as intraoperative, T-tube, transhepatic and endoscopic retrograde cholangiography (ERCP) are still in use. MRCP has replaced ERCP for first-line investigation of the intra- and extrahepatic biliary trees (see Fig. 5.36), with ERCP now largely reserved for interventional procedures. Preoperative MRCP has also replaced intraoperative cholangiography to look for stones in the bile ducts (see earlier for transhepatic cholangiography).

RADIOLOGY PEARLS

- Some intrahepatic ducts, particularly those to the left lobe, have an anterior course and in transhepatic cholangiography, a patient may need to be turned from a supine to a prone position to visualize them. To view anteriorly or posteriorly directed ducts oblique views are taken. The ducts to the quadrate lobe (segment IV) and to the inferior segment of the left lobe (segment III) are most commonly used as afferent ducts to bypass hilar biliary tumours, and their patency should be established in preoperative assessment of these patients.
- The ducts most commonly punctured during percutaneous transhepatic cholangiography are the ducts of segments V and VI on the right and the duct of segment III on the left, as these are the most accessible.
- The extrahepatic bile ducts are anterior to the vertebral column and oblique views are necessary to project them away from the spine on contrast studies.

MR Cholangiography/Cholangiopancreatography (see Fig. 5.36)

Excellent images of the biliary and pancreatic systems are obtained without the use of intravenous contrast using fluid-sensitive MRI techniques. MRCP utilizes the long T2 relaxation time of static fluid. Heavily T2-weighted fat-suppressed sequences produce images where static fluid in the bile ducts and pancreatic duct is hyperintense and background signal is suppressed. Axially acquired images can be postprocessed to offer projection images that resemble direct cholangiograms produced by ERCP, or coronal or sagittal images can be acquired directly to demonstrate sections of the ducts. This technique has replaced ERCP as a first-line investigation of the biliary tree.

Fasting is required for a minimum of 4 hours prior to the procedure to reduce gastroduodenal secretions, minimize peristalsis and promote gallbladder distension.

CT of the Biliary Tree

The intrahepatic bile ducts are seen running with the portal veins. The biliary system is best seen on contrast-enhanced CT, ducts are seen as low-density linear structures running anterior to the portal venous system.

On CT the position of the gallbladder is variable. The position of the neck is constant at the porta, defining the quadrate lobe anteromedially. The body and fundus may lie transversely, closely applied to the visceral surface of the liver, or may hang inferiorly. The CBD is also seen at the level of the porta anterior to the portal vein.

On lower level CT slices the CBD may be seen in a groove or a tunnel posterior to the head of the pancreas. The body of the gallbladder is seen anterior to the duodenum.

Scintigraphy of the Biliary System Using ^{99m}Tc HIDA

^{99m}Tc HIDA is injected intravenously, bound to albumin, transported to the liver and excreted by the biliary system, outlining the intrahepatic right and left ducts, the extrahepatic ducts, the gallbladder and the cystic duct. Radioisotope excreted into the duodenum is also seen on the scan.

The Pancreas

The pancreas (Fig 5.37) is situated on the posterior abdominal wall at approximately L1 level. It is described as having a head, neck, body and tail. It is retroperitoneal with the exception of the tail, which lies within the **splenorenal ligament**. It is over 15 cm long and lies transversely and slightly obliquely, with the tail higher than the head.

The **head** of the pancreas lies in the curve of the duodenum, with the pylorus and the duodenal bulb overlapping it slightly on its upper surface. The **uncinate process** projects posteriorly and to the left from its lower part to lie posterior to the superior mesenteric vessels. The remainder of the pancreatic head lies anterior to the vessels of the posterior abdominal wall, namely, the vena cava and renal veins, the aorta and its coeliac and superior mesenteric branches. The CBD passes posterior to the head of the pancreas in a groove or tunnel towards its termination in the second part of the duodenum.

The **neck** of the pancreas extends from the upper part of the anterior portion of the head. It lies anterior to the union of the splenic vein and the SMV to form the portal vein.

The **body** of the pancreas curves over the vertebrae and great vessels to reach the left paravertebral gutter. The splenic vein passes posterior to the body, where it receives the inferior mesenteric vein. The splenic artery runs along the upper surface of the pancreas in a sinuous course that is intermittently above and behind the pancreas. The body lies anterior to the left kidney and adrenal.

The tail of the pancreas is related to the splenic hilum. Here it lies in the splenorenal ligament.

The lesser sac is anterior to the pancreas and anterior to this lies the stomach and part of the lesser omentum.

The architecture of the pancreas is finely lobulated.

THE PANCREATIC DUCTS AND THEIR DEVELOPMENT (FIG. 5.38, 5.40)

The pancreas first appears at about 5 weeks gestation as two outpouchings (buds) of the endodermal lining of the duodenum just distal to the developing stomach, which arise in common with the biliary duct. The larger dorsal bud grows more rapidly than the ventral bud. Each bud joins the duodenum through a duct. The dorsal pancreatic bud forms the neck, body and tail of the developing pancreas; the ventral bud becomes the head and uncinate process. The ventral bud rotates to the right and posteriorly towards the dorsal division, wrapping around the right side of the superior mesenteric vessels and coming to lie posterior and inferior to the larger dorsal bud. The dorsal and ventral pancreas join and the ductal systems fuse.

The uncinate process secretions drain into its ductal system which joins with the distal CBD to form a common dilated portion called the ampulla (of Vater) before entering the duodenum at the papilla. The **dorsal pancreas** secretions drain to the main duct in the tail and body of the gland. The main duct of the dorsal pancreas normally fuses with the ductal system of the uncinate process, draining to the duodenum with the CBD. Its original ductal opening to the duodenum normally atrophies, leaving one main pancreatic duct draining both embryological parts of the gland but variations are common, see below. Sometimes the original draining duct persists as an **accessory duct (of Santorini)** draining to an accessory papilla proximal to the ampulla of Vater in the duodenum. In this situation the accessory duct lies anterior and superior to the distal main pancreatic duct, traversing the pancreatic head in a more horizontal plane.

The exocrine pancreas is a lobulated serous gland which produces digestive enzymes. It is comprised of up to a million tiny clusters of acini connected by short communicating ducts which unite with ducts of adjacent acini into a network of intralobular collecting ductules. The pancreatic duct begins in the tail by the union of ductules and passes

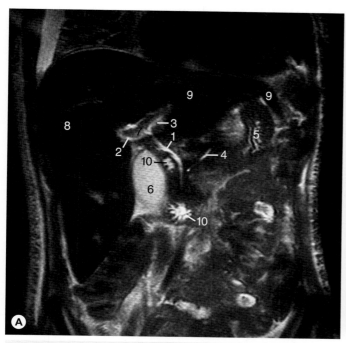 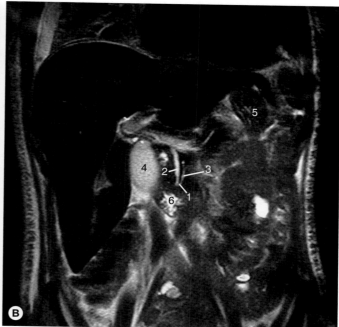

Fig. 5.36 Magnetic resonance cholangiopancreaticogram. Coronally acquired half Fourier single-shot turbo spin-echo (HASTE) images demonstrate parts of the bile duct and pancreatic duct. This is a water-sensitive sequence in which fluid is bright. (A) This section shows the intrapancreatic common bile duct and pancreatic duct. Part of the pancreatic duct is seen in the body of the pancreas. Note – the right lobe of the liver is prolonged inferiorly in a 'Riedel's lobe'. (B) The cystic duct confluence with the common hepatic duct is seen.

(A)
1. Confluence of cystic and bile ducts
2. Right hepatic duct
3. Left hepatic duct
4. Pancreatic duct in the body of the pancreas
5. Stomach
6. Gallbladder
7. Portal vein
8. Right lobe of the liver
9. Left lobe of the liver
10. Duodenum

(B)
1. Confluence of pancreatic and bile ducts
2. Common duct
3. Pancreatic duct
4. Gallbladder
5. Stomach
6. Duodenum

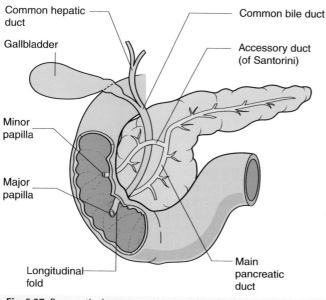

Fig. 5.37 Pancreatic ducts.

transversely towards the head, closer to the anterior than the posterior surface of the gland. It receives smaller ducts along its length at right angles and increases in size as it approaches the head. Secretions into the duodenum are controlled by a muscular layer surrounding the ampulla – the sphincter of Oddi.

Variations in pancreatic ductal anatomy are frequent and are shown in Fig. 5.39 and listed below.

The endocrine component of the pancreas consists of islet cells (islets of Langerhans) that produce and release insulin, glucagon, somatostatin and other hormones.

RADIOLOGY PEARL

The pancreatic and biliary ducts may fuse proximal to the duodenal wall, giving rise to an abnormally long common channel (usually >15 mm). This may allow pancreatic secretions to reflux into the bile duct, giving rise to choledochal cyst formation.

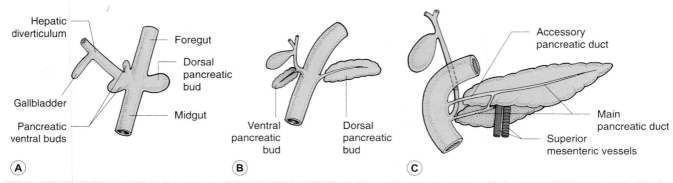

Fig. 5.38 Development of the pancreas. (A) Appearance of two ventral and one dorsal pancreatic buds. (B) Development of one ventral and one dorsal bud. (C) Fusion of the ventral and dorsal buds.

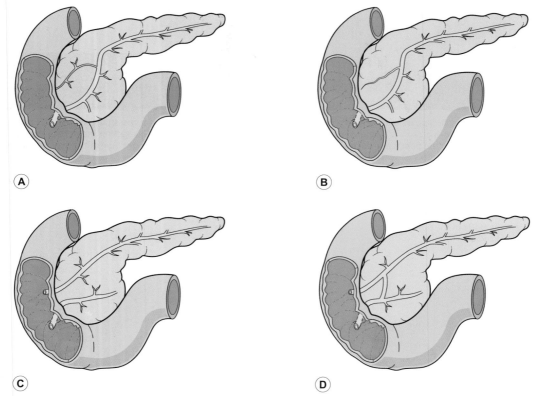

Fig. 5.39 Variation in anatomy of the pancreatic ducts. (A) The atrophic accessory duct persists as a tiny accessory duct in 60%. (B) The accessory (upper) duct atrophies completely – no connection with the duodenum (20%). (C) Major and minor ducts open separately and do not communicate (pancreas divisum) (10%). (D) Both ducts persist, communicate and open separately (10%).

VARIATIONS IN PANCREATIC ANATOMY

These are as follows:

- **Pancreas divisum:** Failure of fusion of the dorsal and ventral moieties results in the anterosuperior part of the head and the body and tail draining via the accessory papilla, while the posteroinferior part of the head drains to the ampulla; this affects about 10% of the population.
- **Annular pancreas:** A rare condition where the ventral pancreatic bud rotates incompletely, leaving a segment of pancreatic tissue surrounding the second part of the duodenum.
- **Agenesis of the dorsal pancreatic moiety:** This results in a pancreas with a head but no body or tail and is very rare.
- **Pancreatic rests/ectopic pancreas** (accessory nodules of pancreatic tissue): This may occur in the wall of the stomach, duodenum, small intestine or within a Meckel's diverticulum. The most common site is in the wall of the duodenum closest to the pancreas and close to the opening of the pancreatic duct.

ARTERIAL SUPPLY OF THE PANCREAS (FIG. 5.40)

The pancreas body and tail is supplied by pancreatic branches of the splenic artery. The head is additionally supplied by the superior and inferior pancreaticoduodenal arteries, which are branches of the gastroduodenal artery and superior mesenteric arteries, respectively. The gastroduodenal artery, arising from the hepatic artery, divides into the right gastroepiploic artery and the **superior pancreaticoduodenal artery**. This latter artery divides early into an anterior branch that lies in the groove between the pancreas and the duodenum and a posterior branch that passes posterior to the head of the pancreas. The **inferior pancreaticoduodenal artery** arises from the right side of the SMA. It divides early into anterior and posterior branches that anastomose with those of the superior pancreaticoduodenal artery.

The splenic artery passes along the upper surface of the pancreas and supplies many small branches to it. One of these is sometimes larger than the others and is called the **pancreatica magna artery**. The **dorsal pancreatic artery** usually arises close to the origin of the splenic artery and passes vertically downwards behind the pancreas. It divides at right angles into a left branch, which passes towards the tail of the pancreas as the transverse pancreatic artery, and a right branch, which passes between the neck and the uncinate process to anastomose with arteries on the anterior surface of the gland.

VENOUS DRAINAGE OF THE PANCREAS

The neck, body and tail of the pancreas drain to the splenic vein. The head drains to the superior mesenteric and portal veins.

LYMPHATIC DRAINAGE OF THE PANCREAS

Lymphatic drainage from the pancreas passes to nodes along the course of the arterial supply, the pancreatic body draining to pancreaticosplenic nodes and the head to pyloric nodes. Subsequently these drain to superior mesenteric and preaortic coeliac nodes.

RADIOLOGICAL FEATURES OF THE PANCREAS

Plain Films of the Abdomen

The pancreas is not visible unless calcified. If calcification is distributed throughout the gland it is seen as a transverse structure at L1 level, with a larger head on the right side and a body and tail extending to the left and upwards.

Ultrasound of the Pancreas (Fig. 5.41)

The gland may be obscured by overlying stomach and transverse colonic gas. It is identified on transverse sections anterior to the splenic vein and has a characteristic sonographic architecture. The splenic vein has a characteristic 'tadpole' appearance at the junction of body and neck which helps to identify the gland on transverse imaging in the midline. The division of the coeliac artery into hepatic and splenic arteries can easily be identified on ultrasound sections just above the pancreas. The hepatic artery and bile duct are seen anterior to the portal vein, also cephalad to the pancreatic head. The antrum of the stomach may be identified anteriorly, with the pylorus and duodenum above and curving around the right side of the head. In the upper part of the head, two round anechoic structures can normally be identified – a cross-sectional view of the gastroduodenal artery anteriorly and the CBD posteriorly. These demarcate the right side of the head of the pancreas from the duodenum. The head and neck of the pancreas are seen in the midline anterior to the confluence of splenic and superior mesenteric veins. Just posterior to this, the left renal vein is usually seen crossing the aorta to drain into the IVC. The uncinate process is identified posterior to the superior mesenteric vessels. The neck of the gland is identified in transverse and sagittal imaging anterior to the confluence of the superior mesenteric and splenic veins. The body runs anterior to the splenic vein across the midline. The tail is viewed by angling the transducer superolaterally from midline towards the splenic hilum, or by oblique views through the spleen.

The pancreatic duct is seen within the gland closer to its anterior surface and it is seen in over 80% of cases. It is best seen in the central portion of the body where it is perpendicular to the plane of imaging. It measures approximately 1.5 mm in the tail, 2 mm in the body and 3 mm in the head. On high-resolution images in slim subjects it can be identified running inferiorly from the neck in the head to the duodenum.

The echotexture of the pancreas is normally homogeneous and iso- or slightly hyperechoic with respect to the liver. With ageing and in obesity it may be hyperechoic due to the presence of fat. When hyperechoic, it can be difficult to distinguish from surrounding fat.

Computed Tomography (Fig. 5.42)

As a result of its oblique position, the pancreas must be studied on sequential CT slices. The tail is visible at the splenic hilum on the highest slices and the uncinate process is the lowest part.

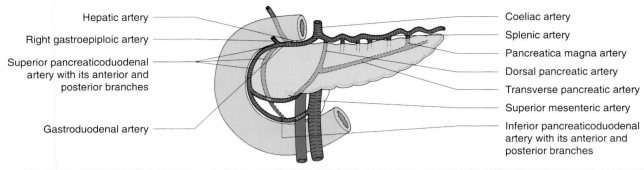

Fig. 5.40 Arterial supply of the pancreas.

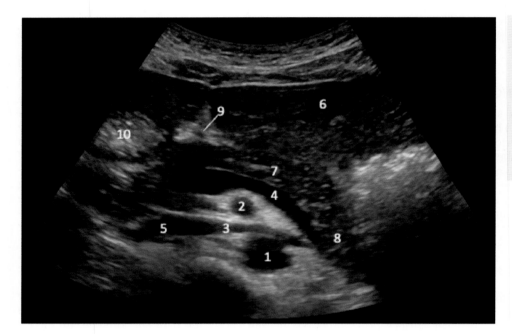

Fig. 5.41 Ultrasound of the upper abdomen: transverse image through the body of the pancreas.

1. Aorta
2. Superior mesenteric artery
3. Left renal vein
4. Splenic vein
5. Inferior vena cava
6. Left lobe of the liver
7. Pancreatic body
8. Pancreatic tail
9. Gastroduodenal artery
10. Duodenum

The normal pancreatic duct is visible in most cases. The CBD and gastroduodenal artery are visible at the pancreatic head. The formation of the portal vein is seen behind the neck and the mesenteric vessels are seen to pass anterior to the uncinate process. A replaced right hepatic artery may be seen arising from the right of the proximal SMA, running towards the liver between the portal vein and the IVC.

MRI of the Pancreas (see Fig. 5.36)

The pancreas has the shortest T1 of the abdominal organs and therefore a higher signal intensity on T1-weighted imaging, equivalent to or slightly higher than that of normal liver. Intrinsic contrast is good on T1 imaging, especially when the surrounding fat is suppressed. The pancreas is also well seen on T2-weighted imaging, and faster sequences, including breath-hold sequences, reduce artefact from breathing. The pancreas is very vascular and enhances intensely during the arterial phase of a gadolinium bolus.

MR pancreatography depicts the normal ductal system as well as congenital variations. The normal pancreatic duct measures 4 mm at the pancreatic head, 3 mm in the body and 2 mm at the tail, and its numerous side branches can be seen draining from the lobules into the duct in a perpendicular fashion.

Endoscopic Retrograde Cholangiopancreatography

ERCP visualizes the pancreatic duct by injection of contrast after cannulation via duodenal endoscopy. The main duct is cannulated in common with the bile duct when the anatomy of the bile duct is normal. The main duct is seen to begin by the union of small ducts in the tail. It passes obliquely downwards and to the right across the L1 vertebra and ends in a dilated ampulla before entering the duodenum. The duct is 16 cm long and measures up to 4 mm in diameter in the head. The accessory duct may be filled via its communication with the main duct and is seen to pass anteriorly and superiorly to the main duct.

Branches join the main duct at right angles. Overinjection of contrast may result in filling of the acini and is normally avoided (possible risk pancreatitis).

The pancreatic duct is foreshortened in PA views on ERCP because of the posterior course of part of the gland

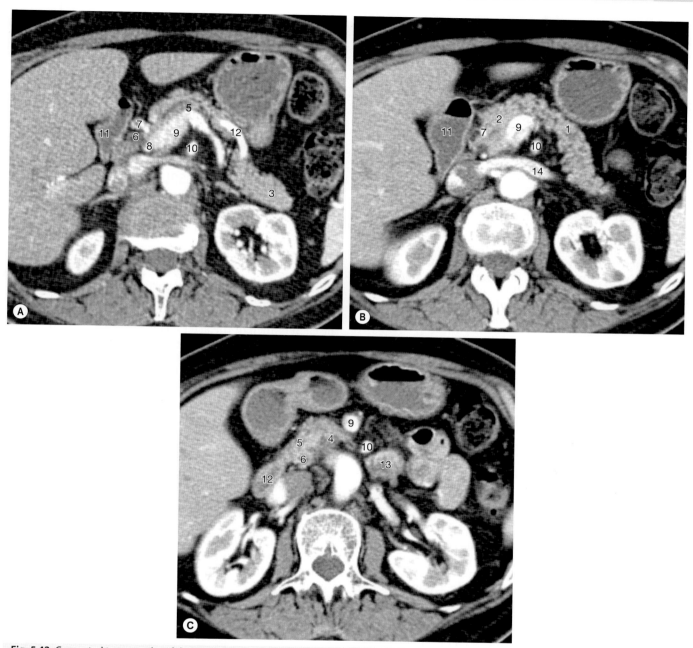

Fig. 5.42 Computed tomography of the pancreas. Images obtained in the portal venous phase after injection of fast bolus of contrast. (A) This level shows part of the tortuous splenic artery and the highest parts of the pancreas – the body anterior to the portosplenic confluence and the tail. A short segment of the duct is visible in this case. (B) Note the position of the gastroduodenal artery relative to the common bile duct in the head of the pancreas. Note the left renal vein passing between the aorta and superior mesenteric artery (SMA). (C) The distal bile duct and distal pancreatic ducts are visible. Note how the uncinate process tucks in behind the superior mesenteric vessels. The duodenum also passes between the aorta and SMA – note the position of the third part. Note the combination of opacified blood (from renal veins) and unopacified blood (from the lower body) in the inferior vena cava, because images are taken before the contrast has had a chance to circulate in the body fully. After a few more cardiac cycles, the contrast will be homogeneously dense, before washing out of the vessels.

1. Pancreatic body
2. Pancreatic head
3. Pancreatic tail
4. Uncinate process
5. Pancreatic duct
6. Common bile duct
7. Hepatic artery

8. Gastroduodenal artery
9. Superior mesenteric vein
10. Superior mesenteric artery
11. Duodenum (first part)
12. Duodenum (second part)
13. Duodenum (third part)
14. Left renal vein

between the head, which lies on the aorta and the IVC, and the tail, which lies in the paravertebral gutter. Right posterior oblique views may be helpful.

Pancreatic duct measurements are higher on ERCP than on MRCP and ultrasound because they distend as they are filled with contrast on ERCP.

Angiography of the Pancreas

This technique shows the vessels as described. Coeliac and superior mesenteric arteries must be opacified as the superior and inferior pancreaticoduodenal branches arise from them. These vessels may also be demonstrated by CT or MR angiography.

Venography of the Pancreas

This technique was performed for venous sampling to identify the site of a hormone-producing islet cell tumour. A transhepatic approach to the portal, splenic and SMVs was used, with samples taken from various sites along these vessels in an attempt to identify a high hormone level at the site of the occult tumour. High-resolution imaging has essentially made this procedure obsolete.

The Spleen

The spleen is found in the left upper quadrant of the abdomen. It arises from a mass of mesenchymal cells located between the layers of the dorsal mesentery, between the aorta and the stomach. As the stomach rotates to the right along its longitudinal axis during development, the spleen and dorsal mesentery are carried to the left along with the greater curvature of the stomach (see section and figures on development of mesentery later in the chapter, p. 208). The base of the dorsal mesentery then fuses with the peritoneum covering the left kidney, giving rise to the splenorenal ligament. A portion of the spleen may be adherent to the anterior surface of the left kidney, giving rise to a 'bare area of the spleen' analogous to the bare area of the liver.

The spleen is the size of a fist, measuring up to 12 cm long, 7 cm wide and 3–4 cm thick. Its long axis is in the line of the tenth rib and its lower pole does not usually extend beyond the midaxillary line.

The spleen has a smooth diaphragmatic surface related through the diaphragm to the costodiaphragmatic recess of the pleura and the ninth, tenth and eleventh ribs. The visceral surface of the spleen faces anteroinferiorly and to the right. Its contours correspond to its relationship to the stomach anteriorly, the splenic flexure of the colon inferiorly and the left kidney posteriorly. The splenic artery enters, and the splenic vein leaves the spleen as four or five branches each at the hilum between the gastric and renal impressions. The tail of the pancreas also lies at the splenic hilum.

The spleen is covered with peritoneum on its visceral and diaphragmatic surfaces. At the hilum it is attached by peritoneum to the posterior abdominal wall – the phrenicosplenic and splenorenal ligaments – and to the greater curve of the stomach – the gastrosplenic ligament. The gastrosplenic ligament is composed of two layers of dorsal mesentery, which separate the lesser sac posteriorly from the abdominal cavity (greater sac) anteriorly. The splenic vessels and the pancreatic tail pass towards the spleen in the former and the short gastric and left gastroepiploic vessels pass in the latter.

The spleen is composed of red and white pulp interwoven with connective tissue (splenic cords). The red pulp consists of blood vessels (splenic sinusoids) which filter the blood removing old and defective blood cells and microorganisms. The white pulp is inside the red pulp and consists of little foci of lymphoid tissue.

BLOOD SUPPLY OF THE SPLEEN

The splenic artery arises from the coeliac trunk. The splenic vein receives the inferior mesenteric vein and joins with the superior mesenteric vein to form the portal vein.

VARIANTS

The spleen develops in many parts in the dorsal mesentery of the stomach at 5–7 weeks of intrauterine life. These parts are represented in the adult by the segments supplied by each branch of the artery. The adult may, however, have **multiple spleens** or may retain some **fetal lobulation**. Up to 10% of normal adults have, in addition to a normal spleen, accessory spleens called **splenules (splenunculi)**. These occur most commonly in the splenic hilum or near the pancreatic tail but may also be found in the mesentery or in the greater omentum. They are identified by the similarity in imaging characteristics and enhancement pattern to that of the spleen and by their typical locations.

Anatomical asplenia (no spleen) **and polysplenia** (several small rudimentary splenic bodies) are associated with congenital heart disease and isomerism (bilateral right- or left-sided anatomy of the heart, bronchi and abdominal structures). This reflects the development of the spleen and the heart at the same period of intrauterine life. **Functional asplenia** occurs where, because of an interruption to the blood supply or diffuse disease, no spleen is seen on scintigraphy, which depends on functioning splenic tissue.

A '**wandering spleen**' is a rare condition characterized by abnormally lax, deficient or long splenic attachment ligaments, which allows the spleen to move in the abdomen and possibly tort on its pedicle.

RADIOLOGICAL FEATURES OF THE SPLEEN

Plain Films of the Abdomen

The spleen is often not visible on plain films, but its lower pole may be outlined by fat. Its size and position may be deduced from the distance between air in the lung and its impression on the gastric or colonic gas shadows. Assessing its size by measurement of its width 2 cm above the splenic tip on plain films is less accurate than measurement of its length from the dome of the diaphragm to the tip. This is usually less than 14 cm.

The relationship of the spleen to the ninth, tenth and eleventh ribs is important in plain films of trauma cases, where fracture of these ribs is associated with splenic rupture.

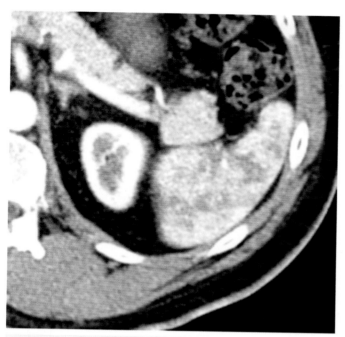

Fig. 5.43 Heterogeneous splenic enhancement caused by rapid enhancement of the vascular sinusoids. (From Zaheer A, Raman SP. *Diagnostic Imaging: Gastrointestinal*, 4th ed. Elsevier; 2022).

RADIOLOGY PEARLS

- Phagocytic cells of the immune system in lymph nodes, the spleen and the Kupffer cells of the liver form the **reticuloendothelial system**. These cells take up iron oxide particles which cause these organs to be very dark on MRI. Abnormal masses stand out as relatively hyperintense areas in a dark background.
- In haemochromatosis, the reticuloendothelial system is a site of iron accumulation also resulting in a dark liver and spleen on MRI.
- Intrapancreatic splenule: A splenule be entirely intrapancreatic or indent the pancreas so that it appears intrapancreatic. In such cases it may appear to be a focal pancreatic mass. However on CT and especially on MRI, its imaging characteristics and enhancement pattern will be exactly the same as the main splenic tissue.
- Splenic volume is calculated using the ellipsoid formula of $L \times W \times H \times 0.52$. This may be a more accurate method to diagnose splenomegaly than length. Various factors influence its size including sex and body habitus. The average volume is about 250 mL; a range of 100–430 mL has been reported in normal individuals.

Ultrasound of the Spleen

The spleen is of similar echogenicity to the liver or even higher, although the liver may appear more echogenic because of the reflectivity of its many vessels. It usually measures less than 12 cm in its long axis but may measure 14 cm in taller males. The splenic vessels are best seen when enlarged.

The spleen enlarges anterior to the colon and becomes easier to see on ultrasound. Retroperitoneal masses, by comparison, may be masked by colonic gas.

Splenules can be identified by ultrasound by demonstrating supply by the splenic artery and drainage by the splenic vein.

Computed Tomography

On CT the spleen is seen as homogeneously enhancing. In the arterial phase a palisading pattern of enhancement of the splenic sinusoids (roughly parallel bands of enhancement separated by nonenhancing connective tissue) may be seen (Fig. 5.43). Its relationship to the diaphragm, pleura and ribs, and to the pancreas, stomach, colon and left kidney can be appreciated. The spleen is enlarged if anterior to the aorta or extending below the ribs.

Magnetic Resonance Imaging

The spleen is readily visible on MRI and its relationships to the diaphragm, left kidney and adrenal gland can be appreciated especially well on sagittal and coronal imaging. Poor differentiation between the normal spleen and tumour may be improved by the use of reticuloendothelial contrast agents.

Scintigraphy

Technetium-labelled sulphur colloid is taken up by the Kupffer cells of the reticuloendothelial system. Activity may be seen in splenules in addition to the normal spleen and the liver.

The Portal Venous System (Figs. 5.44, 5.45)

Blood from the gastrointestinal tract, the spleen, pancreas and gallbladder drains to the liver via the portal venous system. The superior and inferior mesenteric and the splenic veins unite to form the portal vein. There are valves in this system in the fetus and young infant but not in the adult.

SUPERIOR MESENTERIC VEIN

This lies to the right of the SMA and drains the area supplied by this artery. Its branches are similar to the arterial branches, except proximally, and are as follows:
- Right gastroepiploic and inferior pancreaticoduodenal proximally
- Jejunal and ileal branches to its left side
- Ileocolic, right colic and midcolic branches to its right side

INFERIOR MESENTERIC VEIN

This lies to the left of the inferior mesenteric artery and drains its area of supply in the colon via the:
- Left colic, sigmoid and superior rectal veins
- Some pancreatic branches

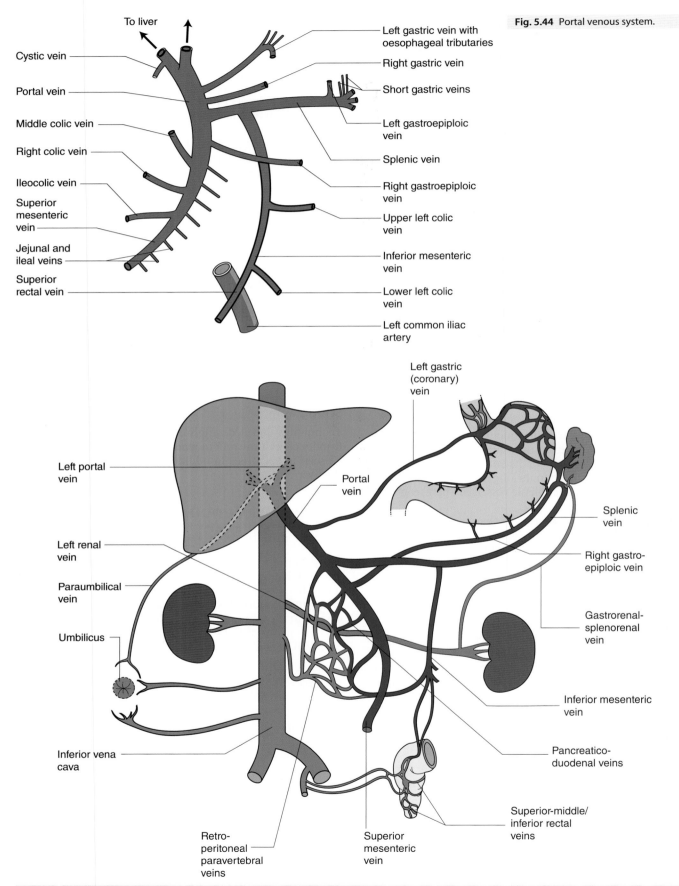

Cystic vein

Portal vein

Middle colic vein

Right colic vein

Ileocolic vein

Superior mesenteric vein

Jejunal and ileal veins

Superior rectal vein

To liver

Left gastric vein with oesophageal tributaries

Right gastric vein

Short gastric veins

Left gastroepiploic vein

Splenic vein

Right gastroepiploic vein

Upper left colic vein

Inferior mesenteric vein

Lower left colic vein

Left common iliac artery

Fig. 5.44 Portal venous system.

Left portal vein

Left renal vein

Paraumbilical vein

Umbilicus

Inferior vena cava

Retro-peritoneal paravertebral veins

Superior mesenteric vein

Left gastric (coronary) vein

Portal vein

Splenic vein

Right gastro-epiploic vein

Gastrorenal-splenorenal vein

Inferior mesenteric vein

Pancreatico-duodenal veins

Superior-middle/inferior rectal veins

Fig. 5.45 Points of communication between the portal and systemic circulations.

THE SPLENIC VEIN

Four or five branches leave the splenic hilum and unite to form the splenic vein. Occasionally, a vein from the upper pole of the spleen joins the splenic vein more proximally (the superior polar vein). Proximally the splenic vein receives the short gastric veins and the left gastroepiploic vein from the stomach. It receives multiple pancreatic branches and the inferior mesenteric vein as it passes posterior to the tail and body of the pancreas. The splenic vein then unites with the SMV to form the portal vein behind the neck of the pancreas.

THE PORTAL VEIN

The portal vein is formed by the union of the superior mesenteric and splenic veins behind the neck of the pancreas at the level of the L1/L2 lumbar vertebra. It then runs to the right behind the neck of the pancreas and receives the superior pancreaticoduodenal vein. It passes behind the first part of the duodenum and receives the right gastric and left gastric (**coronary**) veins. It passes in the **free edge of the lesser omentum** posterior to the CBD and the hepatic artery. Here it is separated from the IVC by the **epiploic foramen**. Its proximity to the IVC at this point is utilized at surgery for portosystemic venous shunting in portal hypertension.

At the porta hepatis the portal vein divides into right and left branches. The right branch receives the cystic vein if one is formed, and the left receives the paraumbilical veins. Attached to the left portal vein is the **ligamentum teres** and its continuation, the **ligamentum venosum**. Within the liver the portal vein is distributed with the branches of the hepatic artery.

PORTOSYSTEMIC ANASTOMOSES (SEE FIG. 5.45)

Portal venous pressure rises when there is obstruction to blood flow in the portal vein, the liver or the hepatic veins. Portosystemic collateral pathways then open where these two systems communicate (Table 5.3).

RADIOLOGICAL FEATURES OF THE PORTAL VENOUS SYSTEM

Ultrasound (Fig. 5.31)

The portal vein is visible on ultrasound as it passes towards the liver posterior to the CBD and hepatic artery.

Its diameter is variable but always greater than that of the normal bile duct.

Portal vein branches in the liver are seen as having echogenic walls.

The splenic vein is an important landmark in ultrasound as it passes posterior to the pancreas (see Fig. 5.41). It helps identify this gland. An abnormality in its course around the vertebrae and prevertebral structures can be an indication of a mass here.

The direction and velocity of blood flow, which is important to evaluate in portal hypertension, can be assessed with pulsed Doppler interrogation of the portal vein. Colour flow Doppler helps in identification of the vessels.

RADIOLOGY PEARLS

- The direction of blood flow in the portal vein should be part of the assessment of the liver in patients with liver disease. Flow should be towards the liver (hepatopedal), with minimal respiratory variation.
- Gas in the portal vein and its radicles may occur in cases of ischaemic bowel where ischaemic mucosal breakdown allows gas to enter the vascular space.
- Portal vein gas may also be seen in well patients after insertion of feeding tubes into the jejunum because of physical mucosal damage caused by tunnelling of the tube.
- Gas in portal vein radicles in the liver it may be distinguished from gas in the bile ducts (pneumobilia) by its more peripheral position.
- The **portacaval space** is the space between the portal vein and IVC. It is the site of normal lymph nodes in the lesser omentum, which may be enlarged in pathological processes.

Computed Tomography

The portal vein is easily identified at the porta hepatis and its branches are seen in the liver, generally posterior to the bile duct and hepatic artery branches. The portal vein is seen posteriorly in the free edge of the lesser omentum. Here it is separated from the IVC by the epiploic foramen.

The splenic vein is seen posterior to the pancreas and unites with the inferior mesenteric vein laterally and the SMV behind the neck of the pancreas. It lies anterior to the left kidney and its hilum, the renal vein and IVC.

The SMV is seen to the right of the artery on lower slices, and together these pass anterior to the uncinate process of the pancreas.

Magnetic Resonance Imaging

MR angiography of the portal system is an excellent method of providing detailed information regarding portal vein anatomy and portosystemic collateral vessels. Information regarding portal blood flow direction and velocity can be obtained using 'time of flight' or phase contrast angiographic techniques without the need for intravenous contrast. With these techniques the background signal is suppressed and flowing blood is bright. The source data can be viewed as MR angiograms.

Table 5.3 Portosystemic Anastomoses

Site	Portal System	Systemic Veins
Gastro-oesophageal junction	Left gastric vein	Oesophageal veins
Rectum	Superior rectal veins	Inferior rectal veins
Retroperitoneum	Tributaries in mesentery	Retroperitoneal, renal, lumbar and phrenic veins
Umbilicus	Paraumbilical veins with ligamentum teres	Veins of the abdominal wall

Portography

Direct Portography. This includes **splenoportography**, where contrast is introduced directly into the spleen and outlines the splenic vein and the portal vein.

A **transhepatic** route can also be used to cannulate the portal vein and via this the splenic or other veins. This can be used to gain access to the system and allow sclerosis of oesophageal varices.

Transumbilical portography can be performed in the neonate by catheterizing the umbilical vein, which drains to the left portal vein.

Indirect Portography. Contrast is injected into the coeliac and superior mesenteric arteries (sequentially or together) and films are taken in the venous phase. To show the inferior mesenteric vein that artery must also be injected. Images can be acquired by film-screen techniques, or more easily using digital subtraction angiography.

If the spleen is very large, the splenic vein may be difficult to visualize by this indirect method because of pooling of contrast in the spleen.

Flow of blood in the portal venous system is slow and there is poor mixing of blood from the splenic and superior mesenteric veins, with the former supplying principally the left lobe of the liver and the latter the right lobe. This should not be misinterpreted when only one artery is injected.

Contrast in the liver preferentially fills the right lobe of the liver in the supine patient because of the more posterior position of this lobe. To overcome this effect of gravity it may be necessary to rotate the patient.

The Kidneys

The kidneys lie retroperitoneally in the paravertebral gutters of the posterior abdominal wall. They lie obliquely with their upper poles more medial and more posterior than their lower. The kidneys measure 10–15 cm in length, the left being commonly 1.5 cm longer than the right. Their size is approximately that of three-and-a-half lumbar vertebrae and their associated discs on a radiograph.

On coronal cross-section (Figs. 5.46 and 5.47) each kidney is seen to have an outer **cortex** and an inner **medulla**. Extensions of the cortex centrally as **columns of Bertin** separate the medulla into **pyramids** whose apices, jutting into the calyces, are called the **papillae**. There are usually seven pairs of **minor calyces**, each pair having an anterior and a posterior calyx, although there is wide variation. Minor calyx pairs combine to form two or three **major calyces**, which in turn drain via their **infundibula** to the pelvis. This arrangement is quite variable, but when there are two infundibula these usually drain four pairs of calyces from the upper pole and three pairs from the lower. When there are three infundibula there are usually three pairs of upper pole calyces, and two sets of two pairs of calyces draining the midpolar region and lower pole. The pelvis may be **intrarenal** or partially or entirely **extrarenal**. The gap between the renal substance and the pelvis is called the **renal sinus** and is filled with fat.

A **simple** calyx has one papilla indenting it; a **compound** calyx has more than one. Compound calyces are said to be less efficient at preventing intrarenal reflux of urine from the calyx and are more common in the upper pole.

The **hilum** of the kidney lies medially at L1 on the left and at L1/L2 on the right, owing to the bulk of the liver above pushing down the right kidney. At the hilum, the pelvis lies posteriorly and the renal vein lies anteriorly with the artery in between. The artery may branch early and a posterior arterial branch may enter the hilum posterior to the pelvis. Lymph vessels and nerves also enter at the hilum.

The functional subunit of the kidney is called the **nephron** and consists of a glomerulus in the cortex and a tubule in the medulla. This drains to a collecting duct, which empties into the calyx at the tip of the medulla. The kidney has approximately 1 million nephrons.

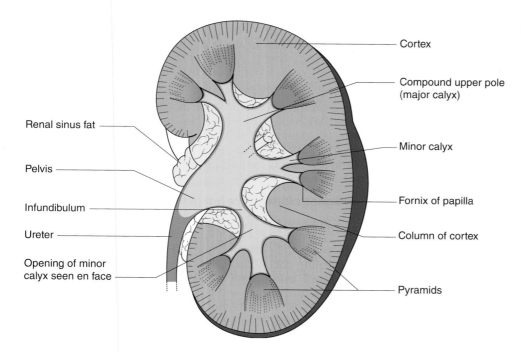

Fig. 5.46 Structure of the kidney.

Cortex

Compound upper pole (major calyx)

Minor calyx

Fornix of papilla

Column of cortex

Pyramids

Renal sinus fat

Pelvis

Infundibulum

Ureter

Opening of minor calyx seen en face

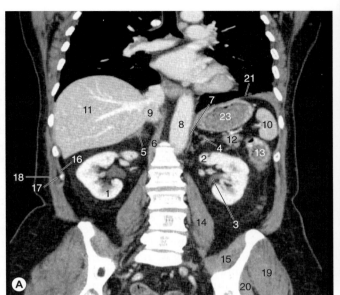
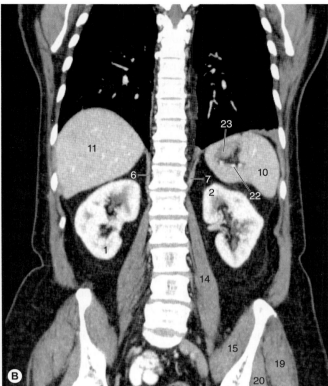

Fig. 5.47 (A and B) Coronal reformatted computed tomography of the abdomen showing the kidneys and their relations.

1. Right kidney (lower pole)
2. Left kidney (upper pole)
3. Renal pelvis
4. Left adrenal
5. Right adrenal
6. Crus right hemidiaphragm
7. Crus left hemidiaphragm
8. Aorta
9. Inferior vena cava
10. Spleen
11. Liver
12. Tail of pancreas
13. Splenic flexure
14. Psoas muscle
15. Iliacus muscle
16. Transversus abdominis muscle
17. Internal oblique muscle
18. External oblique muscle
19. Gluteus maximus muscle
20. Gluteus medius muscle
21. Left hemidiaphragm
22. Hilum of the spleen
23. Fundus of the stomach

RELATIONS OF THE KIDNEYS

These are as follows:
Posteriorly:
- Upper third, diaphragm and twelfth rib and the costo-diaphragmatic recess of the pleura
- Lower third, medial to lateral: psoas, quadratus lumborum and transversus abdominis muscles

Superiorly: the adrenal gland
Anteriorly:
- Right kidney: liver, second part of the duodenum, ascending colon, small intestinal loops
- Left kidney: stomach, pancreas and its vessels, spleen, splenic flexure of the colon, jejunal loops

BLOOD SUPPLY OF THE KIDNEYS

The renal arteries normally arise from the aorta at L1/L2 level. The right renal artery is longer and lower than the left and passes posterior to the IVC. Both renal arteries usually have two divisions: one passes posterior to the renal pelvis and supplies the posterior upper part of the kidney; another anterior branch supplies the upper anterior kidney; a branch of the anterior division passes inferiorly and supplies the entire lower part of the kidney.

Within the hilum the renal arteries divide inconsistently into segmental branches which cross the renal sinus anterior and posterior to the pelvis and pierce the medulla in between the pyramids. These are termed **interlobar arteries**, as they pass between the lobes or pyramids. At the corticomedullary junction and the base of the pyramids the interlobar arteries become the **arcuate arteries**. They do not anastomose, but form arcades around the bases of the pyramids. Branches of the arcuate arteries give off the **interlobular arteries**, which run to the **capsule**. **Afferent arterioles** arise from the interlobular arteries to the glomeruli. Distal to the glomeruli, the **efferent arterioles** supply the **convoluted tubules** of the nephron unit.

VENOUS DRAINAGE OF THE KIDNEYS

There is extensive anastomosis between the veins of the kidney. Five or six **interlobular veins** unite at the hilum to form the renal vein. The renal vein lies anterior to the pelvis at the hilum. The renal veins drain directly to the IVC. The left renal vein is much longer than the right and passes anterior to the aorta to reach the IVC. It also receives the **inferior phrenic**, **adrenal** and **gonadal** veins of that side. The right renal vein receives no extrarenal tributaries.

LYMPHATIC DRAINAGE OF THE KIDNEYS

Lymph drainage follows the arteries to para-aortic nodes.

FASCIAL SPACES AROUND THE KIDNEYS (FIG. 5.48)

A true **fibrous capsule** surrounds the kidney. This, in turn, is surrounded by perirenal fat, which separates the kidney from the surrounding organs including the adrenal gland. A condensation of fibroareolar tissue around the perirenal fat forms the **renal fascia**. Thus the retroperitoneum is divided into three compartments: the **perirenal space** around the kidneys within the renal fascia, and the **anterior** and **posterior pararenal** spaces anterior and posterior to the renal fascia.

The **perirenal space** has an anterior (**Gerota's**) **fascia** and a posterior (**Zuckerkandl's**) **fascia**. These fascial layers are fused laterally as the **lateral conal fascia**, which is continuous with the fascia on the deep surface of the transversalis abdominis muscle, and this defines the lateral limit of the space. Above, the layers do not join but are open to the bare area of the liver on the right and the subdiaphragmatic extraperitonal subdiaphragmatic space on the left. The anterior renal fascia blends with right inferior coronary ligament near the bare area of the liver and the posterior renal fascia blends with the diaphragmatic fascia. Medially, the fascia fuses with the sheaths of the aorta and the IVC, but cadaveric studies have shown a narrow anterior communication across the midline in some cases. The posterior fascia fuses with the psoas muscle. The **perirenal space** contains the kidneys, adrenals and their vessels. Below, the perirenal space is relatively open to the retroperitoneal spaces of the abdomen and pelvis. The anterior layer merges with the areolar tissue that binds the peritoneum with the posterior abdominal wall, preventing communication of the lower perirenal spaces across the midline. The posterior fascial layer becomes continuous with the fascia over the iliacus muscle. The fat within the perirenal space has septa that can lead to loculation of any urine, blood or pus that escapes into this space.

The **anterior pararenal space** lies anterior to the anterior renal fascia and behind the posterior peritoneum. It is continuous across the midline and contains the pancreas, duodenum and ascending and descending colon. It fuses with the lateral conal fascia and peritoneum laterally. Superiorly, the space is limited where the anterior renal fascia blends with the posterior peritoneum, but inferiorly the space is open to the pelvic extraperitoneal spaces. Some anatomists describe the anterior pararenal space as multilaminar rather than a single space.

The **posterior pararenal space** lies posterior to the posterior renal fascia and anterior to the muscles of the posterior abdominal wall. This is limited medially by the attachment of the renal fascia to the psoas muscle but is continuous laterally with the extraperitoneal fatty tissue (properitoneal fat plane), deep to the transversalis fascia. It extends inferiorly to the fat anterior to the iliacus muscle and the pelvic extraperitoneal spaces. It contains only fat.

DEVELOPMENT OF THE KIDNEY

The glomerulus and proximal ductal system of the definitive kidney are derived from the metanephros. The collecting duct, calyces, pelvis and ureter are derived from the metanephric duct.

The kidney is formed in the pelvis from approximately 12 distinct lobules and assumes its adult position by the differential growth of the ureters relative to the trunk. It is supplied first by branches of the iliac artery and subsequently by a series of vessels from the abdominal artery, each of which disappears as the kidney develops a new supply.

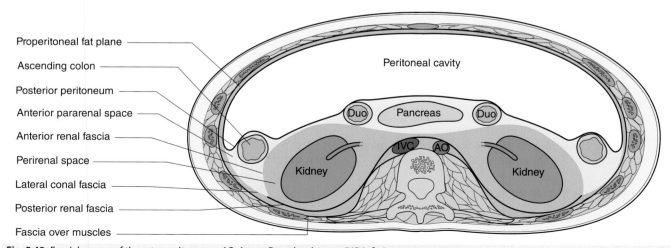

Fig. 5.48 Fascial spaces of the retroperitoneum. *AO*, Aorta; *Duo*, duodenum; *IVC*, inferior vena cava.

Developmental Abnormalities and Variants

- The commonest anomaly of development is duplication of the collecting system, which occurs in 4% of individuals (see section on development of the ureter, below).
- The adult kidney may retain some degree of **fetal lobulation**. This may involve the entire kidney or just the middle and lower thirds. It is frequently bilateral.
- It is common for the kidney to ascend to a normal position but retain a supply from one or more **accessory arteries**, which usually enter the lower pole below the hilum.
- The kidneys may fuse during development and lead to a **horseshoe kidney** (1 in 700 births). In this condition the kidney is fused across the midline in its lower pole. The isthmus, which joins the kidneys, may be fibrous or composed of functioning renal tissue. In this condition the fused kidney must fail to ascend, as branches of the aorta impede its upward movement. Such kidneys are more prone to trauma as they lie across the vertebral column.
- One or both kidneys may fail to migrate cranially, resulting in a persistent **pelvic kidney** supplied by a branch of the internal iliac artery (1 in 1500 births).
- Rarely (1 in 2500 births) one kidney is absent.
- The kidneys may be fused but lie on one side or the other in **crossed fused ectopia**. The lower pole of the normally situated kidney is fused with the upper pole of the ectopic kidney.
- Very rarely both kidneys are completely fused in the pelvis. There is extensive fusion of the upper and lower poles along the medial surface of the kidneys resulting in a flat ovoid fused kidney referred to as **pancake kidney**.
- A very rare anomaly called **thoracic kidney** (although the diaphragm is usually intact) occurs when the kidney is found much higher than its normal position; this may cause an opacity on a chest radiograph.

RADIOLOGY PEARLS

- The adrenal glands, which develop from neural crest cells near the aorta, are situated in their normal location in cases of abnormal renal migration, but their shape may be more discoid because of the absence of moulding by the kidneys during development.
- Fetal lobulation is distinguished from pathological scarring by the position of the surface notches: in fetal lobulation surface notches are between the calyces, whereas scarring occurs directly over the calyces.

RADIOLOGICAL FEATURES OF THE KIDNEY

Plain Films of the Abdomen

Perirenal fat often makes part or all of the renal outlines visible. Renal **size** is variable, with a normal range of 10–15 cm on a radiograph or approximately three-and-a-half vertebral bodies in height. The left kidney is usually larger, but a difference in size of more than 2 cm is abnormal. The kidneys are relatively larger in the child (approximately four vertebral bodies in height).

The kidneys are seen to move with changes from supine to erect positions and, because of their relationship with the diaphragm, to move with respiration. These moves may be more than 5 cm and are generally greater in women than men. As the kidney moves inferiorly its degree of tilt increases, with its lower pole becoming more anterior. It may, as a result, appear foreshortened on an AP radiograph.

Ultrasound Examination of the Kidneys

Renal size is not magnified on ultrasound and so is smaller than on radiographs – normally 9–12 cm. The renal outline is usually smooth. Cortical thickness is uniform but is slightly thicker at the upper and lower poles. Persistent (fetal) lobulation may be seen as cortical indentations but does not narrow the cortical thickness. The cortex is distinguishable from the relatively hypoechoic renal pyramids – a difference that is more marked in the young infant. The cortex is usually less echogenic than that of liver or spleen, but in the young infant is iso- or hyperechoic with respect to these organs.

The renal sinus contains fat, calyces, infundibula and vessels, and is highly echogenic because of the multiple tissue interfaces. The renal pelvis may be intrarenal or extrarenal. When extrarenal, it may appear dilated. Visualization of the collecting system is variable. It is best seen when the subject is well hydrated and/or in a state of diuresis.

The aorta, IVC and renal artery and vein are visible on ultrasound. The structures at the hilum (i.e. the vein, artery, pelvis from anterior to posterior) can also be identified. Blood flow can be assessed with colour flow Doppler and pulsed-wave Doppler. The relationship of the right kidney to the liver and the left to the spleen can be appreciated. Gas in the stomach, duodenum, small intestine and colon, which are anterior to the kidneys, may obscure their view from an anterior scanning approach on ultrasound, but visualization is almost always possible from a posterolateral, lateral or posterior approach.

RADIOLOGY PEARL

On sagittal ultrasound images, the right renal artery is seen as a round hypoechoic structure indenting the anterior surface of the IVC.

RADIOLOGY PEARLS

- A **dromedary** or **splenic hump** is a lateral bulge of the left kidney just below the splenic margin, usually associated with some flattening of the upper pole. It is a variation in the shape of the kidney rather than an area of hypertrophy.
- **Junctional cortical defects** or **junctional parenchymal defects** may be seen as triangular echogenic areas, usually in the upper pole, and represent normal extensions of renal sinus due to partial fusion of the embryonic renunculi. They extend from the outer cortex to the renal sinus and contain fat.
- **The arcuate arteries**, which separate the cortex and medulla, may give rise to small echogenic foci on ultrasound due to reflections of the ultrasound beam and should not be confused with calcifications.

CT and MRI

The kidneys are seen on slices from T12 to L3 vertebral levels.

Posterior relations (i.e. diaphragm, pleura and ribs, psoas, quadratus lumborum and transversus abdominis muscles) and anterior relations (i.e. liver, pancreas, spleen and gastrointestinal tract) can be seen.

The kidney is seen to be surrounded by perinephric fat. This is most abundant medial to the lower pole, and this is a favoured site of accumulation of blood or urine in the ruptured kidney and of pus in a perirenal abscess. The renal fascia is less than 1 mm thick in the normal subject and can generally be seen if it is at right angles to the imaging plane in a subject with adequate fat.

The renal substance is homogeneous on unenhanced CT images. On MRI, the intrinsic contrast between cortex and medulla is seen on T1- and T2-weighted images. On T1-weighted images the renal cortex has a slightly higher signal than the medulla. On T2-weighted images the renal cortex is slightly lower in signal than the medulla and intrinsic renal contrast is superior. Corticomedullary differentiation may be reduced in subjects who are dehydrated, as well as in renal disease. After administration of intravenous contrast, the cortex is opacified first, followed by the medulla and pyramids, making it possible to distinguish between them. On both CT and MRI three phases of enhancement can be appreciated: an arterial corticomedullary phase, where the cortex enhances strongly and contrast between cortex and medulla is greatest; a venous nephrographic phase, where the contrast is homogeneous throughout the kidney; and a delayed excretory phase, where contrast is seen in the collecting system. The pyramids are seen from base to tip at the hilum on axial images and are cut at various degrees of obliquity in other slices but are well seen on coronal MRI or coronal CT reconstructed images. Fetal lobulation and its relationship to the calyces can be appreciated. Prominence of the midportion of the lateral border of the left kidney is a normal variant called a **dromedary hump** or **splenic hump** (because of the proximity of the spleen).

The renal vessels can be identified on unenhanced images but are best seen after contrast. The arteries are best seen early in a contrast bolus (first 25 seconds); the veins are best seen after approximately 60 seconds. With MRI, the renal arteries and veins can also be imaged without intravenous contrast using flow-sensitive imaging sequences.

Arteriography of the Kidneys

Direct arteriography allows assessment of vascular and other lesions of the kidneys, but is primarily used to facilitate interventional procedures such as renal artery angioplasty or stent placement. Aortography is performed prior to selective studies and identifies accessory renal arteries if present. These are found in more than 20% of arteriograms and are even commoner in horseshoe and ectopic kidneys. Aortography also establishes the presence and location of both kidneys.

In selective studies, the upper pole is seen to be supplied by anterior and posterior branches of the renal artery, and the lower pole by an anterior branch. Because of the posterior angulation of the renal artery from the aorta, it is best seen by oblique views with the side of interest uppermost in the supine patient.

Renal Venography

This is performed via the IVC. Although it is rarely used, it may be required to identify the location of a renin-producing tumour. The left adrenal and left gonad are also imaged via left renal venography because of the common drainage of veins from these organs on this side.

The renal veins are seen to have valves. These are more common on the left side.

The right renal vein is multiple in 10% of venograms and receives the right gonadal vein in 6% of cases.

The left renal vein is five times as long as the right. It is multiple in 14% of venograms, has tributaries which surround the aorta in 7% and is retroaortic in 3.5%.

Interventional Procedures in the Kidney

These are performed via fluoroscopy, ultrasound, CT and angiography.

The anatomy and anatomical relations of the kidney are important to consider when planning a site of percutaneous puncture. The midlateral external border is relatively avascular (the vessels are smallest at the periphery and the midplane of the cortex marks the interface of the anterior and posterior arterial supply) and avoids the major hilar structures. This linear safe zone is known as **Brodel's line**.

The diaphragm lies posterior to the kidney; as a result the kidney is seen to move significantly with respiration. Punctures should be performed in suspended respiration.

The close relationship with the pleura posteriorly and superiorly means that a lower pole approach is preferable.

Scintigraphy of the Kidney

This method is used primarily in the study of the physiology of the kidney. Technetium-labelled dimercaptosuccinic acid (^{99m}Tc DMSA) static scans have some anatomical uses. These are used to establish how much of the fused part of horseshoe kidneys is functional renal tissue. Static scans are also useful in the evaluation of pseudotumours of the kidney due to hypertrophy of a column of Bertin. Technetium-labelled diethylene triamine penta-acetic acid (DTPA) or mercaptoacetyltriglycine (MAG 3) are isotopes that are filtered into the urine and can be used to assess overall and split renal function as well as glomerular filtration rate. They also provide structural information regarding the collecting systems and bladder.

The Ureter (Fig. 5.49)

The ureters carry urine from the kidneys to the bladder. Each is 25–30 cm long and is described as having a pelvis and abdominal, pelvic and intravesical parts. The ureter is a retroperitoneal, extraperitoneal structure.

The pelvis has been described with the kidney. The remainder of the ureter has a diameter of about 3 mm but is narrower at the following three sites:
- The junction of the pelvis and ureter
- The pelvic brim
- The intravesical ureter where it runs through the muscular bladder wall

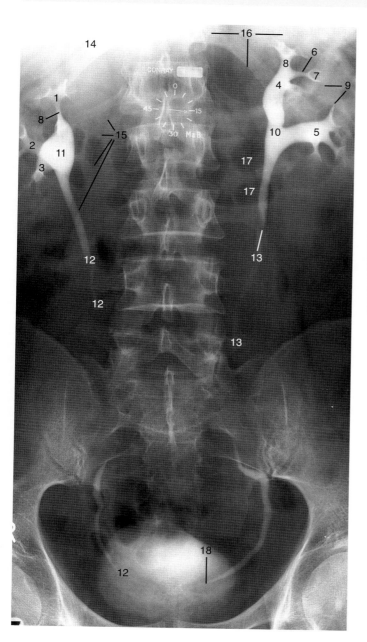

Fig. 5.49 Intravenous urogram. The right kidney has three major calyces. The left kidney has two major calyces, and a bifid pelvis. Note the course of the lower ureters. The distal part of the ureter passes behind the bladder.

1. Right upper pole (major) calyx
2. Right middle (major) calyx
3. Right lower pole (major) calyx
4. Left upper pole (major) calyx
5. Left lower pole (major) calyx
6. Minor calyx (infundibulum of)
7. Papilla
8. Infundibulum
9. Fornix
10. Bifid left renal pelvis
11. Right renal pelvis
12. Right ureter
13. Left ureter: vascular impression
14. Upper pole right kidney
15. Right psoas outline
16. Gas in body of stomach
17. Gas in transverse colon
18. Intravesical ureter

The abdominal ureter passes on the medial edge of the psoas muscle, which separates it from the tips of the transverse processes. On the right side it is related to the second part of the duodenum and is crossed by the gonadal, right colic and ileocolic vessels, and lies lateral to the IVC. On the left side it is crossed by the gonadal and left colic vessels and has jejunal loops anterior to it. It is crossed at the pelvic brim on the left side by the mesentery of the sigmoid colon and is posterior to this part of the colon.

The ureter enters the pelvis at the bifurcation of the common iliac artery anterior to the SI joint. It then lies on the lateral wall of the pelvis in front of the internal iliac artery, at a point just anterior to the ischial spine, where it turns forwards and medially to enter the bladder.

Close to the bladder in the male, the ureter passes above the seminal vesicle and is crossed by the vas deferens. In the female this part of the ureter is close to the lateral fornix of the vagina and 2.5 cm lateral to the cervix. It passes under the uterine artery in the base of the broad ligament.

The intravesical portion of the ureter has an oblique course of 2 cm through the bladder wall. The vesical muscle has a sphincteric action and the obliquity has a valve-like action. The ureter opens into the bladder at the vesicoureteric orifice.

BLOOD SUPPLY OF THE URETER

The ureter is supplied by branches of nearby arteries and drains to corresponding veins, that is, the aorta and IVC, and the renal, gonadal, internal iliac and inferior vesical vessels. Despite the varied arterial supply, the ureter is prone to vascular injury at surgery, which may lead to stricture formation.

DEVELOPMENT OF THE URETER

The ureter develops as a blind diverticulum from the metanephric duct and grows first posteriorly and then cranially to unite with the developing kidney.

Developmental Abnormalities and Variants

Duplication of part or all of the ureter occurs in about 4% of subjects. It is the commonest significant congenital anomaly of the urinary tract. Duplication is two to three times commoner in females. When complete duplication occurs, the ureter serving the upper renal moiety drains fewer calyces and is inserted lower into the bladder than that draining the lower moiety – known as the **Weigert–Meyer law**. The low insertion may extend to the bladder neck or the urethra or, in females, the vestibule or vagina.

Ureteric **ectopy** is most common in association with duplication but may occur in a single ureter.

Ureterocele is a dilation of the intramural portion of the ureter due to narrowing of its orifice. This is most common in a duplicated system, when it occurs in the ureter draining the upper renal moiety that is usually ectopic.

RADIOLOGICAL FEATURES OF THE URETER

Plain Films of the Abdomen

The ureter is not visible, but a knowledge of its course in relation to the skeleton is necessary when looking for radio-opaque calculi. The ureters pass anterior to the tips of the transverse processes of L2–L5 lumbar vertebrae and anterior to the SI joint. They then curve laterally at the ischial spines and medially again to the bladder.

Ultrasound

The proximal and distal ureters may be visible on ultrasound when well distended. Intestinal gas generally obscures the midportion unless it is abnormally dilated.

Computed Tomography

Ureteric calculi are frequently not visible on radiographs but they are readily visible on CT. Noncontrast CT is commonly used for the diagnosis of ureteric calculi. The normal ureter can be identified on noncontrast scans, although it is easier to identify if it contains contrast medium.

CT Urography

The excretory phase, performed after a 5–10-minute delay after intravenous contrast (sometimes with added diuretic to optimize distension), demonstrates the collecting systems outlined by excreted contrast.

In the excretory phase the calyceal system can be seen. Reconstructed images in coronal oblique and other planes can be generated to optimize visualization of the calyces. Minor and major calyces are seen. These are connected to the pelvis of the kidney by **infundibula**, which may be long or short. Occasionally a calyx is connected directly to the pelvis of the kidney. The papillae are conical and indent the calyces with surrounding sharp fornices. Several papillae may indent a single calyx – known as a complex calyx – an arrangement that is more common in the upper pole.

Contrast in the collecting tubules in the papilla causing papillary enhancement is sometimes seen and may be prominent when there is ectasia of the tubules in renal tubular ectasia. The renal pelvis is triangular in shape and lies in the posterior part of the renal hilum surrounded by fat. Arteries may lie anterior and posterior to the hilum with the renal vein anterior. The junction of the pelvis and ureter is the ureteropelvic junction. The ureters are visible medial to the lower pole of the kidney, anterior to psoas. More distally the ureter remains anterior to the psoas muscle and is lateral to the great vessels. Having crossed the bifurcation of the common iliac artery, the ureter in the pelvis is medial to the iliac arteries and veins. It enters the bladder posterolaterally and the ureterovesical junction. The ureter can be seen running obliquely in the bladder wall. Ureteric peristalsis causes variations in the calibre of the ureter and there is the impression of the iliac arteries that may cause a transient hold up of contrast in the ureter. Uretic peristalsis may result in a jet of contrast being observed in the bladder. Variants such as duplication may be easily identified.

The renal pelvis is **bifid** in 10% of cases. This may be associated with complete or partial renal duplication. Partial renal duplication may lead to hypertrophy of septal cortex in the midportion of the kidney – known as hypertrophied **column of Bertin** – causing a pseudomass appearance.

If renal sinus fat is prominent this may cause thinning and elongation of the infundibula on IVU ('spidery' calyces). Cysts at the renal hilum may also elongate and distort the calyces.

MR Urography (Fig. 5.50)

The ureters may be imaged using static fluid MR urography (as for MRCP). However, because they are intermittently collapsed due to peristalsis, parts of the ureter may not be distended with urine and thus not imaged using these techniques. Sequential static images may be acquired (cine MR urography) to demonstrate different parts of the collecting system, but this technique is at its best in obstructed, fluid-filled systems. MR contrast urography can be performed where the ureters are imaged during the excretory phase after intravenous gadolinium and is aided by concurrent administration of a diuretic.

RADIOLOGY PEARLS

- Gadolinium shortens the T1 relaxation time of urine, which initially causes excreted urine to be bright on T1-weighted images. When the subject is well hydrated and a diuretic is used, the excreted gadolinium will be well dispersed, dilute and bright. At standard doses of 0.1 mmol/kg, without the use of a diuretic the gadolinium quickly becomes concentrated in the urine, causing the urine to become dark (T2* effect). There may be layering between concentrated and less concentrated urine.
- In extrarenal pelvis, the renal pelvis protrudes beyond the confines of the renal hilum. As a distensible structure, it may appear relatively dilated when full of urine and may be erroneously interpreted as pathologically dilated.
- MR urography is useful in pregnant patients with suspected ureteric calculi. The right collecting system is physiologically more dilated than the left in pregnant patients.

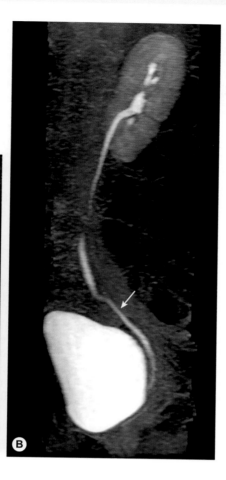

Fig. 5.50 Maximum-intensity projection (MIP) magnetic resonance urogram images in the (A) coronal and (B) sagittal planes. (From Siegelman ES. *Body MRI.* Saundars; 2005.)

The Adrenal Glands

The adrenal glands lie retroperitoneally above each kidney. They are each enclosed within the perirenal fascia but in a separate compartment from the kidney. Each gland is composed of a body with medial and lateral limbs. The adrenal glands have an outer cortex derived from mesoderm and an inner medulla (10% of the weight of the gland), which is derived from the neural crest and is related to the sympathetic nervous system.

The right adrenal gland tends to have a consistent location. It lies posterior to the IVC, medial to the right lobe of the liver and lateral to the right diaphragmatic crus. It is lower and more medial in relation to the spine than the left. On cross-section it is linear or V shaped, with a larger medial limb and a smaller lateral limb.

The left adrenal gland lies posterior to the splenic vein and lateral to the diaphragmatic crus, but its position is less consistent than that of the right side. The left adrenal gland is more semilunar than the right and it extends down the superomedial border of the kidney towards the hilum. On cross-section it is triangular or Y-shaped.

Embryologically, the adrenals do not develop with the kidneys. They develop in the retroperitoneum and descend, whereas the kidneys develop in the pelvis and ascend. In cases where the kidneys fail to ascend normally, the adrenal glands are still found in the expected position although their shape may be more discoid owing to lack of moulding by the kidneys during development.

At birth the adrenal glands are relatively much larger than in the adult – one-third the size of the kidney at birth and one-thirtieth in the adult. The size of the gland is somewhat variable, but as a rule of thumb on cross-sectional imaging the limbs of the adrenal should not be thicker than the diameter of the adjacent crus of the diaphragm.

ARTERIAL SUPPLY

Three arteries supply these glands on each side, namely:
- The superior adrenal artery from the inferior phrenic artery
- The middle adrenal artery from the aorta
- The inferior adrenal artery from the renal artery

VENOUS DRAINAGE OF THE ADRENAL GLANDS

One vein drains the adrenal gland on each side. The right adrenal vein drains to the IVC and the left adrenal vein drains to the left renal vein.

Variants

Small masses of adrenal cortical tissue called cortical bodies or cortical rests are often found near the adrenal glands. These may become attached to other organs early in embryology and migrate with these organs to be found in such places as the broad ligament of the uterus, the spermatic cord and the epididymis.

RADIOLOGICAL FEATURES OF THE ADRENAL GLANDS

Plain Films of the Abdomen

The adrenal glands are visible only if calcified, and they are then seen to be lateral to the spine at the level of the upper pole of the kidneys.

Computed Tomography

The shape of the adrenal gland on CT cuts is variable, with a linear, inverted V shape being commonest on the right and a triangular or Y shape commonest on the left. Its craniocaudal extent is less than 4 cm and limb thickness is usually less than 1 cm.

The right adrenal gland is seen posterior to the IVC. More laterally it lies between the liver and the crura of the diaphragm. The left adrenal is higher and extends more laterally anterior to the kidney, from which it is separated by perirenal fat. Contrast medium may help to distinguish it from the adjacent splenic vessels.

MRI

The adrenals are very well seen on MRI because of surrounding fat (more easily than with CT). They are iso- or slightly hypointense compared to liver on both T1- and T2-weighted images. They lose signal on fat suppression or fat-subtraction techniques, depending on the cholesterol content of the adrenal cortex (cortisol is derived from cholesterol esters).

Ultrasound

In thin individuals the adrenal glands can sometimes be seen between the kidney and liver on the right and between the kidney and pancreatic tail on the left using high-resolution scanning. They are readily seen in neonates and usually seen in children.

Arteriography of the Adrenal Gland

- The superior adrenal artery usually consists of several branches from the inferior phrenic artery. It may arise separately from the aorta, usually above the coeliac artery, but may arise below this or from the renal artery.
- The **middle adrenal artery** arises from the aorta and is multiple in more than 30% of studies.
- The **inferior adrenal artery** may arise from the renal artery directly or with the superior capsular artery.

Other arteries to the adrenal gland may arise from the gonadal arteries.

The Abdominal Aorta (Fig. 5.51)

The aorta enters the abdomen through the aortic hiatus of the diaphragm between the crura at T12 vertebral level. It lies anterior to L1–L4 vertebral bodies, adjacent to the left psoas muscle. The left lumbar veins pass behind it. Anteriorly it is related to the pancreas, which separates it from the stomach; to the third part of the duodenum and to the small intestine.

The abdominal aorta is 12 cm long and ends by dividing into the right and left common iliac arteries at L4 vertebral level.

BRANCHES OF THE ABDOMINAL AORTA

These are as follows:
Three unpaired anterior branches:
- Coeliac trunk at T12/L1
- SMA at L1
- Inferior mesenteric artery at L3

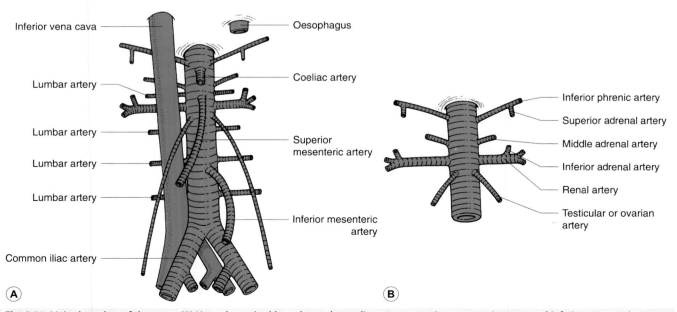

Fig. 5.51 Major branches of the aorta. (A) Ventral unpaired branches – the coeliac artery, superior mesenteric artery and inferior mesenteric artery. Lateral paired branches – the lumbar arteries and the common iliac arteries. (B) Other lateral paired branches.

Three lateral paired visceral arteries:
  - Adrenal arteries at L1
  - Renal arteries at L1/L2
  - Gonadal arteries at L3
Five lateral paired parietal branches:
  - Inferior phrenic arteries at T12
  - Four pairs of lumbar arteries
Terminal arteries:
  - The common iliac arteries
  - Median sacral artery

RADIOLOGICAL FEATURES OF THE AORTA

Plain Films of the Abdomen

The aorta is visible only if calcified. It is seen as linear calcification vertically in the midline and to the left of midline. Tortuosity of the aorta in the elderly may cause considerable variation in the site of this calcification. Aneurysmal dilatation may be detected based on the position of the mural calcification.

Proximity of the vertebral bodies may lead to bony erosion by aneurysms of the aorta, which may be detectable on radiographs.

Ultrasound

This is a useful means of studying the aorta, particularly for aneurysm screening. It can be visualized posterior to the pancreas, where its coeliac and superior mesenteric branches can be easily seen. Where it passes posterior to loops of small intestine it is often obscured by gas. However, by turning the subject on to their right side the length of the aorta can almost always be visualized from the left side of the anterior abdomen (scanning behind the loops of bowel that tend to fall anteriorly and to the right).

The aortic diameter is 2–3 cm depending on age; it diminishes as the aorta progresses caudally. The aorta can be distinguished from the IVC on ultrasound of the upper abdomen by its course near the diaphragm. The aorta remains posteriorly placed to reach the aortic hiatus posterior to the crura of the diaphragm. The IVC, on the other hand, passes ventrally to pierce the central tendon of the diaphragm, hugging the posterior aspect of the liver.

Computed Tomography

A contrast bolus is given at a high rate (e.g. 4–5 mL/s) and rapid scan acquisition is performed in the arterial phase outlining aorta and branches.

Magnetic Resonance Imaging

3D gadolinium-enhanced MR angiography provides high-resolution data that can be used to generate projection angiographic images and multiplanar reformatted images.

Angiography

The anatomy, as described above, is best imaged by aortography or selective arteriography of its branches.

The Inferior Vena Cava

The IVC is formed by the union of the right and left common iliac veins at L5 vertebral level behind the right common iliac artery. It passes superiorly to the right of the aorta as far as T12 level, where it is separated from the aorta by the right crus of the diaphragm. The IVC pierces the diaphragm at T8 level, passes through the pericardium and enters the right atrium. An incomplete semilunar valve is found at its entry to the atrium. Apart from this the IVC has no valves.

The IVC lies on the bodies of the lumbar vertebrae. Part of the right adrenal gland and the right inferior phrenic, right adrenal, right renal and right lumbar arteries pass posterior to it. It is related anteriorly from below upwards, to coils of small intestine and the root of the mesentery, the third part of the duodenum, the head of the pancreas and the CBD, the first part of the duodenum and the epiploic foramen, with the portal vein anterior to it. It then passes in a deep groove in the liver (sometimes a tunnel) before piercing the diaphragm and entering the heart.

TRIBUTARIES OF THE INFERIOR VENA CAVA

These are as follows:
- Third and fourth lumbar veins (upper two to the azygos vein, the fifth to the ileolumbar vein)
- Right gonadal vein
- Right renal vein
- Right adrenal vein
- Small veins from right and caudate lobes of liver
- Right, middle and left hepatic veins
- Right inferior phrenic vein (left drains to left adrenal vein)
- Left renal vein (which has already received the left gonadal and adrenal veins)

EMBRYOLOGY AND VARIANTS

The IVC arises embryologically by a complex series of fusion of primitive veins. As a result of this its lower tributaries lie posterior to the aorta and its upper tributaries lie anterior to the aorta. Variation in this development can give rise to several congenital abnormalities of the IVC. It may, for example, be double below the renal veins owing to persistence of a primitive vein on the left side (**persistent left-sided IVC**). This may be associated with a failure of union of the common iliac veins. Occasionally the IVC is continuous with a much-enlarged azygos vein, which carries all of its blood to the superior vena cava (SVC). The IVC may be left-sided as far as the renal veins and then cross over (behind the aorta as a continuation of the left renal vein) and continue as a right-sided IVC through the liver to the heart.

Radiology of the inferior vena cava

Chest Radiography. The shadow of the IVC can be identified as it pierces the right hemidiaphragm and enters the heart. On a lateral chest radiograph it identifies a hemidiaphragm as being the right-sided one.

Cavography. The IVC can be opacified by contrast medium that is introduced either simultaneously into the dorsal pedal veins of both feet or via both femoral veins, or by a catheter that is introduced into the vessel itself. Some contrast may be introduced into its tributaries by the performance of a Valsalva manoeuvre.

During placement of a caval filter to prevent pulmonary emboli it must be established that there is not a persistence of a left-sided cava, this would require placement of a second filter in that vessel. This can be established by introducing contrast into the left common iliac vein (Valsalva manoeuvre helps). The renal veins should likewise be identified, as the filter should be placed **below** these.

Ultrasound. The IVC can be identified where it is not obscured by intestinal gas. Its hepatic and proximal courses are readily seen with ultrasound. It can be seen posterior to the portal vein at the epiploic foramen. The hepatic veins can be seen draining to the IVC before it enters the right atrium. The IVC curves ventrally just before piercing the diaphragm, unlike the aorta, which passes posterior to the diaphragm.

Computed Tomography. The IVC is seen on the right of the aorta. It is a transverse oval in cross-section but its shape varies from slit-like on inspiration to circular on expiration. The right adrenal gland is seen to be partly posterior to the IVC. Some liver tissue may also be found posterior to it in its upper course. The right aortic branches that pass behind the IVC are usually visible.

The union of the common iliac veins to form the IVC can be identified, and the left common iliac vein is seen to be posterior to the right common iliac artery. In fact, all the pelvic veins are dorsal to the corresponding arteries.

Veins of the Posterior Abdominal Wall (Fig. 5.52)

There is a rich venous anastomosis in the lumbar area between lumbar, sacral, intercostal veins and IVC, via segmental lumbar veins which drain directly into the cava and the ascending lumbar and azygos systems. This system usually has a connection with the left renal vein.

The internal and external vertebral venous plexuses drain via segmental lumbar veins into the IVC. The lumbar veins are joined sequentially on both sides of the vertebral column by an ascending lumbar vein, which also extends inferiorly to the lateral sacral and iliolumbar veins.

The ascending lumbar vein ascends on the vertebral bodies at the root of the transverse processes deep to the psoas muscle and extends superiorly to the azygos system.

The azygos vein is a right-sided structure and may arise in one of three ways:

- It may be simply the continuation of the ascending lumbar vein on the right side entering the thorax with the aorta or by piercing the right crus of the diaphragm.
- It may arise from the left renal vein or from the IVC at the level of the renal veins.
- It may begin as the continuation of the subcostal vein.

Similarly, the hemiazygos vein may arise in different ways:

- It may be the continuation of the left ascending lumbar vein and enter the thorax to the left of the aorta or by piercing the left crus.

- It may arise from the posterior aspect of the left renal vein.
- It may be the continuation of the left subcostal vein.

In congenital absence of the IVC, or following obstruction of the IVC, the ascending lumbar and azygos veins drain blood to the SVC and are enlarged. The role of this system in the spread of malignant and other disease from the pelvis to the spine is controversial. It is said to account for the propensity of prostate cancer to spread to the sacrum and lumbar vertebrae, and for infections arising in the pelvis to seed the intervertebral discs.

RADIOLOGICAL FEATURES OF THE VEINS OF THE POSTERIOR ABDOMINAL WALL

CT and MRI

The ascending lumbar veins, the azygos and hemiazygos veins, may be visible deep to the psoas distally and are identified on either side of the aorta proximally as they pass between the crura of the diaphragm. These veins are much more easily seen if enlarged, as occurs in obstruction of the IVC or SVC.

ABDOMINAL LYMPHATIC SYSTEM (TABLE 5.4)

Lymph channels in the abdomen travel with the arteries. Most lymph drains to nodes around the abdominal aorta. These are arranged into four groups:

- Preaortic
- Right para-aortic
- Left para-aortic
- Retroaortic

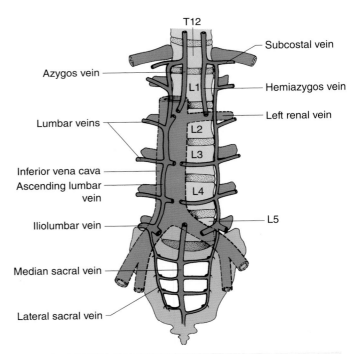

Fig. 5.52 Veins of the posterior abdominal wall.

Table 5.4   Normal Lymph Node Size in the Abdomen

Location of Node	Maximum Short Axis Diameter (mm)
Retrocrural	6
Gastrohepatic ligament	8
Upper para-aortic	9
Porta hepatis	7
Portacaval	10
Lower para-aortic	11

Data from Dorfman, R. E., Alpern, M. B., Gross, B. H., & Sandler, M. A. (1991). Upper abdominal lymph nodes: criteria for normal size determined with CT. *Radiology, 180*(2), 319–322. (A study of 130 patients.)

All of these drain to the **cisterna chyli**, which is an elongated lymph channel that continues in the thorax as the thoracic duct.

Preaortic Nodes

These are arranged around the anterior branches of the aorta (the coeliac trunk and the superior and inferior mesenteric arteries). They drain lymph from the areas supplied by these arteries, that is, the gastrointestinal tract, the liver, gallbladder, pancreas and spleen. Lymph from these viscera passes through visceral nodes (i.e. the nodes at the porta hepatis and nodes of the mesentery), and along the course of the arteries before reaching the preaortic nodes. Lymph from the preaortic nodes passes in the right and left **intestinal trunks** to the cisterna chyli.

Coeliac Nodes

These receive gastric, hepatic and pancreaticosplenic lymph drainage.

The **gastric nodes** have three groups: left gastric, gastroepiploic and pyloric.

- The **left gastric nodes** lie along the lesser curve and drain the lower oesophagus as well as the stomach. These nodes are usually smaller than the para-aortic group; over 8 mm is considered abnormal. The **gastroepiploic group** lie low on the greater curve, near the pylorus, and are related to the right gastroepiploic artery. These drain to the **pyloric group** – a group of approximately five nodes which lie in the bifurcation of the gastroduodenal artery at the junction of the first and second part of the duodenum.
- The **hepatic nodes** are related to the hepatic artery at the porta hepatis in the lesser omentum (gastrohepatic ligament). They are variable in size and number and drain liver, gallbladder and bile ducts, as well as stomach, duodenum and pancreas.
- The **pancreaticosplenic nodes** run with the splenic artery and lie above and behind the pancreas and in the gastrosplenic ligament. These drain the pancreas, spleen and stomach.

Superior and Inferior Mesenteric Nodes

The superior and inferior mesenteric nodes drain the bowel from the duodenojejunal flexure to the anal canal. Lymph drainage from the small bowel is to mesenteric nodes, from the terminal ileum and colon to ileocolic nodes, and from the rectum to pararectal nodes. From here, lymph drains along the arterial supply to nodes at the origins of the superior and inferior mesenteric arteries. All nodes lie on the mesenteric side of the bowel, and lymphatic channels run in the mesentery. Perirectal nodes may lie anywhere around the rectum within the perirectal fat. They drain to a superior rectal group with the superior rectal artery and thence to an inferior mesenteric group. They also drain to the internal and common iliac nodes. The lower part of the anal canal drains to external iliac nodes.

Para-Aortic Nodes

These nodes lie on either side of the aorta in relation to its lateral paired branches. They lie anterior to the medial margin of psoas and the crura of the diaphragm. They receive lymph from the structures supplied by these branches, including the posterior abdominal wall, the diaphragm, the kidneys and adrenals and the gonads. On the right, nodes lie anterior and lateral to the IVC. Nodes lying between the aorta and IVC are referred to as **aortocaval nodes**. A node lying between the IVC and the portal vein is frequently identified and is referred to as the **portacaval node**.

Lymph from the legs drains via the deep inguinal and external and common iliac nodes to the para-aortic nodes. Lymph from the pelvis drains via internal and common iliac nodes to the para-aortic nodes.

Efferent vessels from the para-aortic nodes unite to form the **right and left lumbar trunks**.

Retroaortic Nodes

These nodes represent posteriorly placed nodes of the lateral group. They are worthy of mention because very little else lies between the aorta and the vertebral bodies, and a mass posterior to the aorta is therefore likely to represent lymphatic tissue.

Cisterna Chyli

This thin-walled sac, 6 mm wide and 6 cm long, is the dilated proximal end of the thoracic duct before it passes through the aortic hiatus of the diaphragm. It lies in the retrocrural space, in front of the bodies of L1 and L2 and to the right of the aorta. The cisterna chyli receives the intestinal trunk, the right and left lumbar trunks and paired descending intercostal trunks.

RADIOLOGICAL FEATURES OF THE ABDOMINAL LYMPHATICS

CT and MRI

The 'bean-shaped' appearance of the normal node may be appreciated with its fatty hilum, although the fatty hilum is not always evident. The long axis is parallel to the direction of drainage. Pathologically enlarged nodes tend to be more rounded in shape and may lose their fatty hilum. Normal nodes vary in length from millimetres to several centimetres (see Table 5.4) but are narrow in diameter. In imaging, nodes are measured in their maximum short axis diameter. In the abdomen the normal cross-sectional diameter is variable but should normally be less than 10 mm (this varies by location). On MRI, spatial resolution is less than with CT, but greater contrast resolution allows easier differentiation of lymph nodes from nearby vessels, bowel loops and other retroperitoneal structures.

Lymphography (Fig. 5.53)

There is a recent resurgence in interest in lymphatic imaging because of interventions being offered in various lymphatic disorders. Contrast lymphography is the only imaging technique that can demonstrate lymphatic channels and internal nodal architecture. Oil-based contrast (e.g. lipiodol) is injected directly into lymph nodes, traditionally in the lower limbs to visualize the lymph channels and nodes of the posterior abdominal wall. Lymph channels are visible within hours and should clear in less than 24 hours. Lymph nodes are best seen after 24 hours, when contrast has accumulated within them, and the channels are clear.

Normal lymph nodes have a fine reticular appearance on lymphography. Nodes are normally less than 3.5 cm in length, with their long axis in the line of the lymph vessels.

Lymphography by this method shows the deep inguinal nodes, the external iliac nodes and the common iliac nodes. The para-aortic nodes are seen as right and left lumbar chains of nodes along the tip of the transverse processes of the lumbar vertebrae to L2 level, where they drain to the

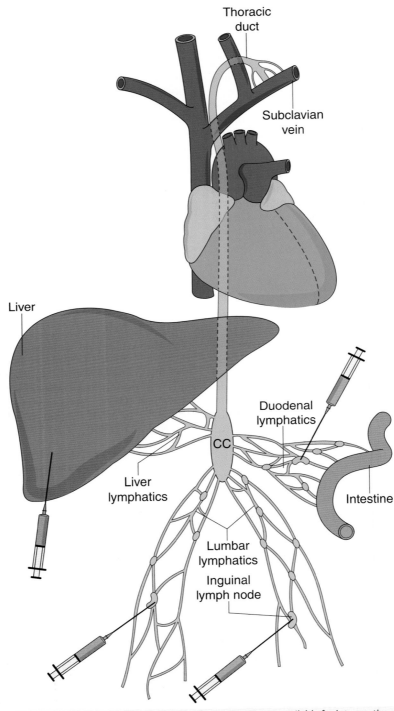

Fig. 5.53 Schematic representation of the lymphatic system showing various injection sites available for intervention

cisterna chyli. In about 60% of cases a middle chain arises from the right chain. Fine, tortuous transverse vessels link the chains. Gaps in the right chain are frequent and associated with bypass vessels, but there are no gaps in the left chain. The upper left lumbar nodes are particularly numerous and are called the 'upper lumbar clump'.

Lymphography using lipiodol is associated with a risk of respiratory compromise due to pulmonary oily contrast emboli. This procedure is contraindicated in patients with poor respiratory reserve.

Transhepatic Lymphangiography. The duodenal and upper jejunal lymphatics may be abnormally dilated in some patients with congenital heart disease, leading to chronic loss of protein through the bowel in a condition known as protein-losing enteropathy. The lymphatics may be accessed retrogradely by transhepatic cannulation of the lymph channels in the hilum of the liver. Lipiodol contrast is injected to demonstrate the fine network of lymphatics. Dilated lymphatics may be sclerosed with a glue.

MR Lymphangiography. Puncture of the lymph nodes at both groins with a 25-gauge needle and slow injection of gadolinium contrast followed by MRI can demonstrate the cysterna chyli and the thoracic duct. This procedure is performed to assess for stenosis in the duct, which may also contribute to protein-losing enteropathy in some patients with congenital heart disease.

Peritoneal Spaces of the Abdomen

DEVELOPMENT AND TERMINOLOGY OF THE MESENTERY AND PERITONEAL SPACES

Most abdominal ligaments and mesenteries are formed from remnants of the ventral and dorsal mesenteries, which suspend the primitive gut (Fig. 5.54).

In the abdomen:
- A **ligament** is formed by two folds of peritoneum that enclose a structure within the peritoneal cavity, and is usually named for the two structures it joins, for example gastrohepatic, splenorenal.

- An **omentum** is a ligament that joins the stomach to another structure.
- A **mesentery** comprises two folds of peritoneum that attach a loop of bowel to the retroperitoneum.

In the embryo the mesenteries divide the coelomic cavity into right and left halves. In the upper abdomen the mesentery suspends the developing stomach and gut in the middle, with the developing liver in the ventral mesentery and the developing spleen in the dorsal mesentery. As development progresses, the organs migrate in an anticlockwise fashion and the liver comes to lie on the right, with the spleen on the left, dragging the mesentery into the position they occupy at maturity (Fig. 5.55). The right coelomic cavity above the transverse mesocolon becomes the perihepatic space and lesser sac, and the left coelomic cavity becomes the left subphrenic space.

The dorsal mesentery gives rise to **ligaments** in the upper abdomen where it is reflected between structures:
- The **gastrophrenic ligament** is the reflection from the stomach to the left hemidiaphragm.
- The **gastrosplenic ligament** is the reflection of the mesentery from stomach to spleen.
- The **splenorenal ligament** is the reflection from the left kidney to the spleen.
- The **phrenicocolic ligament** is the reflection from the splenic flexure to the left diaphragm.
- The **gastrocolic ligament** is the reflection from the stomach to the splenic flexure.

The dorsal mesentery also gives rise to:
- The transverse mesocolon
- The small bowel mesentery
- The sigmoid mesocolon

The ventral mesentery gives rise to:
- The **falciform ligament**, which is the peritoneal reflection from the anterior surface of the liver to the anterior abdominal wall. The falciform ligament has the obliterated umbilical vein running within it, which is known as the ligamentum teres. The leaves of the falciform ligament are continuous with the fissure for the ligamentum venosum.

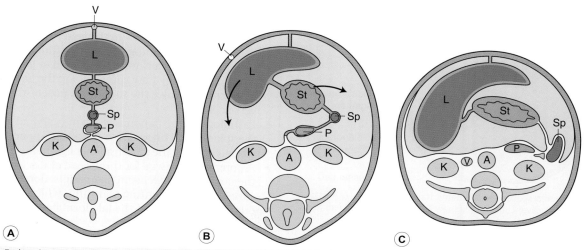

Fig. 5.54 Embryological development of peritoneal spaces. (A) Fetus at fifth week. (B) Fetus at tenth week. (C) Maturity. *A*, Aorta; *L*, liver; *K*, kidney; *P*, pancreas; *Sp*, spleen; *St*, stomach; *V*, vena cava.

- The **gastrohepatic ligament**, which is the reflection of the mesentery from the lesser curve of the stomach to the porta of the liver (and which is the upper part of the lesser omentum).
- The **hepaticoduodenal ligament**, which is the reflection of the peritoneum from the first part of the duodenum to the porta of the liver and also part of the lesser omentum. The lower free edge of this is the free edge of the lesser omentum and forms the entrance to the lesser sac.

The ventral mesentery regresses below the level of the transverse mesocolon.

The Lesser Sac and Associated Ligaments (see Figs. 5.55, 5.56)

The **lesser sac** forms as a result of rotation of the viscera in fetal life and is the remnant of the primitive right coelomic cavity. The posterior wall of the lesser sac is formed by the peritoneum overlying the pancreas, left adrenal and upper pole of the left kidney, whereas its anterior wall is formed by the peritoneum on the posterior wall of the stomach and the lesser omentum. It is limited laterally by the spleen and its gastrosplenic and splenorenal ligaments. The lesser sac is partially divided by the fold of peritoneum over the left gastric artery, the gastropancreatic fold.

The right side of the lesser sac communicates with the general peritoneal cavity via the **epiploic foramen (of Winslow)**.

Boundaries of the Epiploic Foramen

- Posteriorly: IVC.
- Anteriorly: free edge of the lesser omentum, containing the portal vein (posteriorly), hepatic artery (left/medial) and CBD (right/lateral).
- Superiorly: caudate process of the liver.
- Inferiorly: first part of the duodenum.

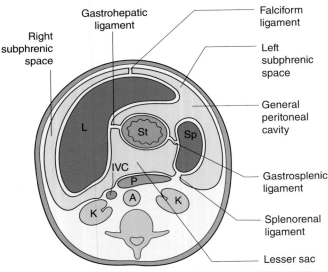

Fig. 5.55 Peritoneal spaces and ligaments: transverse section. *A*, Aorta; *IVC*, inferior vena cava; *L*, liver; *K*, kidney; *P*, pancreas; *Sp*, spleen; *St*, stomach.

Recesses of the Lesser Sac

- The **superior recess** surrounds the medial aspect of the caudate lobe and is separated from the splenic recess by the **gastropancreatic fold** (a peritoneal fold covering the proximal left gastric artery as it runs superiorly). This fold runs from the retroperitoneum to the posterior aspect of the fundus of the stomach and partially divides the superior recess from the splenic recess.
- The splenic recess extends across the midline to the splenic hilum.
- The inferior recess lies between the stomach and the pancreas and transverse mesocolon.

Ligaments of the Lesser Sac

The lesser sac is bounded by remnants of both the dorsal and ventral mesenteries. Anteriorly, the lesser sac is bounded by the lesser omentum. This is a combination of gastrohepatic and hepaticoduodenal ligaments.

- The **gastrohepatic ligament** arises in the fissure for the ligamentum venosum and connects the medial aspect of the liver to the lesser curve of the stomach. It contains the left gastric artery, left gastric vein and lymph nodes.
- The **hepticoduodenal ligament** forms the inferior (free) edge of the lesser omentum and contains the portal vein, common duct and hepatic artery.
- The **gastrosplenic ligament** is a remnant of the dorsal mesentery; it connects the splenic hilum to the greater curve of the stomach and contains the short gastric vessels.
- The **splenorenal ligament**, also a remnant of the dorsal mesentery, forms part of the lateral border of the lesser sac, running from the posterior aspect of the spleen to the anterior pararenal space overlying the left kidney. It encloses the tail of pancreas and the distal pancreatic and proximal splenic arteries.
- The **gastrocolic ligament**, another dorsal remnant, connects the greater curve of the stomach with the superior aspect of the transverse colon and forms part of the anterior border of the lesser sac. It contains the gastroepiploic vessels and also forms the superior aspect of the greater omentum.

RADIOLOGY PEARLS

- Isolated fluid collections in the lesser sac are more likely to occur secondary to local pathology, such as pancreatitis or a perforated duodenal or gastric ulcer.
- Gastric pathology may spread along the gastrocolic ligament to involve the superior aspect of the transverse colon.
- Pathology of the pancreatic tail may spread along the splenorenal ligament to the anterior pararenal space, or along the gastrosplenic ligament.
- A potential pathway for the spread of disease from the porta to the falciform ligament is along the fissure for the ligamentum venosum, which is continuous with the leaves of the falciform ligament.

SUBPHRENIC AND SUBHEPATIC SPACES AND ASSOCIATED LIGAMENTS

The peritoneum over the liver is continuous with that on the abdominal surface of the diaphragm except for a **bare area** posterosuperiorly. The peritoneal reflections that form the boundaries of the bare area are called ligaments:

- The left triangular ligament on the left
- The superior and inferior coronary ligaments on the right
- The right triangular ligament where the superior and inferior coronary ligaments meet laterally

These peritoneal reflections form the boundaries of the **subphrenic** and **subhepatic spaces**, which are common sites for intraperitoneal collections.

The **subphrenic space** lies anterosuperiorly between the diaphragm and the liver. It is incompletely divided by the **falciform ligament** into **right** and **left** parts.

On the **right side** the triangular ligament divides the subphrenic space into two distinct compartments:

- The **subphrenic space** lies between the right hemidiaphragm and the right lobe of the liver. It is limited posteriorly by the right superior reflection of the coronary ligament and the right triangular ligament.
- The **subhepatic space** lies posteroinferiorly between the liver and the abdominal viscera. It is limited superiorly by the inferior reflection of the coronary ligament and the right triangular ligament. It communicates anteriorly and laterally with the subphrenic space, and laterally with the right paracolic gutter. The **posterior part** of the subhepatic space between the liver and the kidney is called the **hepatorenal space (Morrison's pouch)**. The **anterior part** of the right subhepatic space is located just posterior to the porta hepatis and communicates with the lesser sac via the foramen of Winslow.

RADIOLOGY PEARL

Morrison's pouch is the deepest point of the abdominal cavity in a supine patient and is therefore a common site of collection.

On the **left side** there is one large combined subphrenic space comprising three parts:

- The **immediate subphrenic space** lies between the diaphragm and the fundus of the stomach and includes the area anterior to the lateral segment of the left lobe of liver (segments II and III). The **gastrophrenic ligament** runs through this space, suspending the stomach from the dome of the diaphragm.
- The **subhepatic space**, also known as the **gastrohepatic recess**, is situated between the stomach and left lobe of liver.
- The **perisplenic space** surrounds the spleen and is partially separated from the left paracolic gutter by the **phrenicocolic ligament**. This is a major suspensory ligament of the spleen and prevents the passage of fluid from the left paracolic gutter to the left subphrenic space.

The **bare area of the liver** lies between the reflections of the right and left coronary ligaments and is devoid of peritoneum. Intra-abdominal fluid cannot extend medial to the attachments of the right coronary ligament or between the bare area of the liver and the diaphragm. The bare area of the liver is in continuity with the right anterior pararenal space, and pathologic processes can spread via this route.

INFRAMESOCOLIC MESENTERIES AND SPACES

The transverse mesocolon, small bowel mesentery and sigmoid mesentery are all remnants of the dorsal mesocolon. Below the mesocolon (the mesentery of the transverse colon) the **infracolic space** is divided into right and left parts by the root of the mesentery of the small bowel. The attachment of this mesentery runs in an oblique line from the duodenal flexure in the upper left abdomen to the lower right abdomen.

Right and left paracolic spaces (gutters) are found lateral to the ascending and descending colon.

The infracolic and paracolic spaces are continuous with the rectovesical and rectouterine pouches of the pelvis (see Chapter 6).

RADIOLOGICAL FEATURES OF THE PERITONEAL SPACES

Plain Films of the Abdomen

The peritoneum is not visible in the normal abdomen, but in pneumoperitoneum gas may outline the subphrenic space, the falciform ligament, the umbilical ligaments (see section on the anterior abdominal wall at the start of the chapter) or the lesser sac.

Ultrasound

This is a good method of visualizing fluid collections in the right subphrenic and subhepatic spaces. The left subphrenic space between the left lobe of the liver or the spleen and the diaphragm can also be visualized. Gas in the stomach may obscure part of this space. Pelvic ultrasound or transrectal/transvaginal ultrasound may show fluid collections in the pelvic part of the peritoneal cavity.

Gas in the stomach may obscure the lesser sac. Bowel gas generally obscures the remainder of the peritoneal cavity, although if free fluid is present the peritoneal cavity is well seen.

Computed Tomography (Fig. 5.57)

The peritoneal spaces and their ligaments are well seen if free fluid is present. The bare area can be identified as it lies directly on the diaphragm, whereas the remainder of the liver is surrounded with fluid. The ligaments usually contain some fat as well as vessels. The greater omentum can also be seen as a thin fat-filled structure anterior to bowel loops immediately deep to the anterior abdominal wall.

THE MESENTERIC MODEL OF ABDOMINAL ANATOMY

Traditionally abdominal anatomy has been described in peritoneal terms; that is to say that the position the

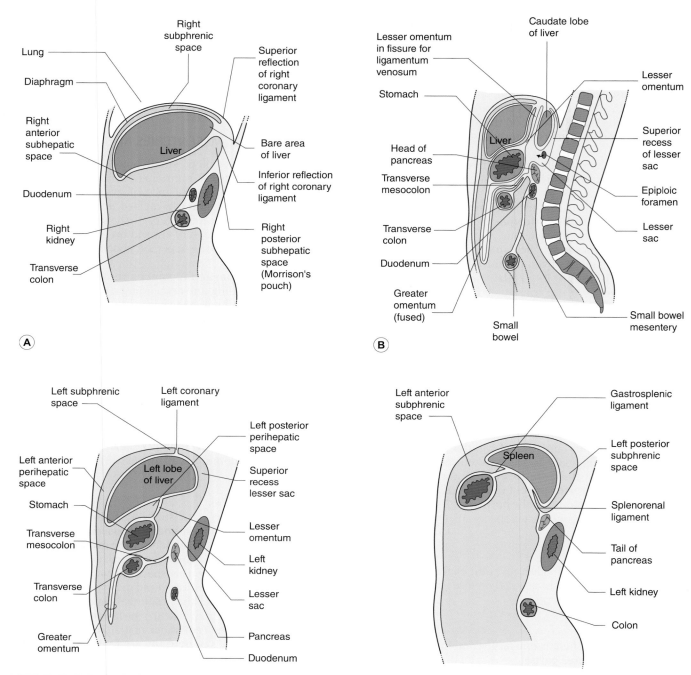

Fig. 5.56 Peritoneal attachments to the posterior abdominal wall and sagittal sections to show peritoneal spaces. (A) This section passes through the right lobe of the liver and right kidney. Note the position of the bare area of the liver, where fluid cannot abut the liver in cases of free intra-abdominal fluid. The right subphrenic space communicates with the right subhepatic space around the front of the liver. (B) This section passes through the liver, stomach, colon with its greater and lesser omenta, and the retroperitoneal duodenum and pancreas. Note that the lesser omentum runs up into the fissure for the ligamentum venosum in the liver. The free lower edge of this contains the vessels running to and from the porta of the liver: hepatic artery portal vein and bile duct. (C) Section through left lobe of liver, stomach with lesser sac behind and colon. Pancreas, duodenum and left kidney are retroperitoneal. Note that the lesser sac extends up to the left subphrenic space. (D) Section through the spleen. Note the splenorenal and gastrosplenic ligaments.

abdominal organs and the means by which these organs are connected are thought of in relation to the peritoneum. In the traditional peritoneal model of anatomy, multiple mesenteries are described. This traditional peritoneal model of abdominal anatomy is currently being superseded by a mesenteric-based model.

In the mesenteric model, described by Coffey et al., 2016 (Lancet; 1:238-47), the mesentery is described as an organ in which all the abdominal digestive organs (liver, spleen, pancreas and intestine) develop. The mesentery remains continuous throughout development from oesophago-gastric to anorectal junction. The organs grow, move and

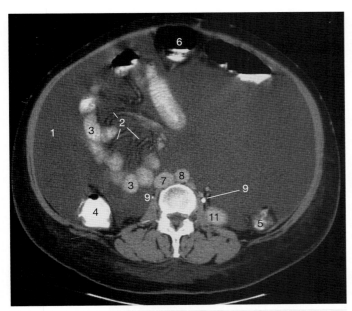

Fig. 5.57 Axial computed tomography of the abdomen. Subject with extensive abdominal fluid. Note the vessels running in the thin mesenteric folds, outlined by fat; and the retroperitoneal location of the ascending and descending colon, the ureters, the aorta and inferior vena cava.

1. Ascites
2. Folds of small bowel mesentery
3. Small bowel loops
4. Ascending colon
5. Descending colon
6. Transverse colon
7. Inferior vena cava
8. Aorta
9. Ureter

rotate as they develop and elongate within the continuous mesentery, creating the spaces described in conventional anatomy descriptions. Separately the genitourinary organs develop on and remain in continuity with the musculoskeletal frame, the separate nonmesenteric domain.

The ex vivo mesentery has been demonstrated to be continuous from oesophagogastric junction to anorectal junction, with all organs of the mesenteric domain connected to the mesentery rather than to the posterior abdominal wall. The mesentery itself is then adherent to the posterior abdominal wall, which provides an anchor between the mesenteric and nonmesenteric domains. This communication between domains is further reinforced by the peritoneal reflections: the visceral peritoneum covering the mesenteric domain and the parietal peritoneum of the nonmesenteric domain.

This model of abdominal anatomy is supported by modern surgical techniques (such as total mesorectal excision/complete mesocolic excision) and modern radiological depictions. It also provides an anatomical framework to understand the physical behaviour of surgical pathologies within the abdomen.

Within this newly described mesenteric model the traditional anatomical terms described in this chapter remain the same, but the development of the mesenteric organs follows an alternative path. The structures of the mesenteric domain are considered to develop beneath the peritoneum. As the mesentery develops during fetal life it displaces the peritoneum anteriorly and moulds the peritoneum into the ligaments, membranes and fossae we have previously described.

Cross-Sectional Anatomy of the Upper Abdomen

AXIAL SECTION THROUGH THE UPPER LIVER AND SPLEEN (FIG. 5.58)

Body Wall

The ribs and intercostal muscles are sectioned obliquely around most of the perimeter of the section. Anteriorly the costal cartilages forming the costal margin are separated by the two **rectus abdominis** muscles and the midline **linea alba** between. Superficial to the ribs and intercostal muscles lie the **serratus anterior** muscles laterally and the latissimus dorsi posterolaterally. The **erector spinae** muscles lie posterior to the vertebra on each side.

Diaphragm

The domes of the diaphragm can be distinguished from the liver and other intra-abdominal viscera only where these are separated by fat. The lung bases lie posteriorly, separated from the liver and spleen by the diaphragm.

The crura are visible anterolateral to the vertebral bodies. With the adjoining diaphragm these form linear structures extending from the posterior aspect of the liver and spleen to the anterior surface of the abdominal aorta. This **retrocrural space** is the lowest recess of the **mediastinum**. In addition to the aorta, it contains the azygos vein on the right side, the hemiazygos vein on the left, the thoracic duct on the right side posterior to the aorta (not usually visible on CT scans unless dilated), lymph nodes and fat. The IVC remains on the abdominal side, that is, lateral to the crura below T8 level, where it pierces the diaphragm.

Liver

The liver occupies most of the right half of this section. Segments II and III are distinguished from segments IVa and IVb by the **fissure for the ligamentum teres** on the anterior surface of the liver. The **fissure for the ligamentum venosum** on the visceral surface separates the caudate lobe (segment I) posteriorly from segments II and IV anteriorly. Branches of the portal veins and bile ducts may be seen, especially on contrast-enhanced scans. This level is above the porta hepatis.

Spleen

Lying posteriorly on the left, close to the diaphragm and the ribs, the spleen has a smooth diaphragmatic surface and a concave visceral surface in axial section.

Other Viscera

The stomach lies deep to the left lobe of the liver. The transverse colon may be seen anterior to the stomach, although its position is variable. The splenic flexure is found anterior to the spleen.

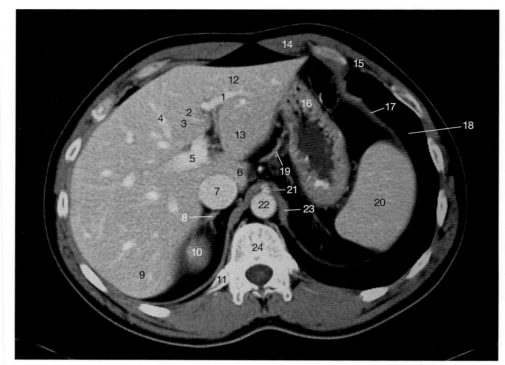

Fig. 5.58 Axial computed tomography, upper liver and spleen (T10/T11 approximately).

1. Left portal vein
2. Left hepatic artery in porta
3. Fissure for ligamentum venosum
4. Middle hepatic vein
5. Right portal vein
6. Caudate lobe (segment I)
7. Inferior vena cava
8. Right adrenal gland
9. Segment VII
10. Upper pole of the right kidney
11. Eleventh right rib
12. Segment II

13. Segment III
14. Rectus abdominis muscle
15. Muscles of the chest wall
16. Stomach with air
17. Anterior left hemidiaphragm
18. Left lung
19. Gastric vessels in the gastrosplenic ligament
20. Spleen
21. Origin of coeliac axis
22. Aorta
23. Left crus of the diaphragm
24. Eleventh thoracic vertebra

AXIAL SECTION AT THE LEVEL OF THE PORTA HEPATIS (FIG. 5.59)

Body Wall

This is as for the level above. The gap between the costal margins becomes progressively wider in lower cuts.

Diaphragm

As above. Usually only the crura and adjacent diaphragm are visible.

Liver

The falciform ligament is **intrahepatic** at this level. On this section, a line dividing the liver that passes through the gallbladder and the IVC defines the morphological right and left lobes (division of segment IV from segments V and VI). This line has to be extrapolated back from the gallbladder, which is seen on lower sections. That part of the anatomical right lobe left of this line and anterior to the porta is the quadrate lobe and the part posterior to the porta is the caudate lobe.

At the porta hepatis the portal veins lie posteriorly with the branches of the hepatic artery and of the bile ducts anteriorly.

Adrenal Glands

The right adrenal gland is a linear structure directly behind the IVC between the crura and the liver. The left adrenal gland extends further in front of the left kidney than does the right. Nearby splenic vessels may be confused for an adrenal abnormality.

Spleen

This section may pass through the splenic hilum. Vessels are seen dividing into branches just medial to the spleen. The splenic vein passes from the spleen posterior to the pancreas and is often visible throughout its length on one or two sections. The splenic artery has a tortuous course and only short segments are visible on axial sections.

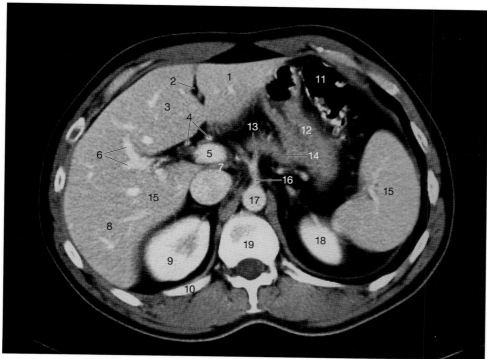

Fig. 5.59 Axial computed tomography through the porta hepatis (T11 approximately).

1. Segment III
2. Ligamentum teres
3. Segment IVb
4. Hepatic artery
5. Portal vein
6. Branches of the right portal vein
7. Papillary process of the caudate lobe
8. Segment VI
9. Upper pole of right kidney
10. Eleventh right rib

11. Transverse colon
12. Stomach
13. Splenic artery
14. Part of the pancreatic body
15. Spleen
16. Coeliac axis
17. Aorta
18. Upper pole of the left kidney
19. T11/T12 disc space

Other Viscera

The aorta lies in the retrocrural space and its coeliac branch may be seen at this level. The IVC lies close to the liver as above.

The stomach and colon are seen as on the higher section.

AXIAL SECTION AT THE LEVEL OF THE BODY OF THE PANCREAS (FIG. 5.60)

Body Wall

The ribs and intercostal muscles are seen as before. The latissimus dorsi is more lateral in position than before and the serratus anterior muscle is seen interdigitating with the external oblique muscle. The internal oblique muscle is seen arising from the deep aspect of the ribs.

Liver

The left lobe of the liver is smaller or not seen at this level. The gallbladder is visible below the porta hepatis.

Pancreas

The tail and body lie higher than the head of the pancreas. The tail of the gland is related to the splenic hilum. The body of the pancreas is seen anterior to the splenic vein and the aorta.

Other Viscera

The adrenal glands are still visible on this section. The upper pole of the left kidney (higher than that of the right) is visible.

The first part of the duodenum lies superior to the pancreatic head. The lower pole of the spleen lies behind the colon and lateral to the left kidney.

AXIAL SECTION AT THE LEVEL OF THE PANCREATIC HEAD AND RENAL HILA (FIG. 5.61)

Body Wall

The abdominal wall proper is now visible with the recti on each side of the linea alba and the three muscle layers of the abdominal wall – the internal and external oblique and transversus abdominis muscles – between the recti and the lower ribs.

Liver

The lower part of the right lobe is seen. A smaller left lobe, which may be completely separate from the right lobe, may be seen. The neck of the gallbladder (its highest part) may be seen. The spleen is not usually seen at this level.

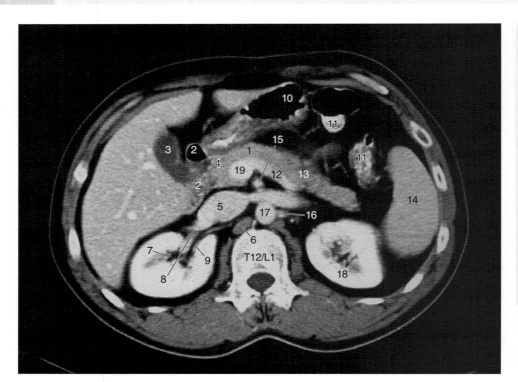

Fig. 5.60 Axial computed tomography at the level of the body of the pancreas (T12/L1).

1. Neck of the pancreas
2. Duodenum
3. Gallbladder
4. Head of the pancreas
5. Inferior vena cava
6. Right crus of the diaphragm
7. Renal sinus fat
8. Right renal vein
9. Right renal artery branch
10. Stomach
11. Splenic flexure
12. Splenic vein
13. Body and tail of the pancreas
14. Spleen
15. Superior mesenteric artery
16. Left renal artery
17. Aorta
18. Left kidney
19. Confluence of splenic and portal veins

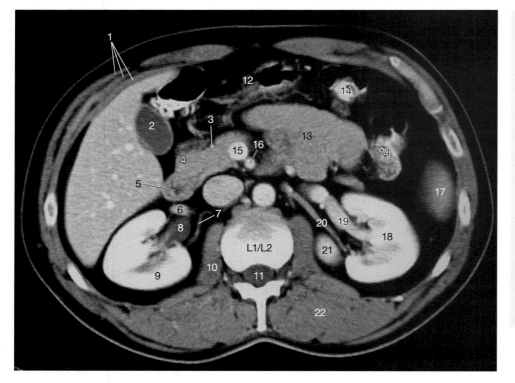

Fig. 5.61 Axial computed tomography at the level of the pancreatic head (L1 approximately).

1. Three layers of the anterior abdominal wall
2. Gallbladder
3. Gastroduodenal artery
4. Head of the pancreas
5. Duodenum
6. Renal vein
7. Branch of the right renal artery
8. Ureter
9. Right kidney
10. Psoas muscle
11. Thecal sac in the spinal canal
12. Transverse colon
13. Small bowel loops
14. Splenic flexure
15. Superior mesenteric vein
16. Superior mesenteric artery
17. Inferior pole of the spleen
18. Left kidney at hilum
19. Left renal vein
20. Left renal artery
21. Renal lobulation
22. Erector spinae muscle

Pancreas

The head of the pancreas is seen at this level. The pancreatic duct may be identified as a thin, hypodense linear structure. The CBD and gastroduodenal artery are seen in cross-section. The bile duct lies in the lateral aspect of the head, close to the duodenal surface. The gastroduodenal artery (a branch of the hepatic artery) lies lateral and more anterior. In slightly lower sections the head of the pancreas is seen to be separated from the uncinate process by the superior mesenteric vessels (the vein lies right of the artery).

Kidneys and Renal Vessels

This section includes one or both renal hila (the left hilum is usually slightly higher than the right). The left renal vein is seen passing to the IVC from the left hilum anterior to the aorta. The renal arteries have frequently divided already into anterior and posterior branches and may lie both anterior and posterior to the vein and pelvis.

Renal medullary pyramids can be demonstrated in their full length at the level of the hilum, whereas above and below this they are intersected at various planes to their long axis because of their orientation towards the hilum.

The Aorta and the Inferior Vena Cava

The aorta remains between the crura. Its superior mesenteric branch is visible at this level. The IVC is separated from the aorta by the crura and, at this level, is free from the liver.

Other Viscera

The second part of the duodenum lies lateral to the pancreatic head. The loops of small intestine lie to the left of the head of the pancreas. Vessels and fat are seen in its mesentery.

AXIAL SECTION BELOW THE KIDNEYS (FIG. 5.62)

Body Wall

The crura of the diaphragm may be seen as muscular columns that are not connected to one another, depending on level (not seen below L3). The right crus is usually larger than the left and extends further caudally.

The psoas muscle lies along the lateral aspect of the vertebral bodies and, although thin here, it increases in bulk in lower cuts. Other muscles are as described in previous sections.

Duodenum

The third part of the duodenum is seen passing between the aorta and the SMA.

Colon and Jejunum

The transverse colon is seen close to the anterior abdominal wall, with the ascending and descending colon laterally. Loops of jejunum and their mesentery occupy most of the anterior part of this section.

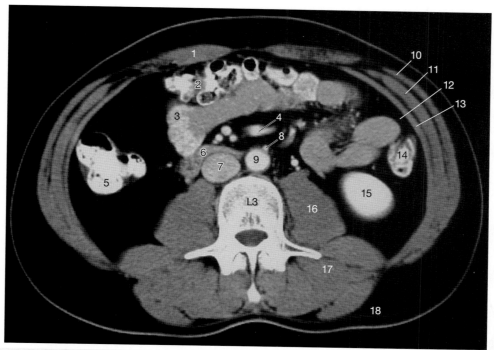

Fig. 5.62 Axial computed tomography through the mid-abdomen (L2/L3).

1. Rectus muscle
2. Transverse colon
3. Small bowel loops
4. Mesenteric vessels
5. Ascending colon
6. Third part of the duodenum
7. Inferior vena cava
8. Inferior mesenteric artery
9. Aorta
10. External oblique muscle
11. Internal oblique muscle
12. Peritoneal fat
13. Transversus abdominis muscle
14. Descending colon
15. Left pole of the left kidney
16. Psoas muscle
17. Erector spinae muscle
18. Subcutaneous fat

Summary of Spinal Levels (Table 5.5)

Table 5.5	Anatomy by Spinal Level
T8	Caval opening in the diaphragm containing the IVC and right phrenic nerve
T10	Oesophagus passes through the diaphragm with branches of the left gastric vessels and vagus nerve
T12	Aortic aperture in the diaphragm containing the aorta, azygos and hemiazygos veins, thoracic duct
	Origin of the coeliac axis
L1	*Transpyloric plane of Addison*
	Origin of the superior mesenteric artery
	Pancreatic neck
	Origin of the portal vein
	Gallbladder fundus Hila of the kidneys
	First part of the duodenum
	Pylorus of the stomach
	Splenic hilum
	Cisterna chyli
L1/2	Origin of the renal arteries
	Termination of the spinal cord in adults
L2	*Subcostal plane*
	Origin of the azygous and hemiazygous veins
	Thoracic duct begins
	Duodenaojejunal flexure
	Ligament of Treitz
L3	Origin of the inferior mesenteric artery
	Spinal cord terminates in infants
L3/4	Umbilicus
L4	*Transtubercular plane*
	Bifurcation of the aorta
L4/5	Inferior vena cava formed by the union of the common iliac veins

The Pelvis

JACK POWER
EDITED BY MICHELLE McNICHOLAS

CHAPTER CONTENTS	The Bony Pelvis, Muscles and Ligaments 245	The Lower Urinary Tract 261
	The Pelvic Floor 248	The Male Urethra 263
	The Sigmoid Colon, Rectum and Anal Canal 250	The Female Urethra 264
		The Male Reproductive Organs 264
	Blood Vessels, Lymphatics and Nerves of the Pelvis 258	The Female Reproductive Tract 272
		Cross-Sectional Anatomy 281

The Bony Pelvis, Muscles and Ligaments

The pelvis (Fig. 6.1) is a bony ring consisting of paired **innominate bones**, the **sacrum** and **coccyx**. The innominate bones articulate with each other anteriorly and with the sacrum posteriorly. Each innominate bone is composed of three parts – the ischium, ilium and pubis – which fuse at the acetabulum, at the Y-shaped **triradiate cartilage**, visible in the immature skeleton (see Fig. 8.9).

The **ilium** is a flat curved bone and bears the **iliac crest** superiorly. The **anterior** and **posterior superior iliac spines** are on either end of the iliac crest, with the anterior and posterior inferior iliac spines below them. The inner surface of the bone is smooth and has a sharp crest at its base – the **arcuate line** – running from the sacroiliac joint to the **iliopectineal eminence**. This line extends anteriorly to the pubic tubercle as the anatomic **iliopectineal line and delineates the inner margin of the pelvic inlet**.

The **pubic bone** consists of a **body**, and **inferior and superior rami**. The body of the pubic bone articulates with its fellow at the **symphysis pubis**. It bears the **iliopectineal eminence** on its superolateral aspect and the **pubic tubercle** on its superomedial aspect. The iliopectineal line is a ridge on the superior pubic ramus. The articular surfaces of the symphysis pubis are covered in hyaline cartilage with a fibrocartilaginous disc between them. The pubic bone is strengthened on all sides by dense ligaments.

The **ischium** is composed of a body and an inferior ramus, which joins the inferior pubic ramus. The body bears the **ischial tuberosity** inferiorly and a spine posteriorly. The **ischial spine** defines the greater and lesser sciatic notches above and below.

The **obturator foramen** is bounded by the body and rami of the pubic bone and the body and ramus of the ischial bone.

PELVIC INLET

The pelvic inlet (also known as the pelvic brim or ring) is the division between the true and false pelvis. It passes through the anterior aspect of the sacral promontory and the upper part of the pubic symphysis. The arcuate and pectineal lines are visible as the **iliopectineal line** on plain radiographs (see Fig. 6.2).

The Sacrum

Five fused vertebrae comprise this triangular bone, which is curved posteriorly. The anterior part of its upper end is termed the sacral promontory. It articulates with the lumbar spine superiorly and with the coccyx inferiorly. Anteriorly the sacrum has four pairs of **sacral foramina**, which transmit nerves from the **sacral canal**. Lateral to these are the **lateral masses** or **alae** of the sacrum. The sacrum also bears four pairs of posterior sacral foramina and the canal ends posteriorly in the **sacral hiatus** – a midline opening that transmits the fifth sacral nerves.

The Coccyx

This is composed of three to five fused vertebrae. The first segment is often separate. It articulates at an acute angle with the sacrum.

The Sacroiliac Joints

The sacroiliac joints are covered with cartilage. The anterior aspect of the joint is lined with synovium. The joint surface is flat and uneven, and this irregularity helps lock the sacrum into the iliac bones. Ligaments support the front and back of the joint. There are dense interosseous **sacroiliac ligaments** (see Fig. 6.3) which further lock the sacrum to the iliac bones, limiting movement in all planes.

The **sacrospinous ligament** runs from the ischial spine to the sides of the sacrum and coccyx. It defines the inferior limit of the **greater sciatic foramen**.

The **sacrotuberous ligament** runs from the ischial tuberosity to the sides of the sacrum and coccyx. It defines the posterior limit of the **lesser sciatic foramen**.

The **iliolumbar ligament** runs from the transverse process of L5 to the posterior part of the iliac crest, further stabilizing the joint.

The pelvic muscles are shown in Figs. 6.4 and 6.5. At the level of the iliac crest the paired **psoas muscles** lie on

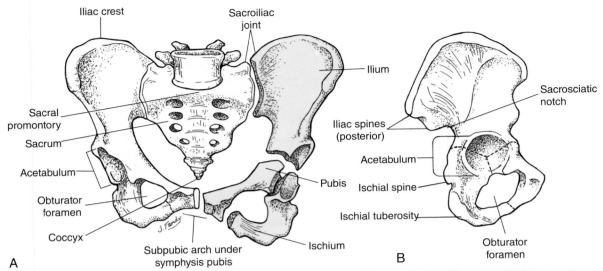

Fig. 6.1 Pelvic bones. (A) Inner and (B) outer surfaces. (From Perry S, et al. *Maternal Child Nursing Care*, 6th ed. Elsevier; 2018.)

either side of the spine (see Fig. 6.4). They descend anteriorly, fusing with the **iliacus muscle**, which arises from the inner surface of the ilium. The fused **iliopsoas muscle** passes anteriorly under the inguinal ligament to insert into the lesser trochanter of the femur.

The aponeurosis of the abdominal wall muscles inserts into the superior surface of the pubic bone. A thickening of the aponeurosis is the **inguinal ligament**, which runs from the pubic tubercle to the anterior superior iliac spine. All the muscles of the anterior, lateral and posterior abdominal walls insert, to some degree, into the iliac crest, inguinal ligament and pubic bone.

The gluteal region is an anatomical area located posteriorly in the pelvic girdle. The muscles of the gluteal region move the lower limb at the hip joint and can be broadly divided into a superficial group that abducts and extends the femur and deep group that laterally rotates the femur (see Fig. 6.6).

Hip muscles: see Figs. 6.6 and 6.7.

The superficial abductors and extenders comprise the glutei and tensor fascia lata (see Figs. 6.6 and 6.7).

The gluteus maximus is the largest, the most superficial and the most posterior gluteal muscle, covering the posterior part of the ilium and the sacroiliac joints. It arises from the posterior ilium, sacrum and coccyx, and inserts into the gluteal tuberosity of the femur. The gluteus medius and minimus are more anteriorly placed, the gluteus minimus being the smallest and the most deeply placed. Both originate from the gluteal surface of the ilium and insert into the greater trochanter; the gluteus medius inserts into the lateral part and the gluteus minimus inserts into the anterior part. The tensor fascia late is a small superficial muscle originating for the anterior superior iliac spine and inserts onto the lateral condyle of the tibia.

The **deep lateral rotators** comprise the piriformis, obturator internus, gemellus superior and inferior and quadratus femoris (see Figs. 6.6 and 6.7). These are smaller muscles that mainly rotate the femur laterally. They also stabilize and help to hold the femoral head in the acetabulum. The

piriformis is the most superior and arises from the anterior surface of the sacrum. It travels inferolaterally through the greater sciatic foramen, inserting into the greater trochanter. The obturator internus forms the lateral wall of the pelvic cavity. It originates from the pubis and ischium around the rim of the obturator foramen as well as from the inner surface of the obturator membrane. It passes through the lesser sciatic foramen, inserting into the greater trochanter. The superior gemellus arises from the ischial spine and the inferior gemellus arises from the ischial tuberosity. The gemelli are two small triangular muscles and insert into the greater trochanter. The quadratus femoris is a flat, square muscle and is the deepest of the gluteal muscles, located below the obturator and gemelli muscles. It arises from the lateral side of the ischial tuberosity and inserts into the intertrochanteric crest of the femur.

RADIOLOGY OF THE PELVIC RING

Plain Films (see Fig. 6.2)

Bony landmarks may be identified on plain radiograph (see Fig. 6.2). The sacral promontory and superior part of the pubic bone define the pelvic inlet and the **iliopectineal line**, running between and separating the true pelvis below from the false pelvis above. The sacroiliac joints are not optimally seen on the frontal view owing to their obliquity. Special views may be performed so that the X-ray beam passes through the joint to demonstrate it clearly.

Anomalous Lumbosacral Anatomy. Some variations of the lower lumbar spine and sacrum occur. The first sacral segment may be partially or completely separate – so-called **lumbarization** of the sacrum. Similarly, the lowest lumbar vertebra may be partially or completely fused to the sacrum – known as **sacralization** of the lumbar spine. The posterior elements of the lower lumbar vertebra or the sacral vertebrae may not be fused in some people, with no apparent sequelae.

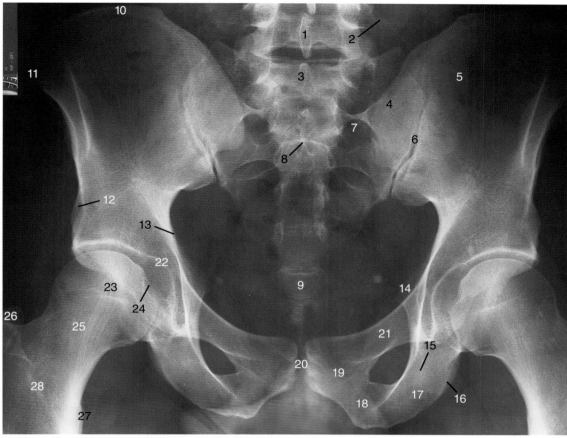

Fig. 6.2 Anteroposterior radiograph of the male pelvis.

1. Spinous process of L5 vertebra
2. Transverse process of L5 vertebra
3. Spinous process of the first sacral segment
4. Lateral sacral mass
5. Ilium
6. Sacroiliac joint
7. Sacral foramen of S2 vertebra
8. Spinous process of S3 vertebra
9. Coccyx: first segment of three
10. Iliac crest
11. Anterior superior iliac spine
12. Anterior inferior iliac spine
13. Pelvic brim
14. Ischial spine
15. Body of ischium
16. Ischial tuberosity
17. Ramus of ischium
18. Inferior pubic ramus
19. Body of pubic bone
20. Pubic symphysis
21. Superior pubic ramus
22. Acetabulum
23. Head of femur
24. Fovea
25. Neck of femur
26. Greater trochanter of femur
27. Lesser trochanter of femur
28. Intertrochanteric femur

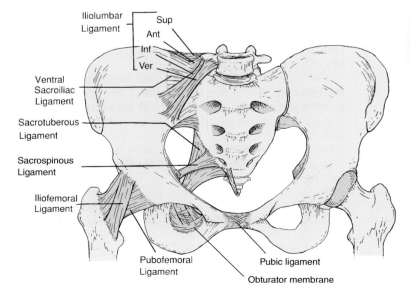

Fig. 6.3 The ligaments of the pelvic girdle from an anterior view. (Modified from Lee 2010, with permission. Lee D. *The Pelvic Girdle: An Integration of Clinical Expertise and Research*, 4th ed. Churchill Livingstone, Edinburgh; 2010.)

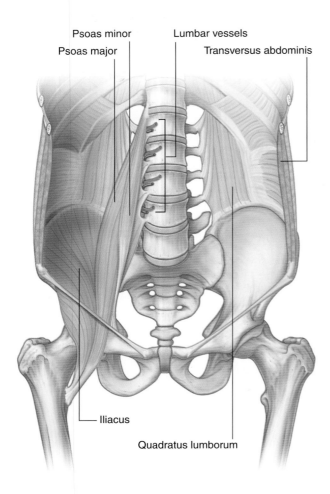

Psoas minor

Psoas major

Lumbar vessels

Transversus abdominis

Iliacus

Quadratus lumborum

Fig. 6.4 Muscles attached to the pelvis. (From Drake RL, Vogl AW, Mitchell AWM. *Gray's Anatomy for Students*, 5th ed. Elsevier; 2024.)

RADIOLOGY PEARL

In radiology reports it is important to identify disc levels clearly. In magnetic resonance imaging (MRI), the usual convention is to count from the lowest disc. The lowest full disc level is designated L5/S1 even if there are six lumbar vertebrae. This must be clearly stated in the report.

Differences between the Male and Female Pelvis.

- The muscle attachments are more prominent in the male.
- The pelvic inlet is heart-shaped in the male and oval in the female.
- The angle between the inferior pubic rami is narrow in the male and wide in the female.

Cross-Sectional Imaging

The muscles of the pelvis may be seen on computed tomography (CT) and MRIs (see Figs. 6.6 and 6.7).

The Pelvic Floor

This is a sling of muscles and fascia attached to the pelvic bones that closes the floor of the pelvis (see Fig. 6.8). It provides static support of the pelvic and abdominal contents against gravity and increased intra-abdominal pressure. It also permits active control of the urethra and rectal sphincters, permitting both continence and evacuation. The urethra and rectum in the male, and urethra, vagina and rectum in the female, pierce the pelvic floor. The floor is composed of two muscular layers, the **levator ani/coccygeus complex** and the **perineum**.

The **levator ani** muscle is the principal support of the pelvic floor. It provides muscular support for the pelvic organs and reinforces the urethral and rectal sphincters (see Fig. 6.9). The levator ani arises in a line from the posterior aspect of the superior ramus of the pubis to the ischial spine. Between these bony points, the muscle arises from the fascia covering the obturator internus muscle on the inner wall of the ilium in an arc known as the **tendinous arch** or **white line**. Its fibres sweep posteriorly, inserting into the **perineal body** (a fibromuscular condensation behind the urethra in males and behind the urethra and vagina in females) (see Fig. 6.10), the **anococcygeal body** (a fibromuscular condensation between the anus and coccyx) and the lowest two segments of the coccyx. The midline raphe (fusion) of the levator ani anterior to the coccyx is also known as the **levator plate**. The fibres of the levator ani sling around the prostate gland or vagina and rectum, blending with the **external anal sphincter**. The components of the levator ani are named according to their attachments. **Pubococcygeus**, the main component, arises from the inner surface of the body of the pubis and the tendinous arch running posteriorly to the sacrum and coccyx. The **puborectalis**, the thickest and most medial aspect of the muscular sling, arises from the inner surface of the pubic bone and forms a sling behind the anorectal junction. The **iliococcygeus** is the posterior part of the muscle and runs from the posterior tendinous arch and the ischial spine to the coccyx.

The **coccygeus muscle** is in the same tissue plane as the levator ani. It arises from the ischial spine and sacrotuberous ligament and inserts into the side of the coccyx and lower sacrum. It aids the levator ani in supporting the pelvic organs.

The **perineum** is the diamond-shaped space between the pubis, the ischial tuberosities and the coccyx. It is divided into two compartments by the **transverse perineal muscles**, which arise from the ischial tuberosity and run medially to insert into the perineal body.

The anterior compartment is the **anterior urogenital triangle**. The anterior urogenital triangle contains a tough sheet of fascia – the **perineal membrane** – which is pierced by the urethra and in females by the vagina as well. The external urethral sphincter is reinforced by this layer. Its **inferior surface** gives attachment to the bulb and crura of the penis or clitoris (**bulbocavernosus** and **ischiocavernosus**).

The posterior compartment is the **anal triangle**. It contains the anus and its sphincters, with the **ischiorectal fossa** on either side. The ischiorectal fossa is the space below and

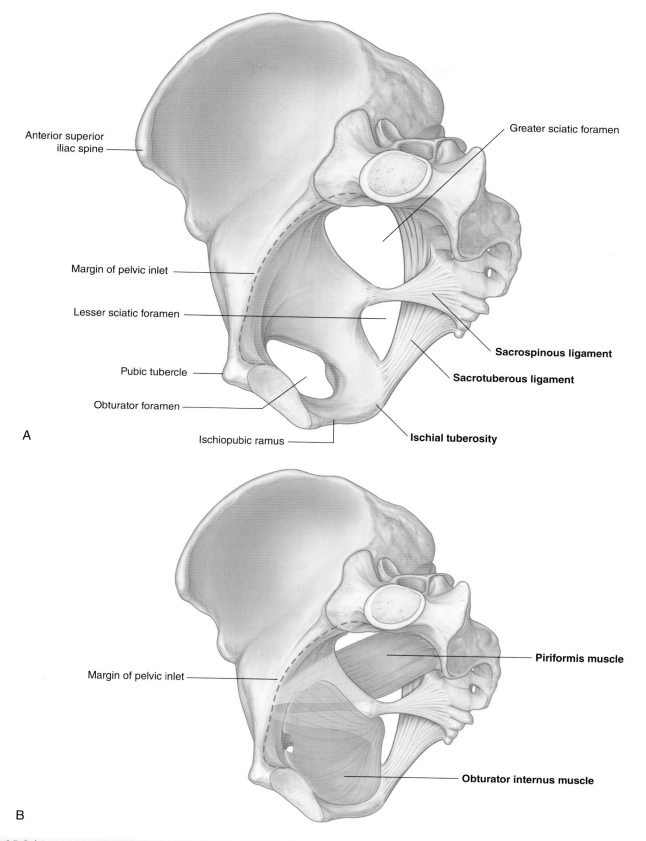

Fig. 6.5 Pelvic muscles and foramina as viewed from inside the pelvis. (From Drake RL, Vogl AW, Mitchell AWM. *Gray's Anatomy for Students,* 5th ed. Elsevier; 2024.)

A — Anterior superior iliac spine, Margin of pelvic inlet, Lesser sciatic foramen, Pubic tubercle, Obturator foramen, Ischiopubic ramus, Greater sciatic foramen, **Sacrospinous ligament**, **Sacrotuberous ligament**, **Ischial tuberosity**

B — Margin of pelvic inlet, **Piriformis muscle**, **Obturator internus muscle**

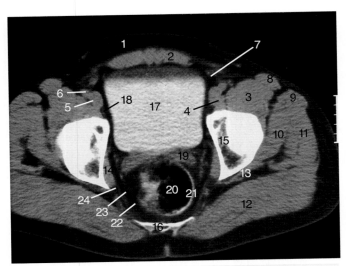

Fig. 6.6 Computed tomography scan of the pelvis: axial section through the male bladder. Intravenous contrast has been given. The full bladder displaces small bowel loops superiorly.

1. Subcutaneous fat
2. Rectus abdominis muscle
3. Iliacus muscle
4. Psoas muscle and tendon
5. External iliac vein
6. External iliac artery
7. Inferior epigastric vessels
8. Sartorius muscle
9. Tensor fasciae latae muscle
10. Gluteus minimus muscle
11. Gluteus medius muscle
12. Gluteus maximus muscle
13. Piriformis muscle
14. Obturator internus muscle
15. Acetabulum
16. Lower sacral segment: S4 vertebra
17. Bladder: full of layering urine and contrast
18. Perivesical fat
19. Seminal vesicle
20. Rectum containing air, faeces and contrast medium
21. Wall of rectum
22. Perirectal (mesorectal) fat
23. Perirectal fascia (known as Denonvillier's fascia anteriorly)
24. Pararectal fat

transverse perineal muscles, external anal sphincters, and the puborectalis and fibres from the external urethral sphincter – insert into this structure.

RADIOLOGY OF THE PELVIC FLOOR

Imaging of the pelvic floor is mostly required for evaluation of excessive pelvic floor laxity, leading to problems with urinary and bowel continence and rectal evacuation. This is most common in women as a result of childbirth injury.

Dynamic Proctography

Indirect imaging of the rectal floor is possible with defecating proctography, where the rectum, bladder and vagina are outlined with contrast and the subject is imaged in the lateral plane. Images are obtained at rest, during a 'clenching' or 'Kegel' manoeuvre to elevate the pelvic floor and during straining/evacuation to evaluate pelvic floor movement and the dynamics of rectal evacuation.

Magnetic Resonance Imaging (see Figs. 6.10, 6.11)

The muscles of the pelvic floor can be directly imaged by MRI. Pelvic floor movement can be assessed dynamically (see section on dynamic MRI).

The Sigmoid Colon, Rectum and Anal Canal

THE SIGMOID COLON

The sigmoid colon is extremely variable in length (12–75 cm, average 40 cm). It is covered by a double layer of peritoneum, supported on its mesentery, which is attached to the posterior and left lateral pelvic wall. It has the same sacculated pattern as the rest of the colon in young people. In older subjects it may appear featureless. The redundant sigmoid lies on the other pelvic structures.

Blood Supply (Figs 5.24, 5.25)

Arterial supply is from the inferior mesenteric artery via the sigmoid arteries, which join in the arterial cascade of the large bowel. Venous drainage is to the portal system via the inferior mesenteric vein.

Lymph Drainage

This is via the blood supply to preaortic nodes around the origin of the inferior mesenteric artery.

THE RECTUM (FIGS. 6.12, 6.13)

The rectum is about 12 cm long. It commences anterior to S3 and ends in the anal canal 2–3 cm in front of the tip of the coccyx. It forms an anteroposterior (AP) curve in the hollow of the sacrum. The rectum has no sacculations or mesentery. Its upper third is covered by peritoneum on its front and sides; its middle third has peritoneum on its anterior surface only, and its lower third has no peritoneum. The lower part of the rectum is dilated into the rectal ampulla. In the resting state, the mucosa of the rectum has three to

lateral to the posterior part of the levator ani and medial to the inner wall of the pelvis. It is bounded posteriorly by sacrotuberous ligaments and the gluteus maximus muscle, laterally by the fascia of the obturator internus muscle and anteriorly by the perineal body. It contains mainly fat and is of importance in pathological conditions of the rectum. The anococcygeal body extends from the anus to the coccyx posteriorly. It receives fibres from the anal sphincter and levator ani muscles.

The **perineal body** (see Fig. 6.10) is a pyramidal fibromuscular structure that is widest inferiorly. It lies between the anus and bulb of the penis in males and between the anus and posterior vagina in females. It is important in maintaining the integrity of the pelvic floor, especially in females. The perineal body is the central crossroad for the intersection of different layers of fascia and muscle insertions. All layers of pelvic floor muscles – the bulbospongiosus, the superficial

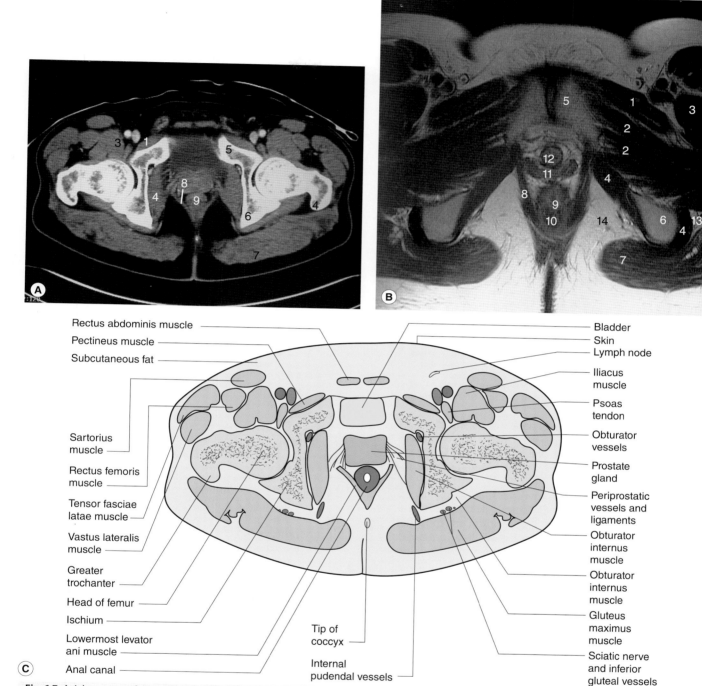

Fig. 6.7 Axial anatomy of the pelvis. (A) Computed tomography section through the male perineum. (B) Magnetic resonance section through the female perineum. (C) Axial diagram of the male perineum.

(A and B)
1. Pectineus muscle
2. Obturator externus muscle
3. Iliacus muscle
4. Obturator internus muscle
5. Pubic bone
6. Ischial tuberosity
7. Gluteus maximus muscle
8. Levator ani
9. Anus
10. External anal sphincter
11. Vagina
12. Urethra surrounded by external urethral sphincter
13. Sciatic nerve and inferior gluteal vessels
14. Ischiorectal fossa

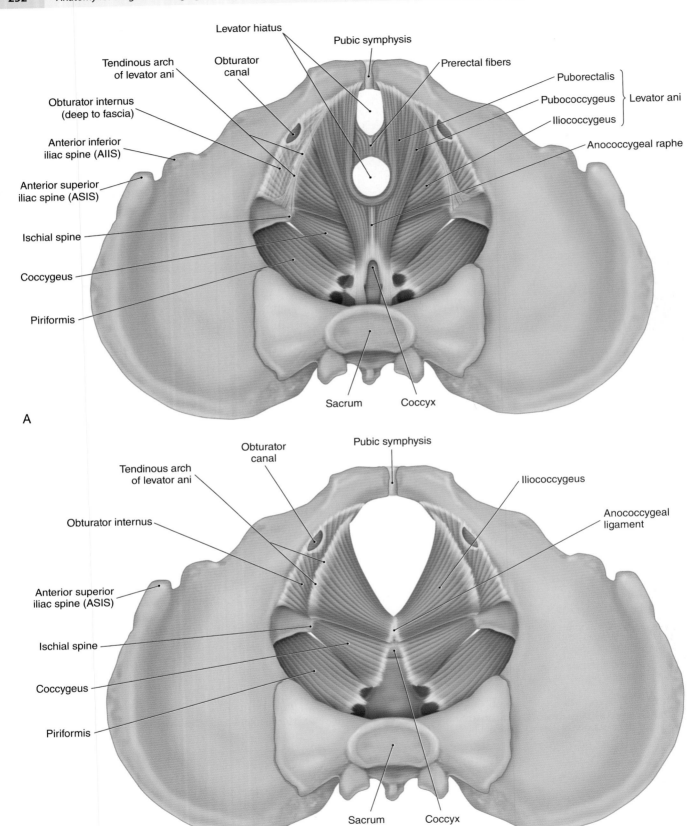

Fig. 6.8 Muscles of the pelvic floor. (A) Superficial view (B) Deep view. (From Muscolino JE. *The Muscular System Manual: The Skeletal Muscles of the Human Body*, 5th ed. Elsevier; 2024.)

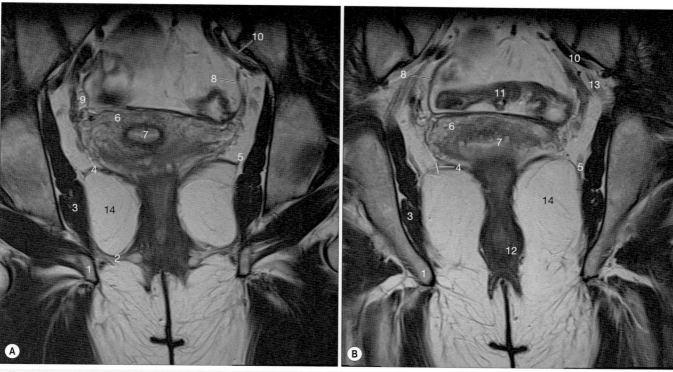

Fig. 6.9 Magnetic resonance image of the pelvis – coronal section through the male pelvis. (A) Anterior section. (B) Posterior section.

1. Ischium
2. Transverse perineal muscle
3. Obturator internus
4. Levator ani
5. Attachment of levator to the tendinous arch of the fascia overlying the obturator muscle
6. Body of the uterus
7. Endometrial cavity
8. Peritoneum reflected to the pelvic side wall

9. Uterine vessels entering the broad ligament (deep to fascia)
10. Internal iliac vessels
11. Sigmoid colon
12. Levator ani contributing to the external anal sphincter
13. Sciatic nerve
14. Ischiorectal fossa

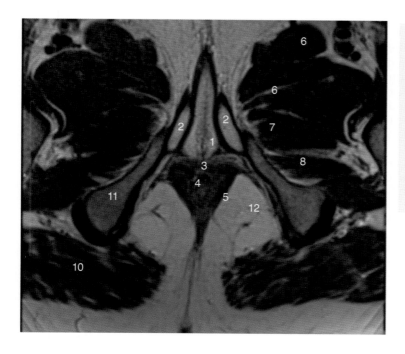

Fig. 6.10 T2-weighted axial magnetic resonance image through the perineal body in a male

1. Bulb of penis
2. Corpus cavernosum
3. Perineal body
4. External anal sphincter
5. Puborectalis
6. Adductor longus
7. Adductor brevis
8. Adductor minimis
9. Obturator externus
10. Gluteus maximus
11. Inferior pubic ramus
12. Ischioanal fossa

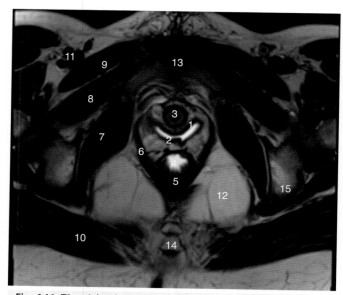

Fig. 6.11 T2-weighted axial magnetic resonance image through the female perineum.

1. Anterior wall of vagina
2. Posterior wall of vagina
3. External urethral sphincter
4. Anal canal
5. External anal sphincter
6. Puborectalis
7. Obturator internus
8. Obturator externus
9. Pectineus
10. Gluteus maximus
11. External iliac vessels
12. Ischioanal fossa
13. Pubic symphysis
14. Coccyx
15. Ischial tuberosity

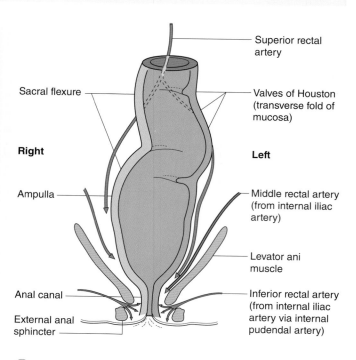

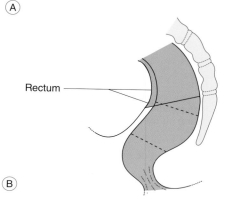

Fig. 6.12 The rectum. (A) Anterior view and blood supply. (B) Lateral view showing peritoneal reflections.

four longitudinal mucosal folds, known as the **columns of Morgagni**. The taenia coli fuse in the rectum. Some longitudinal shortening of the rectum occurs, giving the rectum a slight S shape. This creates three transverse mucosal folds – left, right and left from above downward. These are known as the **valves of Houston**. The lowest part of the rectum, known as the ampulla, relaxes to store faeces until defecation occurs.

Posteriorly are the sacrum and coccyx. Anteriorly, loops of small bowel and sigmoid colon lie in the peritoneal cul-de-sac between the upper two-thirds of the rectum and the bladder or uterus. The lower third is related to the vagina in the female and to the seminal vesicles, prostate and bladder base in the male.

The rectum is surrounded by **perirectal fat**. Fascia known as the **perirectal fascia** surrounds the perirectal fat, and lateral to the perirectal fascia is the **pararectal fat**. The perirectal fascia separates the seminal vesicles and prostate from the rectum anteriorly.

Mesorectal Fascia (see Fig. 6.13)

The mesorectal fascia is a continuation of the fascia of the sigmoid colon at the rectosigmoid junction and surrounds the rectum and perirectal fat, from the origin of the rectum to its lower end at the levator ani. The mesorectal fascia is continuous anteriorly with the rectovesical fascia (Denonvilliers fascia), separating rectum from bladder, seminal vesicles and prostate. Posteriorly it is fused with the presacral fascia (Waldeyer fascia). The mesorectum is perirectal fat surrounding the rectum and carries the vessels and nerves that supply it. It is delineated by the mesorectal fascia.

RADIOLOGY PEARL

The mesorectum and mesorectal fascia can be recognized on MRI. In rectal cancer surgery, the fascia forms the surgical resection margin, which aims for total mesorectal excision. Distance of tumour from the fascia is of prognostic significance.

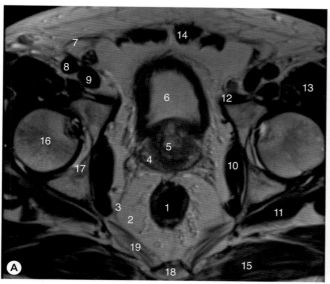 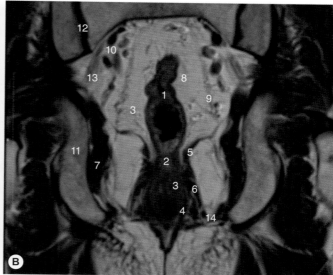

Fig. 6.13 (A) T2-weighted axial MRI rectum in a male. (B) T2-weighted coronal MRI in a male with visualization of the levator ani and anal sphincter.

(A)
1. Rectum
2. Mesorectal fat
3. Mesorectal fascia
4. Peripheral zone prostate
5. Transition zone prostate
6. Bladder
7. Spermatic cord
8. External iliac artery
9. External iliac vein
10. Obturator internus
11. Lower fibres piriformis
12. Pectineus
13. Iliopsoas
14. Rectus abdominus
15. Gluteus maximus
16. Femoral head
17. Acetabulum
18. Coccyx
19. Coccygeus

(B)
1. Rectum
2. Anal canal
3. Internal anal sphincter
4. External anal sphincter
5. Levator ani
6. Puborectalis
7. Obturator internus
8. Mesorectal fat
9. Mesorectal fascia
10. Internal iliac vessels
11. Iliac bone
12. Sacroiliac joint
13. Sciatic nerve
14. Transverse perineal muscles

THE ANAL CANAL (FIG. 6.14)

This is directed posteriorly almost at right angles to the rectum. It is a narrow, muscular canal. It has an **internal sphincter** of **involuntary muscle** and an outer **external sphincter** of **voluntary muscle**, which blends with the levator ani. The internal (smooth muscle, involuntary) sphincter occupies the upper two-thirds of the anal canal. The external (striated, voluntary) sphincter occupies the lower two-thirds. Thus, the sphincters overlap in the middle third, with the internal deep to the external. The junction of the rectum and anal canal is at the pelvic floor where the puborectal sling encircles it, causing its anterior angulation.

Anteriorly, the perineal body separates the anus from the vagina in the female and the bulb of the urethra in the male. Posteriorly, the anococcygeal body is between it and the coccyx, and laterally is the ischiorectal fossa.

The anal canal is lined by **mucous membrane** in its upper two-thirds and by **skin** in its lower third. The mucosa of the anal canal has several vertical folds.

Radiology of the Anal Canal (see Figs. 6.13, 6.14)

MRI, with its excellent soft-tissue resolution, is the imaging modality of choice for anal and perianal abnormalities.

The internal and external sphincters can be identified with the intersphincteric space between them. Images are obtained in the coronal plane and at right angles to the anal canal.

Endoanal ultrasound (Fig. 6.14B) is used to assess the integrity of the sphincters, mainly in the investigation of obstetric injuries. The internal and external sphincters, transverse perineal muscles and puborectalis can be evaluated longitudinally and axially at upper mid- and lower anal canal levels. The test can be combined with endoanal physiology using a pressure-sensitive catheter to assess pressures at rest and during squeezing and bearing-down manoeuvres. In the upper (proximal) anal canal, the U-shaped fibres of the puborectalis muscle may be identified sweeping posteriorly. At mid-anal canal level, where the internal anal sphincter (IAS) and external anal sphincter (EAS) overlap, the following layers can be identified

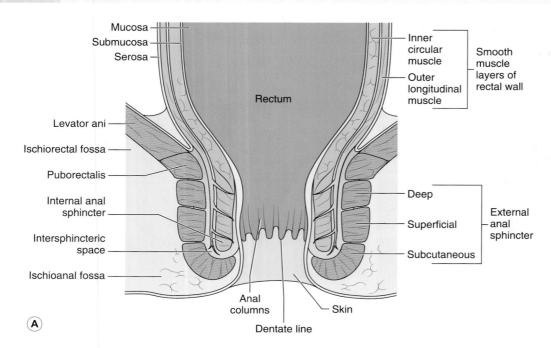

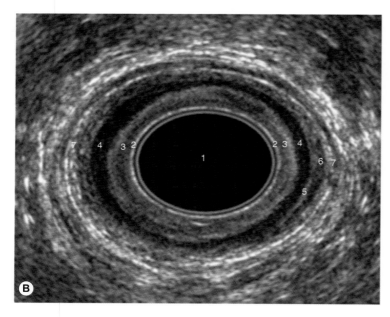

Fig. 6.14 (A) Anatomy of the anal canal and sphincter. (B) Endoanal ultrasound of the anal sphincter. (B)

1. Endoanal probe
2. Thin bright (echogenic) line is mucosal surface interface
3. Subepithelial tissue deep to mucosa – intermediate signal
4. Dark (hypoechoic) line is internal anal sphincter
5. Thin bright (echogenic) line is longitudinal muscle outside the internal anal sphincter
6. Intersphincteric space
7. Striated intermediate signal thick outermost layer is external anal sphincter

from inside out: the echogenic mucosa, the intermediate signal subepithelial layer (submucosa), the hypoechoic internal anal sphincter, a thin higher signal longitudinal muscle layer outside the IAS, the intersphincteric space outside the longitudinal muscle and the striated EAS outermost. At mid-canal level, the EAS forms a complete ring. At distal anal canal level, the IAS has terminated and only the EAS is seen. At this level the EAS does not form a complete ring.

Blood Supply (Figs. 6.15, 6.16)

The superior, middle and inferior rectal (haemorrhoidal) arteries form a rich submucous plexus supplying the

RADIOLOGY PEARL

The mucocutaneous junction is known as the dentate line or Hilton's white line. This defines a division between arterial supply and venous and lymphatic drainage.

Owing to the posterior angulation of the anal canal from rectum to skin, insertion of an endorectal ultrasound probe should be inserted with a slight anterior angulation, to follow the line of the anal canal.

rectum and anal canal. The superior rectal artery is a branch of the inferior mesenteric artery. The middle and inferior arteries arise from the internal iliac artery.

The plexus drains via a superior rectal vein to the inferior mesenteric vein and via middle and inferior veins to the internal iliac vein. This represents communication between the systemic and portal systems.

Lymph Drainage

The rectum and upper anal canal drain to **pararectal nodes**. Lymph from the upper rectum drains to preaortic nodes around the inferior mesenteric artery and from the lower rectum to internal iliac nodes. The lower anal canal drains to superficial inguinal nodes.

RADIOLOGY OF THE SIGMOID AND RECTUM

Plain Films (see Fig. 5.2)

The sigmoid colon and rectum may be identified on plain radiographs outlined by air, faeces or both. The sigmoid colon has a characteristic S-shaped curve as it joins the descending colon to the rectum, which lies anterior to the sacrum.

CT Colonography

The cleansed colon is insufflated with gas (CO_2) to achieve gaseous distension of the entire colon. Ingestion of a cup of contrast such as gastrografin the day before the scan coats residual stool and differentiates it from polyps (faecal tagging). This technique allows examination of the mucosa for polyps through a number of viewing techniques, including surface-rendered imaging, in which the interface between mucosa and air in the lumen is electronically rendered into a surface image of the lumen.

Computed Tomography

The rectum and perirectal tissues are readily assessed by CT. Detail is considerably enhanced by administration of intravenous contrast. The rectal wall, perirectal fat and fascia and pararectal fat may be identified. Images may be reconstructed in multiple planes.

Contrast Enema (see Fig. 5.23)

The best detail is achieved by using a double-contrast barium technique. A small amount of thick barium is used to coat the mucosa, followed by sufficient air or gas to distend the bowel. The patient is rotated to allow the barium and gas to reach and coat all regions of the colon from the rectum to the tip of the caecum. Various projections are required to open up the overlapping loops satisfactorily, especially sigmoid colon, splenic and hepatic flexures. This ensures adequate views of all the large bowel. The valves of Houston are the transverse mucosal folds or indentations of the rectum seen on an anterior view and are usually less than 5 mm thick. The appendix may be seen as a long, blind-ending structure in the right iliac fossa if it fills (50%–70%). Above the appendix, an indentation from the ileocaecal valve may be identified on the medial wall of the right colon. This demarcates the transition from caecum to ascending colon. The longitudinal columns of Morgagni are best identified after evacuation of barium, when the rectum is not distended. These normally measure 3 mm in width. The posterior impression of the pubococcygeal fibres of levator ani may be identified at the lower limit of the rectum. The anal canal may be identified if outlined with contrast after removal of the enema catheter; it makes an acute, posteriorly directed angle with the rectum (see also Chapter 5).

Magnetic Resonance Imaging (Fig. 6.13)

MRI is highly useful for assessing stage and evaluating the mesorectal fat in rectal tumours, both for operative planning and to assess response to chemoradiation. The anal sphincter can also be evaluated for pathology such

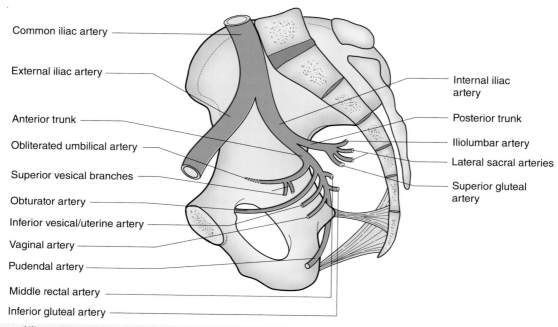

Common iliac artery
External iliac artery
Anterior trunk
Obliterated umbilical artery
Superior vesical branches
Obturator artery
Inferior vesical/uterine artery
Vaginal artery
Pudendal artery
Middle rectal artery
Inferior gluteal artery

Internal iliac artery
Posterior trunk
Iliolumbar artery
Lateral sacral arteries
Superior gluteal artery

Fig. 6.15 Internal iliac artery and branches.

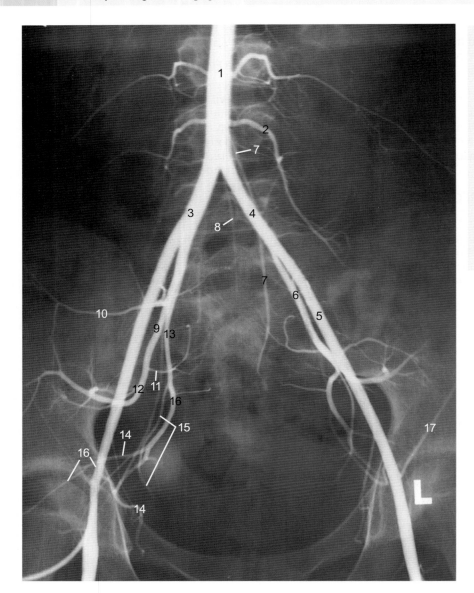

Fig. 6.16 Aortogram: external and internal iliac branches.

1. Abdominal aorta
2. Lumbar artery
3. Right common iliac artery
4. Left common iliac artery
5. Left external iliac artery
6. Left internal iliac artery
7. Inferior mesenteric artery
8. Median sacral artery
9. Posterior trunk of right internal iliac artery
10. Iliolumbar artery (branch of 9)
11. Lateral sacral artery (branch of 9)
12. Superior gluteal artery (branch of 9)
13. Anterior trunk of right internal iliac artery
14. Obturator artery (branch of 13)
15. Vesical artery (branch of 13)
16. Inferior gluteal artery (branch of 13)
17. Deep circumflex iliac artery

as perianal inflammatory conditions leading to fistulae and sinus tracts. It is important to image parallel to and at right angles to the plane of the structure being imaged. The rectum or anal canal are first identified on sagittal images. Coronal and axial images of the rectum and anal canal can then be acquired perpendicular and parallel to the structure being imaged. High-resolution T2 images are best for anatomy detail.

RADIOLOGY PEARL

Heavily T2-weighted sequences that saturate fat (fat becomes dark) and show fluid as bright signal are used to demonstrate sinus tracts and fistulae from the anal canal using a clock face terminology to describe their anal origin (12 o'clock being anterior midline and 6 o'clock being posterior midline).

Dynamic Imaging (Fig. 6.17)

The rectum can be evaluated dynamically during straining or evacuation with dynamic MRI or barium defecography. During defecation, the rectum and anus descend with the pelvic floor and the acute anorectal angle increases (straightens out) as contrast material is evacuated. During contraction of the pelvis the rectum and anus ascend, the anorectal angle narrows and a posterior impression is seen at the lower end of the rectum owing to the action of puborectalis.

Blood Vessels, Lymphatics and Nerves of the Pelvis

OVERVIEW OF THE ARTERIES AND VEINS

The aorta bifurcates at the level of L4 slightly to the left of midline. At the level of the iliac crest the common

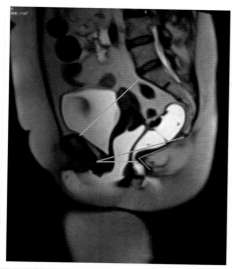

Fig. 6.17 Static T2-weighted sagittal image during a dynamic pelvic magnetic resonance image. There is contrast in the rectum and vagina (sterile gel). The cervix and posterior vaginal fornix are well delineated by gel. *Orange line:* Pelvic inlet – line drawn from superior pubic bone to sacral promontory. *Green line:* Pubococcygeal line – from inferior pubis to last sacrococcygeal joint, representing levator/coccygeus complex. *Yellow line:* H line (hiatus) – anteroposterior dimension of levator hiatus, inferior pubis to puborectalis impression at anorectal junction. *Blue line:* Anorectal angle – line drawn parallel to posterior wall of rectum intersects with line drawn parallel to posterior wall of anal canal. This angle should be 90 degrees or less. This angle opens during passage of contrast.

iliac arteries are slightly anterior to the common iliac veins. Both vessels are located on the medial border of the psoas muscle as this passes anteriorly into the pelvis. The vessels pass behind the distal ureters. At the level of the pelvic inlet the internal iliac vessels run medially and posteriorly towards the sciatic notch, and the external iliac vessels continue down on the medial aspect of the iliopsoas muscle, passing under the inguinal ligament to enter the thigh.

INTERNAL ILIAC ARTERY (FIGS. 6.15, 6.16)

This artery arises in front of the sacroiliac joint at the level of L5–S1 or the pelvic inlet. It descends to the sciatic foramen and divides into an anterior trunk, which continues down towards the ischial spine, and a posterior trunk, which passes back towards the foramen. Anterior to the internal iliac artery are the distal ureters, and in the female the ovary and fallopian tube. The internal iliac vein is posterior and the external iliac vein and psoas muscle are lateral. Peritoneum separates its medial aspect from loops of bowel.

Branches of the Anterior Trunk

These are as follows:

- **Umbilical artery**: Before birth, this carries blood from the internal iliac artery to the placenta. It is obliterated after birth to become the **medial umbilical ligament** and usually gives rise to one or several **superior vesical arteries**.

- **Obturator artery:** Passes anteriorly through the obturator foramen.
- **Inferior vesical artery** (male) or **uterine artery** (female): Supplies the seminal vesicles, prostate and fundus of the bladder in the male. In the female, the uterine artery runs medially in the broad ligament to supply the uterus, cervix and fallopian tubes, with branches to the ovary and vagina.
- **Middle rectal artery**: To inferior rectum with branches to the seminal vesicles, prostate or vagina.
- **Inferior gluteal artery**: Passes through the greater sciatic foramen to supply muscles of the buttock and thigh.
- **Internal pudendal artery**: Passes through the greater sciatic foramen and curves around the ischial spine or sacrospinous ligament to re-enter the pelvis through the lesser sciatic foramen, thence running anteriorly in the lateral aspect of the ischiorectal fossa. It passes through the pudendal canal (a fascial sheath derived from the obturator internus) in the lateral wall of this fossa, exiting the pelvis medial to the ischial tuberosity to form the dorsal and deep arteries of the penis or clitoris.

Branches of the Posterior Trunk

These are as follows:

- **Iliolumbar artery**: This ascends in front of the sacroiliac joint. It supplies the psoas and iliacus muscles and gives a branch to the cauda equina.
- **Lateral sacral arteries**: Usually two. These pass through the anterior sacral foramina and exit through the posterior sacral foramina. They supply the contents of the sacral canal and muscle and skin of the lower back.
- **Superior gluteal artery**: A continuation of the posterior trunk. This passes through the greater sciatic foramen to supply the muscles of the pelvic wall and gluteal region.

EXTERNAL ILIAC ARTERY (FIG. 6.16)

This runs downwards and laterally on the medial border of the psoas muscle to a point midway between the anterior superior iliac spine and the pubic symphysis. At this point it passes under the inguinal ligament to become the common femoral artery. In front of and medial to the vessel, the peritoneum separates it from loops of bowel. Its origin may be crossed by the ureter. In the female it is crossed by the ovarian vessels. In the male it is crossed by the testicular vessels and the ductus deferens. The external iliac vein is posterior to its upper part and medial to its lower part.

Branches of the Iliac Artery

Both branches arise just above the inguinal ligament and are as follows:

- Inferior epigastric artery: This runs superiorly on the posterior surface of anterior abdominal wall to enter the rectus sheath.
- Deep circumflex iliac artery: This ascends laterally to the anterior superior iliac spine behind the inguinal ligament and passes back on the inner surface of the iliac crest, supplying the abdominal wall muscles.

THE ILIAC VEINS (SEE FIG. 6.6)

The external and internal iliac veins accompany the arteries. At the groin, the veins lie medial to the arteries. As the veins ascend, they become posterior to the arteries. The upper part of the left common iliac vein then passes to the right behind its artery to form the inferior vena cava by joining with its fellow to the right of and slightly posterior to the aortic bifurcation.

RADIOLOGY OF THE ILIAC VESSELS (FIG. 6.16)
Conventional Angiography

In conventional angiography contrast medium is injected under high pressure into the distal aorta via a pigtail catheter, which is inserted retrogradely through a common femoral artery. Images may be acquired using plain radiographs or using digital subtraction angiography, where information is acquired on an image intensifier and processed by computer.

CT Angiography

CT following the administration of intravenous contrast gives excellent cross-sectional information about the vessels in the pelvis and their relationship to surrounding structures. Acquisition of images is timed to optimize the contrast opacification of the vessels being imaged. The arteries have a round, even calibre whereas the veins are usually larger and more oval-shaped in the supine position. Reconstructions in coronal, sagittal and various oblique planes may be performed on the raw data to display the vessels optimally.

Magnetic Resonance Imaging

MRI of the iliac vessels can be performed without contrast, although contrast images are diagnostically superior. The vessels may be imaged in any plane.

Venography

The veins are identified on cross-sectional contrast imaging. Direct contrast opacification of the internal iliac veins would require intraosseous injection of contrast into the bodies of the pubic bones.

Ultrasound

Ultrasound may also identify the common and external iliac vessels, although visualization is somewhat dependent on unpredictable factors such as bowel gas and body habitus of the subject. The vessels are seen as anechoic linear structures. Colour and pulsed-wave Doppler techniques demonstrate the direction of blood flow and facilitate identification.

THE LYMPHATICS

Lymph drainage runs in lymphatic channels related to the blood vessels. Three chains accompany the external iliac vessels – one (antero)lateral to the artery, one (postero)medial to the vein, and a variable middle chain anteriorly between the vessels. The obturator node is part of the middle chain. These chains drain to the common iliac and para-aortic nodes. The internal iliac lymph vessels and nodes drain to nodes around the common iliac and from here superiorly to the para-aortic nodes. Sacral nodes drain to the internal chain.

RADIOLOGY OF THE LYMPHATICS
Lymphangiography

Direct lymphangiography can be performed using an oily contrast agent (Lipiodol) which is imaged with fluoroscopy. Lymphangiography is the only radiological method available for direct demonstration of the lymphatics, and the technique has been adapted to allow visualization of the lymphatics on MRI, for example in the study of lymphedema. Lymphatics in the foot can be identified by injecting a blue dye into the web spaces of the toes. A 'blue' lymphatic vessel is cannulated with a very fine cannula and lipiodol contrast injected for direct fluoroscopic imaging. A gadolinium agent may be injected for MR lymphography. The external iliac, obturator, common iliac and para-aortic nodes can be demonstrated. The internal iliac nodes are not visualized using this method as lymph from the lower limb does not drain to the internal iliac nodes (see also lymphography in Chapter 5).

Cross-Sectional Imaging

Lymph nodes are visible on ultrasound, CT and MRI, especially when over 5 mm. Lymph nodes enhance after contrast, aiding their visibility. In a normal node, the cortex should be smooth and uniform, and is usually less than

3 mm. Although a lymph node can be over 2 cm in length, its short-axis measurement should not be more than 1 cm in the abdomen and pelvis. A normal lymph node typically has a fatty hilum and a uniform cortical thickness. Measurements on cross-sectional imaging are always made on the short axis.

In MRI, sequences that suppress fat signal allow easier identification of nodes on conventional MRI. In a further refinement, injected super magnetic iron oxide particles (USPIO) accumulate in the normal reticuloendothelial structure of the lymph nodes, causing them to appear dark (due to iron) on MRI.

IMPORTANT NERVES OF THE PELVIS

The anterior divisions (rami) of the nerve roots from L1 to S3 form the lumbosacral plexus of nerves. The rami divide into several cords which then combine to form the peripheral nerves to the pelvis and lower limbs. The lumbar plexus is formed within the psoas muscles and anterior to the transverse processes by the anterior divisions (rami) of L1–L4. The sacral plexus is formed by the anterior divisions of L4–S3 on the sacrum and piriformis muscle. The lumbar plexus is joined to the sacral plexus by the fourth and fifth anterior lumbar roots, which combine to form the lumbosacral trunk.

The **femoral**, **sciatic**, **obturator** and **pudendal** nerves pass through the pelvis to supply the lower limb. They are formed by the union of various cords of the **lumbosacral plexus** of nerves.

The obturator nerve (ventral divisions of anterior rami of L2–L4 nerves) descends through and emerges medial to the psoas muscle, runs along the lateral pelvic wall and through the upper part of the obturator foramen into the thigh. It passes behind the common iliac vessels to lie posteromedial to the common iliac vein in the pelvis. It provides sensory innervation of the medial thigh and motor innervation of some of the anterior and medial thigh muscles.

The femoral nerve (dorsal divisions of anterior rami of the L2–L4 nerves), surrounded by fat, descends through the psoas, emerging between the psoas and iliacus muscles, passing under the inguinal ligament into the thigh and dividing into anterior and posterior divisions. It is separated from the femoral artery under the inguinal ligament by a portion of psoas muscle. It supplies the skin and muscles in the anterior thigh.

The sciatic nerve (see Fig. 6.7) is the largest in the body. It is formed from the lumbosacral plexus on the anterior surface of the sacrum and piriformis from ventral divisions of L4–S3. It exits the pelvis through the greater sciatic foramen below the piriformis muscle into the gluteal region, then runs down into the back of the thigh. It supplies most of the skin of the leg, the posterior thigh muscles and muscles of the lower leg and foot.

The pudendal nerve arises from the ventral divisions of S2–S4. It passes between the piriformis and coccygeus, and exits the pelvis through the lower part of the greater sciatic foramen. It then hooks around the ischial spine/sacrospinous ligament and re-enters the pelvis through the lesser sciatic foramen, running anteriorly in the lateral aspect of the ischiorectal fossa on the medial surface of the obturator internus muscle. It is accompanied by the pudendal artery and vein in a sheath of obturator fascia called the **pudendal canal**. It supplies the external genitalia in both sexes as well as the urethral and anal sphincters.

Nerves to the organs of the pelvis are also derived from the lumbosacral plexus.

RADIOLOGY OF THE NERVES OF THE PELVIS

The nerves of the pelvis can be identified along with their vessels in CT and MRI. Thin-section, high-resolution images with fat saturation in the coronal plane are used to demonstrate the lumbosacral plexus.

RADIOLOGY PEARL

It is important to avoid the sciatic nerve in transgluteal procedures such as abscess drainage. Since it exits the pelvis through the greater sciatic notch running laterally, keeping the needle below the sacrospinous ligament and medial (close to the lateral border of the sacrum) will avoid risk of nerve injury.

The Lower Urinary Tract

THE PELVIC URETERS

The distal ureters enter the pelvis anterior to the psoas muscle. They pass anterior to the bifurcation of the iliac vessels and run on the lateral wall of the pelvis. Just in front of the ischial spine they turn medially to enter the posterolateral aspect of the bladder. The distal ureter lies above the seminal vesicles in the male and is crossed by the vas deferens. The distal ureter passes above the lateral vaginal fornix in the female, lateral to the cervix and below the uterine vessels in the broad ligament. The intravesical ureter tunnels obliquely through the bladder wall from lateral to medial. The bladder muscle exerts a sphincter-like action on the lower ureter.

THE BLADDER (FIG. 6.18)

This is a pyramidal muscular organ when empty. It has a triangular-shaped smooth-walled base posteriorly, the trigone. The ureters enter the posterolateral angles of the trigone and the urethra leaves inferiorly at the narrow **neck**, which is surrounded by the (involuntary) **internal urethral sphincter**. It has one superior and two inferolateral walls, which meet at an **apex** behind the pubic symphysis. The **trigone** is the triangular inner wall of the bladder between the ureteric and urethral orifices, as seen on cystoscopy. This part of the wall is smooth and relatively fixed; the remainder of the bladder wall is coarsely trabeculated by criss-cross muscle fibres and readily distensible.

The urethra is separated from the pubic symphysis by the **retropubic fatty space** (of **Retzius**), which

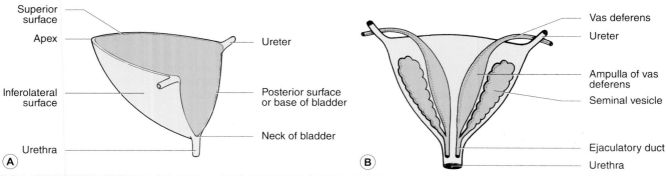

Fig. 6.18 Male bladder and urethra. (A) Lateral view. (B) Diagram of the prostatic urethra to show ducts.

contains a venous plexus as well as nerves and lymphatics. Perivesical fat surrounds the bladder. The obturator internus muscle is anterolateral and the levator ani muscle inferolateral to this. Superiorly it is loosely covered by peritoneum, which separates it from loops of small bowel and sigmoid colon.

In the female, the body of the uterus rests on its posterosuperior surface and the cervix and vagina are posterior, with the rectum behind. In the male, the termination of the vasa and the seminal vesicles are between the posterior bladder and the rectum. In the female, the bladder neck rests on the pelvic fascia. In the male it is fused with the prostate. The bladder is an extraperitoneal structure. As it fills it becomes ovoid and rises into the abdomen, stripping the loose peritoneum off the anterior abdominal wall and displacing the bowel loops superiorly. The peritoneum is loose over the bladder, except posteriorly where the ureters enter. The bladder is relatively fixed inferiorly via condensations of pelvic fascia, which attach it to the back of the pubis, the lateral walls of the pelvis and the rectum. Its continuity with the prostate in the male makes it even more immobile at this point owing to the strong puboprostatic ligaments. Bladder rupture may occur with fractures of the pelvis owing to the rigid fixture of the bladder neck to the pelvis. Such ruptures are usually extraperitoneal; extravasated urine may track into the scrotum and the anterior abdominal wall. Intraperitoneal rupture may occur in blunt trauma to the abdomen when the bladder is full. The point of tear is usually at the junction of the loose and the fixed peritoneum at the posterior part of the bladder.

RADIOLOGY PEARL

The ability of the full bladder to elevate and displace bowel loops is taken advantage of in pelvic ultrasound, where the full bladder provides an acoustic window through which the sound waves can travel.

Peritoneal Reflections (Fig. 6.19)

In the female, the peritoneum is reflected from the superior surface of the bladder to the anterior surface of the uterus. The peritoneum is further reflected from the posterior part of the uterus to the rectum, and this fold is known as the **pouch of Douglas** or **cul-de-sac**. In the male, the peritoneum is reflected off the bladder to the rectum, forming the **rectovesical pouch** or cul-de-sac. These peritoneal pouches usually contain loops of bowel.

Blood Supply

The bladder is supplied via the internal iliac artery, via superior and inferior vesical arteries. Venous drainage is via a venous plexus to the internal iliac vein.

Lymph Drainage

This is along the blood vessels mainly to the external iliac and thence to para-aortic nodes.

RADIOLOGY OF THE BLADDER

Plain Films

The bladder may be identified on plain films, especially when full. It is seen as a round, soft-tissue density surrounded by a lucent line of perivesical fat. It should be smooth and symmetrical.

RADIOLOGY PEARLS

- The urachus is a tubular structure in the fetus running from the apex of the bladder to the umbilicus that normally involutes before birth. It may persist to some degree as an elongated tubular extension of the anterior superior part of the bladder to the umbilicus. A persistent communication between the bladder and umbilicus is usually associated with other anomalies and presents at birth. The urachus may be partially open as a sinus from the bladder, or a cyst may be found along its course if it fails to close completely. A vesicourachal diverticulum may occur at the site of the origin of the urachus. These partial remnants are normally incidental and asymptomatic but may become infected or develop malignancy.
- The median umbilical ligament is a persistent fibrous remnant of the urachus and may be seen outlined by air in the pneumoperitoneum or may be identified incidentally on CT or MRI.

Contrast Studies

The bladder may be filled with contrast either after intravenous injection in intravenous urography or retrogradely via the urethra. The corrugations of the bladder wall are

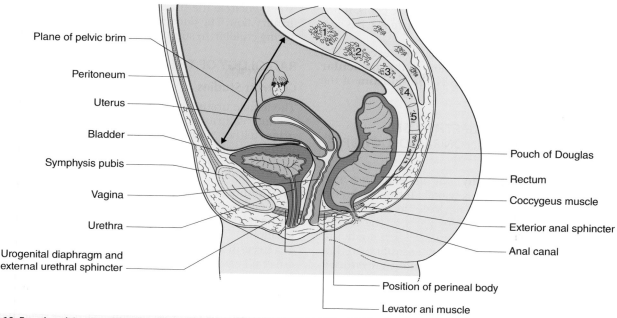

Plane of pelvic brim
Peritoneum
Uterus
Bladder
Symphysis pubis
Vagina
Urethra
Urogenital diaphragm and external urethral sphincter

Pouch of Douglas
Rectum
Coccygeus muscle
Exterior anal sphincter
Anal canal
Position of perineal body
Levator ani muscle

Fig. 6.19 Female pelvis – sagittal view of the female pelvis and peritoneal reflections.

seen. The smooth impression of the uterus may be seen posterosuperiorly. The prostatic impression is seen inferiorly in the male. Irregular collections of contrast may be trapped between muscle fibres after micturition.

Cross-Sectional Imaging

The bladder is readily identified by ultrasound, CT and MRI, especially when distended. Ultrasound is best for assessing its internal anatomy. CT and MRI have the advantage of also being able to assess the surrounding structures.

The Male Urethra (Fig. 6.20)

The male urethra runs from the **internal urethral sphincter** at the neck of the bladder to the **external urethral orifice** at the tip of the penis. In radiological terms it may be divided into posterior and anterior parts. The posterior urethra comprises the prostatic and membranous urethra and the anterior part comprises the bulbous and penile urethra.

The **prostatic urethra** traverses the ventral part of the prostate and is the widest part. It is about 3 cm long. It has a longitudinal midline ridge known as the prostatic crest. Several prostatic ducts open into the prostatic sinus, a shallow longitudinal depression on either side of the prostatic crest. The prostatic crest bears a prominence called the **verumontanum** (also known as the **seminal colliculus**). A small blindly ending sinus – the **prostatic utricle** – opens on to this (this is the vestigial remnant of the uterovaginal canal in the embryo.) On either side of it, or just within the prostatic utricle, the **ejaculatory ducts** open. These are the common terminations of the seminal vesicles and the vasa. The lower part of the prostatic urethra is relatively immobile as the prostate is fixed here by the puboprostatic ligaments.

The **membranous urethra** is so-called as it traverses the **membranous urogenital diaphragm**, which forms

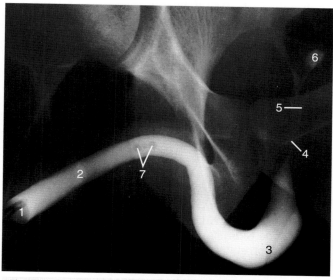

Fig. 6.20 Retrograde urethrogram in the male: oblique view.

1. Balloon of catheter in the navicular fossa
2. Penile urethra
3. Bulbous urethra
4. Membranous urethra
5. Impression of the verumontanum in the prostatic urethra
6. Filling of the utricle (not usually seen)
7. Air bubbles in contrast

the (voluntary) **external urethral sphincter**. It is the narrowest part of the urethra and is about 10–15 mm long. The urethra is quite immobile at this point. A bulbourethral gland is present at either side at this point – **Cowper's gland**. The membranous urethral length is of significance in prostate surgery and can be measured on MRI (see also prostatic MRI).

The **bulbous urethra** lies in the bulb of the penis. It has a localized dilatation called the **intrabulbar fossa**. It is surrounded by the corpus spongiosum.

The **penile urethra** is long and narrow, except for a localized dilatation at its termination – the **navicular fossa**. It is surrounded by the **corpus spongiosum** of the penis.

RADIOLOGY OF THE MALE URETHRA (SEE FIG. 6.20; SEE ALSO SECTION ON RADIOLOGY OF THE PENIS)

In **retrograde urethrography**, the male urethra may be outlined by contrast, which is usually introduced retrogradely via a soft catheter in the navicular fossa. The intrabulbar fossa is seen and the various parts of the urethra are recognized by position and calibre. The verumontanum appears as a posterior filling defect in the prostatic urethra, and the utricle may occasionally fill. In **voiding cystourethrography** contrast in the bladder is voided, outlining the urethra from above. The technique allows better distension of the posterior urethra, which is difficult to achieve with the retrograde approach. **Penile sonourethrography** may be performed with retrograde instillation of saline into the urethra, or during voiding where the distal urethra is clamped with a device or manually. This technique has the advantage of allowing evaluation of all of the structures of the penis.

The urethra may also be identified on MRI (see the section on radiology of the penis).

The Female Urethra

This is 4 cm long. It extends from the **internal urethral sphincter** at the bladder neck through the urogenital diaphragm, ending at the **external urethral meatus** in the cleft between the labia minora (vestibule). The urethra lies on the anterior vaginal wall and curves obliquely downward and anteriorly, posterior to the pubic symphysis. The external urethral sphincter opens anterior to the vaginal opening and approximately 2.5 cm posterior to the clitoris. Multiple tiny **urethral glands** open into the lower urethra draining via **Skene's tubules**. These glands are homologous to the prostate in the male.

URINARY CONTINENCE IN THE FEMALE

There are no true anatomical sphincters in the female urethra. The decussation of vesical muscle fibres at the urethrovesical junction acts as the **involuntary internal urethral sphincter** and is the primary continence mechanism. Involuntary muscles of the urethral wall also provide resistance, keeping the urethra closed except during micturition. There are three muscle layers – innermost longitudinal smooth muscle, middle layer circular smooth muscle and outermost striated muscle (also known as the rhabdosphincter). The outermost layer is the most important urethral continence mechanism. The **external urethral sphincter** is at the urogenital diaphragm but is less well developed than that in the male. It is composed of **voluntary** muscle fibres arising from the inferior pubic ramus,

which encircle the urethra and allow voluntary arrest of urinary flow. The pudendal nerve (which may be damaged during childbirth) supplies the external urethral sphincter.

RADIOLOGY OF THE FEMALE URETHRA

Contrast Studies

The female urethra may be evaluated dynamically during voiding contrast cystourethrography. Contrast-opacified urine (either after intravenous excretion or retrograde instillation of contrast-saline) outlines the urethra.

Ultrasound

The urethra may also be imaged with perineal, endovaginal (EV), endorectal or endourethral ultrasound. It is difficult to see on transabdominal ultrasound because of its retropubic location.

Three-dimensional ultrasound using a perineal transducer allows acquisition of an unlimited number of ultrasound sections, and this data volume may then be viewed in any plane. This is an advantage for urethral imaging because of its obliquity. On 3D EV or endorectal ultrasound the urethra is target-like in cross-section. The outer striated muscle layer is dark (echopoor), while the inner urothelium and smooth muscle layers appear bright (echogenic). The length of the striated layer (rhabdosphincter) can be measured. At the level of the bladder neck, echogenic urothelium is surrounded by an irregular echopoor ring corresponding to the internal urethral sphincter. The external urethral sphincter is not reliably identified as a discrete structure.

Magnetic Resonance Imaging (Fig. 6.21)

On T2-weighted or postcontrast T1-weighted images, it has a target-like appearance in the axial plane. On axial T2-weighted images the muscular layers can be appreciated – there is an outer low-signal striated muscular layer, a middle intermediate-signal layer corresponding to smooth muscle and submucosa, and an inner low-signal layer corresponding to mucosa. Anteriorly, the retropubic space is heterogeneously bright (fat) with dark (hypointense) tubular blood vessels.

The Male Reproductive Organs

THE PROSTATE GLAND (FIGS. 6.22, 6.23)

This gland is shaped like an upside-down truncated cone and surrounds the base of the bladder and the proximal (prostatic) urethra, extending inferiorly to the urogenital diaphragm and external sphincter. It has:

- A base related to the bladder above.
- An apex inferiorly sitting on the pelvic (urogenital) diaphragm.
- An anterior wall which is separated from the pubic symphysis by the retropubic fatty space (of Retzius).
- A posterior wall related to the rectum behind.
- Two inferolateral walls related to the muscles of the pelvic side wall and the anterior part of levator ani on either side.

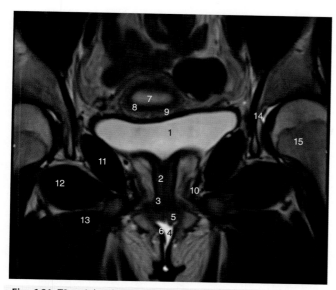

Fig. 6.21 T2-weighted coronal magnetic resonance image showing the urethra.

1. Bladder
2. Urethra
3. External urethral sphincter
4. Gel in the vestibular fossa
5. Labia minora
6. Labia majora
7. Endometrium
8. Junctional zone
9. Myometrium
10. Puborectalis fibres of the levator ani
11. Obturator internus
12. Obturator externus
13. Adductor magnus
14. Acetabulum
15. Femoral head

The urethra enters the upper part of the prostate near its anterior surface and then assumes a somewhat more central position before curving slightly anteriorly again to exit at the apex of the gland.

Posterosuperiorly are the seminal vesicles. Fascia known as **Denonvillier's fascia** separates the prostate and seminal vesicles from the rectum. The **puboprostatic ligament** runs from the antero inferior part of the gland to the pubic bone and provides support. The prostate gland does not have a true capsule but is surrounded by a **fibrous sheath** derived from pelvic fascia and continuous with the puboprostatic ligaments. The **prostatic venous plexus** lies deep to the fibrous sheath.

According to traditional anatomy, the gland is described as having five lobes, which are not well demarcated from one another: anterior, posterior, median and two lateral.

The five lobes can only be differentiated in the fetus up to 20 weeks' gestation. In the mature gland only three lobes – two lateral and one median – can be distinguished, with the fibromuscular stroma anteriorly. These lobes may be palpated through the rectum.

The **rectoprostatic fascia (Denonvillier's fascia)** separates the prostate and seminal vesicles from the rectum and is an important surgical plane. The neurovascular bundles normally run craniocaudally along the posterolateral aspect of the gland anterior to this fascial plane.

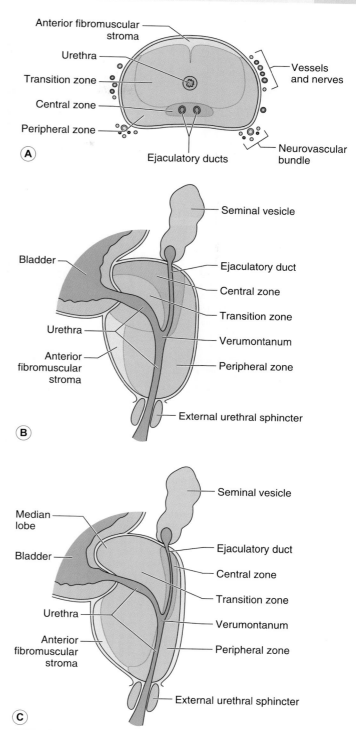

Fig. 6.22 | Prostate gland: zonal anatomy in a young adult in the axial (A) and sagittal (B) plane. With ageing, the transition zone hypertrophies, compressing the peripheral zone (C). The central and transition zones (central gland) cannot be distinguished radiologically.

ZONAL ANATOMY OF THE PROSTATE (FIG. 6.22)

The gland may more usefully be described based on its internal architecture as having three glandular zones with the nonglandular isthmus or fibromuscular stroma anteriorly:

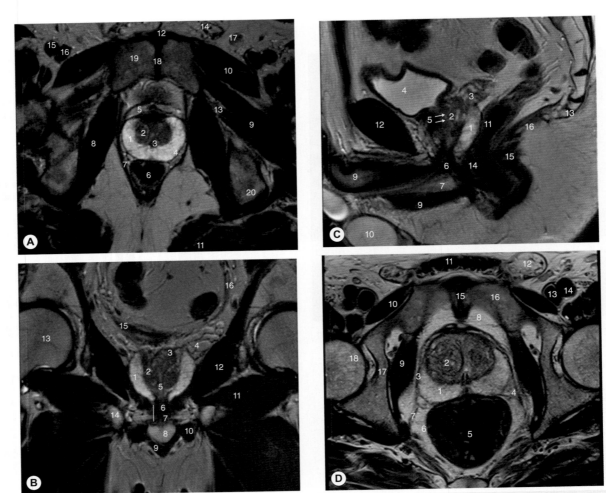

Fig. 6.23 (A) T2-weighted axial prostate magnetic resonance image (MRI). (B) T2-weighted coronal prostate MRI. (C) T2-weighted sagittal prostate MRI. (D) T2-weighted axial MRI of a prostate with benign prostatic hyperplasia.

(A)
1. Peripheral zone of the prostate
2. Transition zone of the prostate
3. Prostatic urethra level verumontanum
4. Prostate capsule
5. Denonvilllier's fascia
6. Lower rectum
7. Levator ani
8. Obturator internus
9. Obturator externus
10. Pectineus
11. Gluteus maximus
12. Rectus abdominis
13. Obturator foramen
14. Inguinal canal
15. Common femoral artery
16. Common femoral vein
17. Inguinal lymph node
18. Pubic symphysis
19. Pubic bone
20. Ischial tuberosity

(B)
1. Peripheral zone of the prostate
2. Transition zone of the prostate
3. Central zone of the prostate
4. Seminal vesicles
5. Prostatic urethra
6. Membranous urethra
7. External urethral sphincter
8. Corpus spongiosum
9. Bulbospongiosus
10. Ischiocavernosus
11. Obturator externus
12. Obturator internus
13. Femoral head
14. Inferior pubic ramus
15. Bladder trigone

16. Ureter
Line: Membranous urethral length (MUL) (C)
1. Peripheral zone of the prostate
2. Transition zone of the prostate
3. Seminal vesicles
4. Bladder
5. Urethra
6. External urethral sphincter
7. Corpus spongiosum
8. Corpus cavernosum
9. Bulbospongiosus
10. Testicle
11. Rectum
12. Pubic symphysis
13. Coccyx
14. Position of the perineal body
15. Puborectalis
16. Levator plate
(D)
1. Peripheral zone of prostate
2. Transition zone of prostate with benign prostatic hyperplasia
3. Capsule of prostate
4. Neurovascular bundle
5. Rectum
6. Mesorectal fat
7. Mesorectal fascia
8. Retropubic space
9. Obturator internus
10. Pectineus
11. Rectus abdominis
12. Inguinal canal
13. External iliac vein
14. External iliac artery
15. Pubic symphysis
16. Pubic bone
17. Acetabulum
18. Femoral head

- The **peripheral zone**, which contains about 70% glandular tissue
- The **central zone**, which contains 25% glandular tissue
- The **transition zone**, which contains 5% glandular tissue in the normal young prostate

The central zone surrounds the urethra above the level of the ejaculatory ducts which pass through it, and roughly corresponds to the median lobe. The transition zone is a narrow area **surrounding the urethra** inside the central zone at the level of the ejaculatory ducts and verumontanum. The peripheral zone makes up the rest, occupying the posterior, lateral and apical parts of the gland. The peripheral zone is separated from the central and transition zones of the gland by a fibrous layer. The prostate is contained within a sheath or pseudo capsule derived from pelvic

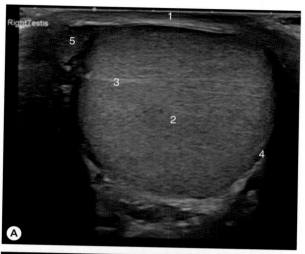

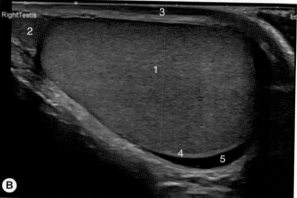

Fig. 6.26 (A) Transverse view of the testis. (B) Longitudinal view of the testis with visualization of the epididymal head.

(A)
1. Scrotal skin
2. Testis
3. Mediastinum testis
4. Tunica albuginea
5. Epididymal head
(B)
1. Testis
2. Epydidimal head
3. Scrotum
4. Tunica albuginea
5. Fluid in scrotal sac

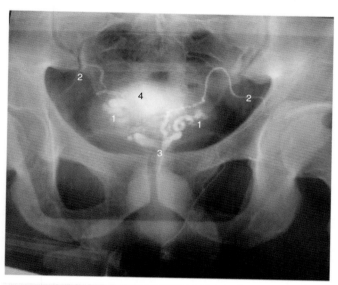

Fig. 6.24 Vasogram. An incision is made in the scrotum with contrast administered through cannulation of the vas deferens.

1. Seminal vesicles
2. Vas deferens
3. Prostatic urethra
4. Bladder

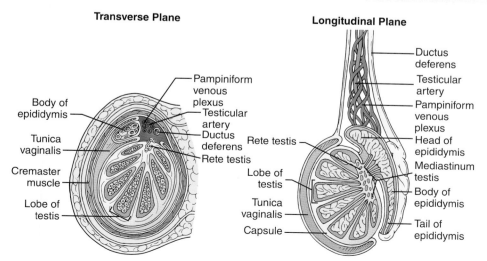

Fig. 6.25 Normal testicular anatomy. Cross sectional anatomy of the testicle in transverse (A) and longitudinal planes (B). (From Soni NJ, Arntfield R, Kory P. *Point of Care Ultrasound*, 2nd ed. Elsevier; 2020.)

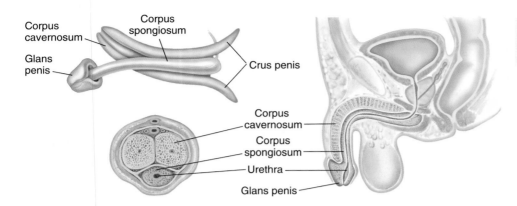

Fig. 6.27 Anatomy of the penis. (From Flynn JA, et al. *Seidel's Guide to Physical Examination: An Interprofessional Approach*, 10th ed. Elsevier; 2023.)

fascia. This sheath is composed of smooth muscle, skeletal muscle and loose connective tissue, and is **penetrated** by numerous vessels and nerves. This is a layer of concentrically orientated fibromuscular tissue that is inseparable from the prostatic stroma histologically, but which contains no glandular elements. This layer is absent at the apex.

The anterior fibromuscular stroma is continuous with the detrusor superiorly and blends with the striated levator muscle and puboprostatic ligaments inferiorly.

Neurovascular Bundles

The cavernosal nerves and prostatic neurovascular supply generally lie on the posterolateral surface of the prostate in a discernible round neurovascular formation, and mediate erectile function and continence. They can be identified on MRI. However, the structures are not always organized into a clearly discernible bundle. In prostate cancer surgery, preservation of the neurovascular bundles is a consideration for the preservation of erectile function and continence.

RADIOLOGY PEARLS

- With ageing, the transition zone hypertrophies and the central zone atrophies.
- The relevance of the zonal anatomy is that more than 70% of prostate cancers occur in the peripheral zone of the gland. Thus imaging of the prostate for local staging of cancer and image-guided biopsies for diagnosis focus on this region.
- Benign prostatic hypertrophy affects the transition zone and, when pronounced, occupies most of the volume of the enlarged prostate, compressing the peripheral and central zones. The hypertrophied transition zone may extend superiorly into the bladder as a 'median lobe'. The median (also called middle) lobe is a cone-shaped part of the prostate between the ejaculatory ducts and the urethra at the upper posterior prostate.

THE SEMINAL VESICLES (FIGS. 6.22–6.24)

These are paired sacculated diverticula that lie transversely behind the prostate and store seminal fluid. These convoluted tubes narrow at their lower end to fuse with the vas deferens to become the **ejaculatory ducts**.

Blood Supply of the Prostate Gland and Seminal Vesicles

Blood supply is from the internal iliac arteries, mainly via branches from the inferior vesical artery. Venous drainage is via the **prostatic venous plexus** (**Santorini venous plexus**), which surrounds the sides and base of the gland, to the internal iliac veins. The prostatic venous plexus communicates posteriorly with the **internal vertebral venous plexus**, providing a potential route for the spread of prostatic cancers.

Nerve Supply

Innervation is from parasympathetic fibres from the pelvic splanchnic nerves (S2–S4).

Lymph Drainage

This is via lymphatic channels that accompany blood vessels to internal iliac and sacral nodes. Positron emission tomography scanning with radiolabelling of prostate specific membrane antigen (PSMA) has demonstrated that lymph drainage may also occur to perirectal nodes.

RADIOLOGY OF THE PROSTATE GLAND AND SEMINAL VESICLES (FIG. 6.23)

Ultrasound

The prostate gland is most frequently imaged by transrectal ultrasound (usually to direct biopsy). This is achieved with an ultrasound probe in the rectum. Inbuilt linear and sector scanners allow longitudinal and transverse imaging of the gland, which lies immediately anteriorly. The prostate gland yields uniform, low-level echoes. The seminal vesicles can be identified as sacculated structures above and lateral to the base of the gland. The urethra is seen as an anechoic central structure with a thin echogenic wall. It is surrounded by a relatively hypoechoic area composed of the smooth muscle, the periurethral glands and the transition zone (in the normal nonhypertrophied gland). The central zone is that part of the gland surrounding and above the ejaculatory ducts. The ejaculatory ducts may sometimes be identified forming a triangular hypoechoic 'beak' as they project into the central zone. The posterolateral peripheral zone can generally be identified and may be separated from the lateral aspect of the gland by a hypoechoic line. The prostatic 'capsule' or outer fibro-muscular layer is not well defined, and prominent vessels in the periprostatic soft tissues may blend with the gland sonographically, making its margin difficult to define. The peripheral zone is isoechoic and the central part of the prostate is relatively hypoechoic, but may contain hyperechoic foci or areas of calcification. Because the anatomical zones cannot be truly differentiated on imaging, it has been suggested that the peripheral zone be referred to as the 'outer gland' and the inner part of the prostate be referred to as the 'central gland'.

Prostatic MRI

MRI is an excellent method of imaging the prostate. It can be adequately imaged at 1.5 Tesla but there is better detail on 3 T imaging. The zonal anatomy is seen on the T2-weighted image. The peripheral zone is of uniformly high intensity and contrasts with the intermediate signal intensity of the transition and central zones. In younger subjects it comprises most of the gland, surrounding the transition zone posteriorly and laterally, extending anteriorly on either side of the transition zone, and it occupies most of the apex of the gland, blending inferiorly with the external urethral sphincter. As the transition zone hypertrophies and compresses the peripheral zone with ageing and with benign prostatic hyperplasia, a low-signal band separates them on T2-weighted images. The central zone can be seen on coronal imaging as a 'seagull-shaped' or wedge-shaped area of low signal at the base between the peripheral and transition zones. The superior extent of the central zone lies above the superior extent of both the transition and peripheral zones. It surrounds the ejaculatory ducts and converges centrally onto the verumontanum. In younger subjects the central zone may not be distinguishable from the transition zone, but as the transition zone hypertrophies it takes on a characteristic appearance and is of higher signal intensity than the low-signal central zone.

The periprostatic venous plexus is of high signal intensity on T2-weighted images, as is the fat in the retropubic space of Retzius, contrasting with the low-intensity puboprostatic ligament and pubococcygeus muscle. The anatomical outer 'capsule' is also seen as a low-signal outer band. Fat-suppressed T2-weighted images improve contrast between the peripheral zone and the surrounding fat. Denonvillier's fascia may be identified as a low-intensity line between the posterior aspect of the prostate and the rectum.

The neurovascular bundles, when identifiable, are identified running posterolaterally, entering the gland as hypointense structures outlined by high-signal periprostatic fat.

The seminal vesicles are seen posterosuperior to the prostate and bladder on axial and sagittal images.

The prostatic urethra is of relatively high signal intensity on T2-weighted images. It enters the gland anteriorly from the bladder neck, curving slightly posteriorly as it passes through the gland, before curving anteriorly and exiting the prostate as membranous urethra. It is surrounded by an inner circular layer and an outer longitudinal layer of smooth muscle. The peripheral zone of the prostate may extend inferior to the lower end of the prostatic urethra. The urethra may be displaced and compressed by asymmetric hypertrophy of the transition zone.

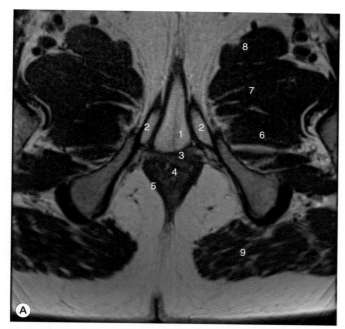
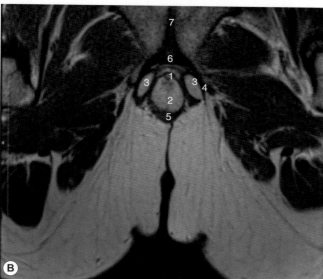

Fig. 6.28 (A) T2-weighted axial magnetic resonance image (MRI) through the male perineum and penis. (B) T2-weighted coronal MRI through the pubic symphysis and bulb of penis.

(A)
1. Corpus spongiosum
2. Corpus cavernosum
3. Perineal body
4. Anus
5. Levator ani
6. Adductor minimus
7. Adductor longus
8. Adductor brevis
9. Gluteus maximus
10. Ischial tuberosity

(B)
1. Urethra
2. Corpus spongiosum
3. Corpus cavernosum
4. Tunica albuginea
5. Bulbospongiosus
6. Inferior pubic ligament
7. Pubic symphysis

Computed Tomography

On CT the gland is seen as a round structure of soft-tissue density inferior to the bladder. Its margin is well seen where outlined posteriorly by fat, and the seminal vesicles are identified as convoluted structures above the prostate between the bladder and rectum. Periprostatic vessels are frequently identified in the surrounding fat. The zonal anatomy is not distinguished, however, and at the apex where it abuts the lower fibres of the levator and is surrounded by the external urethral sphincter, the prostatic margins cannot be distinguished.

Vasography (injection of contrast into the vas) (see Fig. 6.24), occasionally performed in the investigation/treatment of male infertility, fills the seminal vesicles and outlines the ejaculatory ducts, outlining any blockage. This is performed by cutting down on the vas in the groin and injecting contrast retrogradely.

THE TESTIS, EPIDIDYMIS AND SPERMATIC CORD

The Testis (Figs. 6.25, 6.26)

This is an oval sperm-producing gland that is described as having an upper and lower pole (Fig. 6.25). It is suspended by the spermatic cord in the scrotal sac and is covered by a tightly adherent fibrous capsule called the **tunica albuginea**. The tunica is thickened posteriorly and forms a fibrous septum known as the **mediastinum testis**. Multiple fibrous septae divide the testis into lobules. The tunica albuginea, mediastinum and fibrous septae connect to form the support and internal architecture of the testis. Some 250–400 lobules contain sperm-producing cells, which are drained by highly coiled **seminiferous tubules**. The seminiferous tubules then converge on the mediastinum testis, forming 20 or so larger ducts. These enter the mediastinum testis, forming a network of channels within the stroma known as the **rete testis** (rete anastomosing network). From here, 10–15 **efferent ductules** from the superior mediastinum pierce the tunica near the upper pole to convey sperm to the head of the epididymis.

The testis and epididymis are invaginated anteriorly into a double serous covering, the **tunica vaginalis** (analogous to the invagination of bowel into the peritoneum). The tunica vaginalis is continuous with the peritoneum during development via the **processus vaginalis**. This is normally obliterated at birth. This loose covering has visceral and parietal layers.

The outer covering of the testis and epididymis is the thick scrotum, which has a midline **septum** dividing the paired scrotal contents. This has several layers from external to internal. These comprise skin, **tunica dartos** (a thin fibroelastic vascular layer), and **external spermatic,**

cremasteric and **internal spermatic** fasciae derived from the fascial layers of the anterior abdominal wall.

Testicular Size. This depends on age and sexual maturity. At birth the testis is approximately 1.5 cm (length) by 1 cm. In the adult, the dimensions are approximately 5 cm (length) by 3 cm (width) by 2 cm (AP).

The Epididymis

This is a convoluted sperm duct that measures about 6 m when unravelled. It is intimately related to the testis, with its **head** lying on the upper pole, its **body** along the posterolateral aspect of the testis and its **tail** lying inferiorly. From here it turns back on itself at an acute angle to become the vas deferens. The efferent ductules of the testis drain sperm to the head of the epididymis. The epididymis concentrates, stores and transports sperm to the ejaculatory ducts and has a role in its maturation.

The Vas Deferens

This is a sperm duct that extends from the tail of the epididymis through the scrotum, inguinal canal and pelvis to fuse with the duct of the seminal vesicle to form the **ejaculatory duct** in the prostate gland.

The Spermatic Cord

The spermatic cord contains the vas deferens, along with all of the arterial supply, draining veins, lymphatics and nerves of the testis. It is tightly covered by a fibrous sheath composed of internal spermatic, cremasteric and external spermatic fascial layers derived from the transversalis, internal and external oblique abdominal fasciae as it passes through the anterior abdominal wall.

Blood Supply

The testis is supplied by the **testicular artery**, which arises directly from the aorta below the level of the renal arteries. Numerous veins drain from the testis at the mediastinum to a complex plexus of veins called the **pampiniform venous plexus**, which is situated superiorly. The epididymis and scrotum are drained by the **cremasteric venous plexus,** which runs posterior to the testis related to the epididymis. Both plexuses have anastomosing channels and drain superiorly, running with the vas deferens in the spermatic cord. They anastomose to become one **testicular (internal spermatic) vein** at the upper end of the inguinal canal. The right testicular vein drains into the inferior vena cava and the left into the left renal vein.

The vas deferens and epididymis are supplied by branches of the inferior vesical artery (deferential artery) and inferior epigastric artery (cremasteric artery).

The scrotum is supplied by branches from the internal pudendal artery (posterior scrotal artery), external pudendal branches of the femoral artery and branches of the inferior epigastric artery (cremasteric).

Lymph Drainage

The testis drains to para-aortic nodes via the testicular vessels. The scrotum drains to superficial inguinal nodes.

RADIOLOGY OF THE TESTIS

Ultrasound (Fig. 6.26)

The testes may be imaged by ultrasound as oval structures having a homogeneous granular echotexture with uniform medium-level echoes. The mediastinum may be identified as a linear echogenic band running superolaterally. The fibrous septae dividing the lobules may sometimes be appreciated as linear echogenic thin bands running through the testis. On longitudinal scans, the upper and lower poles are identified. Vessels are often identified running through the testis as hypoechoic linear structures. The appendix of the testis may be identified on high-resolution images, especially if outlined by fluid.

RADIOLOGY PEARLS

- The upper pole of the testis has a small sessile projection called the appendix of the testis, which is situated just below the head of the epididymis, also known as the organ of Morgagni. This is present in over 90% of cases and is a remnant of the Müllerian duct. Other testicular appendages may also exist.
- The head of the epididymis may be seen to have one or more small sessile projections superiorly, known as the appendix(ces) of the epididymis. Any of these appendages may tort, cutting off their blood supply and presenting with symptoms and signs suggestive of testicular torsion.
- Occasionally the rete testis is prominent as multiple anechoic structures in the posterosuperior aspect of the testis. This is termed tubular ectasia of the rete testis and represents dilated seminiferous tubules.
- The fibrous septae supporting the testicular architecture may sometimes be appreciated as linear echogenic thin bands running through the testis. These are more readily appreciated if the testis is swollen in pathological conditions, giving rise to a so-called 'zebra pattern' of echogenic stripes contrasting with the hypoechoic swollen testis.

The head of the epididymis is seen to rest on the upper pole posteriorly. The body of the epididymis is seen posterolateral to the testis, and the spermatic cord is medial to the epididymis. The various parts of the epididymis are better seen if outlined by fluid. The scrotal septum is seen between the testes. A small amount of anechoic fluid may surround the normal testis. The appendix of the epididymis may be seen if fluid is present.

The tortuous veins of the pampiniform plexus may be seen related to the cord above the upper pole. Slow venous flow may be demonstrated by colour Doppler techniques.

Magnetic Resonance Imaging

Use of a surface coil improves resolution. The tunica albuginea, mediastinum testis and fibrous septae are of low signal intensity compared with the high signal intensity of normal testicular tissue on T2-weighted imaging. The testis is of homogeneous low-signal intensity on T1-weighted imaging. The epididymis is of variable intensity.

THE PENIS (FIGS. 6.10, 6.27, 6.28)

The anatomy of the penis is described with the penis lying on the anterior abdominal wall; that is, the ventral surface is the surface that normally lies on the scrotum. The penis comprises three cylinders of endothelium-lined erectile tissue which arise from the perineum: a ventral **corpus spongiosum**, which surrounds the penile urethra, and two paired dorsal **corpora cavernosa**, which are the main erectile bodies. The corpora are each surrounded by a thick fibrous capsule, the **tunica albuginea**. Superficial to the tunica albuginea is **Buck's fascia**, which is the deep fascia of the penis. This binds the three corpora together and is a continuation of the **deep perineal fascia**.

The ventral corpus spongiosus is expanded to form the **glans penis** distally and the **bulb** proximally. The enlarged posterior part of the bulb is penetrated by the bulbar part of the urethra, which then runs in the corpus spongiosum to the external meatus. The distal corpus spongiosum expands to form the conical glans penis, which projects beyond the ends of the corpora cavernosa. The dorsal corpora cavernosa are fused in the median plane, but diverge posterosuperiorly to form the **crura**, which attach to the inferior part of the internal surface of the corresponding ischiopubic ramus.

BLOOD SUPPLY

The arterial supply originates from the internal pudendal arteries, arising from the anterior division of the internal iliac artery. **Paired deep dorsal arteries** lie external to the tunica albuginea and course lateral to the deep dorsal vein, supplying the skin and the glans. **Paired cavernosal** arteries run in the corpora cavernosa. The corpora cavernosa are drained through emissary veins of the wall of the corpora and then to the deep dorsal vein.

RADIOLOGY OF THE PENIS (SEE ALSO SECTION ON THE MALE URETHRA)

Ultrasound

The corpora and urethra may be identified by high-frequency ultrasound with the subject in a supine position. The corpora yield mid-level homogeneous echoes in the flaccid state. The paired corpora cavernosa are two rounded structures separated by a hypoechoic penile septum on transverse images. These lie anterior to the more ovoid corpus spongiosum. The corpus spongiosum contains the urethra, which has a circular echogenic wall and an anechoic lumen on transverse images. The tunica albuginea appears as a thin echogenic line surrounding the penile bodies. In the investigation of erectile dysfunction, anatomical and structural changes of the cavernosa and colour Doppler of penile arterial and venous blood flow may be assessed following intracavernosal injection of erectile pharmaceuticals.

Magnetic Resonance Imaging (Fig. 6.28)

The corpora are of high signal intensity on T2-weighted images and of intermediate signal on T1-weighted images. The fascial layers are of low signal on both T1 and T2. The corpora are highly vascular on contrast-enhanced images.

RADIOLOGY PEARL

Contrast MR is the best imaging method to demonstrate fractures of the corpora cavernosa. Extravasation of contrast administered intravenously from the corpora is seen. Such fractures occur secondary to trauma to the erect penis.

The Female Reproductive Tract

THE VAGINA (FIG. 6.29)

The vagina is an extraperitoneal structure. This muscular canal extends from the uterus to the vestibule, opening between the labia minora, behind the urethra and clitoris. It has a rectangular shape, being flattened from front to back. Superiorly the cervix of the uterus projects into its anterior wall at an acute angle. The cervix invaginates the upper vagina and arbitrarily divides it into shallow anterior,

deep posterior and lateral recesses or **fornices**. The ureters pass medially above the lateral fornices. In front of the vagina is the base of the bladder and the urethra. Posterior to the upper vagina is the **pouch of Douglas**, containing loops of bowel. Posteroinferior to this peritoneal reflection is the rectum. On either side are the levator ani muscles and the pelvic fascia, which are slung around the vagina and rectum, supporting these structures. The vagina traverses the levator ani and the urogenital diaphragm, which have a sphincter-like action. The levator muscles insert into a fibromuscular node called the perineal body, which lies between the lower vagina and the anal canal (see below).

Blood Supply

Vaginal branches of the internal iliac and the uterine arteries supply the vagina. Venous drainage is via a plexus on its lateral walls to the internal iliac vein.

Lymph Drainage

The upper two-thirds drain to internal and external iliac nodes. The lower third drains to superficial inguinal nodes.

THE UTERUS (FIGS. 6.29–6.31)

The uterus is extraperitoneal. It is a pear-shaped muscular organ lying between the bladder and rectum. It has a **fundus**, a **body** and a **cervix**. The body narrows to an **isthmus** at its lower end. It lies on the posterosuperior surface of the bladder with its cervix projecting into the anterior wall of the upper vagina. The cavity of the uterus is triangular in coronal section. Its anterior and posterior walls are opposed, separated by the endometrial cavity, giving it a linear appearance of variable thickness in the sagittal plane. The fundus is the broad curved upper part of the uterus where the fallopian tubes insert. The fallopian tubes open into the **cornua** of the fundus in its superolateral aspect. The body is the part of the uterus below the fallopian tubes.

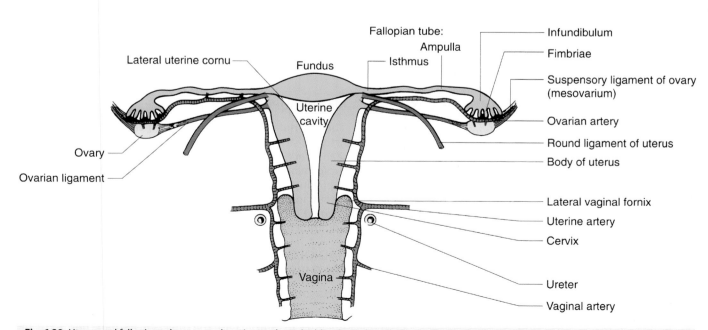

Fig. 6.29 Uterus and fallopian tubes: coronal section to show the blood supply and ureter relative to the uterine artery, cervix and vaginal fornices.

The lowest part of the uterine cavity narrows to an **isthmus** just above the cervical canal. The uterus leads to the vagina via the **cervical canal**. The **internal os** is at the upper end of the cervical canal and the **external os** at its lower end.

The inner lining of the uterus is the **endometrium**, which undergoes cyclical changes of proliferation and desquamation in the premenopausal female.

The **myometrium** is the main muscular layer and consists of smooth muscle arranged in layers, intermixed with areolar tissue, blood vessels, lymphatics and nerves. It has three layers. The external and middle layers are muscular and the inner layer is a greatly hypertrophied muscular mucosa. The external layer fibres are arranged transversely and continue into the fallopian tubes, the ovarian ligament, round ligament and ligament of the ovary. Some lateral uterine fibres run laterally into the broad ligament and some cervical fibres run posteriorly into the sacrouterine fibres. The middle layer has fibres running in all directions and is the most vascular. The internal deep layer consists of circular fibres which surround the openings of the fallopian tubes and form a distinct sphincter at the internal os.

The **serosa** is a thin outer smooth membrane derived from the peritoneum and consists of a layer of cells with a thin layer of connective tissue beneath it, which allows the uterus to move. It covers the fundus and posterior body of the uterus entirely, but only covers the anterior part as far as the junction of the uterine body and cervix.

The peritoneum covers the fundus, body, cervix and upper part of the vagina posteriorly. From here it is reflected onto the anterior surface of the rectum, forming the **pouch of Douglas** or **rectouterine pouch**. Anteriorly the peritoneum is reflected from the junction of the uterine body and cervix upper to the superior surface of the bladder (**vesicouterine pouch**). The rectouterine pouch is deeper than the vesicouterine pouch.

On either side of the uterus the peritoneum is reflected to the lateral pelvic walls covering the fallopian tubes. The fold of peritoneum so formed is called the **broad ligament**. This is a peritoneal fold rather than a true ligament. Several important structures run in this fold.

Variant Anatomy

Uterine development begins with two tube-shaped Müllerian ducts which later come together and fuse in the midline. The fused wall resorbs, leaving one uterine cavity. Various failures of development, fusion and septal resorption may lead to uterine anomalies. The reported prevalence is 2%–4%.

- Uterine agenesis: Both sides fail to develop.
- Unicornuate uterus: One side fails to develop.
- Uterus didelphys: Both sides develop but fail to fuse in the midline resulting in two separate uteri and cervixes.
- Bicornuate uterus: Both sides develop and the cervix fuses but the uterus fails to fully fuse resulting in a 'heart-shaped' separation of the two uterine fundi sharing one cervix.
- Septate uterus: Both sides develop and fuse, but the shared wall does not resorb fully. The uterus is divided by a band of muscle or fibrous tissue.
- Complex uterus: One side may fuse abnormally into the body or fundus of the main uterine cavity.

Normal Variants of Uterine Position

In 80% of women the uterus is anteverted; that is, its long axis is tilted anteriorly with respect to the vagina, and it lies on the bladder. It is frequently also anteflexed with the body of the uterus making an anterior angle with the long axis of the cervix. The uterus is considered retroverted when its long axis lies in a posterior plane to the vagina, directed upwards and backwards. It may also be retroflexed when the uterus is bent backwards on the cervix. These positions are not of clinical importance in most women but retroversion/retroflexion make visualization of the uterus by ultrasound more difficult. The uterus may also lie to the right or left of midline or be somewhat rotated in its axis. The uterus is relatively mobile and changes with the degree of fullness of the bladder, and with pregnancy.

In children the cervix is twice the size of the uterus. The uterus grows disproportionately until they are of equal size at puberty. In adulthood the uterus is twice the size of the cervix.

THE FALLOPIAN TUBES

The fallopian (uterine) tubes lie in an upper 'free edge' of the broad ligament and convey ova from the ovaries to the uterus. They open into the uterine **cornua**. They are described as having five parts as follows:

- Fimbriae: Approximately 25 finger-like projections extend from the outer part of the fallopian tube draping over the ovary. One of the fimbriae is longer than the rest. This is called the **ovarian fimbria** as it is attached to the ovary.
- Infundibulum: This is the outer funnel-shaped extremity of the tube attached to the fimbriae. It extends out beyond the broad ligament. Its distal opening into the peritoneal cavity is known as the abdominal ostium.
- Ampulla: This is the longest section – a dilated tortuous outer part which curves over the ovary, where fertilization of the ovum most commonly occurs.
- Isthmus: This is the narrowest segment, just lateral to the uterus.
- Intramural segment: This is the part that passes through the myometrium of the uterus and opens into it.

BLOOD SUPPLY OF THE UTERUS AND UTERINE TUBES (FIG. 6.30)

The uterine artery, a branch of the internal iliac, runs medially in the base of the broad ligament to reach the lower lateral wall of the uterus. It ascends tortuously within the broad ligament to supply the uterus and tubes, and anastomoses with the ovarian artery.

Venous drainage from the uterus and medial two-thirds of the fallopian tubes is via a venous plexus in the base of the broad ligament to the internal iliac vein. The lateral third of the fallopian tubes drains via the pampiniform plexus to the ovarian veins.

> **RADIOLOGY PEARL**
>
> The fallopian tube is the most common location of ectopic pregnancy (90%). Over 80% are in the distal tube. About 10% occur at the narrow isthmus, with a high rate of haemorrhage and increased morbidity and mortality.

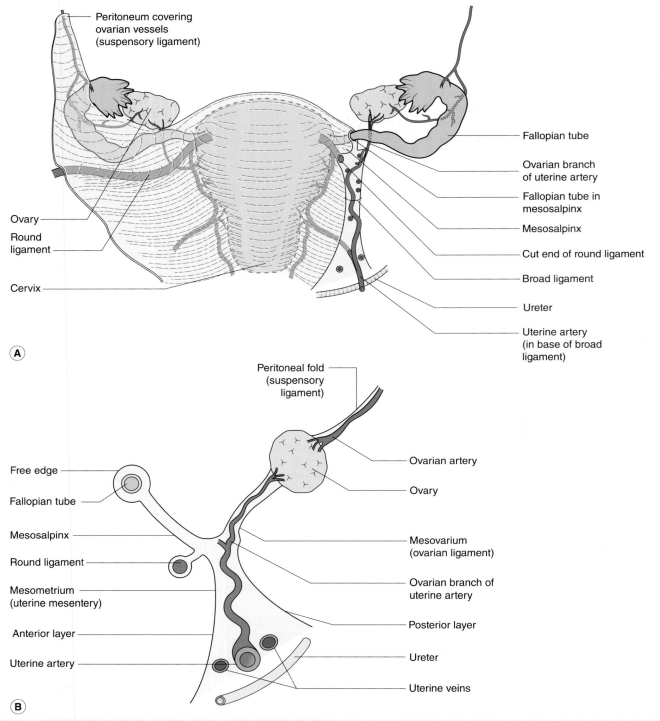

Fig. 6.30 (A) Broad ligament. (B) Sagittal cross-section of the broad ligament.

Lymph Drainage

The fundus drains along ovarian vessels to para-aortic nodes.

The body drains via the broad ligament to nodes around the external iliac vessels and occasionally via the round ligament to inguinal nodes. The cervix drains to external and internal iliac nodes and posteriorly to sacral nodes.

THE BROAD LIGAMENT (FIGS. 6.30, 6.31)

This double layer of peritoneum is a mesentery that encloses the fallopian tubes in its upper part and extends from the sides of the uterus to the pelvic side walls and pelvic floor. The **mesometrium** is that part which supports the uterus. The two layers are continuous with each other laterally at a free edge that surrounds the fallopian tube (**mesosalpinx**)

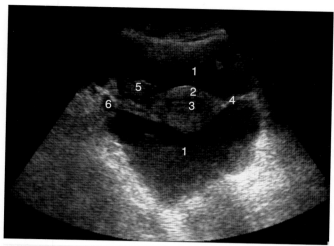

Fig. 6.31 Transverse ultrasound of the uterus and broad ligament. The broad ligament is outlined by fluid, and therefore can be seen. The right ovary lies in its anterior surface. The broad ligament is attached at the internal iliac vessels. The uterine artery runs in the base of the ligament, within its leaves.

1. Free fluid
2. Uterus – body
3. Uterus – endometrium
4. Broad ligament
5. Ovary
6. Internal iliac vessels

where this opens into the abdominal cavity. The uterine artery runs in its base, travelling medially via the transverse cervical ligaments. The ureter loops under the uterine artery within the broad ligament, passing just lateral to the cervix above the lateral vaginal fornix to enter the bladder. The uterine plexus of veins in the base of the broad ligament communicates with the veins of the vagina and bladder via the pelvic plexus of veins. A fold of ligament (**mesovarium**) contains the ovarian branch of the uterine artery running posterosuperiorly to the ovary and the round ligament lies anteroinferiorly within the layers. Both of these structures attach to the uterus close to the attachment of the uterine tubes. The broad ligament helps define the vesicouterine pouch between bladder and uterus and rectouterine pouch (of Douglas) between the uterus and rectum.

THE OVARIES

These are paired intraperitoneal organs measuring approximately 3 cm × 2 cm × 2 cm. They are ovoid structures, usually orientated somewhat vertically and thus can be described as having upper and lower poles. They lie on the posterior surface of the broad ligament in close contact with the infundibulum of the fallopian tube and attached to its ovarian **fimbria**. The fimbriae of the uterine tubes lie superior and lateral. The surface of the ovary is not covered by peritoneum, but by a layer of **germinal epithelium** that becomes continuous with the peritoneum at the hilum of the ovary. The ovary has a tough outer layer of **tunica albuginea** beneath the germinal layer. The anterior surface of the ovary is attached to the posterior surface of the broad ligament by a short **meso-ovarium** that fuses with the surface of the ovary. The lower pole of the ovary is attached

to the uterus by the **ovarian ligament**. A superolateral extension of the broad ligament, the **suspensory ligament of the ovary**, runs from the upper pole of the ovary to the pelvic side wall. The ovarian vessels and nerves run in this, crossing over the external iliac vessels. Despite all its attachments the ovary is very mobile, especially in women who have had children. In nulliparous women it is generally found lateral to the uterus, anterior to the internal iliac vessels and ureter, inferior to the external iliac vessels.

Blood Supply

Arterial supply is via the ovarian artery, which arises directly from the aorta at the level of the renal arteries.

Venous drainage is via the right ovarian vein into the inferior vena cava, and via the left ovarian vein into the left renal vein.

Lymph Drainage

Lymph drainage is along the ovarian vessels to the para-aortic nodes.

ENDOPELVIC FASCIA OF THE FEMALE PELVIS (FIG. 6.32)

The bladder, urethra, uterus and vagina (and prostate and seminal vesicles in the male) are all enveloped in a three-dimensional spider's web of supporting fascia. The fascia is continuous with the fascia investing these organs (visceral fascia) and with the fascia overlying the muscles of the pelvic side wall and pelvic floor (parietal fascia). The fascia is composed of connective tissue that is mostly fatty and avascular, and easily distensible overlying bladder, uterus and rectum. In other parts is much more fibrous containing collagen and elastic fibres described as fascial 'condensations' or ligaments with a more supportive role.

Fascial Ligaments

- **The tendinous arch** is a condensation of fascia overlying the obturator internus muscle that forms a fibrous band running from the inner superior pubic rami to the ischial spine. It is to this layer that much of the lateral fasciae supporting the pelvic viscera is attached. The tendinous arch also gives rise to part of the levator ani muscle and is also known as the tendinous arch of levator ani.
- The **pubourethral and pubovesical ligaments** run from the posterior pubic bones to the urethra and anterior vaginal walls.
- **The pubocervical ligaments** or **fascia** run anteriorly from the cervix, around the base of the bladder to the pubic bone.
- **The transverse cervical** (cardinal) ligaments run laterally from the cervix and lateral aspect of the vaginal fornix to the tendinous arch on the pelvic side wall. This is a substantial ligament, transmitting the uterine arteries with the ureters running below.
- **The uterosacral ligaments** run posterosuperiorly to the midsacrum on the upper surface of the levator ani muscle.
- **The rectovaginal fascia (Denonvillier's fascia)** separates the uterus and vagina from the rectum in the craniocaudal plane. It connects the transverse cervical and uterosacral ligaments to the perineal body inferiorly and the tendinous arch superiorly.

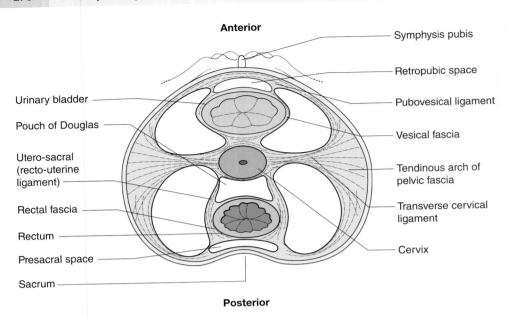

Anterior

- Symphysis pubis
- Retropubic space
- Pubovesical ligament
- Vesical fascia
- Tendinous arch of pelvic fascia
- Transverse cervical ligament
- Cervix

- Urinary bladder
- Pouch of Douglas
- Utero-sacral (recto-uterine ligament)
- Rectal fascia
- Rectum
- Presacral space
- Sacrum

Posterior

Fig. 6.32 Support ligaments of the female pelvis

Other Uterine Supports

The **round ligament** is a fibromuscular band that passes from the upper lateral part of the uterus to the inguinal canal, ending in the labium majoris.

The bladder supports the uterus on its upper surface in the normal anatomic arrangement. This arrangement and the transverse cervical ligaments are the main passive support of the uterus. It is also supported below by the muscles of the pelvic floor, which provide active support by contracting when intra-abdominal pressure is raised. Of the levator ani muscles, the puborectalis and iliococcygeus are the most important uterine supports. At rest, the levator ani muscles are in contraction, keeping the rectum, vagina and urethra elevated and closed.

The **perineal body** is an important structure in the pelvic floor and is described as the central tendon of the perineum. It is critical to the integrity of the pelvic floor in females. It is a wedged-shaped structure whose apex is the lower limit of the rectovaginal septum. It is at the junction of the anus and the urogenital triangle between the external anal sphincter and the lower posterior vaginal wall. Several muscles converge on and insert into the perineal body including the external anal sphincter, bulbospongiosus muscle, superficial and deep transverse perineal muscles and fibres of the external urethral sphincter.

RADIOLOGY PEARL

The perineal body may rupture during childbirth. This leads to a gap between the free borders of the levator ani which may widen over time, leading to pelvic floor prolapse.

RADIOLOGY OF THE FEMALE PELVIS
Ultrasound (Fig. 6.33)

Ultrasound is the most common and accessible radiological method of imaging the female reproductive tract. Transabdominal ultrasound is performed through a moderately full bladder. The urine-filled bladder lifts gassy loops of bowel out of the way and provides an acoustic window through which the pelvic organs may be visualized.

The cervix usually lies in the midline, but the uterus may lie obliquely to either side. The uterine myometrial wall yields uniform low-level echoes. Sagittal images are obtained by scanning in the same plane as the uterus, parallel to its long axis. Transverse images of the uterus are obtained by scanning at a right angle to the sagittal plane. The fundus of a retroflexed or retroverted uterus may be difficult to visualize transabdominally because of its distance from the transducer. The normal ovaries are usually identified lateral or posterolateral to the anteflexed uterus. They commonly lie anterior to the internal iliac vessels, in a somewhat vertical orientation, with their long axis parallel to those vessels. When the uterus is tilted to one side, the ovary on that side is frequently located superior to the fundus. However the ovaries may lie high in the pelvis or may be in the pouch of Douglas. In premenopausal women the normal ovary usually contains small anechoic **follicles**, aiding identification. In the late phase of the menstrual cycle, after ovulation with rupture of the dominant follicle, a small amount of fluid may be seen in the pouch of Douglas.

The myometrium is relatively hypoechoic. The endometrium yields a thin high-level echo that is seen as a long white stripe on longitudinal images and a central echo on transverse images. This is thicker and more obvious perimenstrually. A central sharp echo is caused by the opposing endometrial surfaces. Immediately adjacent to the central echo is the functional layer of endometrium. This is relatively hypoechoic during the proliferative phase and becomes echogenic during the secretory phase, when the entire stripe is thicker and more homogeneous. A narrow hypoechoic layer of myometrium has been noted deep to the endometrium – the **subendometrial halo**. This represents a layer of compact, relatively avascular myometrium and is analogous to the junctional zone on MRI. The vagina is also seen as a white stripe of increased echogenicity on

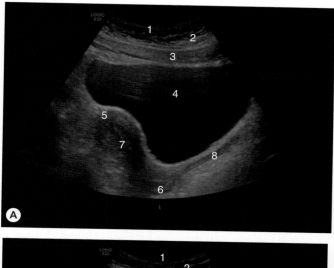

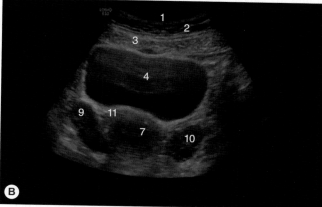

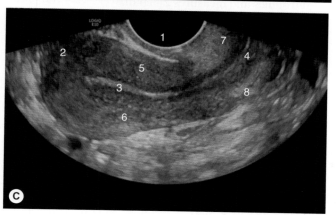

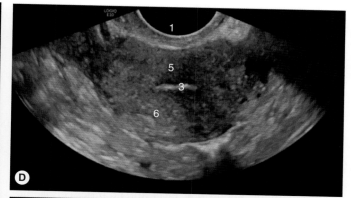

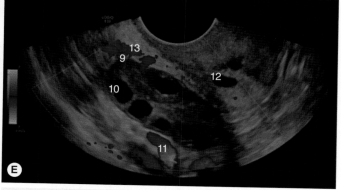

Fig. 6.33 Transabdominal ultrasound of the female pelvis. The ultrasound probe is on the lower abdominal wall. (A) Sagittal view through a full bladder. (B) Transverse view through a full bladder showing the uterus and both ovaries. Transvaginal ultrasound of the pelvis (C-E). The ultrasound probe is in the vagina. (C) Transvaginal ultrasound with a sagittal view of the uterus. (D) Transvaginal ultrasound with an axial view of the uterus. (E) Transvaginal ultrasound imaging of an ovary with overlying colour doppler.

(A and B)
1. Probe skin interface
2. Subcutaneous fat
3. Abdominal wall muscle
4. Bladder
5. Uterine fundus
6. Cervix
7. Endometrial stripe
8. Vagina
9. Right ovary
10. Left ovary
11. Anterior myometrium

(C–E)
1. Endovaginal probe interface with vaginal wall
2. Uterine fundus
3. Endometrial stripe
4. Endocervical canal
5. Anterior myometrium
6. Posterior myometrium
7. Anterior cervix
8. Posterior cervix
9. Sagittal ovary
10. Follicle
11. External iliac vessels
12. Adnexal vessels
13. Nabothian cyst in cervix

longitudinal images. The vaginal stripe makes an acute angle with the body of the uterus. Owing to the rectangular shape of the vagina, it is seen as a transverse line on transverse images.

EV or transvaginal (TV) ultrasound (see Fig. 6.31) is performed with an ultrasound transducer in the vagina. The basic ultrasound features are the same, but the resolution is better. The orientation is different because the transducer is inferior to the uterus at the cervix. There is improved visualization of the adnexal areas and the internal architecture of the ovary, as well as the uterus and uterine cavity. The cervix is also readily imaged and its canal and os

may be demonstrated. Small dilations of cervical glands are frequently seen as small cysts related to the endocervical canal – these are termed **nabothian cysts**.

Dynamic ultrasound – the 'sliding test' – can also be used to assess the normal 'glideability' of the structures of the pelvis when no adhesions are present. Gentle pressure by the probe on the uterus and ovaries should be able to move and deform these structures when healthy. The anterior rectum and sigmoid colon should glide freely across the posterior aspect of the uterus cervix and vaginal wall – this is known as a positive sliding test. It should be possible to move the ovary away from the uterus with gentle probe pressure.

Endometrial Thickness on Ultrasound

The endometrium changes with the ovulatory and menstrual cycle:

- During menstruation it is a thin echogenic line measuring 1–4 mm.
- In the early proliferative phase (day 6–10) it is thin and brightly echogenic, measuring 5–7 mm. Sometimes a little fluid can be seen separating the anterior and posterior endometrium.
- In the late proliferative periovulatory phase (day 10–14) it develops a trilaminar appearance, an outer echogenic layer, a middle hypoechoic layer and an inner echogenic stripe at the central interface, and can measure up to 11 mm.
- In the secretory phase (day 15–28) it is thick and uniformly echogenic and can measure up to 16 mm.

The above measurements are a guide and not a standard. The actual thickness may be very variable between individuals.

In postmenopausal women, the endometrium no longer undergoes cyclical change and should measure less than 5 mm. The thickness should be uniform.

RADIOLOGY PEARLS

- Endometrial thickness is always measured on the sagittal view, at the thickest part of the endometrium. Only the echogenic endometrial stripe is measured. If there is fluid between the layers of the endometrium in the central uterine cavity, the thickness of the fluid is subtracted from the combined thickness of the anterior and posterior layers or echogenic endometrium.
- It is essential to know the menstrual status of the woman when performing gynaecological ultrasound, in order to properly interpret the findings. This is usually the number of days since the last menstrual period and is usually annotated on the ultrasound image. Similarly, if a woman is postmenopausal, this should be indicated.
- The endometrial thickness may be increased in postmenopausal women taking hormone replacement therapy or the drug Tamoxifen.
- Endometrial thickness may be reduced in women taking the oral contraceptive pill and when an intrauterine contraceptive device is in situ.
- A negative sliding test is seen with pelvic adhesions, most commonly from endometriosis.

Sonohysterography

Sonohysterography involves TV imaging of the uterus and adnexae, after saline is introduced into the uterine cavity via a small catheter through the cervix. This distends the cavity and allows evaluation both of the endometrial surface and for tubal patency.

Ovarian Volume (see Fig. 6.33E)

Ovarian volume is an important measurement in many pathologies and can be calculated on ultrasound. There is a significant reduction in ovarian volume with each decade from 30 to 70 years. Volume is calculated by using the formula for an ellipsoid, where three measurements are taken:

$$Sagittal \times transverse \times AP\,dimension \times 0.52$$

The normal mean ovarian volume is 6–7 mL in a nonpregnant, premenopausal female. Ovarian volume varies with differing body weights and heights, and is maximal at 20–40 years of age. Ovarian volumes in fertile years may be up to 24 mL and asymmetry between ovaries is common. In a premenopausal woman, the normal ovary contains simple cysts, or Graafian follicles. Follicles and their maturation may be assessed with ultrasound. Up to 10 follicles may develop during the menstrual cycle, with one of these going on to become the dominant ovarian follicle. The dominant follicle can grow to between 18 and 20 mm in diameter, and when it ruptures it releases the oocyte. After release of the oocyte, the dominant follicle regresses, and the granulosa cells in the inner lining proliferate and swell to form the corpus luteum which secretes progesterone to prepare the endometrium for possible pregnancy. If pregnancy occurs, the corpus luteum remains with an important role in maintenance of pregnancy; if pregnancy does not occur it degenerates into a small scar (corpus albicans).

Ovarian volumes decrease after the menopause and can become difficult to localize with ultrasound.

RADIOLOGY PEARLS

- In the postmenopausal woman the endometrium atrophies and measures 2–3 mm.
- In postmenopausal women who take hormone replacement therapy the endometrium may measure up to 10 mm.
- **Nabothian cysts** may be seen related to the endocervical canal. They represent an accumulation of fluid in the endocervical glands and are usually less than 1 cm in size.
- The corpus luteum is a thick-walled cyst with a highly vascular periphery described as a 'ring of fire' on colour Doppler and has a typically 'crenelated' or wavy inner wall.

Magnetic Resonance Imaging (Fig. 6.34)

MRI is an excellent method to image the uterus because it has superior soft-tissue contrast and has the advantage of being able to image all planes. Sagittal and coronal images are obtained along the long axis of the uterus and axial images perpendicular to the coronal plane. The cervix generally lies in the same sagittal plane as the uterus, but often forms an angle to the body of the uterus, with the uterus lying in a relatively transverse plane and the cervix directed inferiorly towards the vagina. The cervix may be imaged separately in its own coronal plane, with its own transverse images perpendicular to this. It is especially important to image in the correct plane when evaluating for spread of cervical cancer beyond the serosa.

On T2 images the endometrium, endocervical canal and vaginal canal are all of high signal intensity. The inner zone of myometrium is of low signal intensity and is continuous

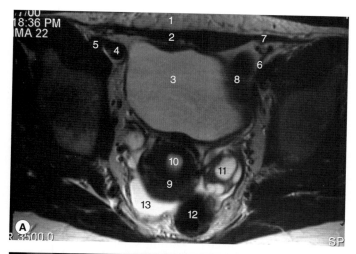

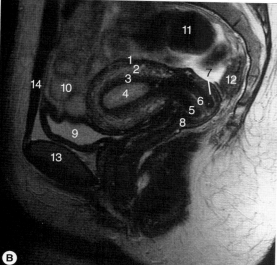

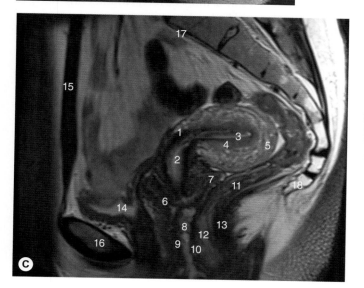

Fig. 6.34 Magnetic resonance image of the female pelvis. (A) Transverse T2-weighted image showing the lower body of the uterus and both ovaries. Note the high signal of endometrium and ovarian follicles. (B) Sagittal section midline. (C) Sagittal view showing a retroflexed uterus.

(A)
1. Subcutaneous fat
2. Rectus muscle
3. Bladder
4. External iliac vein
5. External iliac artery
6. Round ligament
7. Transversus abdominis muscle
8. Small bowel loop
9. Uterus – myometrium
10. Uterus – endometrium
11. Ovary containing follicles
12. Rectum
13. Free fluid in cul-de-sac

(B)
1. Serosa (of uterus)
2. Myometrium
3. Junctional zone of uterus
4. Endometrium
5. Anterior lip of cervix
6. Cervical canal
7. Posterior vaginal fornix
8. Vagina
9. Bladder
10. Small bowel loops
11. Sigmoid
12. Rectum
13. Pubic bone
14. Rectus muscle

(C)
1. Retroflexed uterus
2. Endocervical canal
3. Endometrium
4. Junctional zone
5. Myometrium
6. Anterior vaginal fornix
7. Posterior vaginal fornix
8. Vaginal canal
9. Anterior vaginal wall
10. Posterior vaginal wall
11. Rectum
12. Anal canal
13. Puborectalis
14. Bladder
15. Rectus abdominis
16. Pubic symphysis
17. Sacral promontory
18. Coccyx

with the fibrous stroma of the cervix. This is known as the **junctional zone**. The hypointense signal from this layer, which is histologically similar to the rest of the myometrium, is thought to result from an increased nuclear cellular ratio in the relatively more packed inner myometrial layer. The outer myometrium is of intermediate signal intensity. The outer serosa is a thin hypointense layer. The cervical canal is also of high signal intensity, continuous with the endometrial canal. The narrow **os** may be seen, and occasionally the mucosal folds of the cervix, the **plicae**

palmatae, may be seen as transverse ridges on sagittal images. Dilated glands adjacent to the cervical canal (nabothian cysts) may be seen as hyperintense foci. Outside the high-signal endocervical canal is a low-intensity fibrous stroma continuous with the junctional zone and the myometrium above. The vaginal canal is of high signal owing to secretions. The mucosa is of low signal similar to the cervix and junctional zone, and the muscular vagina wall slightly higher signal than myometrium. The paravaginal and paracervical venous plexuses can be seen as bright structures on axial and coronal T2 images. The ovaries are hypointense on T2 images and the follicles stand out as hyperintense spots in an instantly recognizable pattern surrounded by darker solid ovarian stroma.

On T1 images the uterus and ovaries are of homogeneously intermediate signal intensity with poor intrinsic contrast, but the ligamentous structures are very well seen, being of low signal intensity compared to the surrounding fat. The **round ligaments** are seen coursing anteriorly from the upper lateral part of the uterus to the inguinal canal. The **uterosacral ligaments** can be seen extending back to the sacrum. The peritoneal reflection of the broad ligament and pelvic floor is best appreciated on coronal images, outlined inferiorly by extraperitoneal fat. The muscles of the pelvic floor and side wall are also very well seen. Imaging in the coronal plane allows evaluation of the lymphatic drainage along the internal and common iliac chains.

RADIOLOGY PEARL

Visualization of the vagina and cervix can be improved by the instillation of gel into the vagina. The high signal of the gel on T2 imaging also contrasts with the low signal of the vaginal wall and cervix, and the distension it causes also outlines the structures more clearly. T2 appearances myometrium at different ages.

Dynamic MRI/MR Defecography (see Fig. 6.17)

Ultrafast MRI sequences allow study of the interaction between the pelvic floor musculature and the pelvic organs at rest and during straining (Valsalva). This MR technique allows the acquisition of multiple images at the same location at a rate of one frame per second, thereby capturing the motion of the pelvic floor as it deforms under increasing intra-abdominal pressure in a cine loop. Generally rectal contrast in the form of ultrasound gel is administered prior to imaging and images are acquired at rest, during a 'clenching up' or Kegel manoeuvre, and while bearing down to expel the gel onto a waterproof sheet placed under the subject. Measurements are taken from a line drawn electronically on the viewing screen. Changes in the length and/or orientation of these lines during straining allow for some objectivity in assessing abnormal degrees of pelvic floor movement. A line drawn between the inferior aspect of the pubic bone and the last joint of the coccyx represents the **pubococcygeal line** and defines the expected level of the pelvic floor (pubococcygeus muscle). This is the main line of interest, and descent of any organs such as the uterus or bladder neck are measured in cm perpendicular to the line (e.g. descent might be from 1 cm above the line to 2 cm below the line 0 – a total of 3 cm). A line drawn from the inferior pubic symphysis to the posterior wall of the rectum at the level of the anorectal junction (puborectalis impression) represents the AP dimension of the levator hiatus. The **levator plate** is the midline raphe of the fused fibres of iliococcygeus running from the posterior anorectal junction to the coccyx.

Normal Findings and Measurements. The bladder neck, vaginal fornices and anorectal junction should be above the pubococcygeal line at rest and descend minimally on straining. The AP length of the levator hiatus should measure a maximum of 5 cm in normal women without pelvic floor abnormality at rest (Fielding, 2002). In fact, the anorectal angle is more commonly below the pubococcygeal line in most older women attending for this examination (author experience). The rectum should elevate during the clenching up manoeuvre. During straining, the anorectal angle should straighten (increase) and rectal contrast (ultrasound gel) should be expelled for a properly physiologic evaluation of pelvic floor pathology.

Computed Tomography

On CT the uterus is seen as a round structure of soft-tissue density lying on or behind the bladder. Oral contrast helps to differentiate loops of bowel, which lie on and around it. Intravenous contrast improves contrast between the uterus and surrounding structures, and enhancement may be seen in the myometrium and endometrium, especially mid-cycle. Nonenhancing fluid may also be seen in the uterine cavity during the secretory phase of the cycle. Enhancing vessels may be seen on either side of the lower uterus. The ovaries may usually be identified as small round structures of soft-tissue density, occasionally with small cysts. The broad ligament is not identified, unless abnormal amounts of abdominal free fluid are present to outline it, but the round ligaments can usually be seen running anteriorly to the inguinal ring. The levator ani complex and muscles of the pelvic side wall can be identified.

Hysterosalpingography (Fig. 6.35)

This technique outlines the cavity of the uterus and tubes by injection of water-soluble contrast via the cervical canal. The cervical canal is approximately one-third the length of the entire uterine long axis. **Longitudinal ridges** are seen on the anterior and posterior walls of the cervical canal. In nulliparous women these may have branches running laterally – the **plicae palmatae**. **Cervical glands** may be outlined by contrast as outpouchings from the cervical canal. The **isthmus** is seen as a narrow area above the cervix, and the **internal os** may sometimes be identified as a constriction of the lumen of the isthmus. The uterine cavity is seen to be triangular on the frontal view. It is usually smooth walled. The triangular **cornua** lead to the **fallopian tubes**, which are about 10–11 cm long. The **isthmus** of the tube is uniformly narrow and opens into the wide **ampulla**. Contrast spills freely into the peritoneal cavity.

The walls of the uterus may demonstrate longitudinal folds. Polypoid filling defects may be seen in the secretory phase in normal women. Filling of endometrial glands may also be seen in normal women in the secretory phase.

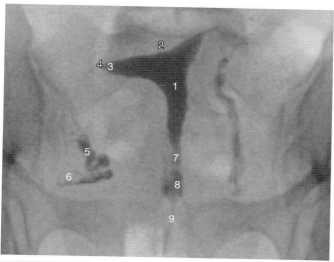

Fig. 6.35 Hysterosalpingogram.

1. Body of the uterus
2. Fundus of the uterus
3. Uterine cornu
4. Isthmus of the fallopian tube
5. Ampulla of the fallopian tube
6. Peritoneal spill of contrast
7. Cervical canal
8. Balloon of catheter in the cervix
9. Catheter in the vagina

RADIOLOGY PEARL

Hysterosalpingography illustrates the connection between the abdominal cavity and the outside via the vagina, uterus and fallopian tubes. Infection may ascend via this route leading to pelvic inflammatory disease. This is a potential complication of hysterosalpingography.

Vaginography

This technique outlines the vagina with contrast. The characteristic rectangular shape of the vagina is demonstrated. It is of utmost importance to recognize this shape in the case of inadvertent filling of the vagina during a barium examination.

Cross-Sectional Anatomy (Fig. 6.36)

The anatomy described can be identified on both CT and MRI images.

MID-SACRAL LEVEL – MALE OR FEMALE (FIG. 6.36A)

This level is above the bladder. The sigmoid colon may be seen close to its junction with the rectum. Loops of small bowel lie in the pelvis, on top of the pelvic organs. Pelvic and mesenteric fat separates the various bowel loops. The sacrum is posterior, with the piriformis muscle arising from its anterior surface. The piriformis muscle passes anteriorly, inferiorly and laterally to insert into the greater tuberosity of the femur. The sciatic nerve lies on the piriformis. The

RADIOLOGY PEARLS

How to differentiate perineal cysts by anatomic location

- A **Gartner's duct cyst** may develop if the remaining parts of Wolffian ducts (embryonic structures that develop in both sexes and go on to form the epididymis, vas and seminal vesicles in males) do not regress completely. They occur in the anterolateral wall of the proximal third vagina and are thus above the perineum and above the level of the inferior part of the pubic bone, higher than other cysts described below.
- A **urethral diverticulum** is a localized out-pouching of the lower urethra into the anterior vaginal wall. It typically forms a horseshoe shape around the posterior urethra between the urethra and anterior vagina.
- **Skene glands** are two pea-sized glands that open onto either side of the urethra close to its orifice and secrete mucoid fluid. A Skene duct cyst occurs when the gland is blocked and will be seen lateral to the distal urethra below the level of the pubic bone. Skene cysts are anterior to the vagina.
- **Bartholin's glands** are two pea-sized glands on either side of the vagina at the posterior introitus that secrete mucoid fluid. A Bartholin's cyst occurs when the gland is blocked and will be seen at the posterior aspect of the vagina below the level of the pubic bone. They are also related to the labia majora.

gluteus muscles are posterior; the gluteus maximus is the largest, most posterior and most superficial. the gluteus minimus is the smallest, most anterior and deepest gluteal muscle. The psoas and iliacus muscles are relatively anterior at this level, with the external iliac vessels lying on them, the artery being slightly anterior and lateral to the vein.

The ureters are lateral on the side wall of the pelvis and are **extraperitoneal** in location. At first they lie anterior to the bifurcation of the iliac artery. At a lower level they are more anteriorly located. In the male, the vasa deferentia pass over the ureters and may be identified by CT or MRI running posteriorly from the inguinal canal, around the side of the bladder to join with the ducts of the seminal vesicles at a lower level.

LOWER SACRAL LEVEL – MALE (FIG. 6.36B)

The bladder has a rather square shape when it contains urine. It extends anteriorly to the anterior abdominal wall. Posteriorly are the seminal vesicles. The rectum is just behind the seminal vesicles, separated from them by the **perirectal fascia**, and is surrounded by **perirectal fat**. Outside the perirectal fascia is the pararectal fat. This is continuous with the fat lining the pelvis above the levator ani muscle. The **obturator internus muscle** is deep to the lateral pelvic wall. It can be seen hooking around the posterior part of the ischium to insert into the greater trochanter of the femur. The ureters insert into the posterolateral aspect of the bladder. They are not seen at the level of the seminal vesicles as they pass over them.

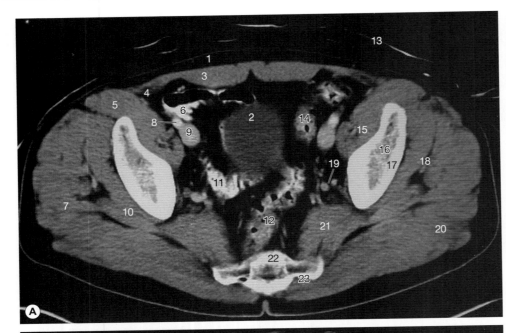

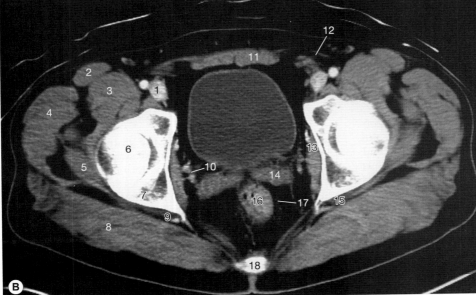

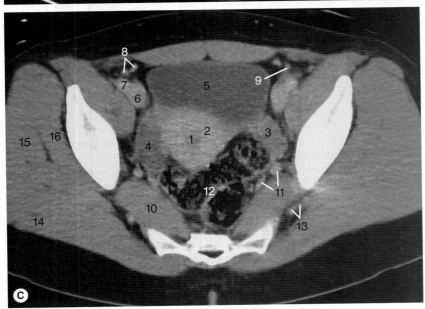

Fig. 6.36 (A) Axial computed tomography (CT) of the male/female pelvis: mid-sacral level. (B) Axial CT of the male pelvis: lower sacral level. (C) Axial CT of the female pelvis showing the uterus and ovaries.

(A)
1. Subcutaneous fat
2. Bladder
3. Rectus muscle
4. Inferior epigastric vessels
5. Iliacus muscle
6. Caecum
7. Gluteus medius muscle
8. External iliac artery
9. External iliac vein
10. Gluteus minimus muscle
11. Small bowel
12. Sigmoid colon
13. Skin
14. Sigmoid colon
15. Psoas tendon
16. Medulla of ischium
17. Cortex of ischium
18. Superior gluteal vessels
19. Internal iliac vessels
20. Gluteus maximus muscle
21. Piriformis muscle
22. Sacrum
23. External sacral neural foramen

(B)
1. Femoral vein, artery and nerve in femoral sheath
2. Sartorius muscle
3. Iliacus muscle
4. Gluteus medius muscle
5. Gluteus minimus muscle
6. Femoral head
7. Acetabulum
8. Gluteus maximus muscle
9. Obturator internus muscle
10. Branches of internal iliac vessels
11. Rectus abdominis muscle
12. Inguinal ligament
13. Obturator internus muscle
14. Left seminal vesicle
15. Obturator internus muscle
16. Rectum
17. Perirectal fat
18. Coccyx

(C)
1. Endometrial cavity
2. Uterus
3. Left ovary
4. Right ovary
5. Bladder
6. External iliac vein
7. External iliac artery
8. Inferior epigastric vessels
9. Round ligament
10. Piriformis muscle
11. Branches of internal iliac vessels
12. Sigmoid colon
13. Inferior gluteal vessels
14. Gluteus maximus
15. Gluteus medius
16. Gluteus minimus

LOWER SACRAL LEVEL – FEMALE (FIG. 6.36C)

The uterus is seen closely applied to the posterior surface of the bladder. The position of the ovaries is variable, and they may be found lateral to the uterus or behind it. The ureters are close to the posterolateral aspect of the bladder at this level. They hook medially in the broad ligament of the uterus (which cannot be identified as a separate structure), passing under the uterine artery and above the lateral vaginal fornix before entering the bladder.

SECTION THROUGH THE PERINEUM – MALE (FIG. 6.10)

The anterior compartment (**urogenital triangle**) is immediately deep to the lower part of the symphysis pubis. It consists of the prostate gland and prostatic urethra. Immediately behind is the anorectal junction in the posterior (anal) triangle. The **ischiorectal fossa** is seen on either side of and behind the anal canal (see earlier discussion for boundaries). Note how far anterior the upper part of the anal canal is. The **puborectalis fibres of levator ani** surround the **external anal sphincter**. Laterally are the obturator internus muscle and the ischial tuberosity. The **sacrotuberous ligament** can usually be identified running laterally from the coccyx and sacrum to the ischial tuberosity. Posteriorly are the gluteus maximus muscle and the coccyx.

SECTION THROUGH THE PERINEUM – FEMALE (FIG. 6.11)

The posterior compartment is the same as that for the male. The anterior compartment has the urethra just behind the pubis, with the vagina immediately behind. These structures are seen more clearly with MRI than with CT.

7 *The Upper Limb*

JOHN HYNES
EDITED BY STEPHEN EUSTACE

CHAPTER CONTENTS

The Bones of the Upper Limb 284
The Joints of the Upper Limb 290
The Muscles of the Upper Limb 308

The Arterial Supply of the Upper Limb 309
The Veins of the Upper Limb 310

The Bones of the Upper Limb

THE SCAPULA (FIGS. 7.1, 7.2)

This flat triangular bone has three processes:
- The glenoid process, which is separated from the remainder by the neck of the scapula. The glenoid cavity forms part of the shoulder joint.
- The spine, which arises from the posterior surface of the scapula and separates the supraspinous and infraspinous fossae. The spine extends laterally over the shoulder joint as the acromion (see Fig. 7.2).
- The coracoid process, which projects anteriorly from the upper border of the neck of the scapula.

RADIOLOGICAL FEATURES OF THE SCAPULA

Plain Radiographs

The inferior angle of the scapula lies over the seventh rib or interspace – this is a useful guideline in identifying ribs or thoracic vertebral levels.

The scapula lies over the ribs and obscures some of the lung on a posteroanterior (PA) chest radiograph (taken through the subject's back with their chest next to the plate), unless the shoulders are rotated forwards. In anteroposterior (AP) views it is not usually possible to rotate the scapulae off the lungs. In AP views of the scapula, the beam is centred over the head of the humerus in order to project the thoracic cage away from the scapula.

In lateral chest radiographs, the lateral border of the scapula may be confused with an oblique fissure. The inferior angle of the scapula may be slightly bulbous and simulate a mass on this view.

> **RADIOLOGY PEARL**
>
> In an isotope bone scan, injected radioactive technetium is taken up by metabolically active bone and emits a signal detectable by a Gamma camera. This is usually done to detect areas of abnormally active bone ('hot spots'), such as in arthritis where there is inflammation or in bony metastases. The inferior angle of the scapula overlying the seventh rib may appear as a 'hot spot' as the isotope signal from both structures is additive.

Ossification

The scapula ossifies in the eighth week of fetal life. An ossification centre appears in the middle of the coracoid process in the first year of life and fuses at 15 years of age. Secondary centres appear in the root of the coracoid process, the medial border and the inferior angle of the scapula between 14 and 20 years, and fuse between 22 and 25 years of age.

> **RADIOLOGY PEARL**
>
> The glenoid is oblique from posterior to anterior, lateral to medial in orientation. This is an anatomic evolutionary feature that prevents posterior dislocation following a fall on an outstretched hand. The same feature leads to the tendency to dislocate anteriorly following a direct fall on the shoulder.

THE CLAVICLE (FIG. 7.3; SEE ALSO FIG. 7.2)

The clavicle lies almost horizontally between the sternoclavicular and the acromioclavicular joints. It is also attached to the first costal cartilage by the costoclavicular ligament, which arises from the rhomboid fossa on its inferomedial surface. It is connected to the coracoid process by the coracoclavicular ligament at the conoid tubercle and the trapezoid line on its inferolateral surface. The subclavian vessels and the trunks of the brachial plexus pass behind its medial third.

RADIOLOGICAL FEATURES OF THE CLAVICLE

Chest Radiograph

The clavicle overlies the apices of the lungs in chest radiographs. Apical or lordotic views are used to project the clavicles above the lungs to evaluate this area further. In portable AP chest radiography, if the patient is inclined backwards from a true vertical position the horizontal beam projects the clavicles above the lungs.

On a chest radiograph, the distance between the medial end of the clavicle and the spine of the vertebrae is equal on both sides unless the patient is rotated.

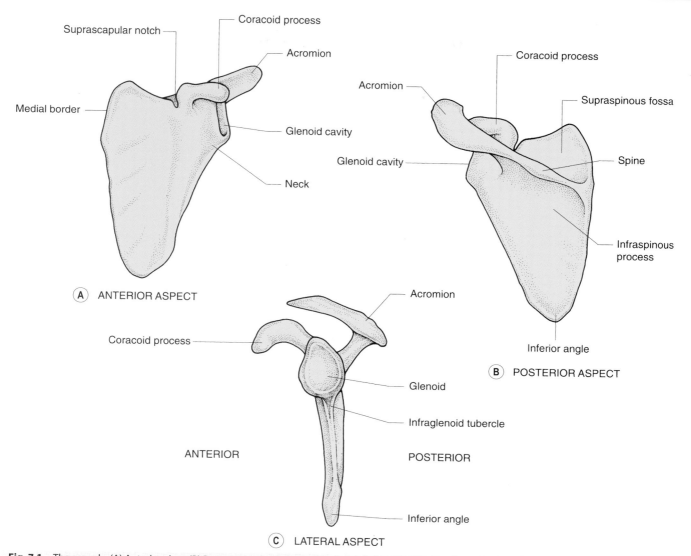

Fig. 7.1   The scapula. (A) Anterior view. (B) Posterior view. (C) Lateral view.

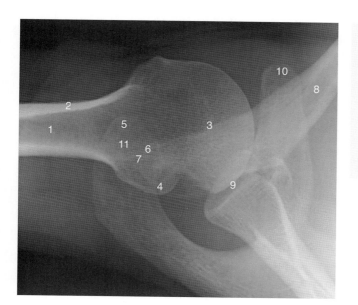

Fig. 7.2   Axial radiograph of the shoulder.

1. Medullary cavity of humeral shaft
2. Cortex
3. Head of humerus
4. Lesser tuberosity
5. Tip of the acromion process
6. Lateral end of the clavicle
7. Acromioclavicular joint
8. Clavicle
9. Glenoid fossa of the scapula
10. Coracoid process of the scapula
11. Acromion process of the scapula

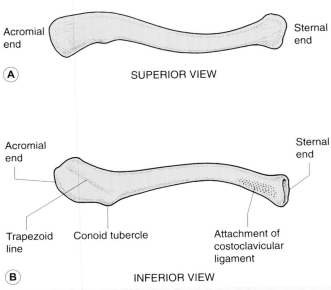

Fig. 7.3   The clavicle. (A) Superior view. (B) Inferior view.

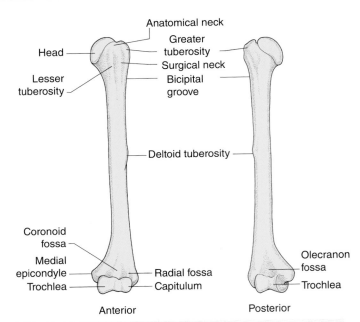

Fig. 7.4   The left humerus: anterior and posterior views.

Ossification

The clavicle begins to ossify before any other bone in the body. It ossifies in membrane from two centres that appear at the fifth and sixth fetal weeks, and fuses in the seventh week. A secondary centre appears at the sternal end at 15 years in females and 17 years in males, and fuses at 25 years of age.

Multislice computed tomography (CT) with reformatted images allows excellent tomographic assessment of the long axis of the clavicle. The articulation with the sternum is best visualized using magnetic resonance imaging (MRI) with a surface coil placed over the anterior chest wall. The width of the acromioclavicular joint can also be measured using high-resolution ultrasound.

THE HUMERUS (FIGS. 7.4, 7.5; SEE ALSO FIG. 7.2)

The hemispherical head of the humerus is separated from the greater and lesser tubercles by the anatomical neck. Between the tubercles is the bicipital groove for the long head of the biceps. The shaft just below the tubercles is narrow and is called the surgical neck of the humerus.

The shaft is marked by a spiral groove where the radial nerve and the profunda vessels run. The deltoid tuberosity on the lateral aspect of the midshaft is the site of insertion of the deltoid muscle.

The lower end of the humerus is expanded and has medial and lateral epicondyles. The articular surface for the elbow joint has a capitellum for articulation with the radial head and a trochlea for the olecranon fossa of the ulna. Above the trochlea are fossae, the coronoid anteriorly and the deeper olecranon fossa posteriorly.

RADIOLOGICAL FEATURES OF THE HUMERUS

Plain Radiographs

The lower epiphysis of the humerus lies at a 25-degree angle to the shaft so that a vertical line down the front of the shaft on a lateral radiograph – the anterior humeral line – bisects the capitellum.

An olecranon foramen may replace the olecranon fossa.

Avulsion of the Medial Epicondyle

The flexor muscles of the forearm arise from the medial epicondyle of the humerus. Repeated contractions or a single violent contraction of these muscles in a child can result

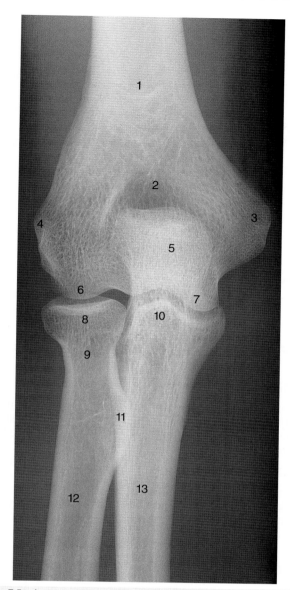

Fig. 7.5   Anteroposterior radiograph of the elbow.

1. Shaft of the humerus
2. Olecranon fossa
3. Medial epicondyle
4. Lateral epicondyle
5. Olecranon process
6. Capitulum
7. Trochlea
8. Head of radius
9. Neck of radius
10. Coronoid process of the ulna
11. Radial tuberosity
12. Shaft of radius
13. Shaft of ulna

in avulsion of the apophysis (a secondary ossification centre occurring outside a joint) of the medial epicondyle.

Ossification

The primary centre for the humerus appears at the eighth week of fetal life. Secondary centres appear in the head of the humerus at 1 year, the greater tuberosity at 3 years, and the

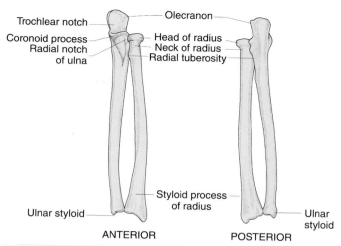

Fig. 7.6   The radius and ulna: anterior and posterior views.

lesser tuberosity at 5 years of age. These fuse with one another at 6 years and with the shaft at 20 years of age. Secondary centres appear in the Capitellum at 1 year, the Radial head at 5 years, the Internal epicondyle at 5 years, Trochlea at 10 years, Olecranon at 10 years and External epicondyle at 10 years (CRITOE). These fuse at 17–18 years of age.

THE RADIUS AND ULNA (FIGS. 7.6, 7.7; SEE ALSO FIG. 7.5)

The radius has a cylindrical head that is separated from the radial tubercle and the remainder of the shaft by the neck. Its lower end is expanded and its most distal part is the radial styloid. The radius is connected by the interosseous membrane to the ulna.

The upper part of the ulna – the olecranon – is hook-shaped, with the concavity of the hook – the trochlear fossa – anteriorly. A fossa found laterally at the base of the olecranon is for articulation with the radial head. The shaft of the ulna is narrow. The styloid process at the distal end is narrower and more proximal than that of the radius.

RADIOLOGICAL FEATURES OF THE RADIUS AND ULNA

Plain Radiographs

The head of the radius has a single cortical line on its upper surface and is perpendicular to the neck in the normal radiograph (see Fig. 7.5). Angulation of the head or a double cortical line are signs of fracture of the radial head.

The triceps muscle is inserted into the tip of the olecranon. Fracture of the olecranon is therefore associated with proximal displacement by the action of this muscle.

The ulnar styloid is proximal to the radial styloid, with a line joining them on an AP radiograph lying at an angle of 110 degrees with the long axis of the radius (see Fig. 7.7). In a lateral radiograph, the articulating surface of the distal radius is angled 10 degrees to a line through the shaft of the radius. Recognition of these normal angles is important in reduction of fractures of the wrist.

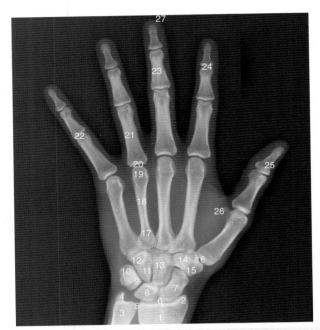

Fig. 7.7   Anteroposterior radiograph of the wrist and hand.

1. Distal radius
2. Styloid process of the radius
3. Distal ulna
4. Styloid process of the ulna
5. Distal radioulnar joint
6. Radiocarpal joint
7. Scaphoid
8. Lunate
9. Triquetral
10. Pisiform
11. Hamate
12. Hook of hamate
13. Capitate
14. Trapezoid
15. Trapezium
16. First metacarpophalangeal joint
17. Base of fourth metacarpal
18. Shaft of fourth metacarpal
19. Head of fourth metacarpal
20. Fourth metacarpophalangeal joint
21. Shaft of the proximal phalanx, ring finger
22. Proximal interphalangeal joint, little finger
23. Middle phalanx, middle finger
24. Distal interphalangeal joint, index finger
25. Distal phalanx, thumb
26. Sesamoid bone
27. Soft tissues overlying the distal phalanx of the middle finger

---

RADIOLOGY PEARL

Failure to restore volar angulation of the distal radius following a fracture of the distal radius often results in loss of grip strength due to impaired flexor function.

The pronator quadratus is a square, flat muscle that arises on the distal ulna and passes to the distal radius. A thin fat pad overlying this muscle is visible as a linear lucency on a lateral radiograph of the wrist. Thickening of the muscle, such as by haematoma in a fracture of the underlying bone, can be detected on a radiograph by bowing of the pronator quadratus fat pad.

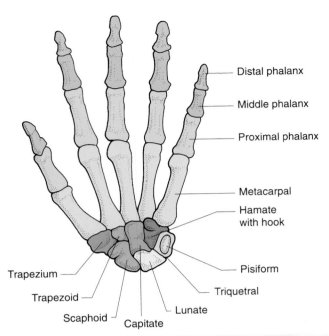

Fig. 7.8   Bones of the hand.

Ossification of the Radius

The primary ossification centre of the radius appears in the eighth week of fetal life. Secondary centres appear distally in the first year and proximally at 5 years of age. These fuse at 20 years and 17 years, respectively.

Ossification of the Ulna

The shaft of the ulna ossifies in the eighth week of fetal life. Secondary centres appear in the distal ulna at 5 years and in the olecranon at 10 years of age. These fuse at 20 and 17 years, respectively.

THE CARPAL BONES (FIG. 7.8; SEE ALSO FIG. 7.7)

The carpal bones are arranged in two rows of four each. In the proximal row, from lateral to medial, are the scaphoid, lunate and triquetral bones, with the pisiform on the anterior surface of the triquetral. The trapezium, trapezoid, capitate and hamate make up the distal row.

Together the carpal bones form an arch, with its concavity situated anteriorly. The flexor retinaculum is attached laterally to the scaphoid and the ridge of the trapezium, and medially to the pisiform and the hook of the hamate. It converts the arch of bones into a tunnel, the carpal tunnel, which conveys the superficial and deep flexor tendons of the fingers and the thumb (except flexor carpi ulnaris and palmaris longus tendons) and the median nerve. The extensor retinaculum on the dorsum of the wrist attaches to the pisiform and triquetrum medially and the radius laterally. Six separate synovial sheaths run beneath it (Fig. 7.9).

RADIOLOGICAL FEATURES OF THE CARPAL BONES

Radiography

These are radiographed in the anteroposterior, lateral and oblique positions (see Fig. 7.7). Carpal tunnel views are

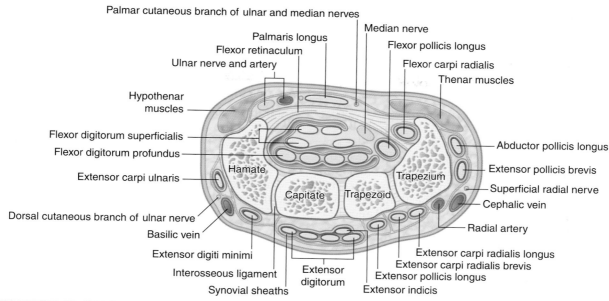

Fig. 7.9 Axial diagram of wrist tendons. (From Waring L, Hall A, Riley S. *Musculoskeletal Ultrasound*. Elsevier; 2022.)

obtained by extending the wrist and taking an inferosuperior view that is centred over the anterior part of the wrist.

Supernumerary Bones

These may be found in the wrist and include the os centrale found between the scaphoid, trapezoid and capitate, which may represent the tubercle of the scaphoid that has not fused with its upper pole, and the os radiale externum, which is found on the lateral side of the scaphoid distal to the radial styloid.

Nutrient Arteries of the Scaphoid

In 13% of subjects these enter the scaphoid exclusively in its distal half. If such a bone fractures across its midportion, the blood supply to the proximal portion is cut off and ischaemic necrosis is inevitable. This occurs in 50% of patients with displaced scaphoid fractures.

Ossification of the Carpal Bones

These ossify from a single centre each. The capitate ossifies first and the pisiform last, but the order and timing of the ossification of the other bones is variable. Excluding the pisiform, they ossify in a clockwise direction from capitate to trapezoid as follows: the capitate at 4 months; the hamate at 4 months; the triquetral at 3 years; the lunate bone at 5 years; and the scaphoid, trapezium and trapezoid at 6 years. The pisiform ossifies at 11 years of age.

THE METACARPALS AND PHALANGES

The five metacarpals are numbered from the lateral to the medial side. Each has a base proximally that articulates with that of the other metacarpals, except in the case of the first metacarpal, which is as a result more mobile and less likely to fracture. The third metacarpal has a styloid process extending from its base on the dorsal aspect. Each metacarpal has a rounded head distally, which articulates with the proximal phalanx.

The phalanges are 14 in number, three for each finger and two for the thumb. Like the metacarpals, each has a head, a shaft and a base. The distal part of the distal phalanx is expanded as the tuft of the distal phalanx.

RADIOLOGICAL FEATURES OF THE METACARPALS AND PHALANGES

Bone Age

A radiograph of the left hand is used in the determination of bone age. Standards of age determined by epiphyseal appearance and fusion have been compiled for the left hand and wrist by Greulich and Pyle, and by Tanner and Whitehouse (TW2 method).

The Metacarpal Sign

A line tangential to the heads of the fourth and fifth metacarpals does not cross the head of the third metacarpal in 90% of normal hands – this is called the metacarpal sign. This line does, however, cross the third metacarpal head in gonadal dysgenesis.

The Carpal Angle

This is formed by lines tangential to the proximal ends of the scaphoid and lunate bones. In normal hands the average angle is 138 degrees. It is reduced to an average 108 degrees in gonadal dysgenesis.

The Metacarpal Index

This is calculated by measuring the lengths of the second, third, fourth and fifth metacarpals and dividing by their breadths taken at their exact midpoint. The sum of these divided by four is the metacarpal index, which has a normal range of 5.4–7.9. An index greater than 8.4 suggests the diagnosis of arachnodactyly.

Sesamoid Bones

Two sesamoid bones are found related to the anterior surface of the metacarpophalangeal joint of the thumb in the normal radiograph. A single sesamoid bone in relation to this joint in the little finger is seen in 83% of radiographs, and at the interphalangeal joint of the thumb in 73%. These are occasionally found at other metacarpal and distal interphalangeal joints. The incidence of sesamoid bones is increased in acromegaly.

Ossification of the Metacarpals and Phalanges

These ossify between the ninth and twelfth fetal weeks. Secondary ossification centres appear in the distal end of the metacarpals of the fingers at 2 years and fuse at 20 years of age. Secondary centres for the thumb metacarpal and for the phalanges are at their proximal end and appear between 2 and 3 years, and fuse between 18 and 20 years of age.

The Joints of the Upper Limb

THE STERNOCLAVICULAR JOINT

Type

The sternoclavicular joint is a synovial joint divided into two parts by an articular disc.

Articular Surfaces

These are the sternal end of the clavicle, the clavicular notch of the manubrium and the upper surface of the first costal cartilage.

Ligaments

These are the anterior and posterior sternoclavicular ligaments, the costoclavicular ligament and the interclavicular ligament.

THE ACROMIOCLAVICULAR JOINT

Type

The acromioclavicular joint is a synovial joint.

Articular Surfaces

These are the outer end of the clavicle and the acromion. In health the undersurface of the acromion will align with the undersurface of the clavicle.

Ligaments

These are as follows:
- Acromioclavicular ligament, which is a thickening of the fibrous capsule superiorly.
- Coracoclavicular ligament, which has conoid and trapezoid parts.

THE SHOULDER (GLENOHUMERAL) JOINT (FIGS. 7.11–7.15)

Type

The glenohumeral joint is a ball-and-socket synovial joint.

Articular Surfaces

These are as follows:
- Head of the humerus.
- The glenoid cavity of the scapula, which is made deeper by a fibrocartilaginous ring – the labrum glenoidale.

The articular surface of the humeral head is four times the area of the glenoid cavity.

Capsule

This is attached to the epiphyseal line of the glenoid and humerus, except inferiorly where it extends downwards on the medial aspect of the neck of the humerus as the axillary pouch.

Synovium

In addition to lining the capsule of the joint, the synovium extends along the tendon of the long head of the biceps and beneath the tendon of subscapularis muscle as the subscapular bursa. The long head of the biceps is therefore extra-synovial but intracapsular attaching to the supraglenoid tubercle.

Ligaments

These are as follows:
- Three glenohumeral ligaments: anterior thickenings of the capsule passing from the upper part of the glenoid to the lesser tuberosity and the inferior part of the head of the humerus. These are weak ligaments and not supported by overlying muscles, unlike the posterior capsule which is reinforced by the infraspinatus muscle.
- The coracohumeral ligament.
- The transverse humeral ligament between the greater and the lesser tuberosities of the humerus which maintains the long head of the biceps tendon within the bicipital groove.

Stability

In addition to ligaments, the stability of the shoulder joint depends upon the surrounding muscles. These are:
- The short muscles known as the rotator cuff muscles (i.e. subscapularis, infraspinatus and teres minor muscles).
- The longer muscles, including the long head of the biceps, pectoralis major, latissimus dorsi, teres major and deltoid muscles.

The inferior part of the joint is least well protected by either ligaments or muscles.

RADIOLOGICAL FEATURES OF THE SHOULDER JOINT

Plain Radiographs

The supraspinatus muscle passes on the superior aspect of the shoulder joint to the greater tuberosity of the humerus.

Calcification occurs in this muscle owing to degenerative change and may be visible on radiographs.

The supraspinatus muscle is separated from the acromion by the subacromial–subdeltoid bursa, the largest bursa in the body. This bursa does not communicate with the shoulder joint unless the supraspinatus is ruptured by trauma or degeneration. This communication is then visible on arthrography. MRI can also be used to detect this rupture.

The capsule of the shoulder joint is lax and relatively unprotected by ligaments or muscles inferiorly. This is the site of accumulation of fluid in effusion or haematoma of the joint.

Arthrography With or Without CT

In the shoulder joint, arthrography is achieved by injection of contrast into the joint below and lateral to the coracoid process. It shows the features of the joint as outlined above. In particular, the axillary pouch can be seen inferior to the humeral head on external rotation of the arm, and the

subscapular (subcoracoid) bursa can be seen on internal rotation of the arm. The subacromial (subdeltoid) bursa is not filled unless the supraspinatus tendon is completely ruptured.

The tendon of the long head of the biceps is seen as a filling defect within the joint and its synovial sheath is opacified outside the joint along the bicipital groove of the humerus.

Subacromial Bursography

Contrast injection to the subacromial bursa with either ultrasound or fluoroscopic guidance is often followed by therapeutic injection of steroid and bupivacaine (Marcaine). Subacromial bursitis or inflammation of the bursa is most frequently secondary to impingement (Fig. 7.10A and B).

Ultrasound

High-frequency linear probes are now often employed as an alternative to MRI to evaluate the rotator cuff (see Fig. 7.10C and D).

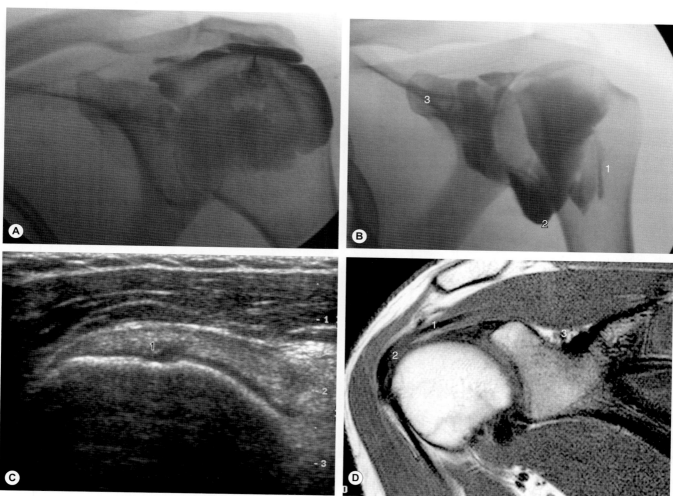

Fig. 7.10 (A) Contrast outlining the subacromial bursa allowing targeted placement of the therapeutic steroid. (B) Shoulder arthrogram showing contrast filling of the joint space. (C) High-frequency ultrasound showing supraspinatus tendon attachment to the humeral head. (D) Corresponding coronal oblique magnetic resonance image.

(B)
1. The biceps sheath
2. The axillary pouch
3. The subcoracoid recess

(C and D)
1. Supraspinatus tendon
2. Supraspinatus tendon attachment
3. The suprascapular notch

Dynamic imaging during movement of the joint can be performed to assess the rotator cuff.

The acromioclavicular distance can be measured to assess for widening.

MRI (see Figs. 7.11, 7.12. 7.14, 7.15)

MRI with surface coils is used increasingly to image the shoulder joint.

RELEVANT ANATOMY – CONTRIBUTORS TO STABILITY

The rotator cuff. Four muscles comprise the rotator cuff: the supraspinatus, the infraspinatus, the teres minor and the subscapularis (pneumonic – SITS) and are readily identified in the coronal oblique (plane parallel to the axis of the supraspinatus tendon), sagittal oblique and axial planes.

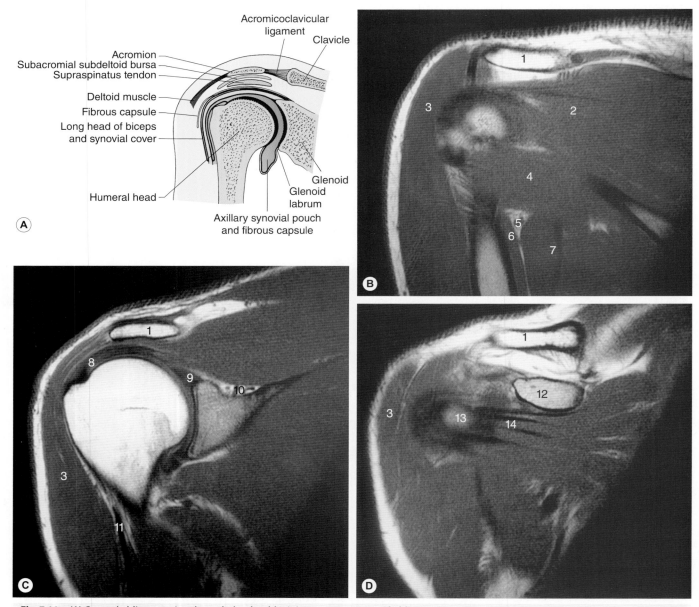

Fig. 7.11   (A) Coronal oblique section through the shoulder joint as seen on coronal oblique magnetic resonance imaging scan. (B–D) Coronal oblique T1-weighted images from posterior to anterior.

(B–D)
1. Acromion process
2. Infraspinatus muscle
3. Deltoid muscle
4. Teres minor muscle
5. Quadrilateral space (containing the circumflex humeral nerve and vessels)
6. Triceps muscle (lateral head)
7. Triceps muscle (long head)

8. Supraspinatus muscle and tendon
9. Superior labrum (and long head of the biceps muscle anchor)
10. Suprascapular notch (containing the suprascapular nerve artery and vein)
11. Biceps tendon
12. Coracoid process
13. Lesser tuberosity of the humeral head
14. Subscapularis muscle and tendon

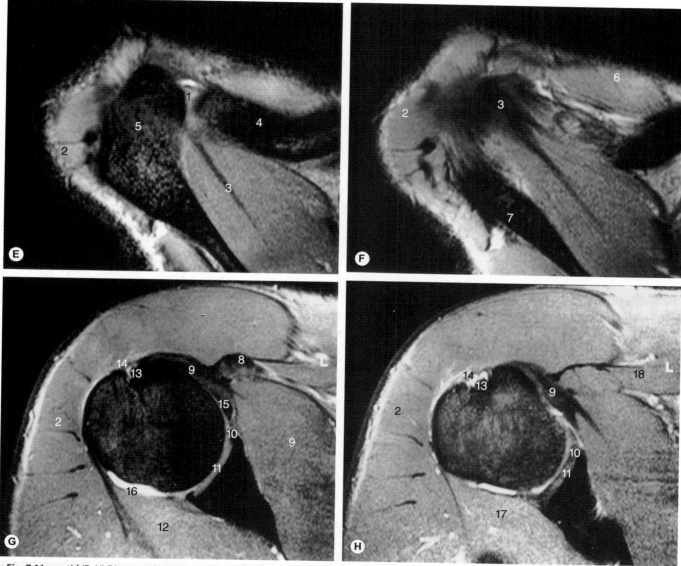

Fig. 7.11, cont'd (E–H) Direct axial images of the shoulder from superior to inferior.

(E–H)
1. Acromioclavicular joint
2. Deltoid muscle, lateral belly
3. Supraspinatus tendon insertion
4. Clavicle
5. Acromion process
6. Deltoid muscle, anterior belly
7. Scapula
8. Coracoid process
9. Subscapularis muscle and tendon
10. Anterior glenoid labrum
11. Hyaline articular cartilage
12. Infraspinatus muscle
13. Long head of biceps tendon and sheath
14. Transverse humeral ligament
15. Middle glenohumeral ligament
16. Posterior glenohumeral joint capsule
17. Teres minor muscle
18. Coracobrachialis

The coracoacromial arch. This represents the osseous, ligamentous arch composed of the tip of the coracoid, the coracoacromial ligament, the acromion and the acromio-clavicular articulation. Three typical acromial shapes are described (see Fig. 7.13A): type 1 curved, type 2 flat and type 3 flat with a marginal hook.

RADIOLOGY PEARL

Type 1 acromion is identified in 75% of the normal population; type 3 is least common but often produces symptomatic impingement of the supraspinatus tendon.

The glenoid labrum. The osseous glenoid is angled 10–20 degrees volarly, preventing posterior dislocation following a fall on the outstretched hand and increasing the likelihood of anterior dislocation following a fall with direct lateral trauma to the shoulder. Hyaline cartilage overlies the osseous glenoid, facilitating smooth articulation. Stability is afforded by the presence of a rim of fibrocartilage, the glenoid labrum, which marginates the osseous glenoid and overlies the hyaline cartilage.

Typically, the glenoid labrum is more rounded posteriorly and more triangular anteriorly.

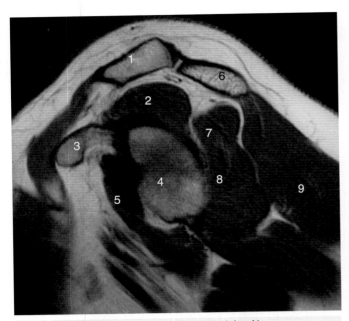

Fig. 7.12   Sagittal oblique proton density-weighted image.

1. Clavicle
2. Supraspinatus muscle belly
3. Coracoid process
4. Glenoid
5. Subscapularis
6. Acromion
7. Infraspinatus muscle belly
8. Teres minor muscle belly
9. Deltoid muscle

The bicipitolabral complex. The configuration of the superior labrum reflects its association with the insertion of the long head of the biceps tendon, the so-called bicipitolabral complex. Three forms of bicipitolabral complex are described (see Fig. 7.13B), which include type 1, in which the long head of the biceps inserts to the osseous glenoid immediately above the labrum; type 2, in which the biceps tendon inserts to the superior surface of the labrum; and type 3, where the long head of the biceps inserts into the labrum to produce a meniscoid-type insertion.

> **RADIOLOGY PEARL**
>
> The type 3 insertion or bicipitolabral complex predisposes to superior labral tears (SLAP: superior labral anteroposterior tear or injury) following applied traction forces.

Coronal MRIs with intra-articular contrast allow the identification of a sulcus along the anterior margin of the superior labrum, the sublabral sulcus, which parallels the configuration of the osseous glenoid in contrast to superior labral tears. The sublabral sulcus becomes more prominent with age.

The Buford complex. A relative deficiency of the anterior labrum is occasionally identified in less than 0.5% of the population between 12 and 3 o'clock on MR arthrography in association with a cord-like middle glenohumeral ligament, the so-called Buford complex (see Fig. 7.14).

In the axial plane it is quite normal to identify hyaline cartilage undercutting the fibrocartilaginous labrum at the level of the coracoid to produce the subcoracoid foramen.

The anteroinferior labrum is identified as a triangular structure in both the coronal and axial planes and is continuous with a fold of the joint capsule termed the inferior glenohumeral ligament.

> **RADIOLOGY PEARL**
>
> Injury to the anteroinferior glenoid following anterior dislocation, with both blunt trauma and traction stresses imposed by the inferior glenohumeral ligament, may result in simple disruption of the labrum (a Perthes lesion), in disruption of the labrum and associated bone (a Bankart lesion), in medialization of the labrum beneath a rind of periosteum (an ALPSA lesion: anterior labral periosteal sleeve avulsion); or merely produce avulsion of the inferior glenohumeral ligament from the humerus, a HAGL injury (humeral avulsion of the glenohumeral ligament).

The anterior capsular attachment. The joint space is enveloped by joint capsule. Posteriorly the capsule is inserted on cortex immediately behind the posterior labrum. Anteriorly three patterns of capsular insertion are described (see Fig. 7.13C): type 1, when the capsule inserts immediately behind the labrum; type 2, when the capsule inserts 1 cm behind the labrum; and type 3, when it inserts more than 2 cm behind the labrum on the neck of the glenoid.

The glenohumeral ligaments. Three folds in the anterior capsule give rise to the superior, middle and inferior glenohumeral ligaments, which result in local strengthening of the capsule and promote stability (see Fig. 7.15).

SHOULDER STABILITY

- Superior stability – of the glenohumeral joint is afforded by the superior labrum, the long head of the biceps, the joint capsule, the supraspinatus tendon, the subacromial bursa, and the structures of the coracoacromial arch.
- Posterior stability – of the glenohumeral joint is afforded by the angulation of the osseous glenoid, the posterior labrum, the capsule, and the posterior tendons of the rotator cuff, the infraspinatus and the teres minor.
- Anterior stability – of the glenohumeral joint is afforded by the labrum, the capsule and its associated folds or glenohumeral ligaments, and the subscapularis muscle.

MARROW PATTERNS

In infancy, marrow in both the axial and the appendicular skeleton is haemopoietic and termed red marrow. During maturation, red marrow converts to yellow marrow in the appendicular skeleton prior to any changes in the axial skeleton. In the extremities, yellow marrow conversion occurs initially in the epiphyses and then in the diaphyses of long bones, with some preservation of red marrow in the metaphyses and at sites of cancellous-type bone (Fig. 7.16).

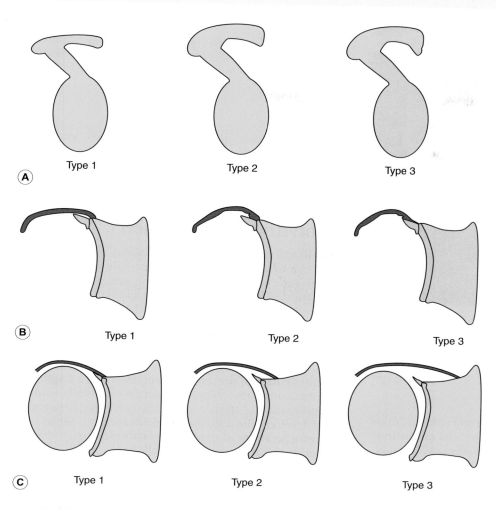

Fig. 7.13 (A) Acromial shapes, types 1, 2 and 3. (B) A diagram of coronal view of shoulder showing variations in the attachment of the long head of the biceps to the superior glenoid (type 1: attachment to glenoid; type 2: attachment to glenoid and labrum; type 3: attachment to labrum). (C) An axial diagram of the shoulder joint showing variations in the attachment of the capsule to the anterior margin of the glenoid (type 1: anterior capsule attachment; type 2: anterior capsule attachment to glenoid; type 3: attachment to medial glenoid).

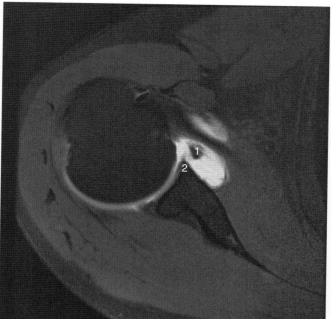

Fig. 7.14 Axial magnetic resonance arthrogram shows Buford complex.

1. Thickened middle glenohumeral ligament
2. Absent anterior glenoid labrum

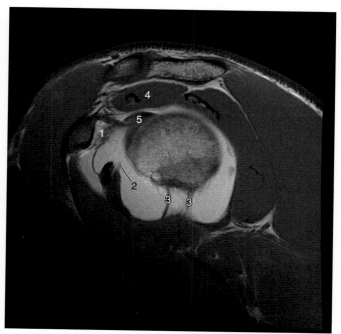

Fig. 7.15 Sagittal magnetic resonance arthrogram.

1. Superior
2. Middle glenohumeral ligaments
3. Inferior glenohumeral ligaments
4. Supraspinatus tendon
5. Biceps tendon

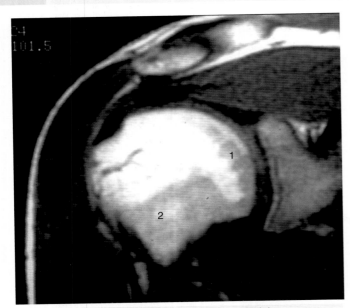

Fig. 7.16   Coronal T1-weighted image in a normal adult.

1. Epiphyseal subarticular red marrow rests
2. Metaphyseal red marrow

RADIOLOGY PEARL

In the shoulder, in adulthood it is normal to identify red marrow in the metaphysis of the humerus and within the glenoid. In the presence of oxygen demand, chronic bronchitis, excessive jogging and cigarette smoking, red marrow reconversion occurs, replacing yellow (fatty) marrow. It is quite normal to identify subarticular red marrow focal deposits within the humeral epiphysis in adulthood (in general there should be no red marrow in the epiphysis of long bones in adulthood), and in the presence of increased oxygen demand these may become more prominent on MRI (see Fig. 7.16). While yellow (fatty) marrow becomes dark on MRI sequences which suppress fat such as STIR, red marrow remains hyperintense (bright).

RADIOLOGY PEARL

Reflecting vascularity and the distribution of red marrow, metastases to bone in adulthood most frequently occur in the glenoid and humeral metaphysis.

THE ELBOW JOINT (FIG. 7.17)

Type

The elbow joint is a synovial hinge joint which incorporates the humeroulnar, the humeroradial and superior radioulnar joints as one cavity.

Articular Surfaces

These are the trochlea and capitellum of the humerus, the head and ulnar notch of the radius and the trochlear fossa, and the radial notch of the ulna.

Capsule

This is attached to the margins of the articular surfaces of the radius and ulna but more proximally on the humerus to include the olecranon, coronoid and radial fossae within the joint.

Ligaments

These are:
- The radial and ulnar collateral ligaments, which are lateral and medial thickenings of the capsule.
- The annular ligament, which surrounds the head of the radius and rotates within it. It is attached to the anterior and posterior edges of the radial notch on the ulna.

THE DEVELOPMENT OF THE ELBOW

At birth, the distal humerus is composed of a single cartilaginous epiphysis separated from the metaphysis by an arched physis. Injury at this time results in complete epiphyseal separations. The primitive epiphysis differentiates into four ossification centres: two epiphyses, the capitellum and the trochlea, and two apophyses, the medial and lateral epicondyles. Following such a division, subsequent injury is usually confined to individual ossification centres, in contrast to the gross injury or displacement that occurs in infancy.

The cartilage of the proximal ulna develops a single ossification centre, the olecranon, which eventually leads to mineralization of the coronoid. The cartilage of the radial head develops into a further single ossification centre.

The appearance of ossification centres occurs 1–2 years earlier in girls than in boys and follows an orderly progression, with appearance of the capitellar ossification centre first at 1–2 years, the radial head at 3–6 years, the inner or medial epicondyle at 4 years, the trochlea at 8 years, the olecranon at 9 years and the external epicondyle at 10 years (Table 7.1).

In adolescence, usually between 10 and 12 years, the three lateral ossification centres fuse, followed by closure of their associated physes at 13–16 years. The medial epicondyle physis is the last to close, at between 16 and 18 years.

Inappropriately treated injury to any of the ossification centres around the elbow may lead to deformity; however as the elbow physes contribute to only 20% of final length, shortening is often subtle.

RADIOLOGICAL FEATURES OF THE ELBOW JOINT

Plain Radiographs (see Fig. 7.17)

The capsule of the elbow joint is lax anteriorly and posteriorly so that effusion within the joint causes distension of the capsule anteriorly and posteriorly. Fat pads anterior and posterior to the joint are displaced away from the joint by an effusion and become visible as linear lucencies that are separated by soft-tissue densities from the bones on a lateral radiograph.

RADIOLOGY PEARL

Since the coronoid fossa is shallow the anterior fat pad can be identified in normality; in contrast the olecranon fossa is deep and therefore the posterior fat pad only becomes visible on a lateral radiograph when elevated by intra-articular fluid/effusion.

Arthrography

Arthrography of the elbow joint is achieved by injection of contrast medium between the radial head and the capitellum. The synovial cavity of the joint is outlined and seen to extend proximal to the articular surfaces on the humerus, with a configuration on AP views that has been likened to rabbit ears and called the 'Bugs Bunny' sign. On lateral views, a coronoid recess is seen anterior to the lower humerus and an olecranon recess posteriorly.

Distally the synovial cavity is seen to extend anterior to the radius as the preradial recess. This is indented where the annular ligament of the radius surrounds it. Air arthrography involves intra-articular injection of up to 10 cc of air prior to multislice CT imaging. This is the optimum method of detecting intra-articular loose bodies.

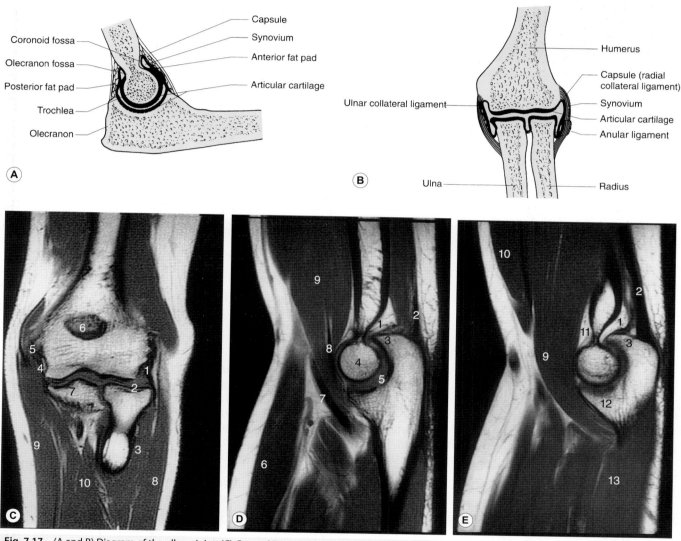

Fig. 7.17 (A and B) Diagram of the elbow joint. (C) Coronal T1-weighted image of the elbow. (D and E) Direct sagittal T1-weighted images: (D) radial side; (E) ulnar side.

(C)
1. Radial collateral ligament
2. Radial head and annular ligament
3. Supinator muscle belly
4. Ulnar collateral ligament
5. Medial epicondyle and common flexor tendon insertion
6. Coronoid fossa
7. Coronoid process
8. Extensor digitorum muscle belly
9. Flexor carpi radialis
10. Pronator teres

(D and E)
1. Olecranon fossa
2. Triceps tendon
3. Olecranon process
4. Trochlea (medial humeral condyle)
5. Trochlear notch
6. Pronator teres muscle belly
7. Biceps tendon
8. Brachialis tendon
9. Brachialis muscle belly
10. Biceps muscle belly
11. Coronoid fossa
12. Coronoid process
13. Flexor carpi ulnaris muscle

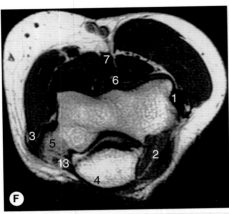 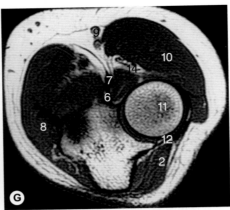

Fig. 7.17, cont'd (F and G) Direct axial proton density-weighted images: (F) from the level of the humeral condyles; (G) to the level of the proximal radioulnar joint.

(F and G)

1. Common extensor tendon insertion
2. Anconeus
3. Common flexor tendon insertion
4. Olecranon
5. Medial epicondyle
6. Brachialis tendon
7. Biceps tendon
8. Flexor carpi ulnaris
9. Brachial artery, vein and median nerve
10. Brachioradialis muscle
11. Radial head
12. Annular ligament
13. Ulnar nerve
14. Radial nerve

Table 7.1   Appearance of Ossification Centres

Capitellum	1–2 years
Radial head	3–6 years
Inner (medial) epicondyle	4 years
Trochlea	8 years
Olecranon	9 years
External (lateral) epicondyle	10 years

MRI (see Fig. 7.17)

Relevant Anatomy

The ulnar collateral ligament. The ulnar collateral ligament (UCL) is responsible for medial elbow joint stability and resistance to valgus strain. It is composed of three discrete tendon bundles:

■ The anterior bundle
■ The posterior bundle
■ The transverse bundle

Despite anatomic complexity, the anterior bundle is the most important contributor to stability and is therefore most frequently injured. The anterior bundle (the A-UCL) is taut in the extended elbow position and is therefore readily visualized on direct coronal images running from the undersurface of the medial epicondyle, just deep to the common flexor tendon origin, distally to its attachment to the medial aspect of the ulnar coronoid process. The anterior bundle blends with the fibres of the overlying flexor digitorum superficialis muscle. The posterior and transverse bundles may be identified in the axial plane forming the floor of the cubital tunnel.

At MRI, similar to other tendons with an organized structure, the UCL is hypointense on all sequences.

The lateral collateral ligament. Injury to the lateral radial collateral ligament occurs less frequently than injury to the medial UCL, complicating either acute varus strain or elbow dislocation.

The lateral collateral ligament has four components:

■ The radial collateral ligament, which is primarily responsible for lateral joint line stability.
■ The lateral UCL, which is primarily responsible for posterolateral stability.
■ The annular and accessory annular ligaments, which are responsible for stability of the proximal radioulnar joint.

At MRI the radial collateral ligament, being taut throughout elbow flexion, is readily identified on coronal images at approximately the same level as the A-UCL. The lateral UCL is identified on posterior coronal images. Being obliquely oriented, running from the lateral epicondyle to the posterolateral aspect of the ulnar, it is identified on serial images. It is taut when varus strain is applied. The annular ligaments, injury to which should be suspected in patients with either acute or repeated radial head subluxation or dislocation, are best visualized in the axial plane.

Similar to the UCL, injury ranges from subtle signal abnormality through peritendinous oedema to complete tendon disruption.

Radial collateral ligament injury, because it often reflects long-term overuse, is commonly accompanied by extensor tendon injury, epicondylitis or tennis elbow (most frequently accompanied by partial tear of the extensor carpi radialis brevis).

Biceps muscle and tendons.
- The biceps brachii muscle is composed of a long head and a short head.
- The two muscle bellies share a single tendon insertion on the bicipital tuberosity of the radius.
- The short head arises from the apex of the coracoid.
- The long head arises from the supraglenoid tubercle of the scapula.

Injury involving the biceps muscle more frequently involves the tendons than the muscle bellies, and, of the tendons, most frequently affects the tendon of the long head.

Injury to the distal biceps tendon is less common, and when it occurs it is usually secondary to acute macrotrauma or eccentric overload, as occurs when attempting to catch or carry a heavy object. In such a way, attempted elbow flexion through the biceps tendon is counterposed by forced extension induced by the object. The resulting tear occurs most frequently at or just proximal to the tendon insertion on the radial tuberosity.

RADIOLOGY PEARL

Although biceps tendon injury is usually clinically apparent, and usually manifests as an obvious mass, compensatory flexion incurred by the brachialis may obscure the diagnosis.

The distal biceps tendon is best visualized in the axial and sagittal planes; the axial images clearly depicting the normal insertion site on the radial tuberosity, the sagittal images allowing an appreciation of the extent of retraction.

Triceps tendon muscle and tendon.
The triceps muscle lies in the posterior compartment of the arm and is composed of three heads:
- The long head arising from the infraglenoid tubercle.
- The lateral head arising from the lateral and posterior aspect of the humerus.
- The medial head arising distally from the medial and posterior aspects of the humerus.

The three heads unite to form the triceps tendon in the midarm, the tendon being composed of a dominant deep component which merges with a superficial component before inserting on the posterosuperior surface of the olecranon.

Triceps tendon injury is extremely uncommon, and most frequently occurs secondary to forced flexion against a contracting muscle (attempting to extend the elbow) as occurs following a fall on an outstretched hand (forced eccentric contraction). Rarely injury may follow a direct blow, or

complicate olecranon bursitis where steroid injections, synovitis and superimposed infection conspire to weaken the tendon.

RADIOLOGY PEARL

In most cases tear of the distal triceps tendon is complete and associated with avulsion of a small fragment of bone from the posterior aspect of the olecranon, readily visualized on conventional radiographs. Rupture of the muscle belly or at the myotendinous junction, in the absence of an avulsion, is extremely uncommon.

LATERAL EPICONDYLITIS

Lateral epicondylitis or 'tennis elbow' is the commonest cause of elbow pain in the adult population. The term epicondylitis is misleading, as the disorder is characterized by soft-tissue changes in the absence of epicondylar bony oedema or inflammation. It is thought to reflect degeneration and tearing of the common extensor tendon as a result of chronic microtrauma secondary to traction forces, as it is most frequently identified in athletes. Resected specimens show fibrillary, hyaline and myxoid degeneration with angiofibroblastic proliferation within the tendon origin and minimal associated inflammatory change.

Medial Epicondylitis

Medial epicondylitis or golfer's elbow is considerably less common than lateral epicondylitis. Like lateral epicondylitis the descriptive term is misleading, as the injury is primarily to the common flexor tendon rather than to the underlying bone.

Repetitive valgus stress at the elbow in overhead racquet games, in golfers and in adolescent baseball pitchers results in chronic microtrauma to the common flexor tendon, with secondary degenerative rather than inflammatory changes. Swelling of the flexor carpi ulnaris within the cubital tunnel may lead to secondary ulnar nerve compression.

RELEVANT NEURAL ANATOMY AND INJURY FOLLOWING ELBOW TRAUMA

Elbow trauma may lead to injury of:
- The median nerve within the anteromedial soft tissues (most frequently following anterior dislocation).
- The radial nerve anterior to the lateral epicondyle (most frequently following lateral epicondylar fracture).
- The ulnar nerve within the cubital tunnel immediately posterior to the medial epicondyle.

Intimately related to the medial epicondyle, the ulnar nerve is the most frequently injured nerve about the elbow. Direct impaction leading to nerve contusion, fracture resulting in nerve compression or traction, and muscle or ligament tear allowing nerve subluxation may all lead to reversible nerve deficit.

'PSEUDOLESIONS' OF THE ELBOW

■ **Pseudodefect of the capitellum**. In the normal elbow there is an apparent osteochondral abnormality (often mistaken as being due to Panner's disease) in the sagittal plane along the posterior half of the perceived articular surface of the capitellum. In cadaveric specimens this has been shown to represent the junction of capitellum and lateral epicondyle.

■ **Pseudodefect of the trochlear groove and ridge**. The junction of the coronoid and olecranon is marked by a ridge 3–5 mm thick, devoid of overlying cartilage, routinely identified on sagittal images of the elbow traversing the joint space. At this junction, bone extends to appose the surfaces created by articular cartilage (ridge), occasionally not quite to the level of the articular cartilage (notch), but never beyond. At the far medial and lateral margins of the ridge the bone flares to form marginal grooves.

■ **The lateral synovial fringe or meniscus**. A triangular circumferential marginal fold of capsule and synovium is interposed between the radial head and the capitellum in the normal elbow. It may become more prominent in patients with Panner's disease secondary to friction imposed by irregular articular surfaces, or in patients with inflammatory arthritis.

■ **Skin thickening over the extensor surface of the elbow**. Skin overlying the olecranon appears thickened on MRI as a result of a paucity of underlying subcutaneous fat, particularly on images acquired in the sagittal plane.

■ **Distal triceps tendon signal heterogeneity**. In the axial plane the fibres of the distal triceps are loosely packed, resulting in signal heterogeneity in the axial plane, even in health. In the hyperextended position sagittal images show triceps tendon laxity and folds, which should not be mistaken for partial tears.

Additional infrequently encountered variants, which include asymptomatic subluxation of the ulnar nerve (secondary to an absent arcuate ligament), an accessory muscle in the region of the cubital tunnel fixing the ulnar nerve termed the anconeus epitrochlearis, an accessory osseous process extending from the anteromedial border of the distal humerus oriented towards the joint, the supracondylar process, or an accessory ossicle in the posterior joint space termed the os supratrochleare, are rarely identified. Each variant is reported to occur in less than 1 in 100 patients (1%).

THE INFERIOR RADIOULNAR (WRIST) JOINT (FIGS. 7.18, 7.19)

Type

The inferior radioulnar joint is a synovial pivot joint.

Articular Surfaces

These are the head of the ulna and the ulnar notch of the lower end of the radius and the upper surface of the articular disc (the triangular cartilage). This is triangular, with its apex attached to the styloid process of the ulna and the base to the ulnar notch of the radius. It separates the inferior radioulnar and radiocarpal joints.

Capsule

This is slightly thickened anteriorly and posteriorly. It is lax superiorly and extends upwards as a pouch, the recessus sacciformis, in front of the lower part of the interosseous membrane.

THE RADIOCARPAL JOINT (SEE FIG. 7.18)

Type

This is a synovial joint.

Articular Surfaces

These are the distal radius and distal surface of the triangular cartilage and the proximal surfaces of the scaphoid, lunate and triquetral bones. The articular surface of the radius is divided into a scaphoid and lunate facet. Following a fall on the outstretched hand, differential shear imposed by impaction of the lunate against the lunate facet results in extension of intra-articular fractures of the distal radius to the junction of the lunate and scaphoid articular facets.

Capsule

This is attached around the articular surfaces, except where it extends proximally as the palmar radial recess over the proximal radius to a variable degree.

Ligaments

These are the:
■ Palmar and dorsal radiocarpal ligaments
■ Palmar ulnocarpal ligament
■ Ulnar and radial collateral ligaments

THE INTERCARPAL JOINTS (SEE FIG. 7.18)

A midcarpal joint is found between the proximal and distal rows of carpal bones. This is separated from the radiocarpal and the carpometacarpal joints by interosseous ligaments between the carpal bones.

The carpometacarpal joint of the thumb between the trapezium and the metacarpal of the thumb is separate from the other carpometacarpal joints.

The carpometacarpal joint of the medial four metacarpals has a single synovial cavity and is also continuous with the intermetacarpal joints of the bases of these bones.

RADIOLOGICAL FEATURES OF THE JOINTS OF THE WRIST AND HAND

Wrist Biomechanics – Stable Versus Unstable Equilibrium

The biomechanics of the wrist are complex and involve the integrated motion of two intercalated segments (carpal bones linked by intercarpal ligaments), the proximal and distal row of carpal bones, which articulate with the bases

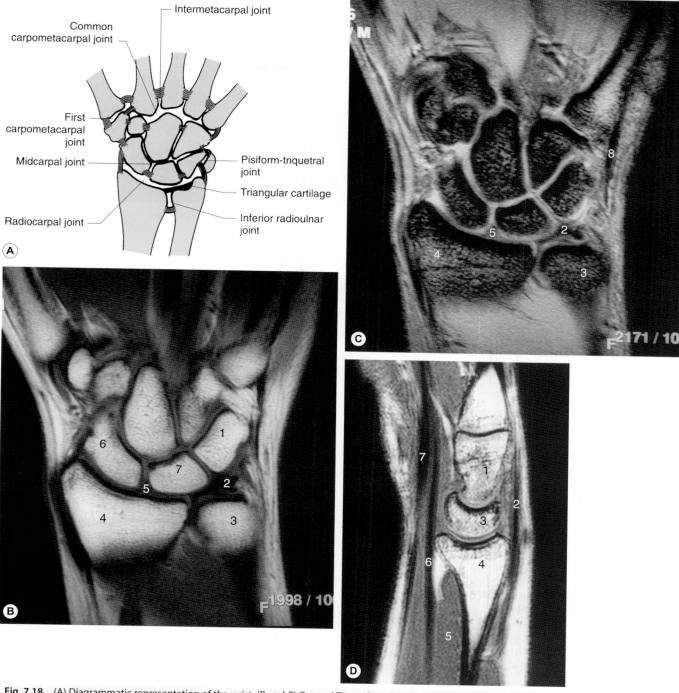

Fig. 7.18 (A) Diagrammatic representation of the wrist. (B and C) Coronal T1- and gradient echo T2-weighted images of the wrist. (D) Sagittal proton density-weighted image.

(B and C)
1. Triquetral bone
2. Triangular fibrocartilage
3. Ulna
4. Radius
5. Scapholunate ligament
6. Scaphoid
7. Lunate
8. Extensor carpi ulnaris tendon

(D)
1. Capitate
2. Extensor tendons
3. Pronator quadratus
4. Flexor digitorum profundus tendons
5. Flexor digitorum superficialis tendons

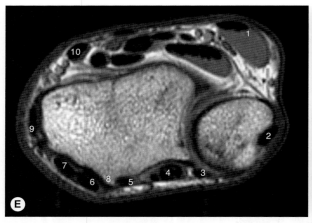 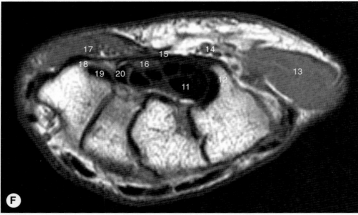

Fig. 7.18, cont'd (E and F) Axial proton density-weighted images at the level of the distal radius and ulna (E); and at the level of the distal pillars of the carpal tunnel (F).

(E and F)
1. Flexor carpi ulnaris muscle belly and tendon
2. Extensor carpi ulnaris tendon
3. Extensor digiti minimi tendon
4. Extensor digitorum tendons
5. Extensor pollicis longus tendon
6. Extensor carpi radialis brevis tendon
7. Extensor carpi radialis longus tendon
8. Lister's tubercle
9. Extensor pollicis brevis tendon
10. Flexor carpi radialis distal muscle belly
11. Flexor digitorum profundus tendons
12. Hook of the hamate
13. Hypothenar eminence
14. Guyon's canal (containing the ulnar nerve artery and vein)
15. Flexor retinaculum
16. Median nerve
17. Thenar eminence
18. Distal tubercle of trapezium
19. Flexor carpi radialis insertion
20. Flexor pollicis longus tendon

of the metacarpals and the distal radius at the radiocarpal articulation, facilitating wrist flexion and extension, ulnar and radial deviation and minimal pronation and supination (although this is most marked at the distal radiocarpal articulation).

Within the proximal carpal row there is a delicate balance between the opposing forces of the volarly angulated scaphoid and the mildly dorsally angulated lunate, transmitted through the scapholunate ligament. Such a balance allows smooth integrated movement of the proximal intercalated segment. In such a way, in the sagittal or lateral plane the scapholunate angle, or the angle between the volarly angulated scaphoid and the mildly dorsally angulated lunate, is 30–60 degrees, whereas that between the lunate and the capitate is 0–30 degrees. The angle of the distal radial articular surface is 10 degrees volar. Although slightly decreasing the range of dorsiflexion at the radiocarpal articulation, this is an evolutionary attempt to stabilize radiocarpal articulation and limit the tendency to dislocate dorsally at the radiocarpal articulation following a fall and dorsally oriented impaction forces (Fig. 7.20A–C).

Plain Radiographs

The normal alignment of the joints of the wrist and hand is visible on PA, lateral and oblique radiographs. Damage to any of the interosseous ligaments can cause displacement of one or more bones. The pisiform is the most anterior carpal bone on a true lateral X-ray of the wrist.

Scaphoid views. Recognizing its volar angulation, direct PA radiographs will project the distal pole of the scaphoid over the midbody and result in foreshortening

and the radiographic ring sign. The scaphoid may be elongated by imaging in ulnar deviation, which minimizes the amount of volar angulation, and by tilting the incident beam to 20–25 degrees. Evaluating the scaphoid in the absence of an angled tube in ulnar deviation is poor practice and likely to lead to erroneous diagnoses.

Arthrography

Arthrography of the radiocarpal or intercarpal or carpometacarpal joints may be achieved by injecting the appropriate space with contrast medium. The synovial cavity extends proximally anterior to the radius as the volar radial recess. The prestyloid recess is medial to the ulnar styloid process.

The inferior radioulnar, the radiocarpal, the midcarpal and carpometacarpal joints are not usually connected to one another. Studies of arthrograms on cadavers have, however, shown communication between the radiocarpal and inferior radioulnar joints in up to 35% of subjects, between the radiocarpal and midcarpal joints in up to 47%, and between the pisiform triquetral joint and the radiocarpal joint in more than 50%. The incidence of these communications increases with age and with force of injection, and probably reflects degenerative change.

MRI (see Fig. 7.18)

Relevant Anatomy

The scapholunate ligament. In health, the scapholunate ligament balances opposing forces of the volarly angulated scaphoid and the dorsally angulated lunate. At MRI, the ligament is delta-shaped in 75% of cases and linear in

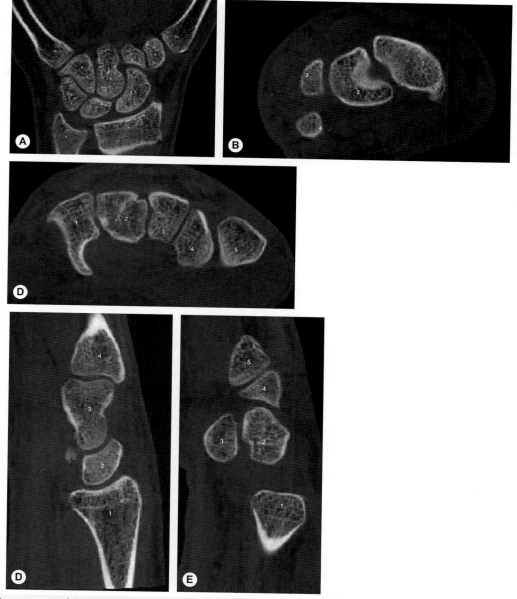

Fig. 7.19 Cone Beam computed tomography of the wrist and carpal bones. (A) Coronal, (B) axial image at the proximal carpal row level. (C) Axial image at the distal carpal row level. (D) Sagittal image through the distal radius. (E) Sagittal image through the distal ulna.

(A)
 1. Distal radius
 2. Ulna
 3. Scaphoid
 4. Lunate
 5. Triquetrum
 6. Trapezium
 7. Trapezoid
 8. Capitate
 9. Hamate
 10. First metacarpal
 11. Fifth metacarpal

(B)
 1. Scaphoid
 2. Lunate
 3. Triquetrum
 4. Pisiform

(C)
 1. Hamate
 2. Capitate
 3. Trapezoid
 4. Trapezium
 5. First metacarpal base

(D)
 1. Distal radius
 2. Lunate
 3. Capitate
 4. Third metacarpal base

(E)
 1. Distal ulna
 2. Triquetrum
 3. Pisiform
 4. Hamate
 5. Fifth metacarpal base

approximately 25%, and is hypointense in approximately 75% versus heterogeneous, with areas of isointensity in 25% of cases. The ligament is usually less than 3 mm in maximal transverse diameter in the coronal plane and is interposed between the scaphoid and lunate in the axial plane as thick dorsal (responsible for stability) and volar fibres, and an interposed membranous portion.

Following a fall on the outstretched hand, impaction forces through the long axis of the capitate are transmitted to the scapholunate interspace and the scapholunate ligament. Under the action of such forces the scapholunate ligament may rupture acutely, most commonly from the proximal pole of the scaphoid, or it may stretch before rupture, in both cases resulting in widening of the scapholunate interspace. In the absence of restraint the scaphoid tilts volarly whereas the lunate tilts dorsally.

On MRI following injury, the delta configuration of an intact ligament is lost as the ligament elongates prior to rupture, and frequently intrasubstance oedema results in apparent swelling or thickening of the ligament. The lunate attachment has more Sharpey's fibres and hence, when it occurs, tear is usually from the base of the scaphoid. Following rupture, hyperintense fluid is noted to pass freely between radiocarpal and midcarpal joint spaces.

Lunotriquetral ligament. The lunotriquetral ligament, similar to the scapholunate, is composed of both volar and dorsal components that attach directly to bone, rather than to hyaline cartilage overlying carpal bones. The ligament establishes continuity between radial and ulnar structures of the proximal carpal row of bones or intercalated segment.

Following a fall in ulnar deviation, impaction forces are transmitted through the ulnar side of the wrist, with acute shear manifesting as rupture of the lunotriquetral ligament, disruption of components of the triangular fibrocartilage complex, as subluxation of the distal radioulnar joint or as fracture.

Triangular fibrocartilage (TFC) complex (Fig. 7.20). The TFC complex is a complex anatomical structure composed predominantly of a triangular wedge-shaped fibrocartilaginous disc bridging the distal radioulnar joint, supported anteriorly and posteriorly by radioulnar ligaments, distally by attachments to the lunate through the volar ulnocarpal ligaments (the ulnolunate and ulnotriquetral ligaments), and laterally by the UCL and the extensor carpi ulnaris. The complex is completed by an additional fold in the lateral capsule interposed between the ulnar styloid and the triquetrum, termed the meniscal homologue. The meniscal homologue is interposed between the prestyloid recess and the triquetropisiform recess (Fig. 7.21).

The TFC is a biconcave disc separating the radiocarpal from the distal radioulnar joint spaces. It has attachments to both the ulnar styloid and the lunate fossa of the radius.

En bloc, the TFC complex functions to buttress forces transmitted to the distal ulnar and distal radioulnar articulations secondary to impaction during ulnar deviation. As such, injury is manifest as atypical pain and tenderness

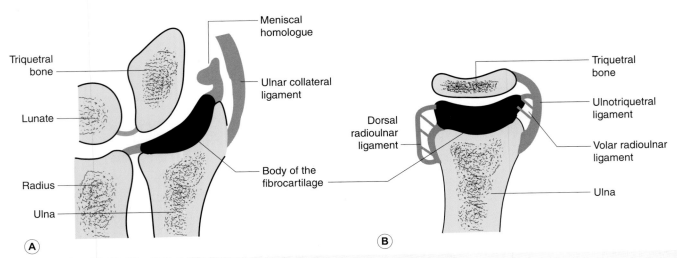

Fig. 7.20   The triangular fibrocartilage complex. (A) is AP, (B) is lateral.

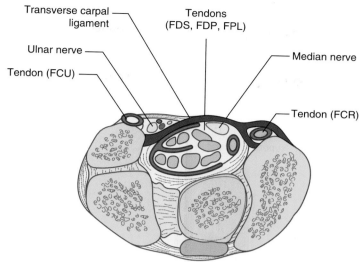

Transverse carpal ligament

Ulnar nerve

Tendon (FCU)

Tendons (FDS, FDP, FPL)

Median nerve

Tendon (FCR)

Fig. 7.21 Structures of the carpal tunnel and Guyon's canal. (Modified from Preston DC, Shapiro BE. *Electromyography and Neuromuscular Disorders*, 3rd ed. Elsevier; 2013:267–288.)

localized to the region of the ulnar styloid, often worse in ulnar deviation. Such discomfort often limits pronation and supination at the distal radioulnar articulations. In old age, as a result of cartilage degeneration, asymptomatic tears of the TFC are common.

At MRI the TFC is the only structure of the TFC complex consistently identified, although three-dimensional gradient echo sequences now allow visualization of both the volar and dorsal radioulnar ligaments.

MRI has a reported sensitivity of between 72% and 100% in the detection of tears, with associated specificities of 89%–100%.

Flexor and Extensor Tendons of the Wrist

There are six extensor compartments at the wrist arising out of the muscles of the extensor compartment of the forearm (see Fig. 7.18). From the ulnar side of the wrist to the radial side they are as follows: the extensor carpi ulnaris compartment, the extensor digiti minimi and the extensor digitorum compartment, the extensor pollicis longus compartment, which is separated from the extensor carpi radialis brevis compartment, the extensor carpi radialis longus compartment and the abductor pollicis compartment by Lister's tubercle. Each tendon is surrounded by a synovial sheath to facilitate tendon gliding.

The flexor tendons of the forearm pass through the carpal tunnel, which contains the flexor carpi radialis tendon, the flexor pollicis longus tendon and the flexor digitorum profundus and superficialis tendons, and the median nerve (interposed between the flexor retinaculum, the flexor pollicis longus tendon and the flexor digitorum tendons) (Fig. 7.22).

Imaging of the Soft Tissues of the Wrist

Both MRI and ultrasound can be used to evaluate the flexor and extensor tendons at the wrist and for assessment of the median nerve in carpal tunnel syndrome.

Tendon Injury at the Wrist

Extensor carpi ulnaris tendon. Extensor carpi ulnaris tenosynovitis usually complicates chronic occupational overuse, presenting as ulnar-sided wrist pain mimicking TFC tear, in chronicity commonly accompanying TFC tear. At MRI the tendon sheath is noted to be thickened, associated with peritendinous hyperintense fluid on T2-weighted sequences. In chronicity, foci of mineralization within the tendon are often noted to be hyperintense. Extension of chronic synovitis at the level of the radiocarpal articulation often leads to TFC degeneration in chronicity.

First extensor compartment syndrome – De Quervain's tenosynovitis. Repetitive wrist flexion and extension, particularly repetitive extension of the thumb, may promote chronic tenosynovitis in the first dorsal compartment or a fibro-osseous tunnel at the level of the radial styloid surrounding the extensor pollicis brevis and abductor pollicis longus tendons.

Intersection syndrome. Two forearm muscles and associated tendons, extensor pollicis brevis and abductor pollicis longus tendons, cross over the wrist tendons, the extensor carpi radialis brevis and longus, at the level of the wrist before attaching to the thumb. When these muscles work, they pull the thumb out and back. The extensor carpi radialis brevis and longus run lengthwise along the back of the forearm and attach on the base of the second and third metacarpal. The action of these two wrist tendons pulls the wrist back, into *extension*. During repetitive wrist flexion and extension, friction at the site of tendon crossing leads to local inflammation.

Scaphoid injury. The scaphoid is the second most commonly fractured bone of the wrist, typically complicating a fall on a dorsiflexed hand. Undisplaced fractures heal without complication in up to 95% of cases. Displaced fractures occur in up to 30% of cases, and when displacement is greater than 1 mm approximately 50% of cases develop either non-union, avascular necrosis or both.

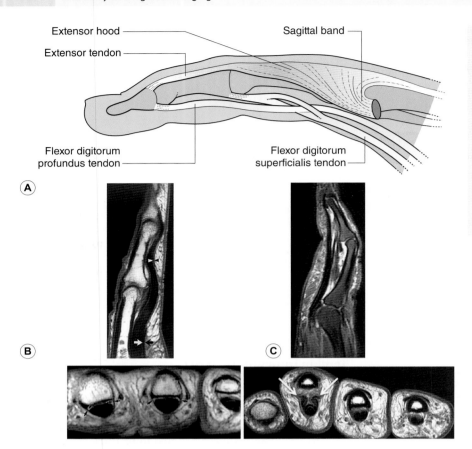

Extensor hood

Extensor tendon

Sagittal band

Flexor digitorum
profundus tendon

Flexor digitorum
superficialis tendon

(A)

(B)

(C)

Fig. 7.22 Sagittal image of the digit. (A) Schematic diagram demonstrating sagittal anatomy of the flexor and extensor tendons of the digit. (B and C) MRI of intact and disrupted pulleys. (B) Sagittal and axial T1-weighted spin-echo images show the A2 and A4 pulleys as focal thickenings of low signal intensity (*arrows* and *arrowheads* in sagittal image) and the osseous insertion of the A2 pulley (*arrows* in axial image), (C) Sagittal fat-saturated proton density and non–fat-saturated axial T1-weighted images in a patient with A2 through A4 ring finger pulley ruptures. The tendon-to-bone distance is increased (bowstringing). The axial image at the level of proximal phalanges demonstrates avulsion of A2 *(white arrows)* from bone. (B and C from *Flexor Pulley System: Anatomy, Injury, and Management*. YJHSU. 0363-5023. 2014.)

Fractures are classified by site and orientation into those affecting the proximal pole, the waist and the distal pole. Fractures of the distal pole rarely develop either non-union or avascular necrosis. In contrast, fractures of the proximal pole develop non-union in almost all cases. Healing of fractures through the midzone or waist is variable. Complications are more common in fractures with displacement or humpback angulation at the fracture margin.

Vascular integrity of fracture fragments. There are three patterns of blood supply to the carpal bones. Single vessels supply the scaphoid, capitate and lunate in 20%. The trapezium, triquetrum and pisiform and 80% of the lunate receive nutrient arteries through two nonarticular surfaces, with a consistent intraosseous anastomosis. The trapezoid and hamate lack an intraosseous anastomosis and after fracture are at risk of ischaemic necrosis.

The proximal 70%–80% of the scaphoid is supplied by the dorsal branch of the radial artery. Disruption of this vessel invariably occurs in fracture through the proximal pole, and occasionally in fracture through the wrist, resulting in ischaemic necrosis (atraumatic interruption of the vascular supply to the proximal pole is termed Preiser's disease). The tuberosity and distal pole are supplied by the volar branches, rarely interrupted by fracture.

The carpal tunnel. This is a fibro-osseous tunnel bounded by carpal bones, medial and lateral bony pillars, the distal pole of scaphoid and the trapezium and the pisiform and the hook of the hamate to which the transverse carpal ligament or retinaculum attaches. The canal contains the flexor tendons and the median nerve. The palmaris longus tendon lies superficial to the retinaculum and is continuous with the palmar fascia.

Guyon's canal. Guyon's canal is a fibro-osseous canal superficial to the flexor retinaculum, intimately related to both the pisiform and the hook of the hamate. The canal contains the ulnar nerve, artery and vein. At the level of the hook of hamate the nerve divides to a superficial palmar branch and a deep motor unit, such that fracture may disrupt either or both branches by direct contusion or persistent compression (see Fig. 7.21).

The Spaces of the Palm of the Hand

The palmar aponeurosis is a continuation of the palmaris longus muscle and associated fascia. It acts to protect underlying palmar structures attaching by a medial septum to the fifth metacarpal bone, by an intermediate septum to the third metacarpal bone and by a lateral septum to the first metacarpal bone.

Spaces and compartments:

- The thenar compartment contains the thenar muscles and is lateral to the septum.
- The hypothenar compartment is medial to the septum and contains the hypothenar muscles.
- The midpalmar space lies between the medial and intermediate septum and contains the flexor digital sheaths of digits 3–5, the lumbricals 2–5 and the digital nerves for digits 3–5.

- The thenar space lies between lateral and intermediate septa and contains the flexor digital sheath for digits 1 and 2, the first lumbrical and digital nerves for digits 1 and 2.

The Intrinsic Muscles of the Hand

- Thenar eminence – abductor pollicis brevis, flexor pollicis brevis, opponens pollicis.
- Hypothenar eminence – abductor digiti minimi, flexor digiti minimi, opponens digiti minimi.
- Central compartment – adductor pollicis, lumbricals, palmar and dorsal interossei.
- The lumbricals insert on the dorsal digital expansion and flex the metacarpophalangeal and extend the proximal interphalangeal articulations.
- The palmar interossei insert on the dorsal digital expansion – these muscles adduct digits.
- The dorsal interossei insert on the dorsal digital expansion – these muscles abduct digits.

Tendons and Soft-Tissue Anatomy of the Digit (Figs. 7.22, 7.23)

The flexor digitorum superficialis tendon splits and forms a sling through which passes the flexor digitorum profundus. The superficialis tendon slips attach to either side of the base of the middle phalanx. The profundus tendon attaches to the base of the distal phalanx.

The extensor digitorum tendons attach to the base of the distal phalanx.

The Volar Plate

The volar plate represents the ligamentous thickening of the volar capsule that bridges and stabilizes the volar aspect of the interphalangeal and metacarpophalangeal joints.

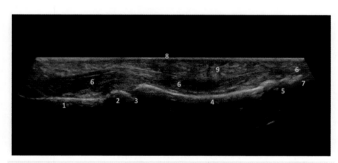

Fig. 7.23 Ultrasound of the flexor tendon of the digit. The ultrasound probe is on the skin of the palmar aspect of the digit. Ultrasound does not penetrate bone, so only the cortex is seen as an echogenic (white) line. However, the shape of the imaged bone is well seen and the gap where the joint is. The linear flexor tendon has lineal striations and its integrity along its length and its insertion into the distal phalanx can be assessed.

1. Proximal phalanx
2. Head of proximal phalanx
3. Proximal interphalangeal joint
4. Middle phalanx
5. Distal interphalangeal joint
6. Flexor tendon
7. Distal phalanx
8. Skin
9. Subcutaneous fat

The volar plate is primarily responsible for passive resistance to hyperextension at these articulations, active resistance being provided by contraction of flexor muscle groups.

The Dorsal Hood

The dorsal hood represents the ligamentous thickening of the dorsal capsule that bridges and stabilizes the dorsal aspect of the interphalangeal and metacarpophalangeal joints. The dorsal hood is responsible for passive resistance to hyperflexion at these articulations, active resistance being provided by contraction of the extensor muscle groups. At the dorsal hood an oblique ligamentous fold contributing to the hood is termed the sagittal band and is responsible for maintaining the central position of the extensor tendon over the metacarpophalangeal joint in flexion. Injury to the sagittal band may follow acute impaction trauma as occurs in boxing.

Collateral ligaments stabilize the ulnar and radial borders of the metacarpophalangeal and interphalangeal articulations.

Applied Anatomy and Digital Injury

Collateral ligament injury. Gamekeeper's thumb derives its name from an injury to the metacarpophalangeal articulation acquired by Scottish gamekeepers attempting to kill rabbits by strangulation. A contemporary term, skier's thumb, is now more frequently employed as it is in this group that the injury is now more frequently recognized. The injury is characterized by disruption of the UCL at the base of the thumb, the integrity of which dictates the ability to successfully appose the thumb and digits. Similar collateral ligaments are responsible for radial and ulnar stability in all the interphalangeal joints and, using MRI, may be imaged following suspected trauma.

Extensor tendon injury – mallet finger. The term mallet finger is used to describe the flexion deformity of the distal interphalangeal joint resulting from loss of extensor tendon continuity to the distal phalanx. The term 'mallet finger of bony origin' is used to describe the same deformity occurring secondary to intra-articular fracture of the dorsal lip of the distal phalanx.

Flexor digitorum profundus tendon injury – jersey finger. Avulsion of the flexor digitorum profundus tendon from its insertion into the base of the distal phalanx is a relatively uncommon injury, usually occurring during active sports, typically when a football or rugby player attempts to tackle the opposition but ends up grabbing a handful of jersey, hence the term 'jersey finger'.

Imaging of the Hand and Wrist

Ligaments are imaged with high-resolution ultrasound and MRI. Ligamentous finger injuries can be diagnosed using ultrasound (Fig. 7.23).

Imaging of the bones is performed by plain X-rays at different obliquity to best resolve the overlapping bony structures.

Cone beam CT (see Fig. 7.19) is a highly accurate method of assessing the bones of the wrist, superior diagnostically to plain X-rays, especially for diagnosis of subtle injuries.

The Muscles of the Upper Limb (Figs. 7.24–7.27)

Modalities such as CT and especially MRI have made imaging of the muscles of the limbs possible. Knowledge of the origin, course and insertion of these muscles is less important in radiology than an understanding of their positions relative to one another in cross-section. A brief description of the cross-sectional layout of muscle compartments is therefore appropriate. Muscles related to the shoulder joint are described in that section.

In the upper arm (see Figs. 7.24 and 7.26) the deltoid muscle covers the upper lateral aspect of the humerus. The flexors of the shoulder – the coracobrachialis and biceps muscles – lie anterior to the humerus in its upper third, and the flexors of the elbow – brachialis and biceps muscles – lie anterior to the lower part of the humerus. Extensors of the elbow joint – the triceps muscle with its long, lateral and medial heads – lie posterior to the humerus.

The neurovascular bundle of brachial artery, basilic vein and median nerve lies superficially, medial to the humerus. The radial nerve and profunda brachii artery lie deeply close to the humerus, at first medially then passing posteriorly close to the lateral side.

In the forearm (see Figs. 7.25 and 7.27) the interosseous membrane unites the radius and ulna and separates anterior and posterior compartments. Anteriorly lie the flexors of the wrist and fingers, flexor digitorum superficialis and profundus. Posteriorly are the extensors of the wrist and fingers and the abductor of the thumb – extensor carpi ulnaris, digitorum and pollicis longus, and abductor pollicis longus. The muscles abducting the wrist – flexor carpi radialis and extensor carpi radialis longus and brevis – lie superficially on the radial side and those that adduct the wrist – flexor carpi ulnaris and extensor carpi ulnaris – lie on the ulnar side.

The interosseous nerves and arteries lie close to the interosseous membrane. The radial nerve and vessels and the ulnar nerve and vessels lie anteriorly on each side, and the median nerve lies in the midline between the superficial and deep flexor muscles.

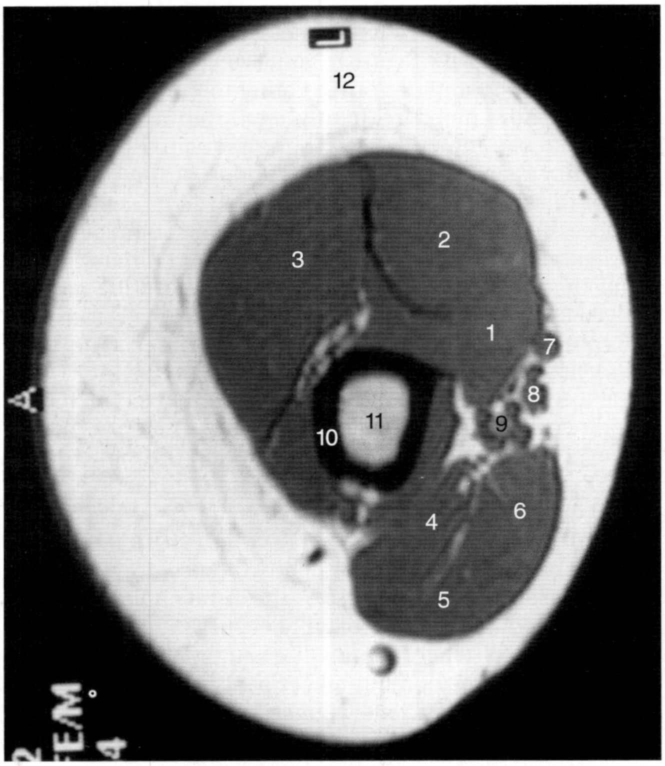

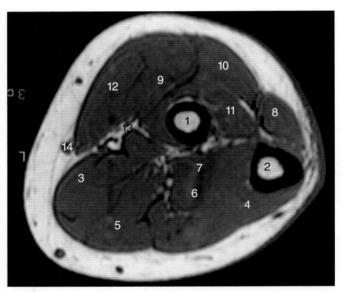

Fig. 7.24 Axial proton density-weighted magnetic resonance imaging section through the upper arm.

1. Biceps muscle – short head (flexor of the elbow)
2. Biceps muscle – long head (flexor of the elbow)
3. Brachialis muscle (flexor of the elbow)
4. Triceps muscle medial head (extensor of the elbow)
5. Triceps muscle lateral head (extensor of the elbow)
6. Triceps muscle long head (extensor of the elbow)
7. Basilic vein (neurovascular bundle)
8. Brachial artery (neurovascular bundle)
9. Median nerve (neurovascular bundle)
10. Cortex of the humeral shaft
11. Medullary cavity
12. Subcutaneous fat in the anterior aspect of the upper arm

Fig. 7.25 Axial proton density-weighted magnetic resonance imaging scan through the forearm. The scan was obtained with the palm facing up. Extensive fat allows easier visualization of the muscle groups. The flexors are anterior and the extensors posterior.

1. Radius
2. Ulna
3. Extensor carpi radialis muscle (longus and brevis)
4. Extensor carpi ulnaris muscle
5. Extensor digitorum muscle
6. Extensor pollicis longus muscle
7. Abductor pollicis longus muscle
8. Flexor carpi ulnaris muscle
9. Flexor carpi radialis muscle
10. Flexor digitorum superficialis muscle
11. Flexor digitorum profundus muscle
12. Brachioradialis muscle
13. Position of radial artery and vein
14. Cephalic vein

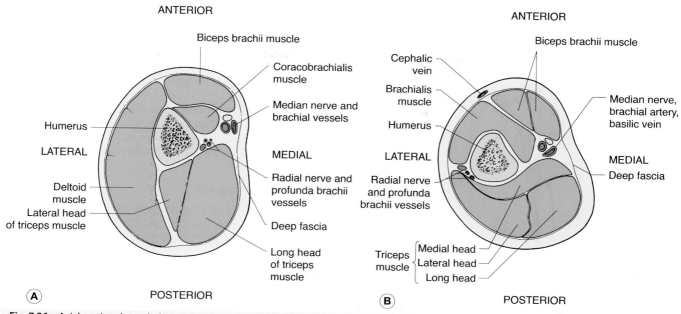

Fig. 7.26 Axial section through the upper arm showing muscle compartments. (A) Upper humeral level. (B) Midhumeral level.

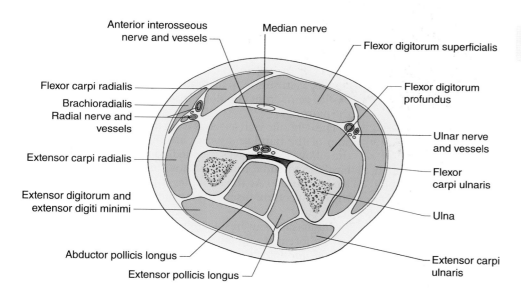

Fig. 7.27 Axial section through the lower arm showing muscle compartments.

The individual muscles may be difficult to distinguish on axial CT because of the lack of fat in the forearm. MRI is the superior method in this respect and has the added advantage of allowing direct imaging in many planes.

The Arterial Supply of the Upper Limb (see Fig. 7.28)

The upper limb receives its supply from the subclavian artery. This has four branches, namely:
- The vertebral artery
- The thyrocervical trunk, which supplies the inferior thyroid, suprascapular and transverse cervical arteries
- The internal thoracic artery
- The costocervical trunk, which divides into the superior intercostal and the deep cervical arteries

The subclavian artery becomes the axillary artery at the outer border of the first rib. The axillary artery lies with the brachial plexus and the axillary vein. It supplies six arteries to the chest wall and the shoulder (SALSA):
- The superior thoracic artery
- The acromiothoracic trunk
- The lateral thoracic artery
- The subscapular artery
- The anterior and posterior circumflex humeral arteries

The brachial artery begins at the lower border of the teres major. Its branches are:
- The profunda brachii artery (which arises medially)
- The nutrient artery to the humerus
- The muscular branches
- The branches to the elbow joint

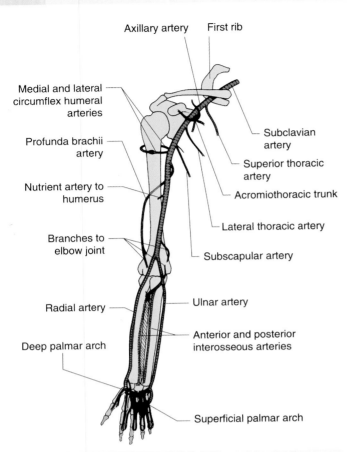

Fig. 7.28 Arteries of the upper limb.

At the level of the radial head (but sometimes much more proximally) the brachial artery divides into the radial and ulnar arteries. The radial artery passes on the lateral side of the forearm to the wrist, where it gives a branch to the superficial palmar arch and then passes via the floor of the anatomical snuffbox to the dorsum of the hand. It passes between the first and second metacarpals to form the deep palmar arch.

The ulnar artery is larger and deeper than the radial artery. It gives rise to the common interosseous artery, which in turn divides into the anterior and posterior interosseous arteries, the latter passing over the top of the interosseous membrane to supply the muscles of the dorsum of the forearm. Close to the wrist the ulnar artery becomes superficial and, having crossed the wrist, becomes the superficial palmar arch and sends a branch to the deep palmar arch.

RADIOLOGICAL FEATURES OF THE ARTERIAL SUPPLY OF THE UPPER LIMB

Arteriography (see also Chapter 1)

Arteriography of the aorta or of its coronary or other branches can be achieved via the arteries of the upper limb. Percutaneous puncture of the axillary artery carries the risks of brachial plexus damage, either directly or

by haematoma formation. The brachial artery, although smaller, is easier to puncture because of its superficial location over a bone. Damage to the nearby median nerve may occur, as may embolism distally to the radial or ulnar arteries.

Arteriography of the upper limb is achieved usually via the aortic arch by a femoral approach. The vessels and their branches already described are seen. Direct puncture of the subclavian, axillary or brachial arteries is occasionally used, particularly for interventional work such as embolization of arteriovenous malformations of the forearm or hand.

CT and MR Angiography

CT angiography of the upper limb provides excellent and rapid evaluation of the arterial system, particularly in the setting of trauma or other emergencies. The patient is generally positioned supine with the affected arm raised over the head. Images are acquired from the aortic arch to the fingertips. Magnetic resonance angiography, with or without gadolinium, also provides excellent image quality without the need for ionising radiation exposure.

The Veins of the Upper Limb (Fig. 7.29)

Superficial and deep veins drain blood from the upper limb. The superficial veins commence in the hand, where smaller veins unite to form three veins – the cephalic and basilic veins from the dorsum and the median vein from the palm.

The cephalic vein ascends from the radial side of the dorsum of the hand and winds around the forearm towards the elbow. Here it gives the median cubital vein to join the basilic vein and it then continues on the lateral side of the biceps muscle. At the shoulder it passes medially, pierces the clavipectoral fascia to become deep and joins the axillary vein.

The basilic vein has a similar course on the medial side of the forearm and elbow. At midhumeral level it passes deeply and joins the brachial vein to become the axillary vein.

The median vein of the forearm passes from the palm along the volar aspect of the forearm to join either the basilic or the cephalic veins at the elbow.

The deep veins of the upper limb are usually paired venae comitantes, which accompany the arteries. The axillary veins are usually double, whereas the subclavian vein is usually single.

RADIOLOGICAL FEATURES OF THE VEINS OF THE UPPER LIMB

Venography

Venography of the upper limb is achieved by injection of the superficial veins of the dorsum of the hand. To visualize the deep veins, films are taken with and without inflation of a tourniquet on the arm above the elbow.

Superior venacavography is achieved by simultaneous injection of veins of both arms. If thrombosis of the superior vena cava is suspected and extension into the axillary

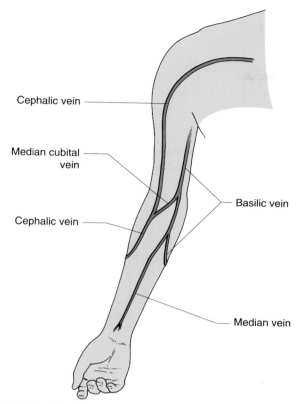

Cephalic vein

Median cubital vein

Cephalic vein

Basilic vein

Median vein

Fig. 7.29 Superficial veins of the upper limb.

veins is a possibility, then cannulation of the basilic veins is preferable to cannulation of the cephalic veins, as the latter bypass the proximal part of the axillary veins.

Intravenous Injection of Contrast or Radionuclides in Dynamic Studies

Blood flow in the cephalic vein may be held up at the site where it passes through the clavipectoral fascia. This makes this vein less suitable than the basilic vein for intravenous injection of contrast or radionuclides in dynamic studies.

Ultrasound

The upper limb veins can be assessed with Doppler ultrasound if upper extremity deep venous thrombosis is suspected. Typically, a 5- or 7.5-MHz probe is utilized and placed in a transverse orientation. The basilic vein lies superficially and medially and is usually single. The brachial vein may be paired and lies deeper, close to the brachial artery. These vessels may be followed proximally to their union forming the axillary vein. Both compressibility and colour Doppler flow should be assessed.

CT and MR Venography

CT and MR venography both allow evaluation of upper limb venous anatomy and latency. These are particularly useful both in situations where ultrasound is equivocal and in cases involving complex anatomy or collateral circulation.

8 The Lower Limb

JOHN HYNES
EDITED BY STEPHEN EUSTACE

CHAPTER CONTENTS

The Bones of the Lower Limb 312
The Joints of the Lower Limb 318
The Muscles of the Lower Limb 337

The Arteries of the Lower Limb 340
The Veins of the Lower Limb 343

The Bones of the Lower Limb

THE FEMUR (FIG. 8.1)

The femur is the longest and the strongest bone of the body. It has a head, neck, shaft and an expanded lower end.

The head is more than half of a sphere and is directed upwards, medially and forwards. It is intra-articular and covered with cartilage apart from a central pit called the fovea, where the ligamentum teres is attached. The blood supply of the femoral head is derived from three sources as follows:

- Vessels in the cancellous bone from the shaft
- Vessels in the capsule of the hip joint, which reach the head in synovial folds along the neck
- A negligible supply via the fovea from vessels in the ligamentum teres

> **RADIOLOGY PEARL**
>
> Reflecting the significance of vascular supply to the femoral head from vessels in the capsule of the joint, avascular necrosis in childhood is thought to be secondary to disruption of capsular supply due to compression by a distended joint effusion.

The neck of the femur is about 5 cm long and forms an angle of 125 degrees in females to 130 degrees in males with the shaft. It is also anteverted, that is, it is directed anteriorly at an angle of about 10 degrees with the sagittal plane.

> **RADIOLOGY PEARL**
>
> A femoral neck angle of less than 120 degrees is termed coxa varus and should be contrasted with a femoral neck angle greater than 135 degrees, termed coxa valgus.

Its junction with the shaft is marked superiorly by the greater trochanter and inferiorly and slightly posteriorly by the lesser trochanter. Between these anteriorly is a ridge called the intertrochanteric line, and posteriorly a more prominent intertrochanteric crest. The capsule of the hip joint is attached to the intertrochanteric line anteriorly but at the junction of the medial two-thirds and the lateral third of the neck posteriorly.

The shaft of the femur is inclined medially so that whereas the heads of the femurs are separated by the pelvis, the lower ends at the knees almost touch. It also has a forward convexity. The shaft is cylindrical with a prominent ridge posteriorly, the linea aspera. This ridge splits inferiorly into medial and lateral supracondylar lines, with the popliteal surface between them. The medial supracondylar line ends in the adductor tubercle.

The lower end of the femur is expanded into two prominent condyles united anteriorly as the patellar surface but separated posteriorly by a deep intercondylar notch. The most prominent parts of each condyle are called the medial and lateral epicondyles. Above the articular surface on the lateral side is a small depression that marks the origin of the popliteus muscle.

RADIOLOGICAL FEATURES OF THE FEMUR (SEE FIG. 8.1)

Plain Radiographs

A **line along the upper margin of the neck** of the femur transects the femoral head in anteroposterior (AP) and lateral radiographs. This alignment is changed when the epiphysis is slipped.

A **line along the inferior margin of the neck** of the femur forms a continuous arc with the superior and medial margin of the obturator foramen of the pelvis. This line, known as Shenton's **line** (see Fig. 8.8), is disrupted in congenital dislocation of the hip.

On an AP radiograph **a line between the lowermost part of each condyle**, although parallel to the upper tibia, lies at an angle of 81 degrees to the shaft of the femur. This amount of genu valgum is normal.

Radiography

The neck of the femur is **anteverted** approximately 10 degrees. In **AP radiography of the neck**, therefore, the leg must be internally rotated 10 degrees to position the neck of the femur parallel to the film.

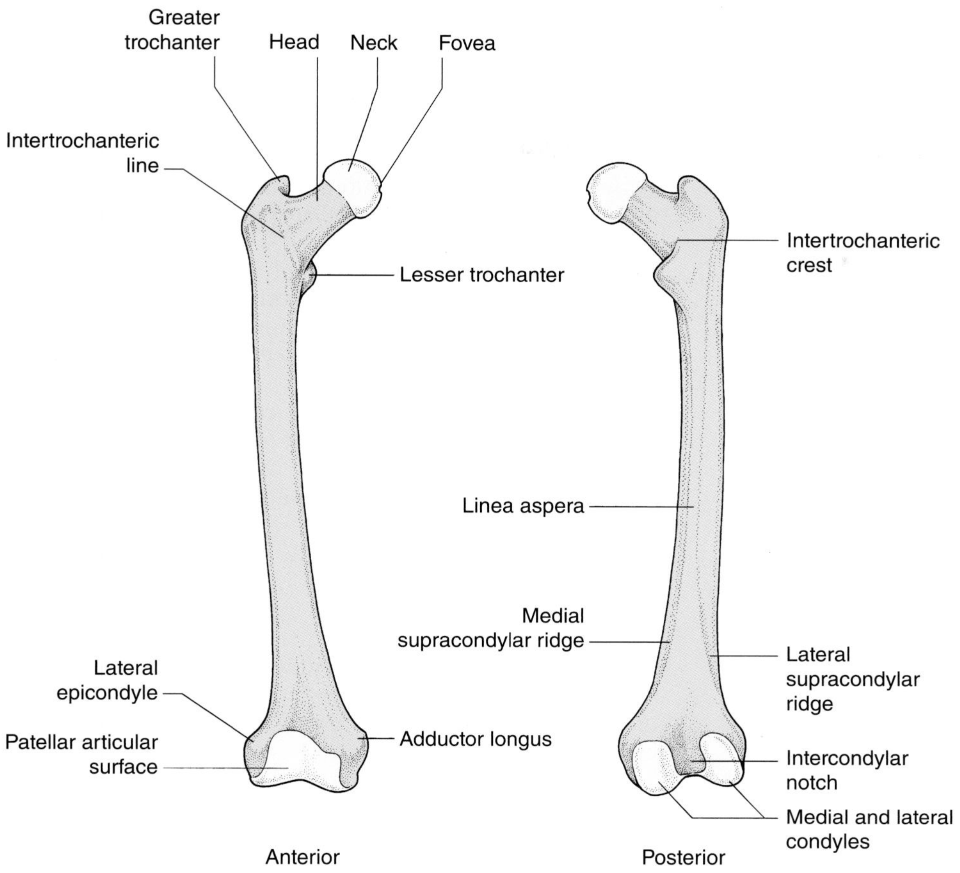

Fig. 8.1 Femur: anterior and posterior views.

Greater trochanter · Head · Neck · Fovea · Intertrochanteric line · Lesser trochanter · Intertrochanteric crest · Linea aspera · Medial supracondylar ridge · Lateral epicondyle · Patellar articular surface · Adductor longus · Lateral supracondylar ridge · Intercondylar notch · Medial and lateral condyles · Anterior · Posterior

RADIOLOGY PEARL

In clinical practice, **femoral neck version** is assessed using computed tomography. An angle is created between the long axis of the femoral neck and a line drawn between the posterior margins of the two femoral condyles at computed tomography (CT).

In a **lateral view of the neck**, a film and grid placed vertically and pressed into the patient's side must be positioned at an angle of 127 degrees to the shaft of the femur because of the angulation of the neck to the shaft.

Views of the intercondylar fossa (tunnel views) are taken with the knee flexed at an angle of about 135 degrees with a vertical beam and with a beam angled at 70 degrees to the lower leg.

Sesamoid Bones

A sesamoid bone called the **fabella** is frequently seen in the lateral head of the gastrocnemius muscle. On radiographs, this is projected on the posterior aspect of the lateral femoral condyle.

Blood Supply of the Head of the Femur

The head of the femur receives its blood supply mainly via the neck, as described above. Thus fracture of the neck, especially **subcapital fracture**, disrupts this blood supply and results in ischaemic necrosis of the head in 80% of cases.

Ossification of the Femur

The primary centre in the shaft appears in the seventh fetal week. A secondary centre is present in the lower femur at birth (this is a reliable indicator that the fetus is full term) and another appears in the head between 6 months and 1 year of age. Secondary centres appear in the greater trochanter at 4 years and in the lesser trochanter at 8 years of age. All fuse at 18–20 years of age.

Trabecular Markings in the Neck of the Femur and Bone Density

Additional biomechanical integrity of the neck of the femur is provided by an ordered internal trabecular network with a combination of primary compressive trabeculae, primary tensile trabeculae and secondary compressive trabeculae. These trabeculae, readily identified on conventional radiographs, surround a triangular area where there is a relative paucity of trabecular markings, termed Ward's triangle. The integrity of these described trabeculae reflects relative osteoblastic activity and stress. In osteoporosis, the disappearance of secondary compressive trabeculae prior to the disappearance of primary tensile trabeculae prior to subsequent disappearance of primary compressive trabeculae forms the basis of the Singh index (Fig. 8.2).

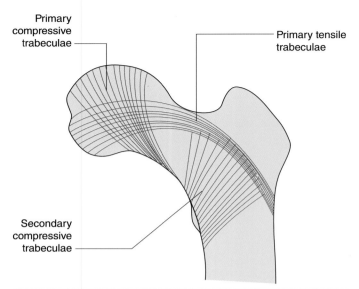

Fig. 8.2 Diagrammatic representation of the trabecular markings of the femoral neck.

THE PATELLA

This is a sesamoid bone in the quadriceps tendon that continues at its apex as the ligamentum patellae. The upper two-thirds of the posterior surface is covered with articular cartilage and is entirely within the knee joint, and its anterior surface is covered by the prepatellar bursa. The lateral articular surface is usually larger than the medial surface.

RADIOLOGICAL FEATURES OF THE PATELLA

Plain Radiographs

The outer surface of the patella as seen on **tangential (skyline) views** is irregular owing to the entry of nutrient vessels here.

Occasionally, the upper outer segment of the patella is separate from the remainder of the bone. Such a patella is called a **bipartite patella** and must be recognized as normal and not fractured.

Dislocation of the Patella

Lateral dislocation of the patella is more common than medial dislocation and occurs following valgus injury with associated imposed bowstringing of the extensor mechanism over the knee joint. Anatomical structures have evolved to prevent dislocation, including relative hypertrophy of the vastus medialis muscle and overgrowth of the lateral femoral condyle.

Wiberg describes three shapes of the patella:
- Type 1, in which the medial and lateral articular facets of the patella are equal in size and dimension.
- Type 2, in which the lateral facet is slightly larger than the medial facet.
- Type 3, in which the lateral facet is dominant and the medial facet is atretic and redundant. The type 3 configuration is more commonly associated with tracking disorders and transient subluxation.

Evaluation of patellofemoral alignment is routinely achieved using the skyline position with the beam centred on the patellofemoral joint from below. Patellofemoral tracking is best achieved using the Merchant views, with the beam directed from above down to a cassette held over the tibia. The Merchant views can therefore be acquired in weightbearing and in varying degrees of flexion and extension.

Ossification

This begins at 3 years and is complete by puberty.

THE TIBIA (FIG. 8.3)

The upper end of the tibia is expanded as the tibial plateau. This has an articular surface with a large medial and a smaller lateral condyle, which articulate with the condyles of the femur. Between the condyles is the intercondylar eminence or the tibial spine, which has medial and lateral projections – the medial and lateral intercondylar tubercles.

Anteriorly, at the upper end of the shaft of the tibia is the tibial tubercle into which the ligamentum patellae is inserted. The anteromedial surface of the shaft of the tibia is subcutaneous. The posterior surface of the shaft has a prominent oblique ridge – the soleal line.

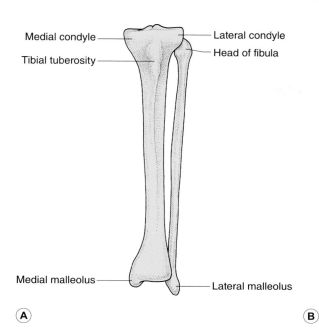

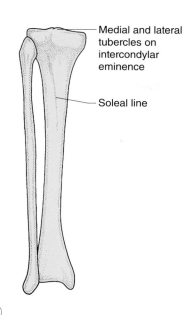

Fig. 8.3 Tibia and fibula. (A) Anterior view. (B) Posterior view.

The lower end of the tibia has the medial malleolus medially and the fibular notch for the inferior tibiofibular joint laterally. Its inferior surface is flattened and articulates with the talus in the ankle joint.

THE FIBULA (SEE FIG. 8.3)

Apart from its role in the ankle joint, the fibula is mainly a site of origin of muscles and has no weightbearing function. It has a head with a styloid process into which the biceps femoris is inserted, a neck, a narrow shaft and a lower end expanded as the lateral malleolus. Proximal and distal tibiofibular joints unite it with the tibia and it articulates with the talus in the ankle joint.

The lateral malleolus is more distal than the medial malleolus. The calcaneofibular ligament is attached to its tip. This may be damaged in inversion injuries.

The fibula is proportionately thicker in children than in adults.

RADIOLOGICAL FEATURES OF THE TIBIA AND FIBULA

Plain Radiographs

The **tibial tuberosity** is very variable in appearance, particularly during the growth period. Asymmetry and irregularity on radiographs may be quite normal.

Some irregularity of the tibia at the upper part of the **interosseous border** may simulate a periosteal reaction here.

Ossification of the Tibia

The primary ossification centre for the shaft of the tibia appears in the seventh fetal week. A secondary ossification centre is present in the upper end at birth and in the lower end at 2 years. The upper centre fuses with the shaft at 20 years, the lower sooner at 18 years.

Ossification of the Fibula

Ossification of the primary centre in the shaft begins in the eighth fetal week, in the lower secondary centre in the first year and in the upper at 3 years. The lower epiphysis fuses with the shaft at 16 years and the upper at 18 years.

The tibia in adulthood. In adulthood, the tibia, like all other long bones, is characterized by thick compact bony cortex in the tubulated diaphysis, in contrast to cortical thinning in the flared metaphysis. Biomechanical integrity of the tibial metaphysis, in contrast to the diaphysis, is provided by an additional internal ordered trabecular network, cancellous bony matrix.

RADIOLOGY PEARL

Reflecting a lack of cancellous matrix and vascular supply, healing of distal tibial shaft fractures is often delayed and so requires stabilization, internal fixation and bone grafting.

THE BONES OF THE FOOT (FIGS. 8.4, 8.5)

In addition to metatarsals and phalanges, there are seven tarsal bones in the foot. These are the talus, calcaneus, navicular, cuboid and three cuneiform bones. Of these, the talus and calcaneus are the most important radiologically.

The Talus

The long axis of the talus points forwards and medially so that its anterior end is medial to the calcaneus. The talus has a:

- **Body** between the malleoli, with a superior articular surface called the trochlear surface;
- **Neck** grooved inferiorly as the sulcus tali which, with the sulcus calcanei, forms the sinus tarsi;
- **Head** anteriorly that articulates with the navicular;
- **Posterior process**, which is sometimes separate as the os trigonum.

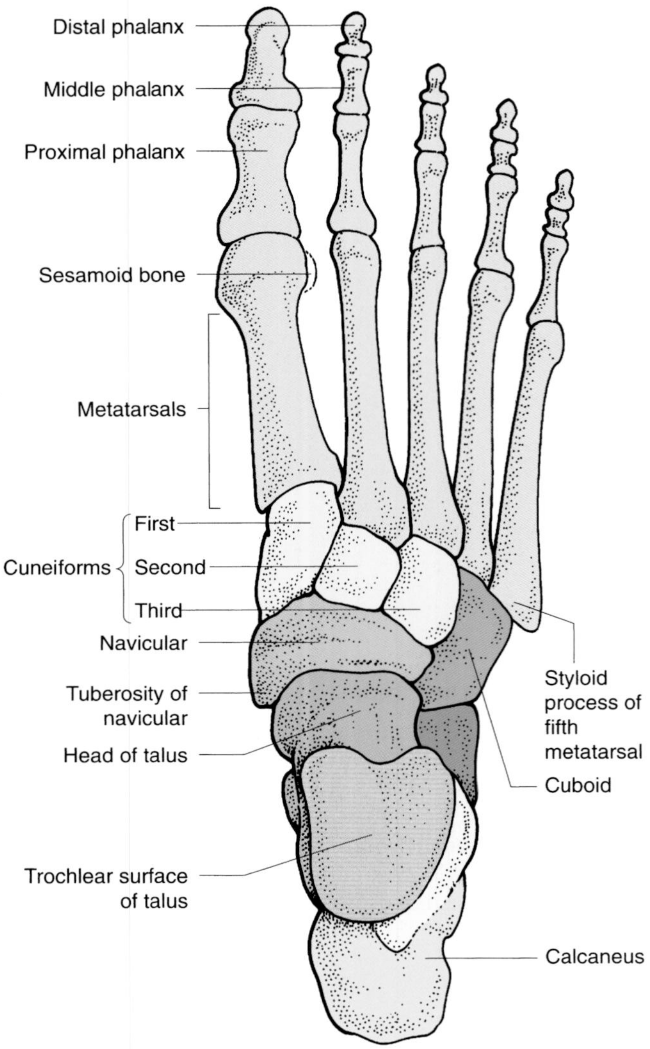
Distal phalanx
Middle phalanx
Proximal phalanx
Sesamoid bone
Metatarsals
Cuneiforms
First
Second
Third
Navicular
Tuberosity of navicular
Head of talus
Trochlear surface of talus
Styloid process of fifth metatarsal
Cuboid
Calcaneus

Fig. 8.4 Bones of the foot: dorsal view.

RADIOLOGY PEARL

Fracture of the posterior talar process may occur following acute ankle trauma and lead to posterior ankle impingement and pain. This fracture, termed a shepherd fracture, is often overlooked or misinterpreted as being an os trigonum.

The **inferior surface** of the talus (see also the subtalar joint) has a large facet posteriorly for articulation with the calcaneus. Separated from this by the sinus tarsi are three facets, separated by ridges, as follows:

- The middle talocalcaneal facet for the sustentaculum tali of the calcaneus
- A facet for the plantar ligament
- The anterior talocalcaneal articular surface

These, in turn, are continuous with the talonavicular facet on the head of the talus. The talus has no muscular attachments.

The Calcaneus

This is the largest tarsal bone. It lies under the talus with its long axis pointing forward and laterally. It is irregularly cuboidal in shape with a shelf-like process anteromedially to support the talus – known as the sustentaculum tali. Its upper surface has three facets for the talus (the middle one is on the superior surface of the sustentaculum tali), which correspond with the facets under the talus.

The plantar surface has a large calcaneal tuberosity posteriorly which has medial and lateral tubercles. There is a small peroneal tubercle on the lateral surface.

RADIOLOGY PEARL

The calcaneus has an outer cortical frame supported by an ordered arrangement of internal trabeculae or cancellous bone. This fact, in association with its superficial position, lends itself to evaluation with high-frequency ultrasound. Decreased acoustic impedance is a marker of decreasing bone density.

The Arches of the Foot

The longitudinal arch is more pronounced medially. It has two components:

- The medial arch, formed by the calcaneus, the talus, the medial three cuneiforms and the first three metatarsal bones.
- The lateral arch, formed by the calcaneus, the cuboid and the fourth and fifth metatarsals.

A series of transverse arches are formed and are most marked at the distal part of the tarsal bones and the proximal end of the metatarsals. Each foot has one half of the full transverse arch.

The arches are maintained by the shape of the bones of the foot, the ligaments and muscles, particularly of the plantar surface.

RADIOLOGY PEARL

The medial longitudinal arch is supported by the plantar fascia. Prolonged stress imposed to the medial arch leads to intrasubstance microtears in the fascia particularly at its attachment to the calcaneus, resulting in local inflammation, termed plantar fasciitis.

RADIOLOGICAL FEATURES OF THE BONES OF THE FOOT (FIG. 8.6)

Plain Radiographs

Boehler's critical angle of the calcaneus (see Fig. 8.6A) is the angle between a line drawn from the posterior end to the anterior end of its superior articular facet and a second line from the latter point to the posterosuperior border of the calcaneus. It is normally 30–35 degrees, with an angle less than 28 degrees occurring when there is significant structural damage to the bone.

Heel pad thickness (see Fig. 8.6A) is measured on a lateral radiograph of the calcaneus between the calcaneal tuberosity posteroinferiorly and the skin surface. Normal thicknesses are 21 mm in the female and 23 mm in the male. Thickening of the heel pad occurs in patients with gigantism or acromegaly.

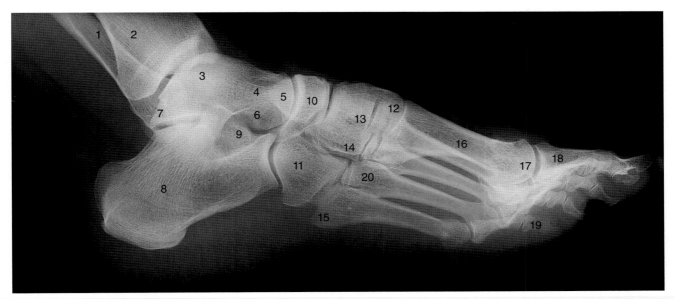

Fig. 8.5 Oblique radiograph of the foot.

1. Fibula
2. Tibia
3. Talus
4. Neck of talus
5. Head of talus
6. Sinus tarsi
7. Posterior process of talus
8. Calcaneus
9. Sustentaculum tali
10. Navicular

11. Cuboid
12. Medial cuneiform (superimposed)
13. Intermediate cuneiform (superimposed)
14. Lateral cuneiform (superimposed)
15. Styloid process of fifth metatarsal
16. Shaft of first metatarsal
17. Head of first metatarsal
18. Proximal phalanx, first toe
19. Distal phalanx, fifth toe
20. Base of fourth metatarsal

On a lateral radiograph of the foot **in children** over 5 years old the **long axis of the talus** points along the shaft of the first metatarsal. In the younger child the talus is more vertical and its long axis points below the first metatarsal (see Fig. 8.6B and C).

RADIOLOGY PEARL

The peroneus brevis tendon is attached to the **styloid process of the base of the fifth metatarsal**. The oblique epiphyseal line here should not be confused with a fracture of the styloid process, which is usually transverse, termed a **Jones fracture** (see Fig. 8.6D and E).

RADIOLOGY PEARL

On a lateral radiograph, the **medial longitudinal arch angle** is measured between a line along the inferior border of the os calcis and a line along the inferior border of the first metatarsal. This angle normally measures 115–125 degrees. An angle greater than 125 degrees is a marker of pes cavus, *which is occasionally a marker of* posterior column neurological insult. An angle less than 115 degrees is termed pes planus, and in the acquired form is usually a marker of disruption of the **plantar fascial aponeurosis** or the tibialis posterior tendon.

Sesamoid Bones

The commonest sesamoid bones seen in foot radiographs (see Fig. 8.6F and G) are as follows:

- Two sesamoids are found in the tendon of flexor hallucis brevis at the base of the metatarsophalangeal joint of the hallux. These may be bipartite. The sum of the two parts in a bipartite patella is larger than the size of the associated unipartite sesamoid, in contrast to a fracture where the sum of the two parts equals the size of the associated intact sesamoid.
- Sesamoid bones are often found at other metatarsophalangeal joints or at the interphalangeal joints of the first and second toes.
- Os trigonum posterior to the talus.
- Os vesalianum at the base of the fifth metatarsal.
- Os peroneum between the cuboid and the base of the fifth metatarsal within the tendon of the peroneus brevis muscle.
- Os tibiale externum medial to the tuberosity of the navicular within the tendon of the tibialis posterior muscle.

Ossification of the Bones of the Foot

Except for the calcaneus, the tarsal bones ossify from one centre each – the calcaneus and talus ossify in the sixth fetal month and the cuboid is ossified at birth; the cuneiforms and navicular ossify between 1 and 3 years of age.

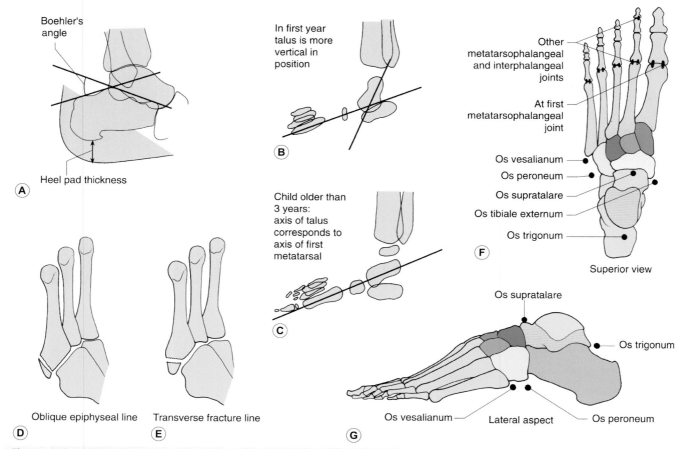

Fig. 8.6 Radiological features of the bones of the foot. (A) Boehler's calcaneal angle and heel pad thickness. (B and C) Orientation of the talus in a child. (D and E) Styloid process of the fifth metatarsal: epiphyseal line and fracture. (F and G) Sesamoid bones of the foot.

The **secondary centre of the calcaneus** ossifies in the posterior aspect of the bone at 5 years and its density may be very irregular in the normal foot. It fuses at puberty.

The **navicular** may ossify from many ossification centres. This should not be confused with fragmentation of osteochondrosis or with fracture. Similarly, the **epiphysis at the base of the proximal phalanx of the hallux** may be bipartite in the normal foot.

Coalition of the bones of the foot. Tarsal coalition represents abnormal fusion between two or more tarsal bones and is a frequent cause of foot and ankle pain. Coalition results from abnormal differentiation and segmentation of primitive mesenchyme preventing the development of a normal joint.

RADIOLOGY PEARL

Approximately 90% of tarsal coalitions involve the talocalcaneal or calcaneonavicular joints with either fibrous, cartilaginous or osseous bridging. Pain develops in the second decade as bone growth is impaired and the abnormal segment becomes mineralized.

The Joints of the Lower Limb

THE HIP JOINT (FIG. 8.7)

Type

The hip joint is a synovial ball-and-socket joint, the femoral head functioning as a ball with the acetabular cavity or socket. The normal acetabulum is obliquely oriented from lateral to medial, from front to back and is inclined such that the outer margin of the roof is lateral to the outer margin of the floor. Such acetabular angulation is an evolutionary modification to accommodate bipedalism without repeated dislocation. Loss of normal acetabular obliquity and inclination in acetabular dysplasia predisposes to repeated subluxation and abnormal stress on the acetabular labrum, which becomes degenerate and torn. Similar to angulation of the acetabulum, the femoral neck is anteverted to 10 degrees relative to the shaft, which decreases the likelihood of posterior hip subluxation and leads to further stability at the hip joint.

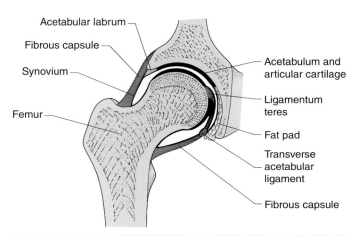

Acetabular labrum
Fibrous capsule
Synovium
Femur

Acetabulum and
articular cartilage
Ligamentum
teres
Fat pad
Transverse
acetabular
ligament
Fibrous capsule

Fig. 8.7 Hip joint: coronal section.

RADIOLOGY PEARL

Abnormal obliquity and inclination of the acetabulum can lead to overcoverage of the femoral head at the ball-and-socket articulation, and this leads to impingement of both periarticular soft tissues and bone termed pincer-type femoro-acetabular impingement.

Articular Surfaces

These are the head of the femur apart from the fovea, which is a horseshoe-shaped articular surface on the acetabulum. The articular surface is deepened by a fibrocartilaginous ring, the acetabular labrum. The acetabulum has a central nonarticular area for a fat pad and the ligamentum teres and an inferior notch bridged by the transverse acetabular ligament, from which this ligament arises.

Capsule

This is attached to the edge of the acetabulum and its labrum and the transverse acetabular ligament; at the femoral neck it is attached to the trochanters and the intertrochanteric line anteriorly; posteriorly it is attached more proximally on the neck at the junction of its medial two-thirds and its lateral third. From its insertion on the femoral neck, the capsular fibres are reflected back along the neck as the retinacula along which blood vessels reach the femoral head.

Synovium

Synovium lines the capsule and occasionally bulges out anteriorly as a bursa in front of the psoas muscle where this muscle passes in front of the hip joint.

Ligaments

These are as follows:
- The iliofemoral ligament (Y-shaped ligament of Bigelow) is an anterior thickening of the capsule between the anteroinferior iliac spine and the neck of the femur to the intertrochanteric line.
- The ischiofemoral ligament is a posterior thickening of the capsule.

- The pubofemoral ligament is a thickening of the capsule inferiorly.
- The transverse acetabular ligament bridges the acetabular notch.
- The ligamentum teres lies between the central nonarticular part of the acetabulum and the fovea of the head of the femur.

RADIOLOGICAL FEATURES OF THE HIP JOINT

Plain Radiographs

On radiographs of the hip joint **pads of fat**, seen as linear lucencies, outline the capsule of the hip joint and closely applied muscle. Bulging of these is an early sign of joint effusion.

A small **accessory ossicle**, the os acetabuli, is sometimes seen at the superior margin of the acetabulum and should not be confused with a fracture here.

Similarly, irregularity of the superior margin of the acetabulum in children is a normal variant.

In assessment of radiographs of the hip in **infants** (Fig. 8.8), the following lines and angles are as described:
- The **Y line** between the unossified centre of each acetabulum, that is, the Y-shaped cartilage between the pubis, ischium and ilium or the triradiate cartilage.
- The **acetabular angle**, normally 15–35 degrees.
- The **iliac angle**, normally 44–74 degrees.
- **Shenton's line** along the inferior margin of the femoral neck and along the superior and lateral margins of the obturator foramen of the pelvis should form a continuous arc.
- Lines along the femoral shafts in **Von Rosen's view** (legs abducted at least 45 degrees and internally rotated) should meet in the midline at the lumbosacral junction.

In assessment of radiographs of the **adult** hip, routine frontal radiographs allow the identification of six lines (see Fig. 8.8). The continuation of the inferior margin of the superior pubic ramus superiorly to the upper outer margin of the acetabular roof forms the outer margin of the anterior column or wall of the acetabulum (line 1). The continuation of the inferior margin of the inferior pubic ramus superiorly to the upper outer margin of the acetabular roof forms the outer margin of the posterior column or wall of the acetabulum (line 2). The continuation of the superior margin of the superior pubic ramus superiorly forms the iliopectineal line (line 3). The continuation of the superior margin of the inferior pubic ramus superiorly forms the ilioischial line (line 4). The roof of the acetabulum forms line 5. The 'tear drop' is formed by the reflections of the cotyloid fossa and quadrilateral plate and represents line 6. Disruption of any of the described lines is employed in the localization of disease processes on conventional radiographs.

Radiography

The hip joint is usually investigated by AP and frog lateral (oblique) radiographs. Visualization of the anterior or posterior margins of the acetabulum may be enhanced by oblique or Judet views. The joint space anteriorly, superiorly and posteriorly may be visualized by the false profile lateral view.

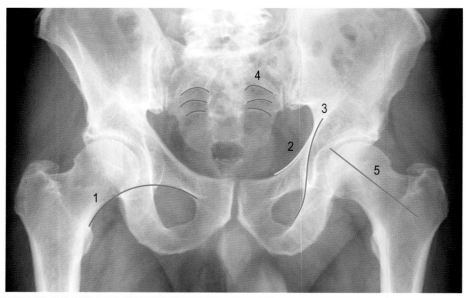

Fig. 8.8 Anteroposterior pelvic X-ray: lines used in assessment *(1–4)*. (From Carver E, Carver B, Knapp K. *Carvers' Medical Imaging*, 3rd ed. Elsevier; 2021.)

Arthrography

Arthrography of the hip joint is achieved by injection of contrast anteriorly just below the head of the femur. The synovial cavity, as described above, is outlined. The ligamentum teres is seen as a filling defect within the joint and the transverse ligament of the acetabulum is seen as a defect near the inferior part of the acetabulum. The labrum is visible as a triangular filling defect around the acetabular rim. A superior acetabular recess is found external to the labrum superiorly. An inferior articular recess is seen at the base of the femoral head.

The synovial cavity is seen to extend along the neck of the femur as described above, and superior and inferior recesses of the neck are seen in the synovial cavity at the upper and lower ends of the intertrochanteric line.

Ultrasound of the Infant Hip (Fig. 8.9)

This is useful as visualization of the as-yet unossified femoral head is possible. The ossified parts of the acetabulum, including its roof and the shaft of the femur, are seen as echoic areas, whereas the cartilage of the acetabulum (the triradiate cartilage) and the head of the femur are hypoechoic. The labrum is also visible at the edge of the acetabulum.

CT of the Hip Joint

In the axial plane, CT allows direct visualization of the margins of the acetabulum. CT scanning allows evaluation of the anterior and posterior walls of the acetabulum, and also allows visualization of the fat-filled cotyloid fossa and of the associated quadrilateral plate.

Axial images are routinely employed to determine the axis of the neck of the femur relative to the shaft (normally anteverted to 10 degrees). This can only be achieved by combining axial imaging of the neck and proximal shaft with axial imaging through the condyles of the distal femur. The angle

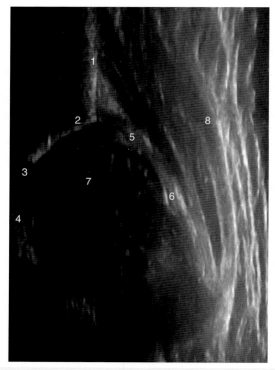

Fig. 8.9 Ultrasound scan of the infant hip: coronal view in standard plane.
1. Iliac wing
2. Acetabulum (iliac part)
3. Triradiate cartilage
4. Acetabulum (ischial part)
5. Labrum of acetabulum
6. Lower limit of joint capsule as it merges with the femoral neck (echogenic focus)
7. Cartilage of the femoral head
8. Gluteal muscles

of anteversion is the angle created by the intersection of a line along the neck of the femur and a line drawn between the two distal femoral condyles.

Magnetic Resonance Imaging of the Hip (Fig. 8.10)

Magnetic resonance imaging (MRI) of the hip may be performed using a body coil and a wide 25–30-cm field of view, allowing simultaneous visualization of both hips and comparison of the normal and abnormal sides. Dedicated imaging of a single hip, to identify the labrum, requires the use of a phased array quadrature surface coil.

The acetabular labrum. The acetabular labrum represents a discontinuous semilunar ring of fibrocartilage marginating the anterior, superolateral and posterior columns

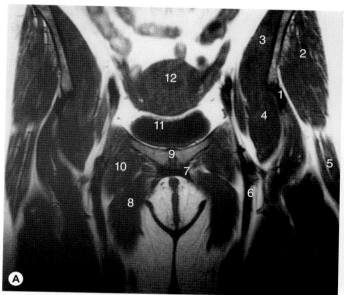
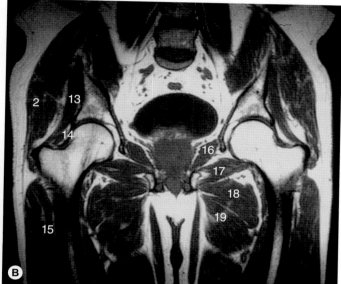
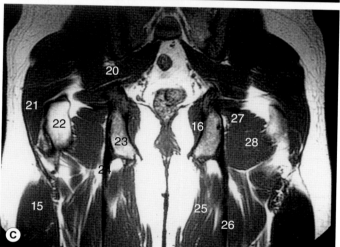

Fig. 8.10 Magnetic resonance image (MRI) of the hip. (A–C) Coronal T1-weighted scans from anterior to posterior.

(A–C)
1. Rectus femoris insertion
2. Gluteus medius muscle
3. Iliacus muscle
4. Iliopsoas muscle belly
5. Tensor fascia lata
6. Femoral vessels
7. Conjoined insertion of gracilis and adductor longus muscles
8. Adductor longus
9. Pubic symphysis
10. Pectineus muscle
11. Bladder
12. Uterus
13. Gluteus minimus
14. Capsule (iliofemoral ligament)
15. Vastus lateralis muscle
16. Obturator internus muscle
17. Obturator externus muscle
18. Adductor brevis muscle
19. Adductor longus muscle
20. Piriformis muscle
21. Gluteus maximus muscle
22. Greater trochanter
23. Ischium
24. Conjoined tendon of long head of semimembranosus and long head of biceps femoris
25. Adductor magnus muscle
26. Semitendinosus muscle
27. Inferior gemellus muscle
28. Quadratus femoris muscle

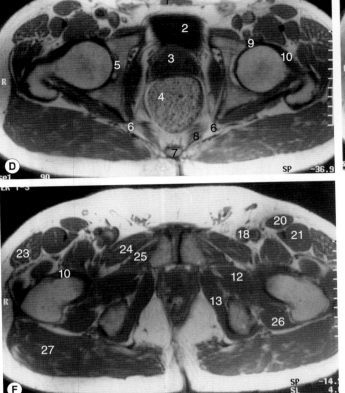

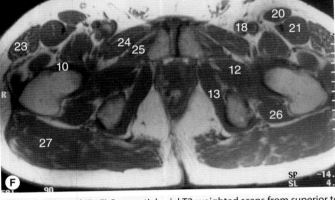

Fig. 8.10, cont'd (D–F) Sequential axial T2-weighted scans from superior to inferior

(D–F)
1. Rectus abdominis muscle
2. Bladder
3. Prostate
4. Rectum
5. Quadrilateral plate of the acetabulum (and cotyloid fossa)
6. Sciatic nerve
7. Coccyx
8. Piriformis
9. Anterior labrum
10. Ileofemoral ligament (anterior fold of the capsule)
11. Posterior wall of the acetabulum
12. Obturator externus muscle
13. Obturator internus muscle
14. Ischiorectal fossa
15. Natal cleft
16. Gluteus medius
17. Cotyloid fossa
18. Femoral vein
19. Femoral artery
20. Sartorius
21. Rectus femoris
22. Iliopsoas
23. Tensor fascia lata
24. Adductor longus
25. Adductor brevis
26. Quadratus femoris
27. Gluteus maximus

of the acetabulum. The inferior margins of the acetabulum are bridged by the transverse acetabular ligament. The fibrocartilaginous labrum is triangular in cross-section, is most frequently inverted in orientation, and is usually thicker posterosuperiorly than anteroinferiorly, reflecting its function to provide stability and prevent subluxation. The synovium-lined capsule of the hip joint arises from bone adjacent to the outer attachment of the labrum. In such a way a sulcus, termed the paralabral sulcus, is created between the labrum and capsule, lined by synovium, from which vascularity to the labrum is derived.

Articular hyaline cartilage extends to the inner or medial margin of the labrum but does not extend between the labrum and underlying bone.

RADIOLOGY PEARL

Hyaline cartilage undercutting the attachment of the fibrocartilagenous labrum to the acetabulum produces localized linear signal alteration often incorrectly thought to represent a labral tear.

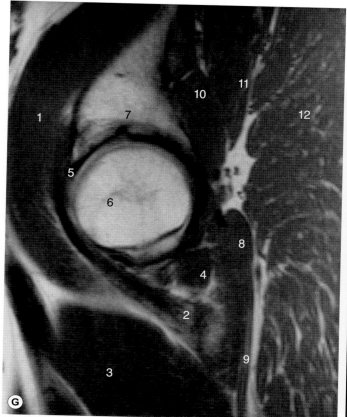
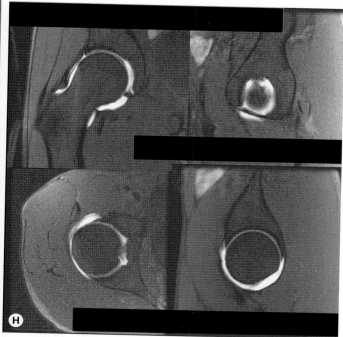

Fig. 8.10, cont'd (G) Sagittal T1-weighted image of the hip. (H) MR arthrographic images showing labral anatomy in coronal (top left), sagittal (right side) and axial (bottom left) planes.

(G)
1. Iliopsoas muscle
2. Iliopsoas tendon
3. Pectineus
4. Obturator externus
5. Anterior labrum
6. Femoral head

7. Roof of the acetabulum
8. Quadratus femoris
9. Sciatic nerve
10. Glutei minimus
11. Gluteus medius
12. Gluteus maximus

RADIOLOGY PEARLS

- Morphologic variants in the configuration of the labrum (such as the glenoid labrum) may lead to diagnostic error. In a study of 200 asymptomatic volunteers the labrum was triangular in shape in two-thirds of patients, round in 10%, flat in 10% and absent in 14%, with variations increasing with age.
- Variations in intralabral signal correlate poorly with histological evidence of degeneration. Although some authors conclude that cartilage does not extend beneath the labrum, and that linear signal at this site indicates a tear, others report that cartilage may extend beneath the labrum and that discrimination between sublabral cartilage and tear can only accurately be made using intra-articular gadolinium-enhanced arthrography.

THE SYMPHYSIS PUBIS (FIG. 8.11)

The symphysis pubis represents a nonsynovial joint specifically adapted to accommodate impaction and shear forces directed at the pelvis from the upper body and lower extremities during twisting and turning of gait, locomotion and sport. It is composed of a fibrocartilagenous disc interposed between hyaline cartilage overlying the bony articular margins of the pubic rami. In adulthood, a physiological linear cleft develops in the centre of the fibrocartilagenous disc.

The symphysis, specifically the fibrocartilagenous disc, is supported superiorly by the superior pubic ligaments, inferiorly by the arcuate ligaments and anteriorly by an aponeurosis created by the adductor longus and gracilis conjoined tendon from the legs and the merged tendons of the oblique and rectus abdominis musculature.

RADIOLOGY PEARLS

- Tear of the combined adductor longus and rectus abdominis tendon at the pubic symphysis manifests at symphysography and MRI as the 'superior cleft sign' (see Fig. 8.11D and E).
- The 'secondary cleft sign' is a similar entity occurring at the attachment of the short adductors (gracilis, adductor brevis and pectineus) at the inferior margin of the inferior pubic ramus. These are both common causes of groin pain in sportspeople.

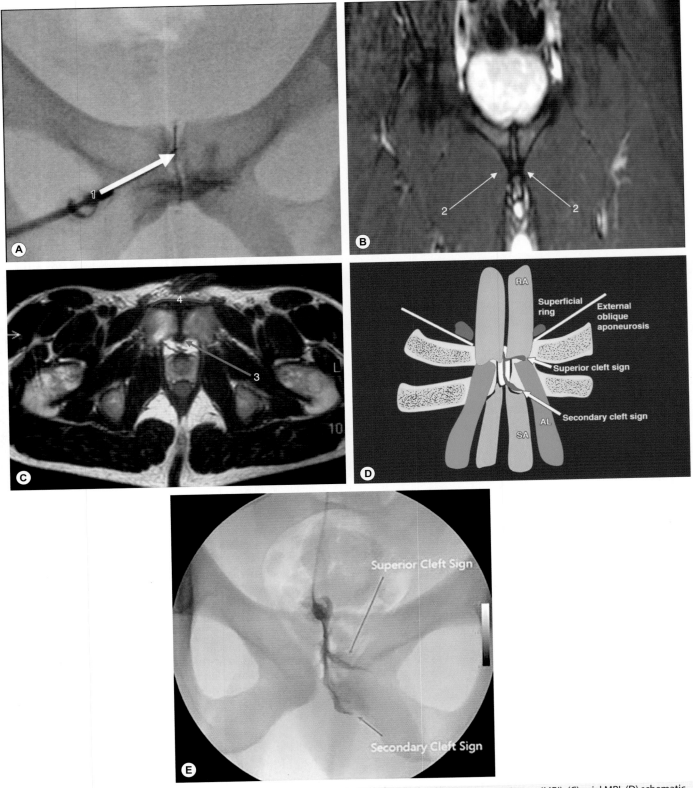

Fig. 8.11 (A) Symphyseal contrast injection, symphysography, with matching (B) coronal magnetic resonance image (MRI), (C) axial MRI, (D) schematic, and (E) fluoroscopic image post contrast injection demonstrating superior and secondary cleft. *AL*, adductor longus; *RA*, rectus abdominis; *SA*, short adductors.

(A–C)
1. Normal symphyseal cleft
2. Normal adductor attachments

3. Posterior bulge of fibrocartilage
4. Anterior rectus abdominis and adductor aponeurosis

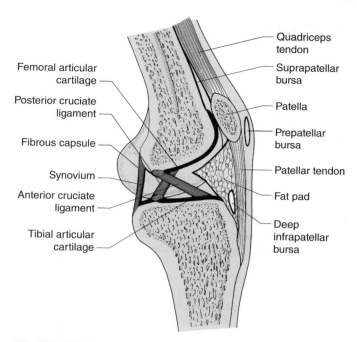

Fig. 8.12 Knee joint: sagittal section.

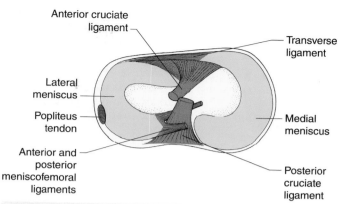

Fig. 8.13 Upper end of the tibia: axial section showing menisci and attachments of the cruciate ligaments.

Symphysography is the term used to describe diagnostic and therapeutic contrast and steroid injection to the cleft in the symphyseal fibrocartilage.

THE KNEE JOINT (FIG. 8.12)

Type

The knee joint is a synovial hinge joint.

Articular Surfaces

These are the condyles and the patellar surfaces of the femur, the tibial articular surfaces on the tibial plateau, and the deep surface of the patella.

Capsule

This is attached at the margins of the articular surface, except superiorly where the joint cavity communicates with the suprapatellar bursa (between the quadriceps femoris muscle and the femur) and posteriorly where it communicates with the bursa under the medial head of the gastrocnemius (semimembranosus bursa). Occasionally the joint cavity is also continuous with the bursa under the lateral head of the gastrocnemius muscle (popliteal bursa). The capsule is perforated by the popliteus muscle posteriorly.

Synovium

The synovium lines the capsule and its associated bursae. A fat pad in the joint deep to the ligamentum patellae is called the infrapatellar fat pad. The synovium covering this fat pad is projected into the joint as two alar folds.

Ligaments

These are as follows:
- The medial (tibial) collateral ligament may be separated from the capsule by a bursa; the deep part of the ligament is attached to the medial meniscus.

- The lateral collateral ligament is attached to the fibula and always clear of the capsule.
- The ligamentum patellae and medial and lateral patellar retinacula.
- The oblique popliteal ligament posteriorly.

Internal Structures (Fig. 8.13)

Anterior and posterior cruciate ligaments arise from the anterior and posterior parts of the intercondylar area of the tibia and are named by their tibial origin. They are inserted into the inner aspect of the lateral and medial femoral condyles, respectively. The anterior cruciate ligament resists hyperextension of the knee and the posterior cruciate resists hyperflexion.

The medial and lateral menisci (or semilunar cartilages) are two crescentic structures, triangular in cross-section, which slightly deepen the articular surface of the tibia. Each is attached peripherally to the tibia and to the capsule. The upper and lower surfaces of the menisci are free. Each is described as having an anterior and posterior horn attached to the intercondylar area of the tibia.

The medial meniscus is bigger, less curved and thinner. Its posterior horn is thick (14 mm) but it thins progressively to the anterior horn, which is 6 mm thick.

The lateral meniscus is smaller, more curved (nearly circular rather than semicircular) and more uniform in thickness (10 mm). The lateral meniscus is less well attached to the capsule than the medial and is grooved posterolaterally by the tendon of popliteus, which passes between it and the capsule. (The tendon of the popliteus is not attached to the lateral meniscus.)

The transverse ligament passes between the anterior horns of the menisci. The meniscofemoral ligament passes between the posterior horn of the lateral meniscus and the medial femoral condyle. This latter ligament has anterior and posterior parts that pass in front of and behind the posterior cruciate ligament, termed the meniscofemoral ligaments of Humphrey (anterior) and Wrisberg (posterior).

RADIOLOGICAL FEATURES OF THE KNEE JOINT

Plain Radiographs of the Knee Joint (Fig. 8.14)

Subcutaneous and intra-articular fat (the infrapatellar fat pad) outlines some of the soft tissues around the joint. The ligamentum patellae is made visible this way.

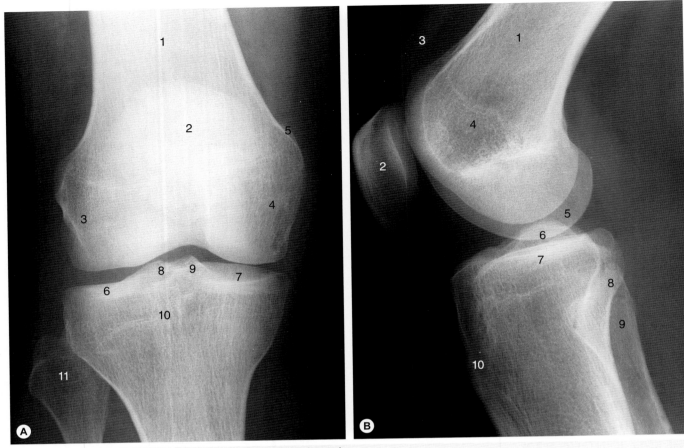

Fig. 8.14 The knee. (A) Anteroposterior radiograph. (B) Lateral radiograph.

(A)
1. Femur
2. Patella
3. Lateral epicondyle
4. Medial epicondyle
5. Adductor tubercle
6. Lateral tibial plateau
7. Medial tibial plateau
8. Lateral tibial spine (intercondylar eminence)
9. Medial tibial spine (intercondylar eminence)
10. Fused growth plate, proximal tibia
11. Head of fibula

(B)
1. Distal femur
2. Patella
3. Quadriceps tendon
4. Epicondyles (superimposed)
5. Femoral condyle
6. Tibial spines (superimposed)
7. Tibial plateaux (superimposed)
8. Head of fibula
9. Neck of fibula
10. Tibial tuberosity

The suprapatellar bursa is best seen on radiographs when distended with fluid. It is then seen as a soft-tissue density above the patella. Routine imaging includes AP, semiflexed lateral, tunnel and skyline views.

Arthrography of the Knee Joint

Contrast medium and air are introduced into the joint deep to the patella and allow visualization of the synovial cavity of the joint as described above, including the suprapatellar bursa and some or all of the associated bursae that may be connected with the joint cavity.

Occasionally, a posterior pouch from the synovium is seen to extend into the popliteal fossa. If such a diverticulum becomes inflamed or its neck becomes obstructed it is referred to as a **Baker's cyst**. Baker's cyst represents a medial out-pouching between the medial head of the gastrocnemius and the semimembranosus and semitendinosus tendons.

The **menisci** are seen as filling defects, triangular in cross-section, whose upper and lower surfaces are outlined by contrast. Their bases are attached to the capsule (some contrast may pass lateral to the lateral meniscus, which is less firmly attached to the capsule). The tendon of popliteus is seen to groove the lateral meniscus posterolaterally.

A **discoid meniscus** is a variant that extends far into the joint space.

MRI of the Knee (Fig. 8.15)

MRI is used in the evaluation of internal derangements of the knee. Using a dedicated quadrature surface coil images are acquired in the coronal plane to evaluate the collateral and cruciate ligaments, in the sagittal oblique plane to evaluate the cruciates and menisci, and in the axial plane to evaluate patellofemoral cartilage. It is crucial that sagittal images are acquired in the sagittal oblique plane parallel to the axis of the anterior cruciate ligament prescribed off an axial localizer.

Ultrasound of the Knee

The superior and posterior joint can be assessed for effusions. The quadriceps and patellar tendons can be evaluated.

RELEVANT MRI ANATOMY

The Menisci

Anatomy. The menisci are C-shaped semilunar rings interposed between the articular surfaces of the femoral condyles and the tibial plateau. They act as a buffer between the two surfaces, protecting articular cartilage, distributing the strain of weightbearing (they support 50% of load sharing), improving stability and providing lubrication to facilitate joint flexion and extension.

The menisci have an organized structure composed of an outer circumferential zone and an inner transverse zone divided by a middle perforating collagen bundle to superior and inferior leaves. Menisci are poorly vascularized, only the outer third being vascularized in adulthood via a perimeniscal plexus derived from branches of medial and lateral geniculate arteries, and therefore following injury meniscal healing is poor.

The medial meniscus has an open C shape and is attached to the intercondylar notch of the tibia both anteriorly and posteriorly, to the anterior horn of the lateral meniscus through the transverse meniscal ligament in 40%, to the posterior capsule and to the medial collateral ligament. The lateral meniscus is more circular in shape, has anterior and posterior intercondylar notch attachments, transverse meniscal attachment to the anterior

horn of the medial meniscus, meniscofemoral ligament attachments to the inner aspect of the medial femoral condyle (Wrisberg posteriorly, Humphrey anteriorly), and is loosely attached to the capsule but not the lateral collateral ligament. It is separated from the posterior capsule by the popliteus tendon.

Menisci are repeatedly subjected to rotational forces on flexion and extension. In extension, the femur internally rotates as a locking screw home mechanism. In flexion, the opposite occurs under the influence of the popliteus tendon. As the popliteus contracts, the posterior horn of the lateral meniscus is pulled posteriorly to accommodate the posterior shift in load bearing as part of flexion.

Meniscal tears. On MRI the compact menisci are hypointense on all sequences. Traditionally sagittal images are used to evaluate their integrity. In the sagittal plane the posterior horn of the medial meniscus is typically twice the size of the anterior horn. In contrast, the anterior and posterior horns of the lateral meniscus are equal in dimensions. Typically the bodies of the menisci are seen on only the outer two slices.

Menisci may tear both in the setting of acute trauma or in the setting of minor trauma superimposed on meniscal degeneration.

Following repetitive trauma, as part of the ageing process the central portion of the meniscus undergoes first globular and then progressive linear mucoid degeneration. Such changes have led to the application of a universally accepted grading system in which intrasubstance focal signal change (slight T1 and T2 hyperintensity) is classified as grade 1, linear or diffuse globular signal abnormality not extending to a surface is classified as grade 2, and signal abnormality, either linear or globular with definite extension to a surface, is classified as grade 3.

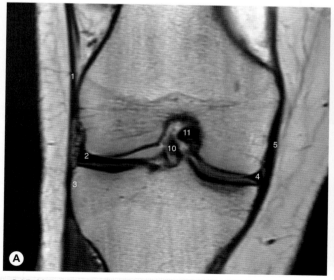 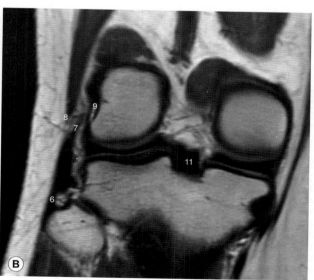

Fig. 8.15 Magnetic resonance scan of the knee. Coronal T1-weighted images of (A) the anterior knee and of (B) the posterior knee.

(A and B)
1. Iliotibial band
2. Lateral meniscus
3. Gerdy's tubercle
4. Medial meniscus
5. Medial collateral ligament (superficial component)
6. Conjoined tendon
7. Fibular collateral ligament
8. Biceps femoris tendon
9. Popliteus insertion, notch
10. Anterior cruciate ligament
11. Posterior cruciate ligament

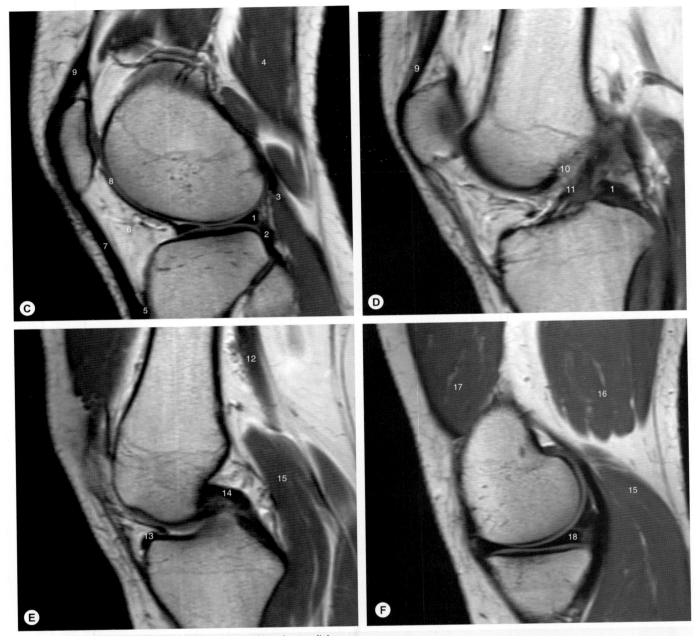

Fig. 8.15, cont'd (C–F) Sequential sagittal scans from lateral to medial

(C–F)
1. Lateral meniscus (posterior horn)
2. Popliteus tendon
3. Lateral head of the gastrocnemius
4. Biceps femoris, muscle belly
5. Tibial tuberosity
6. Hoffa's fat pad
7. Patella tendon
8. Articular cartilage (of the lateral femoral condyle)
9. Quadriceps tendon

10. Intercondylar notch (Blumensaat's line)
11. Anterior cruciate ligament
12. Popliteal vessels
13. Medial meniscus (anterior horn)
14. Posterior cruciate ligament
15. Medial head of the gastrocnemius
16. Semimembranosus muscle belly
17. Vastus medialis muscle belly
18. Medial meniscus posterior horn

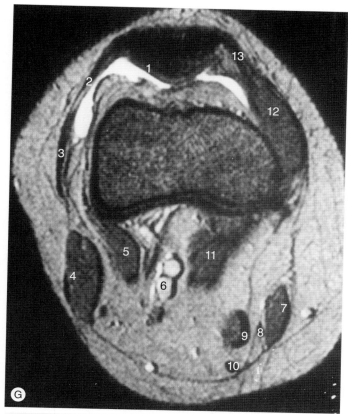

Fig. 8.15, cont'd (G) Axial image at the level of the patellofemoral articulation.

(G)
1. Lateral articular facet of the patella
2. Lateral retinaculum
3. Iliotibial band
4. Biceps femoris muscle
5. Lateral head of the gastrocnemius muscle
6. Popliteal vessels
7. Sartorius muscle
8. Gracilis muscle
9. Semimembranosus muscle
10. Semitendinosus muscle
11. Lateral head of the gastrocnemius
12. Vastus medialis muscle
13. Medial retinaculum

RADIOLOGY PEARLS

• Extension of signal abnormality to a meniscal surface is the hallmark feature allowing diagnosis of meniscal tear.
• Recognizing that extension of signal to multiple surfaces or in multiple planes reflects a more serious tear with surgical implications, some advocate use of the term grade 4 to accommodate this scenario, although this is currently not widely employed.

RADIOLOGY PEARL

Grade 2 signal abnormality may be misinterpreted in the periphery of normal menisci in children secondary to the presence of perforating vessels.

RADIOLOGY PEARL

Lateral meniscal injury is less common than medial, as the meniscus is more mobile and has fewer osseous or capsular attachments.

A discoid meniscus is an anatomical variant in which the normal open configuration of the meniscus is absent and the meniscus acquires a solid appearance. The configuration lacks normal biomechanical integrity and is predisposed to tears and occasionally a painful 'snapping knee syndrome'.

Criteria for diagnosis on MRI include identification of the body of the meniscus on more than three contiguous sagittal 4-mm slices, lack of rapid tapering from the periphery to the free edge of the meniscus and an abnormally wide meniscal body on coronal images, encroaching farther into the femorotibial compartment without the normal triangular configuration (Fig. 8.16).

Collateral Ligaments

The lateral collateral ligament complex. Lateral knee stability is through the joint capsule and structures of the lateral collateral ligament complex. Traditional descriptions divide the lateral collateral ligament into three layers, including an outer layer, comprising the iliotibial band anteriorly, continuous posteriorly with the biceps femoris tendon; the middle layer, which is composed of the posterolateral fibular collateral ligament; and the deep layer composed of the popliteus tendon.

RADIOLOGY PEARL

Injury to the lateral collateral ligament is uncommon and usually accompanies acute varus, either secondary to a motorcycle accident in which the motorcycle falls on the knee, or less commonly complicating an awkward fall.

The Medial Collateral Ligament

Medial knee stability is through subcutaneous fascial investment, the distal sartorius and the medial collateral ligament.

The medial collateral ligament is composed of deep fibres which are essentially meniscofemoral and meniscotibial ligamentous attachments separated from a thick superficial meniscotibial ligament by the medial collateral ligament bursa.

RADIOLOGY PEARL

Medial collateral ligament injury usually accompanies an acute valgus injury, and therefore while valgus strain widens the medial joint space it narrows the lateral space and leads to lateral femoral condylar impaction.

Cruciate Ligaments (see Fig. 8.16)

The Anterior Cruciate Ligament. The anterior cruciate ligament (ACL) is an intracapsular extrasynovial ligament that is primarily responsible for restraining anterior

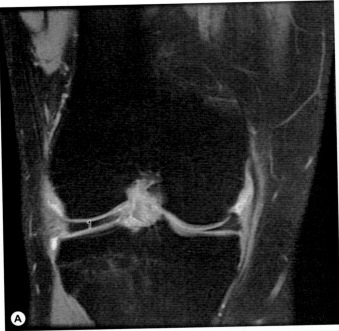
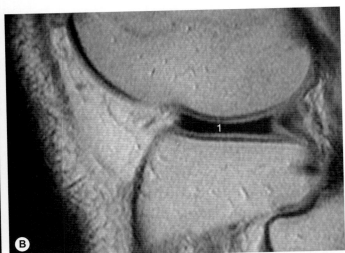

Fig. 8.16 (A) Coronal fat-suppressed magnetic resonance image and (B) sagittal T1-weighted image of the knee showing a discoid lateral meniscus *(1)*.

displacement of the tibia on flexion–extension. The ligament runs in a 'hand in pocket' axis from medial to lateral and from anterior to posterior, from the intercondylar notch hugging the inner aspect of the lateral femoral condyle.

The ligament has two identifiable bands, the anteromedial (AMB) and the posterolateral (PLB), according to insertion on the tibial spine. The AMB is stronger and being taut resists anterior displacement in flexion. The PLB is taut in extension, resisting hyperextension and hence posterior femoral displacement. Being taut throughout the gait cycle, both flexion and extension, the ACL maintains functional isometry.

> **RADIOLOGY PEARL**
>
> Disruption of the ACL most frequently follows a rotational torque injury. Acute stretching, particularly of the AMB, which resists anterior tibial displacement in 30 degrees of flexion, leads to ligamentous disruption. Although the AMB is most frequently disrupted in partial tears, most partial tears progress to complete tears within a year. In addition, when a partial tear is suspected on the basis of MR appearances, cadaveric studies indicate that in most cases both bundles are disrupted but retained within an intact synovial sleeve.

Posterior Cruciate Ligament. The posterior cruciate ligament (PCL), like the ACL, is an intrasynovial extracapsular ligament primarily responsible for resisting posterior translation of the tibia. The ligament is on average 13 mm long and is composed of a dominant anterolateral bundle and a smaller posteromedial band. Arising from the inner aspect of the medial femoral condyle the ligament

runs posteriorly in a C-shaped configuration to attach in a midline depression in the posterior margin of the tibial plateau.

Being tightly bound, the PCL is uniformly hypointense, although some signal hyperintensity is often seen at the apex of the C where fibres run at the magic angle (55 degrees to the Z-axis).

> **RADIOLOGY PEARL**
>
> Injury to the PCL is uncommon and best visualized in the sagittal plane when it occurs. Because it functions to resist posterior translation of the tibia, injury most frequently occurs when posterior tibial translation is forced by impaction injury to the shin or patella, as occurs in a motor vehicle dashboard injury.

The Extensor Mechanism

Extension of the knee occurs through contraction of the quadriceps muscle group, forces of which are translated though the quadriceps tendon, the patella and the patellar tendon. Injury of any of the components manifests as impaired extensor function. Although complete disruption is clinically evident as a result of incurred loss of function, most injuries are partial and clinically occult, and only diagnosed at MRI.

> **RADIOLOGY PEARL**
>
> Injuries of the extensor mechanism may be divided into those occurring in young patients, which tend to be complete and damage the patella tendon, and those occurring in older patients, which are often incomplete and damage the quadriceps tendon.

Popliteus Tendon

The popliteus muscle extends from its inferomedial insertion in the Achilles tendon superiorly through the calf and laterally to buttress the posterolateral aspect of the knee at its tendinous insertion in the popliteus recess of the posterolateral aspect of the lateral femoral condyle. Two additional insertion sites are the posterior fibular head (popliteofibular ligament) and the posterior horn of the lateral meniscus. Electromyography studies have determined that the popliteus is the primary internal rotator of the tibia on the femur in the non-weightbearing state. In the weightbearing state it rotates the femur externally on the leg.

> **RADIOLOGY PEARL**
>
> Popliteal injury usually reflects gross rotational torque injury with varus and is therefore rarely identified as an isolated entity but commonly accompanies complex disruption of the lateral collateral ligament, the ACL and the menisci.

Plantaris Tendon

Like the popliteus tendon, the plantaris tendon extends superiorly from the Achilles to insert on the posterior aspect of the lateral femoral condyle adjacent to the lateral head of the gastrocnemius. Rupture often manifests as haemorrhage and oedema adjacent but deep to the medial head of the gastrocnemius in the calf. Its slender muscle belly, which is approximately 5–10 cm long, lies deep to the lateral head of the gastrocnemius. The thin and long plantaris tendon crosses down between the medial head of the gastrocnemius and soleus muscles. The plantaris is absent in 7%–10% of the population.

> **RADIOLOGY PEARL**
>
> Reflecting rotational torque mechanism of injury, plantaris rupture is often accompanied by disruption of the ACL.

THE TIBIOFIBULAR JOINTS

The proximal tibiofibular joint is a synovial plane joint that is strengthened anteriorly and posteriorly by ligaments. The distal tibiofibular joint is a syndesmosis, which is united by an interosseous ligament that is continuous superiorly with the interosseous membrane. The interosseous membrane acts as an accessory ligament to both joints.

THE ANKLE JOINT (FIG. 8.17)

Type

The ankle joint is a synovial hinge joint.

Articular Surfaces

These are:
- The lower tibia and the inner surface of the medial malleolus
- The medial surface of the lateral malleolus of the fibula
- The trochlear surface of the head of the talus

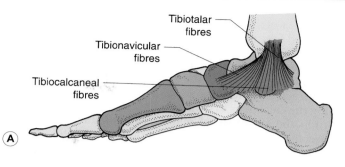

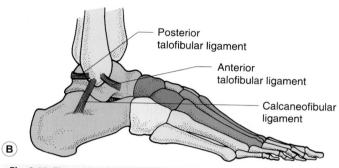

Fig. 8.17 The ankle. (A) Medial view: deltoid ligament. (B) Lateral view.

The articular surface of the talus is broader anteriorly than posteriorly. This makes the ankle more stable in dorsiflexion (i.e. standing) and more mobile in plantar flexion.

Capsule

This is attached to the margins of the articular surfaces, except where it extends distally to the neck of the talus.

Synovium

This lines the capsule and frequently passes up between the lower ends of the tibia and the fibula.

Ligaments

The capsule of the ankle joint is thickened with ligaments medially and laterally but is weak anteriorly and posteriorly.

The **deltoid ligament** is a triangular ligament on the medial aspect of the ankle. It is attached to the apex of the medial malleolus and inferiorly to the medial aspect of the talus, the sustentaculum tali of the calcaneus and the tuberosity of the navicular.

Laterally, the ankle is strengthened by three ligaments:
- The **posterior talofibular ligament**, which passes medially from the lowest part of the malleolar fossa of the fibula to the posterior process of the talus.
- The **calcaneofibular ligament**, which passes from the apex of the lateral malleolus to the calcaneus.
- The **anterior talofibular ligament**, which passes anteromedially from the lateral malleolus to the lateral aspect of the neck of the talus.

BIOMECHANICS OF THE FOOT AND ANKLE

The biomechanics of the foot are complex, involving the integrated motion of 57 articulating surfaces during normal locomotion. In health, the gait cycle is divided into weightbearing and non-weightbearing phases in which impaction forces are distributed either to one or both feet.

The weightbearing cycle is divided into heel-strike, planted-foot and toe-off phases. On heel-strike the hind-foot is everted, the midfoot articulations are aligned and mobile, allowing even distribution of impaction forces. As the foot is planted, the long flexors of the calf begin to contract, elevating the medial longitudinal arch and drawing the calcaneus to neutral or varus. Such movement disrupts the alignment of midfoot articulations and the foot becomes rigid or locked in preparation for the final toe-off phase, in which all forces are transmitted to the base of the first toe, propelling the foot forward.

RADIOLOGICAL FEATURES OF THE ANKLE JOINT

Plain Radiographs (see Fig. 8.17)

On AP radiographs of the ankle joint the tibiotalar surfaces are seen to be parallel to each other and perpendicular to the shaft of the tibia. The articular surfaces of the malleoli on each side are symmetrical about a line through the shaft of the tibia, each making an equal angle with the inferior surface of the tibia.

The **medial and lateral ligaments of the ankle joint** are not visible on plain radiographs but their integrity can be deduced from normal joint alignment in standard views and, where appropriate, stress views. Where the distance between the medial malleolus and the talus is increased then disruption of the deltoid ligament can be diagnosed, and where there is increased distance between the lateral malleolus and the talus without bony injury this is due to disruption of the lateral ligaments. In general, loss of parallelism of the articular surface is significant.

The term **trimalleolar fracture** is sometimes used, although there are only two malleoli. The third 'malleolus' is the posterior lip of the tibial articular surface.

Arthrography

The synovial cavity is outlined by injection of contrast and the integrity of the medial and lateral ligaments can be assessed. The normal articular surfaces are seen to be smooth and parallel. Recesses of the synovial cavity are sometimes prominent anterior and posterior to the tibia and anterior to the inferior tibiofibular joint.

> **RADIOLOGY PEARL**
>
> At ankle arthrography filling of the synovial sheaths around the tendons of flexor hallucis longus or flexor digitorum longus is considered normal – both are filled in 20% of arthrograms. The posterior subtalar joint is filled in 10% of normal studies. All other extravasations are abnormal.

CT

This can be combined with arthrography to assess the bony components of the ankle joint.

Direct coronal and axial images are routinely acquired in slices 2 mm thick.

MRI (Fig. 8.18)

This technique is particularly useful for soft tissues, especially ligaments and tendons. The Achilles tendon can be seen inserting into the posterior aspect of the calcaneus, separated from the posterior surface of the tibia by a fat pad. The cartilaginous surface of the articulating bones can be visualized directly, as can the deltoid and talofibular ligaments. Tendons of tibialis anterior, extensor hallucis longus, extensor digitorum longus and peroneus tertius muscles pass deep to the extensor retinaculum on the anterior aspect of the joint, and the tendons of peroneus longus and brevis pass beneath the peroneal retinaculum on the lateral aspect of the ankle. The tendons of the flexor digitorum longus, flexor hallucis longus and tibialis posterior pass deep to the flexor retinaculum in separate fibro-osseous tunnels on the medial aspect of the ankle.

Ultrasound (Fig. 8.19)

More readily available than MRI, in experienced hands high-resolution imaging of the muscles and tendons can examine their integrity. Images can be acquired to provide an extended field of view and display the entire length of a muscle or tendon on one image.

RELEVANT MRI ANATOMY (SEE FIG. 8.18)

The Ankle Ligaments

There are four major ligamentous stabilizers in the foot and ankle: the lateral collateral ligament, the medial collateral ligament (the deltoid ligament), the syndesmotic complex and the interosseous ligament (talocalcaneal ligament) in the sinus tarsi.

The lateral collateral ligament. The lateral collateral ligament, providing lateral stability to the tibiotalar articulation, is composed of five components, the anterior and posterior talofibular ligaments, the calcaneofibular ligament and the anterior and posterior tibiofibular ligaments. (In fact, the anterior and posterior tibiofibular ligaments are considered to be a part of the syndesmosis, but such a description allows one to consider five components in both the medial and lateral collateral ligaments.)

> **RADIOLOGY PEARL**
>
> Following inversion injury to the lateral collateral ligament, rupture of the anterior talofibular ligament is followed by rupture of the calcaneofibular, and then extremely rarely by the posterior talofibular ligaments. If the calcaneofibular ligament is ruptured, it is always accompanied by rupture of the anterior talofibular ligament.

Anterior talofibular ligament. The normal anterior talofibular ligament is readily visualized in the direct axial plane running anteromedially from the tip of the lateral malleolus (at the level of the malleolar fossa identified on the inner aspect of the malleolus) to the anterolateral aspect of the talus. In health, the ligament is a fine linear structure, homogeneously hypointense on all sequences. Following injury, intrasubstance haemorrhage may result in ligamentous swelling and signal abnormality, often accompanied by incomplete tear of superior fibres. Complete rupture with retraction is always accompanied by joint effusion and leakage of fluid to neighbouring soft tissues. The partially retracted ligament is often noted to billow freely within adjacent joint effusion.

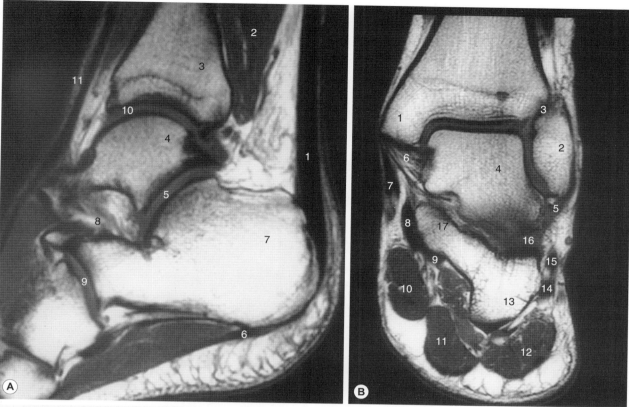

Fig. 8.18 Magnetic resonance image (MRI) of the ankle. (A) Sagittal T1-weighted image. (B) Coronal T1-weighted image.

(A)
1. Achilles tendon
2. Flexor hallucis muscle belly
3. Tibia
4. Talus
5. Posterior subtalar joint
6. Plantar aponeurosis
7. Calcaneus
8. Sinus tarsi and interosseous ligament
9. Calcaneocuboid articulation
10. Tibiotalar articulation
11. Tibialis anterior tendon

(B)
1. Medial malleolus
2. Lateral malleolus

3. Inferior tibiofibular articulation
4. Talus
5. Fibulocalcaneal ligament
6. Tibiocalcaneal ligament
7. Tibialis posterior tendon
8. Flexor digitorum longus
9. Flexor hallucis longus tendon
10. Abductor hallucis muscle
11. Flexor digitorum brevis
12. Flexor digiti minimi
13. Calcaneus
14. Peroneus longus tendon
15. Peroneus brevis tendon
16. Posterior subtalar joint
17. Sustentaculum talus

The calcaneofibular ligament. The normal calcaneofibular ligament is readily visualized on images acquired in an axial oblique plane perpendicular to the posterior subtalar joint, or in the axial plane acquired in a plantarflexed foot. The ligament is identified as a fine linear structure deep to the peroneal tendons and is uniformly hypointense on all sequences. Following injury, intrasubstance haemorrhage and oedema produce swelling and signal abnormality in the ligament, enhancing its conspicuousness. Communication with peroneal tendon sheaths results in frequently identified associated peroneal tendon sheath fluid, and occasionally subluxation.

The posterior talofibular ligament. This is a fan-shaped isointense structure, usually identified on the same image as the anterior talofibular ligament in the direct axial plane. The ligament runs from the malleolar fossa on the inner aspect of the lateral malleolus to the posterior tibial tubercle of the calcaneus. Because of its fan-shaped configuration the ligament is extremely strong and rarely injured.

The medial collateral ligament (the deltoid ligament). The medial collateral ligament has five components, including the anterior and posterior tibiotalar, the tibiocalcaneal, the tibiospring and the tibionavicular ligaments. Classically the ligament is divided into deep and superficial components, the superficial layer arising from the anterior margin of the medial malleolus and branching to the navicular, the sustentaculum, the calcaneus and to the medial tubercle of the talus; the deep layer arises from the posterior margin of the malleolus and attaches to the medial aspect of the talus.

Using MRI, the fan-shaped components of the superficial medial collateral ligament are only visualized in multiple

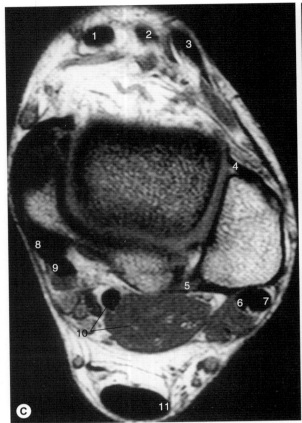

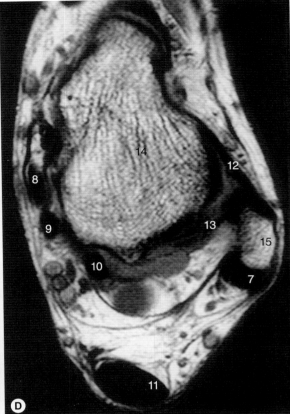

Fig. 8.18, cont'd (C and D) MRI of the ankle: axial proton density image. (E) Axial oblique proton density image.

(C and D)
 1. Tibialis anterior tendon
 2. Extensor hallucis tendon
 3. Extensor digitorum tendon
 4. Anterior tibiofibular ligament
 5. Posterior tibiofibular ligament
 6. Peroneus brevis tendon
 7. Peroneus longus tendon
 8. Tibialis posterior tendon
 9. Flexor digitorum tendon
10. Flexor hallucis longus tendon and muscle belly
11. Achilles tendon
12. Anterior talofibular ligament
13. Posterior talofibular ligament
14. Talus
15. Lateral malleolus

(E)
 1. Tibialis posterior tendon
 2. Flexor digitorum tendon
 3. Flexor hallucis tendon
 4. Peroneus brevis tendon
 5. Peroneus longus tendon
 6. Extensor hallucis tendon
 7. Extensor digitorum tendon
 8. Tibialis anterior tendon
 9. Tarsal tunnel
10. Quadratus plantae muscle
11. Medial plantar nerve, artery and veins
12. Lateral plantar nerve, artery and veins
13. Talus
14. Sustentaculum talus
15. Posterior subtalar joint

oblique planes. In contrast, the deep component is routinely identified on direct coronal images as a short, striated structure. In general, injury to the medial collateral ligament accompanies complex ankle trauma, invariably associated with disruption of the lateral collateral ligament or the syndesmosis.

The syndesmosis. Syndesmosis is the term used to describe the three stabilizing components of the inferior tibiofibular articulation: the anterior and posterior tibiofibular ligaments and the interosseous membrane. Injury to the syndesmosis is extremely uncommon in the absence of a fracture.

The ligaments of the syndesmosis are readily visualized on direct axial images just proximal to the tibiotalar articulation (identification of the malleolar fossa on the inner aspect of the lateral malleolus is used to differentiate between the anterior and posterior talofibular and anterior and posterior tibiofibular ligaments when any doubt exists).

The anterior tibiofibular ligament is a linear hypointense structure running from the anterior tibial tubercle laterally along the anterior margin of the inferior tibiofibular articulation to the fibula. Often the ligament courses slightly inferiorly and therefore can only be fully appreciated by reviewing serial images. The posterior tibiofibular ligament has both similar signal characteristics and orientation to the anterior tibiofibular ligament and runs along the posterior margin of the tibiofibular articulation.

RADIOLOGY PEARL

Injury to the syndesmosis usually involves rupture to the anterior tibiofibular ligament and spares the posterior. The posterior ligament is stronger, and therefore when stressed results in an avulsion fracture at its insertion rather than soft-tissue rupture.

The ligaments of the sinus tarsi. The sinus tarsi is a cone-shaped space interposed between the inferolateral border of the talus and the superolateral surface of the calcaneus. In health, the sinus tarsi is predominantly filled with fat, allowing the space to narrow slightly on eversion. On inversion, widening of the space and hence stability between the talus and calcaneus is maintained by both the cervical and interosseous ligaments. Minor trauma – either inversion or eversion – may manifest as haemorrhage, oedema and secondary compression of neurovascular structures within the space, and hence acute pain. Acute inversion may occasionally result in disruption of ligamentous structures and gross subtalar instability. Occasionally disruption of the ligaments precedes or is a part of subtalar dislocation.

Because the sinus tarsi is richly vascularized, ruptured ligaments readily heal without surgical intervention, although scarring and persistent laxity may result in long-term instability.

At MRI the sinus tarsi is readily visualized on direct coronal images, fat-suppressed inversion recovery images facilitating the detection of oedema and haemorrhage, and turbo spin echo T1-weighted images allowing the evaluation of interosseous and cervical ligaments.

Impingement syndromes. Three impingement syndromes are described that cause chronic pain following ankle trauma: the anterolateral, syndesmotic and posterolateral impingement syndromes. **Anterolateral impingement syndrome** is a soft-tissue impingement with associated pain between anterolateral osseous structures of the ankle joint (the lateral gutter). Most commonly, fibrous overgrowth or synovitis following chronic tear of the anterior talofibular ligament is responsible, and rarely a tear resulting in a hyalinized connective tissue meniscoid lesion. **Syndesmotic impingement syndrome** describes the acute pain incurred when soft tissue is impinged between the osseous structures of the syndesmosis, usually manifest by thickening and synovitis at the site of a chronic tear of the anterior tibiofibular ligament. **Posterior impingement syndrome** describes impingement of the posterior soft-tissue structure between the posterolateral osseous structures of the ankle. In most cases the syndrome reflects impingement of a hypertrophied posterior inferior tibiofibular ligament or the posterior intermalleolar ligament.

The Achilles tendon. Formed by merging of the gastrocnemius and soleus tendons, the Achilles tendon extends inferiorly to insert on the dorsal margin of the calcaneus. It is readily visualized on both ultrasound and MRI in the sagittal plane. Injury occurs either at the insertion of the Achilles in association with retrocalcaneal synovitis and bursitis or at the musculotendinous junction 6 cm proximal to the insertion on the calcaneus, where tendon fibres intertwine and create a zone of relative ischaemia.

Peroneal tendons. The peroneal muscle bellies within the lateral compartment of the thigh give rise to the peroneus brevis and longus tendons at the ankle. The peroneal tendons, peroneus brevis anterior to the peroneus longus, course around the lateral malleolus within its slightly concave aspect called the fibular groove.

The peroneus brevis tendon passes along the lateral margin of the foot to insert at the base of the fifth metatarsal; the peroneus longus tendon courses beneath the cuboid to insert at the base of the first metatarsal and medial cuneiform.

Functioning to plantarflex and evert the foot, the tendons, if unrestrained, would freely bowstring at the lateral malleolus. In health, position within the fibular groove is maintained by a tight retinaculum which prevents both tendon subluxation and dislocation or bowstringing.

Reflecting primary functions of eversion and plantar flexion, it is not surprising that injury is usually a sequel to forced dorsiflexion or forced inversion.

RADIOLOGY PEARL

Peroneus brevis tendon injury is more common than injury to the peroneus longus. It is postulated that laxity of the superior peroneal retinaculum allows the brevis tendon to sublux and interpose between the longus and the fibrous edge of the fibula, resulting in shear-induced longitudinal tendon splits.

Tibialis posterior tendon. The tibialis posterior tendon is the second most commonly injured tendon in the foot (after the peroneus brevis). The tendinous continuation of the muscle belly within the deep posterior compartment of the calf rounds the medial malleolus and passes forward to a dominant insertion at the base of the navicular, and six further lesser insertions in the forefoot, at the bases of the cuneiforms and the bases of metatarsals two to four. The tibialis posterior tendon provides major support to the medial longitudinal arch during the planted-foot phase of the gait cycle and is responsible for both plantar flexion and inversion.

RADIOLOGY PEARL

Although acute injuries to the tibialis posterior tendon have been described following forced dorsiflexion with eversion in young athletes, in most cases injury occurs as a result of chronic overuse or trauma in middle-aged females and leads to the development of pes planus or an acquired flat foot.

Chronic tear results in collapse of the medial arch or acquired flatfoot with progressive hindfoot valgus, posterior subtalar joint subluxation and arthritis. Medial arch collapse may result in impaction bone bruising between the anterior talar process and the navicular or between the calcaneus and the cuboid.

Flexor hallucis longus. The flexor hallucis is a dominant flexor and inverter of the foot, with an extensive course to insert at the base of the distal phalanx of the great toe.

Injury to the flexor hallucis may occur proximally, usually secondary to chronic overuse at the level of the medial malleolus or the musculotendinous junction, as occurs in ballet dancers, or distally, which is usually acute and secondary to stubbing the toe when attempting to kick a football, hence the term 'turf toe'.

Like other tendon or ligamentous injuries, intrasubstance rupture initially leads to tendon swelling prior to attenuation and rupture.

The flexor hallucis tendon runs in a fibro-osseous tunnel along the posterior aspect of the talus, which may be a site of friction leading to tear in ballet dancers, accentuated by an accessory os trigonum.

Although peritendinous fluid is a useful marker of tendon insult and tenosynovitis, communication to the tibiotalar articulation in up to 20% of the normal population may account for this observation in the absence of symptoms.

Tibialis anterior tendon. The tibialis anterior muscle arising in the anterior compartment of the calf gives rise to its tendon at the level of the tibiotalar articulation, which passes to the foot deep to the extensor retinaculum before inserting on the medial cuneiform and the medial base of the first metatarsal. As such the tibialis anterior is a dominant flexor and inverter of the foot, and injury is therefore induced acutely by forced extension and eversion. In most cases rupture is the sequel of chronic trauma, with repeated encroachment of the tendon by the extensor retinaculum over time.

RADIOLOGY PEARL

The os trigonum represents a congenital nonunion of the lateral tubercle of the posterior process of the talus, to which it remains intimately related in adulthood. During flexion and extension, synovial tissue may interdigitate between it and the posterior tibia, resulting in capsular entrapment, local pain and inflammation.

THE SUBTALAR JOINT

This synovial joint is responsible for inversion and eversion of the ankle. It has two parts, each with its own capsule and synovial cavity as follows:
- The **talocalcaneal joint** between the posterior facet on the inferior surface of the talus and the corresponding facet on the calcaneus.
- The **talocalcaneonavicular joint** has four contiguous parts (see also the inferior surface of the talus):
  - Between the inferior surface of the talus and the sustentaculum tali of the calcaneus.
  - The plantar calcaneonavicular (spring) ligament and the anterior talocalcaneal facet.
  - Between the head of the talus and the navicular bone.

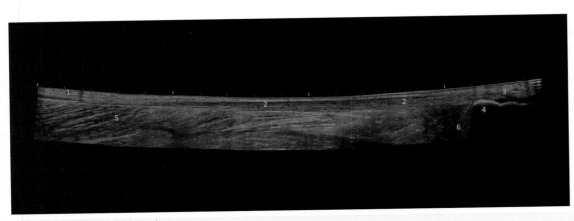

Fig. 8.19 Sagittal ultrasound of Achilles tendon.

1. Skin
2. Achilles tendon. This is thinner superiorly where it blends with muscle
3. Insertion of the Achilles into the calcaneus
4. Calcaneus
5. Gastrocnemius muscle
6. Fat pad (of Kagar)

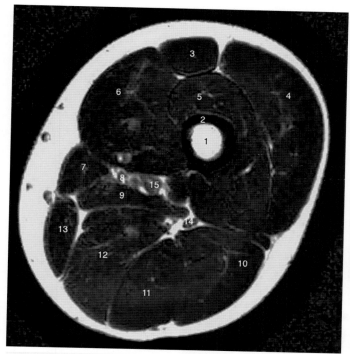

Fig. 8.20 Axial proton density-weighted magnetic resonance scan of the thigh.

1. Medullary cavity of the femur
2. Cortex of the femur
3. Rectus femoris muscle
4. Vastus lateralis muscle
5. Vastus intermedius muscle
6. Vastus medialis muscle
7. Sartorius muscle
8. Superficial femoral vessels in the adductor canal
9. Adductor magnus
10. Biceps femoris muscle (long head)
11. Semitendinosus muscle
12. Semimembranosus muscle
13. Gracilis muscle
14. Position of sciatic nerve
15. Deep femoral vessels

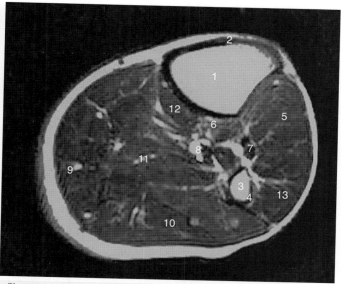

Fig. 8.21 Axial proton density-weighted magnetic resonance scan of the calf.

1. Medulla of tibia
2. Cortex of tibia
3. Medulla of fibula
4. Cortex of fibula
5. Muscles of the anterior tibial compartment
6. Tibialis posterior muscle
7. Anterior tibial artery, vein and nerve
8. Posterior tibial artery, vein and nerve
9. Medial head of the gastrocnemius muscle
10. Lateral head of the gastrocnemius muscle
11. Soleus muscle
12. Flexor digitorum longus muscle
13. Peroneus longus

RADIOLOGICAL FEATURES OF THE SUBTALAR JOINT

Plain Radiography

In radiography of the subtalar joint oblique views of the ankle with the foot internally rotated 45 degrees are used. Films are exposed with tube angulations of 10, 20, 30 and 40 degrees for complete visualization of the complex articular surfaces.

CT

The three components of the talocalcaneal joint, the posterior, the sustentaculum tali and the anterior components, can be seen by coronal imaging with CT.

In addition to bones, MRI can identify the peroneal muscles which contribute to the stability of the joint as well as ligaments, such as:
- The interosseous talocalcaneal ligament.
- The plantar calcaneonavicular 'spring' ligament from the sustentaculum tali to the navicular.

- The short plantar ligament from the calcaneus to the cuboid.
- The long plantar ligament from the calcaneus to the base of the metacarpals.

OTHER JOINTS OF THE FOOT

The intertarsal, tarsometatarsal, metatarsophalangeal and interphalangeal joints of the foot are synovial joints, each with its own capsule and synovial cavity.

The Muscles of the Lower Limb

In the **upper thigh** (Figs. 8.20 and 8.22), muscles that flex the hip and extend the knee are found anteriorly, that is, the quadriceps femoris muscle, made up of the rectus femoris and vastus lateralis, medialis and intermedius muscles. Sartorius, a thin flat strap muscle with a similar action, is also found superficially in the anterior compartment.

The adductor muscles are found medially. These are, from anterior to posterior, the adductor longus, brevis and magnus muscles, with the adductor gracilis lying superficially.

Posteriorly lie the extensors of the hip, the glutei and the flexors of the knee – the hamstrings, that is, the biceps femoris, semimembranosus and semitendinosus muscles.

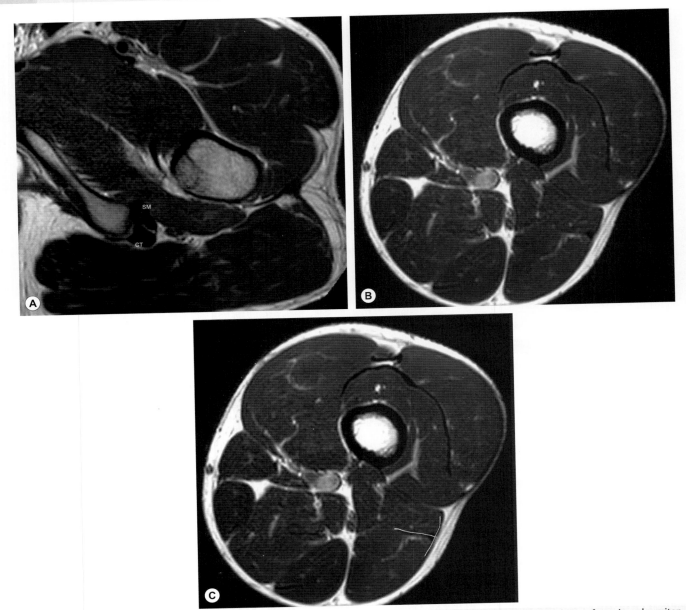

Fig. 8.22 Axial T2-weighted magnetic resonance image depicting hamstring anatomy. (A) The conjoint tendon *(CT)* of the biceps femoris and semitendinosus arising posteriorly to the semimembranous tendon *(SM)*. (B and C) The distal biceps femoris T junction, outlined in (C).

The femoral artery, vein and nerve lie superficially between the anterior and adductor compartments, with the profunda femoris vessels lying deeply close to the femur in the same plane.

At **midthigh level** (Figs. 8.20 and 8.23) the shaft of the femur is surrounded by the rectus femoris and vastus muscles medially, anteriorly and laterally. The shaft of the femur is surrounded posteromedially by the adductors and posterolaterally by the biceps, semitendinosus and semimembranosus.

The femoral vessels lie in the adductor canal deep to the sartorius muscle and between the anterior and adductor compartments. The profunda vessels lie almost posterior to the femur, also between these compartments. The sciatic nerve lies between the muscles of the adductor compartment and the hamstring muscles.

The proximal hamstring origin is an important structure prone both to acute tear injuries in the athletic population and degenerative tendinopathy in older patients. The biceps femoris and semitendinosus muscles arise posteriorly from the ischial tuberosity as a conjoint tendon, with the semimembranosus tendon arising just anteriorly and laterally (Fig. 8.24A).

The distal myotendinous junction of the biceps femoris is the most commonly injured component of the hamstring complex. The long and short heads of biceps femurs combine to form a T-shaped structure on axial MRI (Fig. 8.24B and C). Injury to this distal 'T junction' of the biceps femoris behaves differently to other hamstring injuries with high recurrence rates.

In the **lower leg** (see Figs. 8.21 and 8.25) the tibia lies anteromedially subcutaneously. The fibula lies laterally

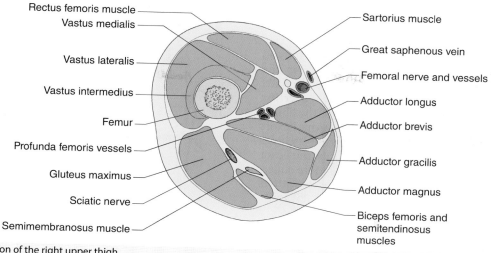

Rectus femoris muscle
Vastus medialis
Vastus lateralis
Vastus intermedius
Femur
Profunda femoris vessels
Gluteus maximus
Sciatic nerve
Semimembranosus muscle

Sartorius muscle
Great saphenous vein
Femoral nerve and vessels
Adductor longus
Adductor brevis
Adductor gracilis
Adductor magnus
Biceps femoris and semitendinosus muscles

Fig. 8.23 Axial section of the right upper thigh.

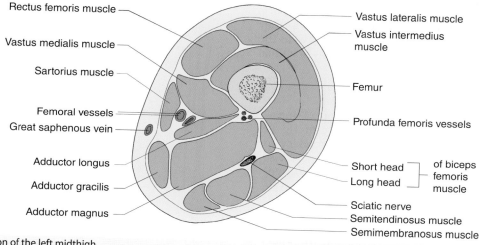

Rectus femoris muscle
Vastus medialis muscle
Sartorius muscle
Femoral vessels
Great saphenous vein
Adductor longus
Adductor gracilis
Adductor magnus

Vastus lateralis muscle
Vastus intermedius muscle
Femur
Profunda femoris vessels
Short head ⎤ of biceps
Long head ⎦ femoris muscle
Sciatic nerve
Semitendinosus muscle
Semimembranosus muscle

Fig. 8.24 Axial section of the left midthigh.

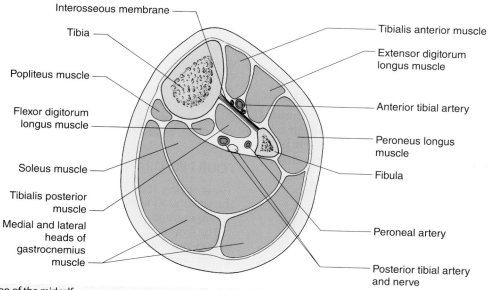

Interosseous membrane
Tibia
Popliteus muscle
Flexor digitorum longus muscle
Soleus muscle
Tibialis posterior muscle
Medial and lateral heads of gastrocnemius muscle

Tibialis anterior muscle
Extensor digitorum longus muscle
Anterior tibial artery
Peroneus longus muscle
Fibula
Peroneal artery
Posterior tibial artery and nerve

Fig. 8.25 Axial section of the midcalf.

and is more centrally placed. The interosseous membrane between these separates anterior and posterior compartments.

Anterior to the interosseous membrane lie the extensors (dorsiflexors) of the ankle and toes: tibialis anterior and extensor digitorum longus. Peroneus tertius is also part of this group (it extends the ankle in addition to everting the ankle) and is found below the lower third of the fibula.

Posterior to the interosseous membrane lie the flexors (plantar flexors) of the ankle and toes. A deep group includes the tibialis posterior and, in the lower two-thirds, the flexor digitorum and flexor hallucis longus muscles. More superficially lie the soleus and the gastrocnemius muscle with its medial and lateral heads. These latter two muscles unite inferiorly to form the calcaneal (Achilles) tendon.

A lateral compartment contains two peroneal muscles: peroneus longus and, in the distal two-thirds, peroneus brevis. These are evertors of the ankle.

The anterior tibial vessels lie anterior to the interosseous membrane deep to the muscles of this compartment. The posterior tibial and peroneal vessels lie between the deep and the superficial muscles of the posterior compartment. At first close together, these vessels separate as they descend and the peroneal vessels come to lie closer to the fibula in the same muscle plane, while the posterior tibial vessels become closer to the tibia.

RADIOLOGY PEARL

Compartment syndrome describes elevation of intracompartmental pressure greater than 10 mm Hg in the calf muscular compartments either secondary to trauma, thrombosis or tumour, or secondary to exercise when it is termed chronic exertional compartment syndrome. As pressures rise above 50 mm Hg capillary vessels occlude and impair exit of fluid from the calf further elevating pressures, leading to accumulation of lactates and neuropraxia. Anterior compartment syndrome results in flexor paresis, and deep peroneal neuropraxia with loss of sensation between the first and second toes. Lateral compartment syndrome leads to loss of peroneal function. Deep posterior compartment syndrome is characterized by deep extensor muscle paresis and an inability to plantar flex the foot.

The Arteries of the Lower Limb (Figs. 8.26–8.28)

The external iliac artery becomes the **common femoral artery** where it crosses under the inguinal ligament midway between the anterior superior iliac spine and the pubic symphysis. The common femoral artery has three superficial branches at this point, namely:

- The superficial circumflex iliac artery
- The superficial inferior epigastric artery
- The superficial pudendal artery

The **profunda femoris artery**, its biggest branch, arises 5 cm distal to the inguinal ligament and has six branches as follows:

- Medial and lateral circumflex femoral arteries
- Four perforating arteries

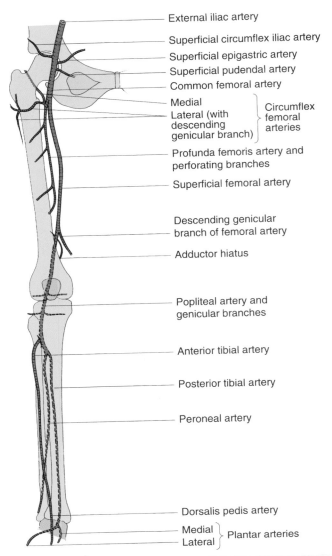

Fig. 8.26 Arteries of the lower limb as seen on angiography.

MEDIAL AND LATERAL CIRCUMFLEX FEMORAL ARTERIES

These arteries form a ring around the upper femur. The lateral circumflex femoral artery has an ascending branch that anastomoses with a branch of the superior gluteal artery and it also sends a descending branch to the knee. Thus it can provide a route of collateral supply capable of bypassing an obstructed common femoral artery or an obstructed superficial femoral artery.

FOUR PERFORATING ARTERIES

These supply the muscles of the thigh (the last of these is the continuation of the profunda) and surround the femur on angiography.

The femoral artery continues as the **superficial femoral artery** and has few branches in the thigh. It passes in the adductor canal between the vastus medialis, the adductors and sartorius. At the junction of the upper two-thirds and the lower third of the femur it passes through the adductor hiatus close to the femur and into the popliteal fossa to become the popliteal artery. Just before it does this it supplies a descending branch to the genicular anastomosis.

The **popliteal artery** (see Fig. 8.28) supplies branches to the genicular anastomosis, branches to the knee joint and divides at the lower border of the knee joint into anterior and posterior tibial arteries.

The **posterior tibial artery** is the larger of the two terminal branches. Its proximal part is sometimes called the **tibioperoneal trunk**. It gives rise to the peroneal artery 2.5 cm from its origin. The posterior tibial artery then passes between the superficial and deep muscles of the posterior compartment of the lower leg. As it descends it becomes more medial.

The posterior tibial artery supplies branches to the genicular anastomosis, to the muscles, the skin and the tibia. At the ankle it supplies a medial malleolar branch to the ankle anastomosis and then passes posterior to the medial malleolus (halfway between the tip of the malleolus and the midline posteriorly) to divide into the medial and lateral plantar arteries, the principal supply to the foot. The lateral plantar artery is the main contributor to the plantar arch.

The **peroneal artery**, as it descends, comes to lie close to the medial aspect of the posterior of the fibula. It runs behind the distal tibiofibular joint and ends as calcaneal branches supplying the superior and lateral aspects of that bone. Its other branches are the:

- Muscular branches.
- Nutrient artery to the fibula.
- Perforating branch, which perforates the interosseous membrane about 5 cm above the lateral malleolus and descends anteriorly to supply branches to the tarsus.

- Communicating branch, which joins a similar branch from the posterior tibial artery as part of the circle of vessels around the ankle.

The **anterior tibial artery**, after it arises from the popliteal artery, passes above the upper margin of the interosseous membrane and descends anterior to this membrane until it becomes superficial at the ankle midway between the malleoli.

This continues as the **dorsalis pedis artery** which, having supplied the arcuate artery for the metatarsal and digital arteries, passes between the first and second metatarsals to join the plantar arch.

RADIOLOGICAL FEATURES OF THE ARTERIES OF THE LOWER LIMB

Arteriography of the Lower Limb (see Figs. 8.27–8.29)

This is performed by catheterization of the femoral artery or, in special circumstances, by translumbar aortography or even by approaching the aortic arch from one of the upper limb arteries.

In arteriography, the femoral artery is projected over the lower part of the head of the femur. The superficial femoral artery has a vertical course, whereas the shaft of the femur lies obliquely. The artery, as a result, is medial to the upper shaft but posterior to the lower shaft as it approaches the popliteal fossa. The profunda femoris artery lies closer to the femur and is also distinguished from the superficial

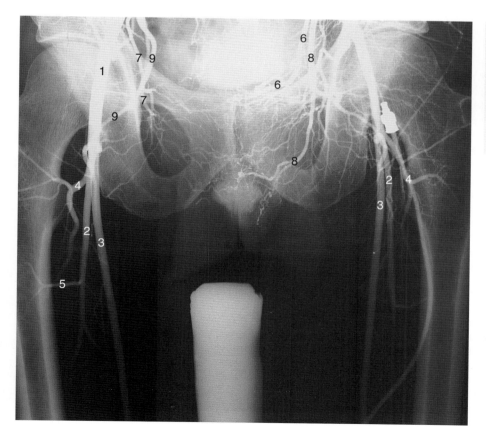

Fig. 8.27 Femoral artery angiogram.

1. Common femoral artery
2. Profunda femoris artery
3. Superficial femoral artery
4. Lateral circumflex femoral artery
5. Perforating artery
6. Superior vesical artery
7. Obturator artery
8. Internal pudendal artery
9. Inferior gluteal artery

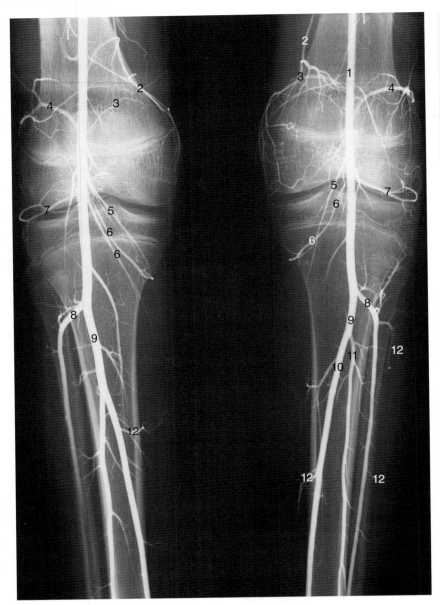

Fig. 8.28 Femoral angiogram: popliteal arteries.
1. Popliteal artery
2. Descending genicular artery
3. Medial superior genicular artery
4. Lateral superior genicular artery
5. Middle genicular artery
6. Medial inferior genicular artery
7. Lateral inferior genicular artery
8. Anterior tibial artery
9. Tibioperoneal trunk
10. Posterior tibial artery
11. Peroneal artery
12. Muscular branches

femoral artery by its numerous branches – the superficial femoral artery has no significant branch in the thigh. The origin and proximal part of the profunda tend to overlie the superficial femoral artery in AP views and are best seen in oblique views.

The division of the popliteal into anterior and posterior tibial arteries (called the trifurcation because the posterior tibial artery soon gives rise to the peroneal artery) lies over the proximal tibiofibular joint. The anterior tibial artery arises at an angle, whereas the posterior tibial (the tibioperoneal trunk) is a more direct continuation of the popliteal artery.

The three main vessels of the lower leg lie over and between the shafts of the tibia and fibula. Slight internal rotation of the foot helps to project the tibia away from the fibula and allows the vessels to be seen between them.

The dorsalis pedis artery is best seen on lateral views of the foot, and the medial and lateral plantar arteries and the plantar arch are seen on dorsoplantar views of the foot.

CT Angiography

CT angiography of the lower limb utilizes iodinated contrast and provides an excellent overview of the lower limb vasculature. The rapidity of acquisition is critical in emergency scenarios or following trauma, where an acute occlusion or other vascular injury is suspected. Lower limb CT angiography is also common in the outpatient setting for evaluating chronic peripheral vascular disease.

MR Angiography

Gadolinium contrast bolus chasing is now routinely performed by combining moving table-top acquisition with coronally acquired datasets. With this approach the lower extremity vascular tree can be examined completely by three to four coronal acquisitions. Acquired images now compete with diagnostic catheter angiograms and in many centres have replaced catheter diagnostic angiography, catheter studies now only undertaken for interventional purposes (Fig. 8.29).

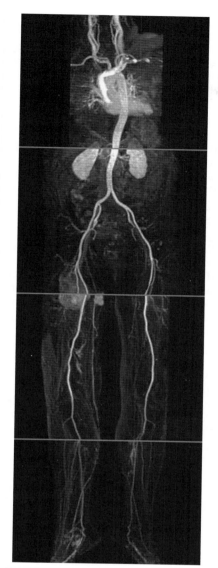

Fig. 8.29 Coronal lower limb gadolinium-enhanced magnetic resonance angiogram.

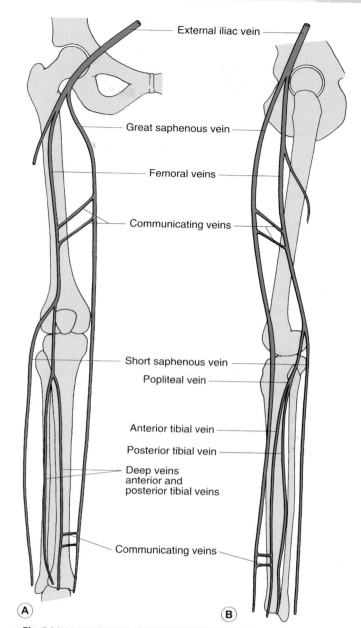

Fig. 8.30 Veins of the lower limb as seen on venography.

Ultrasound

These arteries can be imaged using ultrasound and Doppler ultrasound, especially where they are superficial, that is, the common femoral artery in the inguinal region, the popliteal artery in the popliteal fossa and the dorsalis pedis on the dorsum of the foot.

COLLATERAL ARTERIES

Complete occlusion of a major artery in the leg does not always lead to loss of arterial supply to the limb because of the establishment of collateral supply via alternative routes. Thus occlusion of the common femoral artery can be overcome via branches of the superior and inferior gluteal arteries, which anastomose with branches of the lateral circumflex branch of the profunda femoris artery. Obstruction of flow in the superficial femoral artery can be bypassed by descending branches of the lateral circumflex

artery and of the perforating branches of the profunda artery anastomosing with branches of the distal superficial femoral artery and of the popliteal artery in the genicular anastomosis.

The anastomosis between all the anterior tibial, posterior tibial and peroneal arteries around the ankle joint allows any artery reaching the ankle to supply the foot.

The Veins of the Lower Limb (Fig. 8.30)

Venous blood is drained from the lower limb by a system of deep and superficial veins. The normal direction of flow is from superficial to deep veins. Valves are more numerous in the superficial than in the deep system, and more numerous distally than proximally. The valves and the deep fascia of the lower limb help to propel the blood towards the heart.

The **superficial veins** are the long and short saphenous veins. The **long saphenous vein** starts on the medial side of the dorsum of the foot and passes anterior to the medial malleolus. It ascends vertically so that it lies posterior to the medial side of the knee and anterior to the upper thigh, where it receives the anterior femoral cutaneous vein on the anterior surface of the thigh. The long saphenous vein drains into the femoral vein via the saphenous opening in the deep fascia in the lower part of the inguinal triangle.

The **short saphenous vein** begins on the lateral side of the dorsum of the foot and passes posterior to the lateral malleolus. It ascends on the back of the calf and pierces the deep fascia over the popliteal fossa to enter the popliteal vein.

The **deep veins** of the lower limb accompany the arteries, as described above. They are usually paired, although more than two veins may accompany one artery.

Perforating (communicating) veins carry blood from superficial veins to the deep veins and are variable in site and number. At least two occur in the medial aspect of the lower leg above the ankle. Perforating veins are also found in the medial aspect of the lower thigh.

RADIOLOGICAL FEATURES OF THE VEINS OF THE LOWER LIMB

Venography

Venography of the lower limb is usually performed in cases of suspected thrombosis of the deep veins and is achieved by injection of contrast medium into the veins on the dorsum of the foot. If a tourniquet is applied to the leg just proximal to the first perforating veins, contrast will pass into the deep veins and not into the superficial veins. If both superficial and deep veins are filled these are easily distinguished by their different anatomies, as already described.

The introduction of Doppler venography has almost completely replaced the need for contrast venography, which is now only performed in complex or atypical clinical circumstances.

Retrograde venography is performed by injecting contrast into the femoral vein. Retrograde flow of contrast, and especially from deep to superficial veins, only occurs if valves are defective.

Ultrasound

Flow of blood in the veins of the leg can be detected by **Doppler ultrasound**. Deep veins tend to occur in pairs. Care must be taken in the interpretation of normal flow in the deep veins because the absence of thrombus in a deep vein may be accompanied by thrombus in another vein running in parallel with the patent one.

CT and MR Venography

Indirect CT venography may be useful in assessing the lower limb veins, particularly where there is complex anatomy or an equivocal ultrasound. In addition, CT venography and MR venography are excellent for diagnosing nonvascular deep vein thrombosis mimics such as muscular injury or haematoma.

9 *The Breast*

MICHELLE McNICHOLAS

CHAPTER CONTENTS

General Anatomy 345
Lobular Structure 345
Blood Supply 345
Lymphatic Drainage 345
Axillary Lymph Nodes 346

Lymph Node Imaging 346
Radiology of the Breast 347
Radiological Significance of Breast
  Density and Parenchymal Pattern 350
Age Changes in the Breast 353

General Anatomy

The breast (Fig. 9.1) overlies the second to sixth ribs on the anterior chest wall. It is hemispherical with an axillary tail (of Spence) and consists of fat and a variable amount of glandular tissue. It is entirely invested by the fascia of the chest wall, which splits into anterior and posterior layers to envelop it. The fascia forms septa called **Cooper's ligaments**, which attach the breast to the skin anteriorly and to the fascia of pectoralis posteriorly. They also run through the breast, providing a supportive framework between the two fascial layers. The pigmented **nipple** projects from the anterior surface of the breast. It is surrounded by the pigmented **areola** and its position is variable, but it usually lies over the fourth intercostal space in the nonpendulous breast.

Lobular Structure (Fig. 9.2)

The internal architecture of the breast is arranged into 15–20 **lobes**, each of which is drained by a single major lactiferous **duct** that opens on to the nipple. Each lobe is made up of several **lobules**, each of which drains several **acini**. The lobules drain via a branching arrangement of ducts to the single lobar duct. Each lobule drains several acini – these are blind saccules into which milk is secreted during lactation. The glandular tissue of the acini and the ductal tissue draining them comprise the breast **parenchyma**. The fat surrounding the parenchymal structures and the fibrotic framework of the breast constitute the **stroma**. The relative abundance of parenchyma and stroma varies according to age, parity and other factors.

The breast may be described as having three anatomical zones – premammary, mammary and retromammary – consisting of fatty tissue, fibroglandular tissue, and fat and muscular tissue from superficial to deep.

Blood Supply (Fig. 9.3)

The blood supply to the breast is composed of the following:
- Branches of the internal mammary (thoracic) artery pierce the intercostal spaces and traverse pectoralis muscle to supply approximately 60% of the breast – mainly medial and central.
- The lateral thoracic branch of the axillary artery supplies 30%, mainly the upper outer quadrant.
- Perforating branches of the anterior intercostal arteries.

Venous drainage accompanies the arteries to the axillary and subclavian veins and the azygos system.

Lymphatic Drainage (Figs. 9.3, 9.4)

Lymphatics originate in the walls of the lactiferous ducts in the interlobular tissue of the breast. Lymph drains from the breast lobules to a rich subareolar plexus (Sappey's plexus). Lymphatic vessels are elastic in structure with valves preventing backflow, and have small nodes along their paths, including within the breast tissue. The lymph drainage of the breast in complex with approximately:
- 75% drainage to axillary nodes (mostly outer breast)
- 20% drainage to internal mammary nodes (mostly inner breast)
- 5% drainage to deep channels leading to subclavicular plexus (mostly deep tissues)

RADIOLOGY PEARLS

- Whilst the axilla receives most of its lymph from the outer breast, and the internal mammary chain receives most of its lymph from the inner breast, all parts of the breast may drain to any nodal station.
- Internal mammary nodes may receive lymph from the contralateral breast. Lymph from the inferior breast may communicate with subdiaphragmatic or subperitoneal lymph channels.
- The significance of identifying the nodal groups is that breast cancer is thought to spread in a sequential fashion, initially to the level I nodes. If the level I nodes are not involved, then it is unlikely that other 'higher level' nodes will be involved. This forms the basis for sentinel node mapping techniques (see following).
- If lymph node channels are blocked by disease, surgery or radiotherapy, lymph is more likely to flow through alternative channels to the contralateral breast, the neck, the liver and peritoneal space and the groin via the rectus sheath.

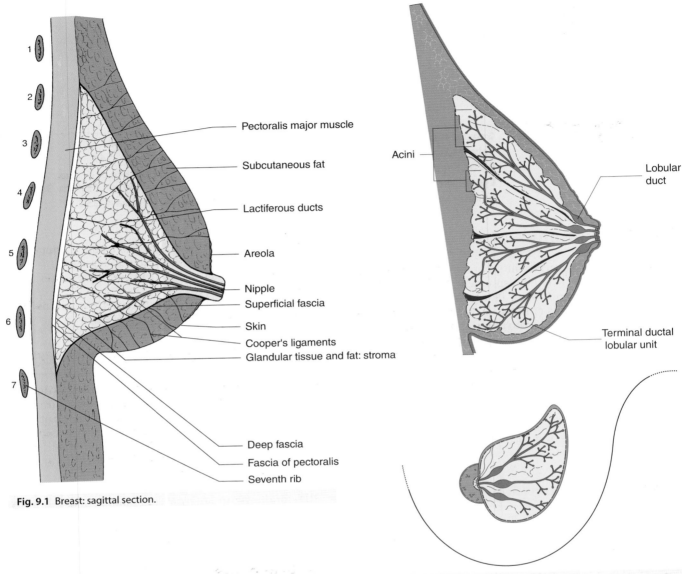

Fig. 9.1 Breast: sagittal section.

- Pectoralis major muscle
- Subcutaneous fat
- Lactiferous ducts
- Areola
- Nipple
- Superficial fascia
- Skin
- Cooper's ligaments
- Glandular tissue and fat: stroma
- Deep fascia
- Fascia of pectoralis
- Seventh rib

Acini — Lobular duct — Terminal ductal lobular unit

Fig. 9.2 Lobular structure of the breast.

Axillary Lymph Nodes

The axillary nodes are the most important to consider in detail as they are of major significance in breast cancer and may be removed surgically.

There are 20–30 axillary nodes arranged into five groups:
Anterior: deep to pectoralis major muscle at its lower border
Posterior: along the subscapular vessels at the posterior axilla
Lateral: along the axillary vein
Central: in the axillary fat
Apical: at the apex of the axilla medial to the axillary vein and above pectoralis minor.
All groups drain to the apical group.

The axillary nodes may also be divided into three levels with respect to pectolaris minor.
Level I: below pectoralis minor (includes anterior, lateral and central groups)
Level II: deep to pectoralis minor (posterior group)
Level III: above pectoralis minor (apical group)

Lymph Node Imaging

Axillary lymph nodes are best seen on MRI with its wide field of view. Axillary, intramammary and internal mammary nodes may be identified. Normal nodes enhance with contrast and have an ovoid or 'bean' shape, with a fatty hilum. They vary in length mm to several cm. On mammograms, lymph nodes are often seen in the axilla on oblique views. Intramammary nodes may be seen if outlined by fat. Ultrasound may also identify lymph nodes by their smooth ovoid appearance and fatty hilum. The axilla is assessed along with the breast tissue in breast ultrasound.

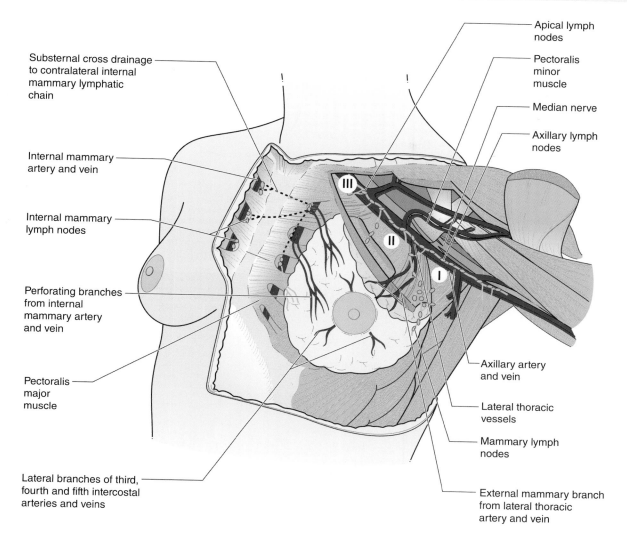

Level I lymph nodes lateral to lateral border of pectoralis minor muscle
Level II lymph nodes behind pectoralis minor muscle
Level III lymph nodes medial to medial border of pectoralis minor muscle

Fig. 9.3 Breast: anterior view demonstrating the relationship with the chest wall, blood supply and lymph drainage.

LOCALIZATION OF BREAST LESIONS USING THE CLOCK FACE (FIG. 9.5)

The breast is frequently described as a clock face with respect to the nipple, with the site of any finding localized by its position on the clock face and its distance from the nipple, for reproducibility. Thus the outer right breast in line with the nipple is the 9 o'clock position; the outer left breast at the level of the nipple is described as the 3 o'clock position. It is important to localize lesions accurately so that palpable lesions can be correlated with imaging findings.

Radiology of the Breast

Mammography (Figs. 9.6–9.8)

This dedicated radiographic technique uses a low-energy X-ray beam to maximize differences in soft-tissue density and demonstrates the internal architecture of the breast. Compression of the breast, a short exposure time and the use of high-quality digital improves the quality of the mammogram. Digital detector plates convert X-ray photons travelling through the breast to an electronic signal, which is then processed and displayed on reading monitors. Mammography monitors are of higher resolution than for all of the rest of radiology to enhance detection of the subtle findings that may indicate underlying disease.

The technique of mammography is highly important for diagnostic quality. Two views are acquired of each breast; a mediolateral oblique (MLO) view and a craniocaudal (CC) view, to ensure that all the breast tissue is imaged. Two views help differentiate abnormality from overlapping normal structures.

There are several criteria that should apply to a quality mammogram (which offers the best chance of detecting

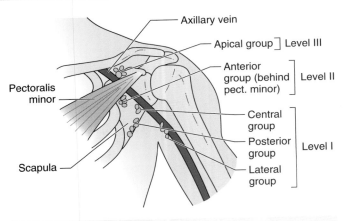

Fig. 9.4 Axillary lymph nodes groups.

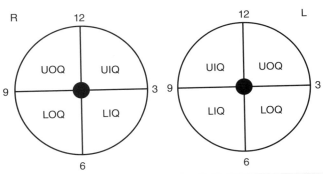

Fig. 9.5 Clockface view of breast to localize breast lesions. Any lesion detected is described by its location in the breast with reference to a clock. Note the 3 o'clock on the right breast is medial; on the left it is lateral. Lesions are then described by how far they are from the nipple, as two lesions could both be on the same 'o'clock', but will be at different distances from the nipple. Accurate localization is important to correlate palpable lesions with imaging findings.

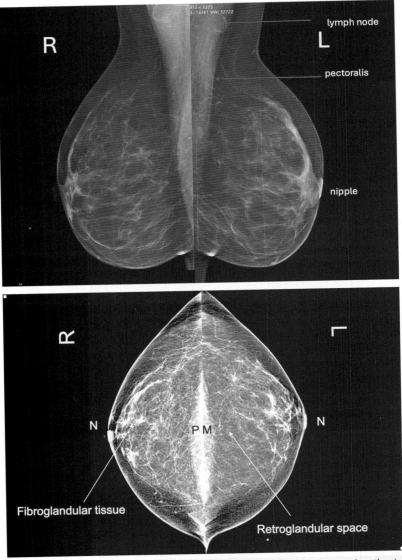

Fig. 9.6 Two-view mammogram. (A) Mediolateral Oblique (MLO) view. Moderately dense breast. By convention, the right breast is on the left and the left on the right. The side marker is at the upper part of the breast and is orientated vertically in the MLO view. (B) Craniocaudal (CC) view. By convention, the left breast is displayed to the right. The side marker is always at the outer (lateral) breast and orientated horizontally for a CC view. The glandular tissue is concentrated mainly in the retroareolar region. There is a retroglandular fatty area between the glandular tissue and the pectoralis muscle on both views. The inframammary fold between breast and the skin below should be included on the MLO view. Note the sliver of pectoralis (PM) on the CC view, which should be evident on a technically well-executed mammogram.

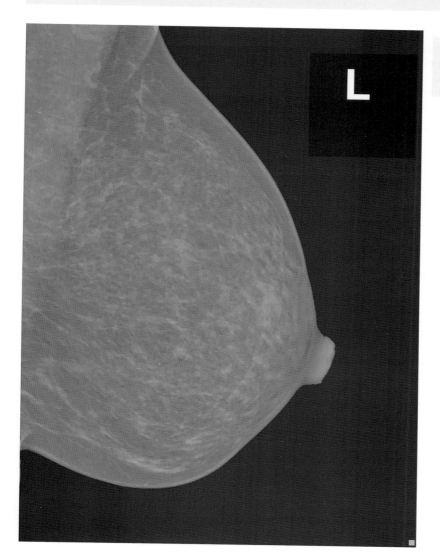

Fig. 9.7 Mediolateral oblique view of left breast with scattered areas of density from stromal and fibroglandular tissue. There is a moderate amount of fat. The entire breast has the same pattern with no concentrated glandular area or retroglandular fat.

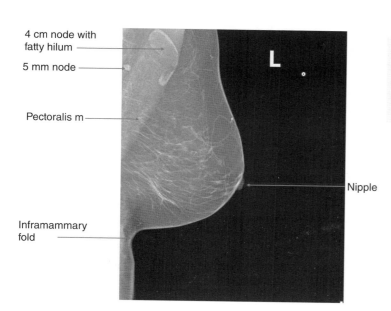

4 cm node with fatty hilum

5 mm node

Pectoralis m

Inframammary fold

Nipple

Fig. 9.8 Mediolateral oblique view of mostly fatty breast. Most of the density in this breast is due to blood vessels and fibrous septae. There is a small amount of glandular tissue. Any change or abnormality would be easy to detect in this breast. In the axilla is an elongated lymph node measuring 5 cm in length and up to 2 cm in short-axis diameter. However, it has a fatty hilum and a uniform thin cortex and is not abnormal.

subtle early signs of potential malignancy), especially in the setting of breast screening. All the glandular tissue should be included on each image; there must be no motion of the breast during the exposure; there should be no skin folds included on the image; and all the necessary annotations should be present (patient ID, side, etc.). The pectoralis muscle should be included on the images (especially MLO) to ensure all of the glandular tissue is being shown. Ideally the nipple should be in profile on both views (not always possible in certain breast shapes) and on MLO view the pectoral shadow should be seen down to the level of the nipple or below.

Mammograms are normally viewed back-to-back – right opposite left for both views – and are always compared with old mammograms, if available. Viewing the images back-to-back allows a comparison of sides in a mirror image fashion, aiding detection of abnormalities on one or other side. Hence the mammograms should be taken in a symmetric fashion and be of a similar size to match up. This may be aided by digital manipulation of the image.

Digital Tomosynthesis

Digital tomosynthesis (three-dimensional mammography) is an advance on digital mammography, which is now widely available. It generates several tomographic images which may be scrolled through, analogous to computed tomography (CT) or magnetic resonance imaging (MRI). Tomosynthesis improves the demarcation of structures and abnormalities by reducing overlap by surrounding structures.

Workflow Differences in Breast Screening and Diagnostic Mammography

Screening mammography is offered in many counties through government or regional health agencies. In screening mammography, the entire target population (e.g. 50–70-year-old women) is invited to undergo a regular (e.g. two-yearly) mammography with the aim of detecting breast cancer in its early stages. Mammograms are read electively and results are sent to the individual. If there is an abnormality, the individual is recalled for further assessment to a clinic.

Diagnostic mammography is performed in women (occasionally men) of all ages who are referred with breast symptoms.

Because mammography involves radiation (even though the dose is very small), and because of the very low risk of breast cancer in this group, diagnostic mammography is not the first line of investigation in women under 35 years. Under 35 years of age, ultrasound is the main imaging tool. Mammography is performed if there is any suspicion of cancer on ultrasound or clinical examination.

In the symptomatic service mammograms are frequently performed and immediately reviewed at clinic by the radiologist, who may request additional mammographic views to demonstrate or characterize a location. Ultrasound is normally also performed.

Radiological Significance of Breast Density and Parenchymal Pattern

There is a wide variation in the density of the breast on mammogram, determined mostly by the percentage of adipose tissue relative to glandular and stromal elements. Although the tendency is for increasing fat and diminishing glandular tissue with ageing and after menopause especially, it is possible for younger women to have quite fatty breasts and for older women to display dense breasts. Women who have very dense breasts before menopause continue to have dense breasts after menopause, although the trend is for a reduction in density. There is a range of mammographic patterns that can be seen, which observers have attempted to classify, notably Wolfe who first classified mammographic breast patterns in 1976 into four categories ranging from primarily fatty to densely fibrous. This categorization is not in use today, but it is of relevance because abnormalities are much more difficult to detect in dense or fibrous breasts. The American College of Radiology's Breast Imaging Reporting and Data System (BI-RADS) recommends that every mammography report start with a description of breast density to inform the referring clinician about how the mammographic density of the patient may affect the sensitivity of the examination.

BI-RADS classification of breast density:
- Type A: Mostly fatty (approximately 10% women)
- Type B: Scattered areas of density (approximately 40%)
- Type C: Consistently dense (approximately 40%)
- Type D: Extremely dense (approximately 10%)

Digital software may also be used to measure breast density.

Digital mammography has improved the quality of mammographic examination in women with dense breasts (who generally tend to be younger).

Contrast Mammography

Contrast-enhanced mammography (CEM) is an emerging technology in breast imaging. It is a relatively fast breast-imaging technique which combines three-dimensional tomosynthesis digital mammography with an intravenous contrast agent and can detect cancers that may not be visible on a standard mammogram. Studies have demonstrated that CEM, alone or in combination with standard mammography, is as accurate as MRI for lesion detection. Intravenous iodinated contrast materials are used in CEM to enhance the visualization of tumour neovascularity. After injection, imaging is performed with dual-energy digital mammography, which helps provide a low-energy image and a recombined or iodine image that depicts enhancing lesions in the breast. CEM capitalizes on neovascularity associated with developing malignancy.

Ultrasound (Fig. 9.9)

Ultrasound of the breast may be performed by direct contact scanning using a high-frequency linear probe.

The skin is hyperechoic (bright). The subcutaneous fat is relatively hypoechoic (dark). The breast parenchyma (glandular and fibrous tissue) is hyperechoic. Fat behind the breast parenchyma is hypoechoic and the muscle underneath is echogenic in a typical linear striated configuration. A dense linear echo may be seen from underlying ribs, and the lung may be seen moving with respiration deep to the

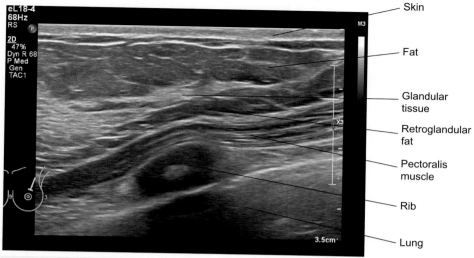

Fig. 9.9 Ultrasound of the breast. The diagram bottom left indicates that it is a sagittal oblique image of the left breast. The left side of the image is the central part of the breast just above the nipple The right side of the image is the axillary tail of the breast.

RADIOLOGY PEARLS

- Breast density is a risk factor for breast cancer as well as making cancers more difficult to detect on mammography.
- Many breast screening programmes report on breast density.
- Hormone replacement therapy increases breast density.

intercostal spaces. Neither air nor bone can transmit ultrasound waves, so all the sound signal is reflected by the lung or the ribs, and nothing can be detected deep to these structures. Linear reflections of Cooper's ligaments may be seen traversing the fat. In young women with glandular breasts the parenchyma is of homogeneously high echogenicity. With increasing age, the pattern is less homogeneous, with increasing deposits of fat showing as hypoechoic lobules separated by echogenic fibrous strands. The lactiferous ducts may be seen as small tubular anechoic structures radiating from the nipple. Deep to the breast parenchyma, an anechoic area of retromammary fat is seen anterior to the echogenic pectoralis muscle.

Technology in Breast Ultrasound

Radiology probes used for breast imaging are typically 7.5–23 MHz. Digital manipulation of the image such as harmonic imaging may improve the image.

MRI (Fig. 9.10)

This technique is performed with the subject prone and the breasts suspended in a dedicated breast coil. Images acquired include T1 and T2 imaging, and T1 imaging acquired dynamically during intravenous contrast (gadolinium). T1 images may be acquired with or without fat suppression. Diffusion-weighted imaging may also be used to improve tissue characterization. Acquisition of all of these sequences which include anatomic, contrast and diffusion imaging is known as multiparametric MRI. In contrast to

mammography and ultrasound, multiparametric MRI is a functional imaging technique. Contrast MRI evaluates the permeability of blood vessels – this is increased in cancer due to tumour angiogenesis. T1 contrast MRI is the most essential of all sequences in the diagnosis of cancer. Diffusion-weighted imaging quantifies the random movement of water molecules in tissue. Cancer shows decreased (restricted) water diffusion because of its increased cell density.

The breast composition is variable from person to person. MRI can assess the amount of fibroglandular tissue that exists relative to fat. The composition may be described as:

a. Almost entirely fatty
b. Scattered fibroglandular tissue
c. Heterogeneous fibroglandular tissue
d. Extreme fibroglandular tissue

The normal background breast parenchyma enhances after contrast injection. The amount of background parenchyma in enhancement may be described as minimal, mild, moderate or marked. The more the background parenchymal enhancement, the harder it is to detect cancer, which also enhances.

Technology in Breast MRI

Breast MRI should be performed on MRI machines that are at least 1.5 Tesla in strength, with resolution improved at 3 Tesla imaging. A breast coil should have at least eight channels. Modern MRI machines have 16 or more channels, resulting in better quality images with improved signal-to-noise ratio, and allowing faster acquisition of images. Although the section thickness of T1 images is 2.5 mm, the in-plane pixel size of the resultant images is 1 mm or lower in modern units (isotropic), allowing reconstruction of images in any plane with no loss of resolution.

Abbreviated MRI protocols have been described that are aimed at lesion detection, which might allow broader access to MRI at a lower cost; the basis of this is a pre- and postcontrast T1-weighted acquisition. Lesions so detected

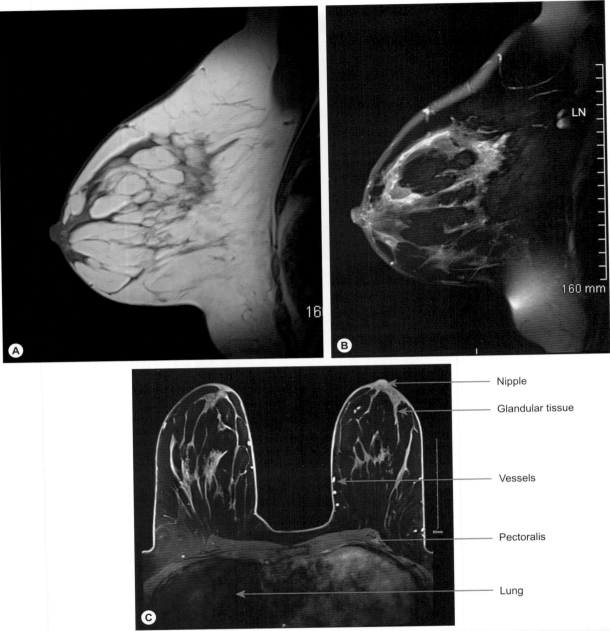

Fig. 9.10 Magnetic resonance image of the breast. (A) Sagittal T1 image without fat saturation. Fat is hyperintense (bright) on T1 and T2 images unless it has been nullified using special fat-saturation sequences. Fibroglandular and stromal elements are hypointense (dark) on T1 images. (B) Sagittal T2-weighted image with fat saturation. Fat is hypointense because it has been saturated out. Glandular elements are relatively hyperintense. Lymph nodes in the axilla are hyperintense. (C) Axial view of both breasts. A T1 image with fat saturation after intravenous contrast. There is mild enhancement of skin and glandular elements. Fat is hypointense as it has been saturated.

could then undergo more extensive protocols to characterize them. Abbreviated MRI offers the potential to be offered more widely as a screening test. MRI is already offered as a screening test in some young women with a strong genetic predisposition to developing breast cancer.

Sentinel Node Mapping (Fig. 9.11)

The sentinel node is the first node to receive lymph drainage directly from a tumour. If the sentinel node is negative, axillary dissection is not required, minimizing morbidity associated with this procedure. Sentinel node mapping is now standard surgical practice in breast and other cancers.

This technique is performed by injecting a technetium colloid into the region of abnormality of the breast or into the periareolar dermal tissue. Imaging after 2 hours demonstrates the 'sentinel node or nodes' – that is, the first 'port of call' for the lymphatic drainage. The nodes can also be identified intraoperatively by a gamma ray detection probe, which can detect the higher concentration of radioactivity. If this node is normal, the likelihood is that the disease process has not spread from the breast.

'Blue dye mapping' involves injection of methylene blue dye into the tumour at the time of surgery and identification of the first 'blue node' visually after approximately centrally if dilated. When fat predominates the ducts may be seen. When fibrotic and glandular tissue predominate, the ducts are difficult to see. Blood vessels may be distinguished from ducts as they run more haphazardly through the breast and have a more uniform calibre, whereas ducts increase in calibre as they converge onto the nipple.

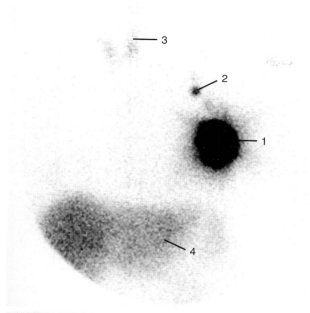

Fig. 9.11 Lymphoscintigram of breast. Technetium sulphur colloid has been injected around a tumour in the left breast. Uptake is seen in the first draining node in the axilla. Uptake is also seen in the thyroid gland and liver.

1. Radioisotope in the tumour
2. Uptake in the sentinel node
3. Uptake in the thyroid gland
4. Uptake in the liver

10 minutes. Blue-coloured lymphatic channels can be identified and followed to the blue-stained sentinel node.

Mammographic Patterns

Depending on the parenchymal pattern, that is, the relative composition of ductal, fatty and fibrotic or glandular tissue, the following may be seen on the mammogram. The ducts radiate out from the nipple and may be seen

---

> **RADIOLOGY PEARLS**
>
> • Since almost all the lymph drainage in the breast passes centrifugally to the periareolar plexus before draining to the sentinel nodes, injection of isotope may be performed into the peri-areolar region. It is important to administer the injection intradermally in order to achieve high pressure and aid efficient passage into the lymphatic system.
> • Tumours located anywhere in the breast may drain to the internal mammary chain, but *isolated* drainage to the internal mammary chain is unusual and occurs in less than 2% of large published series.
> • Methylene blue dye is not injected intradermally as it may lead to a permanent tattoo of the skin.

Age Changes in the Breast

During adolescence the growing breast becomes increasingly glandular. During pregnancy and breastfeeding the number of acini increases, with glandular tissue predominating. When lactation stops, the glandular tissue involutes so that the breast is even less glandular than it was prior to pregnancy. Thus the breast of a parous woman is less glandular than that of a nulliparous woman of the same age. Apart from the situation during pregnancy and lactation, parenchymal atrophy starts in early adulthood and is accelerated at the menopause, with diminishing amounts of glandular tissue and an increasing amount of fat.

Index

Page numbers followed by *f* indicate figures; *t*, tables, *b*, boxes.

A

abdomen, 184–244
  cross-sectional anatomy of, 239–244
  lymphatic drainage of, 232–233, 233*t*, 234*f*
  plain films of, 185, 185*f*
abdominal aorta, 258*f*
abdominal wall
  anterior, 184–185, 242*f*
    computed tomography of, 185, 186*f*, 187*f*, 188*f*
    fascial layers of, 184
    muscle layers of, 184
    properitoneal fat, 184
    radiological features of, 185
    umbilical ligaments of, 185
  musculature, 185*f*, 277*f*
  posterior, veins of, 232–235, 232*f*
abducent (VI) nerve, 71*f*, 76, 77*f*
abductor hallucis muscle, 333*f*–334*f*
abductor pollicis longus muscle, 308*f*, 309*f*
abscess, formation of, 198*b*
absent ribs, 125–126
accessory arteries, 225
accessory duct (of Santorini), 212, 213*f*
accessory fissure, 144–145
accessory hemiazygos vein, 174, 175*f*
accessory meningeal artery, 52
accessory (XI) nerve, 71*f*
accessory ossicle, 319
acetabular labrum, 319*f*, 321–322
acetabular margin, 246*f*, 252*f*
acetabular notch, 246*f*
acetabulum, 246*f*, 247*f*, 250*f*, 255*f*, 265*f*, 266*f*, 282*f*, 319*f*, 320*f*
  labrum of, 320*f*
  posterior wall of, 321–322
  root of, 321–322
Achilles tendon, 333*f*–334*f*, 335, 336*f*
acini (breast), 345, 346*f*
acoustic nerve, 23
acromial artery, 55*f*
acromioclavicular joint, 285*f*, 290, 292*f*–293*f*
acromioclavicular ligament, 292*f*–293*f*
acromion, 284, 285*f*, 292*f*–293*f*, 294*f*
acromion process, 285*f*, 292*f*–293*f*
acromiothoracic trunk, 310*f*
adductor attachments, normal, 324*f*
adductor brevis muscle, 253*f*, 269*f*, 321–322, 321*f*–323*f*, 339*f*
adductor canal, superficial femoral vessels in, 337*f*
adductor gracilis muscle, 339*f*
adductor hiatus, 340*f*

adductor longus muscle, 253*f*, 269*f*, 313*f*, 321–322, 321*f*–323*f*, 339*f*
  conjoined insertion of, 321*f*–323*f*
adductor magnus muscle, 265*f*, 321*f*–323*f*, 337*f*, 339*f*
adductor minimus, 253*f*, 269*f*
adductor tubercle, 326*f*
adenoids, 28, 29*f*
aditus ad antrum, 22, 25*f*
adnexal vessels, 277*f*
adrenal artery
  inferior, 230, 230*f*
  middle, 230, 230*f*
  superior, 230*f*
adrenal gland, 187*f*, 192*f*, 223*f*, 225*b*, 229–230, 240*f*
  arterial supply of, 229
  axial section of, level of porta hepatis, 240
  radiological features of, 230
  variants of, 229
  venous drainage of, 229–230
afferent arterioles, 223
air-filled trachea, 178*f*
airways, 140, 140*b*
ala, of sacrum, 102, 105*f*, 245
alar ligament, 110
ALPSA lesion, 294*b*
alveolar border, 14
alveolar process, 11*f*, 12
alveus, 75*f*
ambient cisterns, 61*f*, 77*f*, 85
ampulla, 26*f*
  of fallopian tube, 272*f*, 280, 281*f*
  of rectum, 254*f*
  of vas deferens, 262*f*
  of Vater, 210, 212
amygdala, 68, 75*f*
anal canal, 251*f*, 254*f*, 255–257, 255*f*, 263*f*, 279*f*
  blood supply, 256–257
  lymph drainage, 257
  mucosa of, 256*f*
  radiology of, 255–256, 256*b*
  submucosa of, 256*f*
anal columns, 256*f*
anal sphincter, subepithelial tissue of, 256*f*
anal triangle, 248–250
anastomotic artery, 119*f*
anastomotic vein
  inferior (of Labbé), 97, 98*f*, 100*f*
  superior (of Trolard), 97, 98*f*, 100*f*
anatomical asplenia, 218
anconeus, 297*f*–298*f*
angiography
  of abdominal aorta, 231
  of cerebral vein, 99–100, 100*f*
  coronary catheter, 166, 168*f*
  of large intestine, 201

angiography (*Continued*)
  of pancreas, 218
  of small intestine, 195*f*, 196
  spinal, 121–122, 122*f*
  subclavian vessels, 56
  upper limb, 310
  of vertebral system, 93–94
angular artery, 91, 94*f*
angular vein, 19
ankle joint, 331, 331*f*
  articular surfaces, 331
  biomechanics, 331–332
  capsule, 331
  ligaments, 331
  magnetic resonance imaging of, 332–336, 333*f*–334*f*
  radiological features, 332, 333*f*–334*f*, 336*f*
  synovium, 331
  type, 331
ankle ligaments, 332–336
annular ligament, 297*f*–298*f*
annular pancreas, 214
annulus fibrosus, 113–114
annulus of Zinn, 18
anococcygeal body, 248
anomalous lumbosacral anatomy, 246–248
anorectal hiatus, 252*f*
anterior adductor aponeurosis, 324*f*
anterior band of disc, 15*f*
anterior capsular attachment, 294
anterior cardiac veins, 161*f*
anterior cerebral artery, 91, 93*f*
  A1 segment, 94*f*
  right, 72*f*
anterior cerebral vein, 99*f*
anterior cervical space, 45
anterior cervix, 277*f*, 279*f*
anterior chamber, 18*f*, 19*f*
anterior choroidal artery, 90–91, 93*f*, 94*f*
anterior commissure, 35*f*, 36*f*, 37*f*, 38, 62, 62*f*, 63*f*, 64*f*, 74*f*, 75*f*
anterior communicating artery, 91, 93*f*
  anteromedial central branches of, 93*f*
anterior cruciate ligament, 325, 325*f*, 327*f*–329*f*, 329–330, 330*b*
anterior cusp, of aortic valve, 168*f*
anterior fibromuscular stroma, of prostate gland, 265*f*
anterior fontanelle, 3*f*
anterior glenoid labrum, 292*f*–293*f*
anterior gluteal line, 246*f*
anterior inferior cerebellar artery (AICA), 23, 92, 93*f*, 95*f*
anterior inferior iliac spine, 246*f*, 247*f*, 252*f*
anterior interosseous nerve, 309*f*
anterior interosseous vessels, 309*f*

anterior jugular vein, 36*f*
anterior junction line, 178
anterior labrum, 321–322
anterior median sulcus, 121*f*
anterior myometrium, 277*f*
anterior pararenal space, 224, 224*f*
anterior perforated substance, 71*f*
anterior pontomesencephalic vein, 98, 99*f*
anterior rectus abdominis, 324*f*
anterior sacral foramina, 252*f*
anterior sacrococcygeal ligament, 252*f*
anterior spina bifida, 108
anterior spinal artery, 92
anterior superior iliac spine, 245, 246*f*,
    247*f*, 249*f*
anterior talofibular ligament, 331–332,
    331*f*, 333*f*–334*f*
anterior temporal artery, 91, 96*f*–97*f*
anterior tibial artery, 337*f*, 339*f*, 340*f*,
    341, 342*f*
anterior tibial compartment, muscles of,
    337*f*
anterior tibial nerve, 337*f*
anterior tibial veins, 337*f*, 343*f*
anterior tibiofibular ligament, 333*f*–334*f*
anterior urogenital triangle, 248
anterolateral central artery, 93*f*
anterolateral impingement syndrome, 335
anteromedial central artery, 93*f*
antimesenteric border, 194
antrum, 188*f*
anus, 251*f*, 269*f*
aorta, 119*f*, 130*f*, 134*f*, 155*f*, 187*f*, 188*f*,
    189*f*, 190*f*, 195*f*, 200*f*, 216*f*, 223*f*,
    239*f*, 240*f*, 241*f*, 242*f*, 243*f*
   abdominal, 192*f*, 230–231
      branches of, 230–231
      radiological features of, 231
   ascending, 167, 168*f*, 175*f*, 181*f*, 182*f*
   axial section of, level of pancreatic head
      and renal hila, 243
   descending, 157*f*, 168*f*, 169, 169*f*,
      181*f*, 182*f*, 183*f*, 191*f*
   radiograph, 178
   thoracic, 167–169, 168*f*, 169*f*
aortic arch, 44–45, 52*f*, 138*f*, 147*f*, 153*f*,
    167–169, 169*b*, 178*f*, 181*f*
   branches, 168–169
aortic isthmus, 169
aortic knuckle, 132*f*
aortic valve, 165*f*
aortocaval nodes, 233
aortograms, 52*f*
aortopulmonary mediastinal stripe, 179
aortopulmonary node, 173
aortopulmonary window, 132*f*
apical ligament, 110
apical lymph nodes, 347*f*
appendiceal orifice, 197*f*
appendices epiploicae, 198–199
appendicitis, acute, 197*b*
appendicular artery, 197*b*
appendix, 194*f*, 197–198, 197*f*, 198*f*
   artery to, 194*f*
   radiological features of, 197–198
   variation in position of, 197*f*
aqueduct of Sylvius, 61*f*, 63*f*, 77*f*, 80*f*, 82*f*
aqueous humour, 20

arachnodactyly, 290
arachnoid granulations
   calcification, 7
   pits, 9
arachnoid mater, 87–88, 117*f*, 118
arch of aorta, 153*f*, 180*f*
arcuate arteries, 223, 225*b*
arcuate eminence, 22
arcuate ligament, 130*f*
arcuate line, 245, 246*f*, 252*f*
   of Douglas, 184
areae gastricae, 186, 191*f*
areola, 346*f*
arteria radicularis magna, 118, 119*f*
arteriography
   of adrenal gland, 230
   of kidneys, 226
   of lower limb, 341–342, 341*f*, 342*f*,
     343*f*
artery of Adamkiewicz, 118
arthrography
   of ankle joint, 332, 332*b*
   of elbow joint, 297
   of hip joint, 320
   of knee joint, 326
   of wrist joint, 302
articular cartilage, 297*f*–298*f*
   of hip joint, 319*f*
   of knee, 327*f*–329*f*
articular facets, 101, 102*f*, 103*f*, 104*f*,
    105*f*, 106*f*, 111*f*–112*f*, 124*f*
articular processes, 101, 104*f*, 105*f*, 108*f*,
    120*f*
articular surfaces
   ankle joint, 331
   hip joint, 319
   knee joints, 325
articular tubercle, 15, 15*f*, 124*f*
aryepiglottic folds, 29*f*, 33*f*, 34, 35*f*, 37*f*,
    39*f*
arytenoid cartilages, 29*f*, 33, 35*f*, 37*f*
   vocal process of, 36*f*
ascending colon, 188*f*, 194*f*, 198*f*, 200*f*,
    224*f*, 239*f*, 243*f*
   attachment of, 194*f*
ascites, 239*f*
asterion, 1, 3*f*
atlantoaxial distance, 110
atlantoaxial joint, 104*f*, 110
atlanto-occipital joint, 109–110
atlas, 101, 103*f*, 104*f*, 108
   anterior arch of, 104*f*, 106*f*
   dens of, 5*f*, 103*f*, 104*f*, 106*f*, 110*f*
   ossification for, 110*f*
   posterior arch of, 106*f*
atrial appendage, 132*f*, 182*f*
   left, 165*f*
   right, 161*f*
atrioventricular groove, 157*f*
atrium
   left, 134*f*, 157*f*, 158, 165*f*
   right, 153*f*, 156–158, 157*f*, 158*b*
attic, 22
atypical ribs, 124–125
auditory artery, internal, 5
auditory canal
   external, 15*f*, 22
   internal, 5

auditory cortex, 59
auditory meatus
   external, 2*f*, 4*f*, 15*f*, 22, 25*f*, 31*f*, 54*f*
   internal, 5, 6*f*, 7*f*, 8*t*, 23, 25*f*
auricle, 153*f*
auricular artery, posterior, 51*f*, 52, 52*f*, 53*f*
auricular surface, 105*f*
auricular vein, posterior, 54, 54*f*
axilla, fat in, 180*f*
axillary artery, 310*f*, 345, 347*f*
axillary lymph nodes, 345, 347*f*
axillary nerve, 56
axillary pouch, 291*f*, 292*f*–293*f*
axillary veins, 310, 347*f*
axis, 101, 104*f*, 108
   body of, 102*f*, 104*f*, 106*f*
azygo-oesophageal line, 136*f*, 178–179,
    178*f*
azygo-oesophageal recess, 178–179, 181*f*,
    182*f*
azygo-oesophageal stripe, 178*f*
azygos fissure, 144, 144*f*
azygos lobe, 144*f*
azygos node, 173
azygos system, 174–175, 175*f*, 176*f*
azygos vein, 56*f*, 132*f*, 144*f*, 147*f*, 157*f*,
    169*f*, 174, 175*f*, 178*f*, 180*f*, 181*f*,
    182*f*, 191*f*, 232*f*
   arch of, 153*f*, 181*f*

B

Baker's cyst, 326
barium enema examination
   of appendix, 197
   of ileocaecal valve, 197
barium follow-through, 195
barium studies
   of duodenum, 191*f*, 192–193, 193*f*
   of small intestine, 193*f*, 195
barium-meal examination, double-
    contrast, 188, 191*f*
Bartholin's glands, 281
basal ganglia, 66–69, 69*f*, 70*b*
   calcification, 7
   radiological features, 67–69
basal vein (of Rosenthal), 98, 99*f*, 100*f*
basilar artery, 61*f*, 77*f*, 92, 93*f*, 95*f*,
    96*f*–97*f*
   with flow artefact, 26*f*
basilic vein, 308*f*, 309*f*, 310, 311*f*
basivertebral vein, 109*f*, 111*f*–112*f*
biceps brachii muscle, 309*f*
biceps femoris muscle, 327*f*–329*f*, 337*f*,
    339*f*
   belly of, 327*f*–329*f*
   long head of, 339*f*
   short head of, 339*f*
biceps femoris tendon, 327*f*–329*f*
biceps muscle, 299, 299*b*, 308*f*
   belly, 297*f*–298*f*
   long head of, 292*f*–293*f*
biceps sheath, 291*f*
biceps tendons, 292*f*–293*f*, 295*f*,
    297*f*–298*f*, 299, 299*b*
bicipital groove, 286*f*
bicipitolabral complex, 294

bifid rib, 125, 126f
bile duct, 202f, 210–211, 210f, 213f
    common, 207f, 209f, 210, 211b, 213f,
        217f
    extrahepatic, 211b
    intrahepatic, 211b
    variation of, 209f
biliary duct, 213b
    variation in, 210–211
biliary system, 208–212
    radiological features of, 211–212
        contrast and cross-sectional
            examinations, 211–212
        CT of biliary tree, 212
        MR cholangiography/
            cholangiopancreatography, 212,
            213f
        plain films, 211
        scintigraphy, 212
        ultrasound, 211
    relations of, 209f
biliary tree, computed tomography of, 212
bipartite patella, 314
bladder, 195f, 250f, 255f, 262b, 263f,
    265f, 266f, 267f, 276f, 277f, 279f,
    282f, 321–322, 321f–323f
    apex of, 261, 262f
    base of, 262f
    inferolateral surface of, 262f
    neck of, 261, 262f
    radiology of, 262–263
        contrast studies, 262–263
        cross-sectional imaging, 263
        plain films, 262, 262b
    superior surface of, 262f
bleeding, diagnosis and characterization
    of, 206b
blood vessels, of pelvis, 258–261
Blumensaat's line, 327f–329f
body wall, axial section of
    below kidneys, 243
    level of pancreatic body, 241
    level of pancreatic head and renal hila,
        241
    level of porta hepatis, 240
    level of upper liver and spleen, 239
Boehler's critical angle, of calcaneus, 316,
    318f
bone age, 289
bones, of lower limb, 312–318
    femur, 312, 312b, 313f, 314f
    fibula, 315, 315f
    foot, 315–316, 316b, 316f, 317f, 318f
    patella, 314
    tibia, 314–315, 315f
bony labyrinth, 22
bony pelvis, 245–248, 246f, 247f, 249f
    coccyx, 245
    pelvic inlet, 245–246
    pelvic ring, radiology of, 246–248
    sacroiliac joints, 245–246
    sacrum, 245
brachial artery, 308–310, 308f, 309f
brachial median nerve, 297f–298f
brachial plexus, 56, 57f, 124f
    radiology of, 56, 56b
    roots of, 57f
brachial vein, 297f–298f

brachial vessels, 309f
brachialis muscle, 297f–298f, 308f, 309f
brachialis tendon, 297f–298f
brachiocephalic artery, 51f, 55f, 138f,
    168f
brachiocephalic trunk, 52f
brachiocephalic vein, 54, 54f, 55f, 56,
    138f, 153f, 175f, 179f, 180f
    left, 175f
    right, 175f
    tributaries of, 170
brachiocephalic vessels, 132f
brachioradialis muscle, 297f–298f, 308f,
    309f
brain
    globe of, 61f
    venous drainage of, 95–100, 98f, 99f,
        100f
brainstem, 68f, 71f, 74–78
    medulla oblongata, 76–78, 78b
    midbrain, 74–76
    pons, 76
branching ductules, normal, 47f
breasts, 345–353
    age changes in, 353
    blood supply of, 345, 347f
    fat in, 351f
    general anatomy of, 345, 346f, 347f
    lobular structure of, 345, 346f
    localization of breast lesions, clock face
        for, 347, 348f
    lymphatic drainage, 345, 345b, 347f
    mammographic patterns of, 353
    radiological significance of density and
        parenchymal pattern, 350–353,
        351b
    radiology of, 347–350
        contrast mammography, 350
        digital mammography, 350
        magnetic resonance imaging, 346,
            351, 352f
        mammography, 347–350, 348f, 349f
        sentinel node mapping, 352–353,
            353b, 353f
        ultrasound, 346, 350–351, 351f
    skin of, 346f, 351f
bregma, 1, 2f, 4f
broad ligament, 273–275, 274f, 275f
    anterior layer of, 274f
    free edge of, 274f
    posterior layer of, 274f
Broca's speech area, 58, 59f
Brodel's line, 226
bronchi, 132f, 138f, 181f, 182f
    blood supply, 142–143
    left main, 141, 141b
        lower lobe, 139f, 182f
        upper lobe, 139f
    radiological features, 143, 148–151,
        149b, 151b, 151f
    relations of, 140–141
    right main, 140–141
        lower lobe, 139f
        middle lobe, 139f
        upper lobe, 139f
    variant anatomy, 141–142, 142b, 142f
bronchial angiography, 121b
bronchial arteries, 147–148

bronchial tree, 139f, 148–152
bronchial veins, 143, 143b
bronchopulmonary nodes, 147f
bronchopulmonary segment, 145, 145b,
    149, 149b
bronchus intermedius, 148f
buccal space, 44
buccinator muscle, 28f, 46f
buccopharyngeal fascia, 26, 27b, 46f
Buck's fascia, 271
Buford complex, 294, 295f
Bugs Bunny sign, 297
bulbocavernosus muscle, 248
bulbospongiosus muscle, 266f, 269f
bulbous urethra, 263f, 264

C

C1/C2 articulation, 111
caecal pole, 198f
caecum, 194f, 198f, 282f
calcaneocuboid articulation, 333f–334f
calcaneofibular ligament, 331, 331f, 333
calcaneus, 316, 316b, 317f, 333f–334f,
    336f
calcar avis, 81
calcarine artery, 93, 95f, 96f–97f
calcarine sulcus, 60, 68f
callosomarginal artery, 91, 94f
calvarium, 1
calyces, 222, 222f, 227f
Cantlie's line, 203
capitate, 288f, 301f–302f, 303f
capitellum, pseudodefect of, 300
capitulum, 286f, 287f
capsular arteries, 90
cardia, 185, 188f
cardiac chambers, orientation of, 154f
cardiac contour, 164
cardiac orifice, 189f
cardiac valves, 156
cardiac vein, 161f, 162
carina, 138, 140, 140b, 181f
carinal nodes, 147f, 173
carotid arteries
    common, 50, 50f, 51f, 53f, 55f
        anatomical relations in the carotid
            sheath, 50
        left, 52f, 55f
        right, 52f
    external, 46f, 50, 53f
        anatomical relations in the carotid
            sheath, 50–51
        branches, 51–53, 51f, 52f, 53f
        right, 52f
    internal, 46f, 50, 51f, 53f
        anatomical relations in the carotid
            sheath, 50
        calcification, 7
    medial deviation of, 45f
    in neck, 50–53, 50f, 51f, 52f, 53f, 54f,
        55f, 56f
    radiology of, 53–54
        angiography, 53–54
        computed tomography and magnetic
            resonance imaging, 54
        ultrasound, 53

carotid artery, 72*f*, 138*f*, 153*f*, 179*f*, 180*f*
carotid canal, 6*f*, 24*f*
carotid foramen, 32*f*
carotid sheath, 48, 48*f*, 109*f*
carotid siphon, 94*f*
carotid space, 44–45, 44*f*, 45*b*
carotid sulcus, 6*f*, 7*f*
carpal angle, 289
carpal bones, 288, 288*f*
    ossification of, 289
    radiological features of, 288–289
    supernumerary, 289
carpal tunnel, 305*f*, 306
carpometacarpal joints, 300
    common, 301*f*–302*f*
    first, 301*f*–302*f*
cartilaginous endplates, 113
catheter, 146*f*
cauda equina, 121*f*
    nerve roots, 111*f*–112*f*
    nerves of, 120*f*
caudate nucleus, 67
    body of, 69*f*
    head of, 64*f*, 65*f*, 66–69, 69*f*
    tail of, 69*b*, 69*f*, 75*f*
caudate process, of caudate lobe, 203, 240*f*
cavernosal arteries, paired, 271
cavernous sinus, 19, 61*f*, 71–72, 72*f*, 96–97, 98*f*, 100*f*
cavography, 231–232
cavum septum pellucidum, 68*f*, 85*f*
cavum velum interpositum, 81, 82*f*, 83*f*, 86
central canal, of spinal cord, 81*f*, 115*f*, 116
central echo complex, 121*f*
central lobule, 79*f*
central nervous system, arterial supply of, 89*f*, 90–95, 93*f*, 94*f*, 95*f*, 96*f*–97*f*
    radiological features, 93–95
central retinal artery, 18*f*, 19
central sulcus (of Rolando), 58, 59*f*, 61*f*
central tegmental tract, 77*f*
central tendon, 131
central zone, of prostate gland, 265*f*, 266*f*, 267
cephalic vein, 308*f*, 309*f*, 310, 311*f*
cerebellar hemisphere, right, 61*f*
cerebellar tonsil, right, 77*f*
cerebellopontine angle cistern, 26*f*
cerebellum, 78–80, 79*f*, 80*f*
    function of, 79, 80*b*
    nodule, 79*f*
    radiological features, 79–80
    subdivision of, 79
    tonsil of, 63*f*
    vermis of, 61*f*, 63*f*, 68*f*, 78
cerebral aqueduct, 82–83, 83*f*
cerebral cortex, 58–60, 59*f*
    computed tomography of, 60
    insula (of Reil), 60
    magnetic resonance imaging of, 60, 61*f*
    radiological features, 60
    ultrasound, 60
cerebral hemispheres, 58
cerebral peduncles, 75

cerebral vein, radiological features, 98–100
cerebrospinal fluid, production and flow, 80–87
    radiological features, 87
cerebrospinal tract, 115*f*
cervical artery, 119*f*
cervical canal, 272–273, 279*f*, 281*f*
cervical cord, 85*f*
cervical glands, 280
cervical ribs, 125, 125*f*
cervical spine
    magnetic resonance imaging of, 109*f*
    myelographic appearance of, 119
    ossification of, 110*f*
    radiograph of, 106*f*, 107
cervical subarachnoid space, 83*f*
cervical vertebrae, 85*f*, 101–102, 102*f*
    ossification of, 108–109
    seventh, 108
    typical, 101
cervix, 272–273, 272*f*, 274*f*, 276*f*, 277*f*
Chamberlain's line, 107
chest radiography
    of inferior vena cava, 231–232
    of lungs, 148–149
    of mediastinum, 177–179
    of thymus, 173
chest wall, muscles of, 240*f*
Chilaiditi's syndrome, 201*b*
chondroglossus, 24
chordae tendineae, 158
choroid, 18*f*, 20
choroid plexus, 7, 81
    in atrium, 68*f*
    of lateral ventricle, 81–82
choroidal vein, 98, 99*f*
ciliary body, 18*f*, 20
ciliary muscle, 20
cingulate gyrus, 59*f*, 60, 68*f*, 74, 74*f*
circle of Willis, 93, 96*f*–97*f*
    commonest variants of, 93
circumflex coronary artery, 159, 161*f*, 164*f*
    left, 161
circumflex femoral arteries, 340*f*
circumflex humeral arteries
    lateral, 310*f*
    medial, 310*f*
cisterna chyli, 233
cisterna magna, 63*f*, 80*f*, 82*f*, 83*f*, 84, 85*f*
claustrum, 61*f*, 64*f*, 67, 69*f*
clavicle, 55*f*, 124*f*, 132*f*, 284, 285*f*, 286*f*, 292*f*–293*f*, 294*f*
    acromial end, 286*f*
    lateral end of, 285*f*
    medial end of, 106*f*
    ossification, 286, 286*b*
    radiological features of, 284–286
    sternal end, 286*f*
clinoid process
    anterior, 4*f*, 6*f*, 7*f*
    posterior, 4*f*, 6*f*, 7*f*
clivus, 3, 4*f*, 6*f*, 7*f*, 63*f*
coccygeus, 248, 252*f*, 255*f*, 263*f*
coccyx, 102, 245, 247*f*, 254*f*, 255*f*, 266*f*, 279*f*, 282*f*, 321–322
    tip of, 251*f*

cochlea, 22, 24*f*, 26*f*
cochlear aqueduct, 22
cochlear duct, 25*f*, 26*f*
cochlear implant, 23*b*
cochlear nerve, 23
cochlear turns, 25*f*
coealic axis, 240*f*, 241*f*
    angiogram of, 189*f*
coeliac artery, 189*f*, 190*f*, 216*f*, 230*f*
coeliac nodes, 233
coeliac trunk, 187, 189*f*
colic artery
    left, 200*f*
    middle, 194*f*, 195*f*
    right, 194*f*, 195*f*
colic vein
    left, 220*f*
    middle, 220*f*
    right, 220*f*
collateral air drift, 145
collateral arteries, 343
collateral ligaments
    injury, 307
    lateral, 298, 332, 332*b*
    medial, 327*f*–329*f*, 333
    radial, 299*b*
collateral sulcus, 75*f*
Colles' fascia, 184
colliculi of tectum, of midbrain, 79*f*
colon. *See also* large intestine; small intestine
    axial section of, below kidneys, 243
column of Bertin, 222, 228
columns of Morgagni, 250–254
comminuted fractures, 314*b*
commissural fibres, 62
    radiological features, 64–66
common carotid artery, 36*f*
    left, 37*f*
    right, 37*f*
common extensor tendon insertion, 297*f*–298*f*
common femoral artery, 266*f*, 340, 340*f*, 341*f*
common femoral vein, 266*f*
common flexor tendon insertion, 297*f*–298*f*
common iliac artery, 257*f*
    left, 258*f*
    right, 258*f*
communicating artery
    anterior, 91, 93*f*
        anteromedial central branches of, 93*f*
    posterior, 90, 93*f*
communicating veins, 343*f*, 344
compartment syndrome, 340*b*
computed tomography (CT)
    of ankle joint, 332
    of anterior abdominal wall, 185, 186*f*, 187*f*, 188*f*
    of basal ganglia, 67–69
    of biliary tree, 212
    of cerebellum, 79–80, 80*b*
    of cerebral cortex, 60
    of cerebral vein, 100
    of corpus callosum, 65–66, 65*b*
    of diaphragm, 135, 135*b*

computed tomography (CT) *(Continued)*
  of heart, 164–166, 164*f*, 165*b*, 165*f*
  of hip joint, 320–321
  of intracranial arteries, 94–95
  of kidney, 185*f*, 187*f*, 226
  of large intestine, 201
  of liver, 187*f*, 188*f*, 191*f*, 192*f*, 205–
    206, 206*f*
  of lungs, 151–152, 151*b*
  of pancreas, 187*f*, 215–216, 217*f*
  of sigmoid and rectum, 257
  of small intestine, 196
  of spinal cord, 108*f*, 120
  of spleen, 187*f*, 191*f*, 192*f*, 219, 219*f*,
    223*f*
  of stomach, 188, 191*f*, 192*f*
  of ventricular system, 83–84
  of vertebrae, 107, 108*f*
computed tomography (CT) angiography
  of iliac vessels, 260
  of lower limb, 342
Computed tomography (CT)
    cisternography cervical
    myelography, 86
computed tomography (CT) colonography
  of large intestine, 201
  of sigmoid and rectum, 257
computed tomography (CT) urography, of
    ureter, 228
computed tomography (CT) venography
  of cerebral vein, 98
  of lower limb, 344
conchae, 12
condylar (mandibular) canal, 4*f*, 17*f*
condylar fossa, 31*f*
condylar neck, 14*f*
condylar process, 14, 14*f*
condyloid canal, 6*f*
conjoined tendon, 327*f*–329*f*
conjunctiva, 18
conjunctival membrane, 18*f*
conoid tubercle, 286*f*
constrictor muscles, pharyngeal, 26
contrast enema, of sigmoid and rectum,
    257
conus, 111*f*–112*f*, 121*f*
convoluted tubules, 223
Cooper's ligaments, 345, 346*f*
coracoacromial arch, 293, 293*b*
coracobrachialis muscle, 292*f*–293*f*, 308,
    309*f*
coracoid process, 284, 292*f*–293*f*, 294*f*
cornea, 18, 18*f*
corniculate cartilage, 29*f*, 34, 35*f*
cornu ammonis, 75*f*
cornua, 34, 273
coronal suture, 2*f*, 3*f*, 4*f*, 6*f*
coronary arteries, 157*f*, 158–159, 182*f*
  dominance, 159
  left, 159, 161*f*
  origin, 164*f*
  right, 159, 160*f*, 161*f*, 182*f*
coronary catheter angiography, 166, 168*f*
coronary dominance, 159
coronary ligament, 202*f*, 238*f*
coronary sinus, 159, 161*f*, 162
coronary veins, 158–159, 159*f*, 160*f*,
    161*f*, 221

coronoid fossa, 297*f*–298*f*
coronoid process, 9, 14, 14*f*, 285*f*, 287*f*,
    297*f*–298*f*
corpora quadrigemini, 74
corpus callosum, 59*f*, 62, 64*f*, 68*f*, 74*f*, 85*f*
  body of, 65*f*, 75*f*
  computed tomography of, 65–66, 65*b*
  genu of, 62*f*, 68*f*, 75*f*
  magnetic resonance imaging of, 65–66,
    65*b*, 65*f*
  rostrum of, 63*f*, 75*f*
  splenium of, 61*f*, 63*f*, 75*f*
  trunk of, 62
corpus cavernosum, 253*f*, 266*f*, 268*f*,
    269*f*, 271
corpus spongiosum, 264, 266*f*, 268*f*,
    269*f*, 271
corpus striatum, 67
cortical bodies, 229
cortical rests, 229
corticospinal tract, 77*f*, 115*f*
costal cartilages, 124*f*, 126–127, 126*b*,
    126*f*, 179*f*
costocervical artery, 55–56
costocervical trunk, 309
cotyloid fossa, 321–322
Couinaud classification, 203
Cowper's gland, 263
cranial fossae, 4
  anterior, 4, 4*f*
  middle, 4, 19*f*, 25*f*
  posterior, 25*f*
cranial nerves. *See also specific nerves*
  in medulla oblongata, 76–78
  in midbrain, 75–76
  in pons, 76
cranial ultrasound, 86
craniopharyngioma, 71
cremaster muscle, 267*f*
cremasteric fasciae, 270
cremasteric venous plexus, 270–271
cribriform plate, 3, 6*f*
cricoid cartilage, 29*f*, 35*f*, 36*f*, 37*f*, 39*f*,
    171*f*
cricoid impression, 171*f*
cricopharyngeus muscle impression,
    171*f*
cricothyroid cartilage, 48*f*
cricothyroid membrane, 29*f*, 33, 35*f*,
    36*f*, 48*f*
cricotracheal membrane, 33, 48*f*
crista falciformis, 23, 25*f*
crista galli, 1, 5*f*, 6*f*, 20*f*, 21*f*
crista terminalis, 157*f*
crossed fused ectopia, 225
cruciform ligament, 110
crus cerebri, 71*f*, 74, 77*f*
crus penis, 268*f*
crypts of Lieberkühn, 201*b*
CT. *See* computed tomography (CT)
cuboid, 316*f*, 317*f*
culmen, 79*f*
cuneatus, 115*f*
cuneiform cartilages, 34, 35*f*
cuneiforms, 316*f*
cystic artery, 189*f*, 190*f*
cystic duct, 210–211, 213*f*
cystic vein, 220*f*

D

dacryocystography, 22
danger space, 44
de Quervain's tenosynovitis, 305
deciduous tooth, resorbing roots of,
    17*f*
declive, 79*f*
deep cerebral vein, 97–98, 99*f*
deep cervical fascia, layers of, 41, 41*f*
deep circumflex iliac artery, 258*f*
deep fascia, 309*f*, 346*f*
deep femoral vessels, 337*f*
deep infrapatellar bursa, 325*f*
deep lateral rotators, 246
deep middle cerebral vein, 99*f*
deep palmar arch, 310*f*
deep perineal fascia, 271
deep veins, 344
deltoid ligament, 331, 333
deltoid muscle, 180*f*, 292*f*–293*f*, 294*f*,
    308, 309*f*
  anterior belly, 292*f*–293*f*
  lateral belly, 292*f*–293*f*
deltoid tuberosity, 286*f*
demifacet, 104*f*
Denonvilliers fascia, 265, 266*f*
dens, of atlas, 5*f*, 103*f*, 104*f*, 106*f*,
    110*f*
dental pantomography, 17–18, 17*f*
dentate gyrus, 74*f*
dentate line, 256*f*
dentate nucleus, 7
denticulate ligament, 118, 121*f*
dentine, 16*f*
depressor anguli oris, 28*f*
dermatome, 116*b*, 116*f*
descending artery
  anterior, 159–161
    branches of, 160–161
    left, 161*f*, 164*f*
  posterior, 160*f*, 161*f*
descending colon, 187*f*, 188*f*, 194*f*, 198*f*,
    200*f*, 239*f*, 243*f*
  attachment of, 194*f*
descending genicular artery, 342*f*
diagnostic mammography, breast
    screening *vs.*, 350
diagonal coronary artery, 164*f*
diaphragm, 129–135, 130*f*, 153*f*, 171*f*,
    191*f*, 192*f*, 238*f*, 240*f*, 242*f*
  axial section of
    level of porta hepatis, 240
    level of upper liver and spleen, 239
  blood supply, 131
  crura of, 130*f*
  nerve supply, 131, 131*b*
  openings in, 131, 131*b*
  pedicle, 130*f*
  radiological features, 130*f*, 131–135
    computed tomography, 135, 135*b*
    curvature of dome, 134
    fluoroscopy, 134, 134*b*
    frontal chest radiograph, 131–132,
      132*f*
    lateral chest radiograph, 132–134,
      134*b*, 134*f*

diaphragm *(Continued)*
　　magnetic resonance imaging, 135
　　ultrasound, 134
　structures that pierce, 131
diaphragma sellae, 71, 87
diaphragmatic hiatus, 171*f*
diencephalon, 69
digastric line, 107
digastric muscle, 48*f*
　anterior belly of, 25, 28*f*
　posterior belly of, 25, 34*f*, 46*f*
digital mammography, 350
digitorum profundus tendons, 305*f*
digitorum superficialis tendons, 305*f*
digits, tendons and soft-tissue anatomy,
　　306*f*, 307, 307*f*
diploic markings, 8
diploic space, 1, 5–7
diploic vein, 1, 4*f*
diploic venous confluence, 4*f*
direct portography, of portal venous
　　system, 222
discography, 114
discoid meniscus, 326
dislocation, of patella, 314, 314*b*
distal femur, 326*f*
distal interphalangeal joint, 288*f*, 307*f*
distal phalanx, 316*f*, 317*f*
　soft tissues overlying, 288*f*
distal radioulnar joint, 288*f*
distal radius, 288*f*, 303*f*
distal triceps tendon signal heterogeneity,
　　300
distal ulna, 288*f*, 303*f*
Doppler ultrasound, of lower limb, 344
dorsal hood, 307
dorsal nerve root, 121*f*
dorsal pancreatic moiety, agenesis of, 214
dorsal radioulnar ligament, 304*f*
dorsal ramus, 117*f*
dorsal root ganglion, 108*f*, 115*f*
dorsalis pedis artery, 341
dorsum sellae, 3, 4*f*, 6*f*, 7*f*
dromedary hump, 225*b*, 226
ductus deferens, 267*f*
ductus reuniens, 26*f*
ductus venosum, 203
duodenal bulb, 190, 191*f*, 193*f*
duodenum, 189–193, 194*f*, 209*f*, 213*f*,
　　216*f*, 217*f*, 224*f*, 238*f*, 242*f*
　arterial supply of, 191, 192*f*
　axial section of, below kidneys,
　　243–244
　first part of, 190, 192*f*
　fourth part of, 191
　lymphatic drainage of, 192
　radiological features of, 192–193
　　barium studies, 191*f*, 192–193, 193*f*
　　ultrasound, 193*f*
　second part of, 187*f*, 190, 192*f*
　third part of, 188*f*, 191, 192*f*, 243*f*
　venous drainage of, 192
dura mater, 85*f*, 87, 117*f*, 121*f*
dural calcification, 7
dural sinuses, 8
dynamic imaging, of sigmoid and rectum,
　　258, 258*b*, 259*f*
dynamic proctography, of pelvic floor, 250

E

ear, 22–23, 24*f*
　development of, 23
　external, 22–23
　inner, 22–23
　middle, 22–23, 22*b*
　radiology, 23
　　computed tomography, 23
　　magnetic resonance imaging, 23
　　plain films, 23
ear lobe, 17*f*
echocardiography, 166
efferent arterioles, 223
efferent ductules, 270
ejaculatory ducts, 262*f*, 263, 265*f*, 268,
　　270
elbow joint, 296, 297*f*–298*f*
　branches to, 310*f*
　capsule, 297*f*–298*f*
　development of, 296, 298*t*
　pseudolesions, 300
　radiological features of, 296–299, 296*b*
　　arthrography, 297
　　magnetic resonance imaging, 297*f*–2
　　98*f*, 298–299
　skin thickening over the extensor surface
　　of, 300
　trauma, 299
enamel, 16*f*
endoanal probe, 256*f*
endocervical canal, 277*f*, 279*f*
endolymphatic duct, 23, 26*f*
endolymphatic sac, 23, 26*f*
endometrial cavity, 253*f*, 282*f*
endometrial stripe, 277*f*
endometrial thickness, 278, 278*b*
endometrium, 265*f*, 273, 275*f*, 279*f*
endopelvic fascia, of female pelvis, 275–
　　276
endoscopic retrograde
　　cholangiopancreatography (ERCP),
　　216–218
endosteum, 1
enteroclysis, 195
epicondyle, 326*f*
　lateral, 287*f*
　medial, 287*f*, 297*f*–298*f*
epicondylitis
　lateral, 299
　medial, 299
epididymis, 270
　body of, 267*f*, 270
　head of, 267*f*, 270
　tail of, 267*f*, 270
epidural fat pad, anterior, 111*f*–112*f*
epidural injection, 119, 122
epidural space, 117*f*, 119–120
　posterior, 111*f*–112*f*
epidural veins, 108*f*, 119
epiglottic cartilage, 29*f*
epiglottis, 29*f*, 33*f*, 34, 35*f*, 36*f*, 37*f*
　base of, 29*f*
epiphyseal subarticular red marrow rests,
　　296*f*
epiploic appendagitis, 199*b*
epiploic foramen (of Winslow), 221, 236

epistaxis, embolization for, 14*b*
epitympanic recess, 22, 25*f*
epitympanum, 24*f*
equator, 18
erector spinae muscle, 108*f*, 111*f*–112*f*,
　　180*f*, 187*f*, 188*f*, 191*f*, 239, 242*f*,
　　243*f*
ethmoid air cells, 5*f*, 19*f*, 21*f*
ethmoid bone, 1, 2*f*, 10*f*
　perpendicular plate of, 5*f*
ethmoid infundibulum, 11*f*
　draining to middle meatus, 21*f*
ethmoid sinuses, 11*f*, 12, 61*f*
ethmoidal air cells, 12
ethmoidal foramen, posterior, 6*f*
ethmoidal nerve, groove for anterior, 9*f*
Eustachian tube, 22
　cartilaginous end of, 30*f*
　opening of, 29*f*, 30*f*, 31*f*
exomphalos, 200
extensor carpi radialis brevis tendon,
　　301*f*–302*f*
extensor carpi radialis longus tendon,
　　301*f*–302*f*
extensor carpi radialis muscle, 289*f*, 308*f*,
　　309*f*
extensor carpi ulnaris muscle, 289*f*, 308*f*,
　　309*f*
extensor carpi ulnaris tendon, 301*f*–30
　　2*f*, 305
extensor digiti minimi muscle, 289*f*, 309*f*
extensor digiti minimi tendon, 301*f*–302*f*
extensor digitorum longus muscle, 289*f*,
　　309*f*, 339*f*
extensor digitorum muscle, 297*f*–298*f*,
　　308*f*
extensor digitorum tendons, 301*f*–302*f*,
　　333*f*–334*f*
extensor hallucis tendon, 333*f*–334*f*
extensor hood, 306*f*
extensor mechanism, 330–331, 330*b*
extensor pollicis brevis tendon, 301*f*–302*f*
extensor pollicis longus muscle, 289*f*,
　　308*f*, 309*f*
extensor pollicis longus tendon, 301*f*–302*f*
extensor tendons, 301*f*–302*f*, 306*f*
external acoustic foramen, 6*f*
external anal sphincter, 248, 251*f*, 253*f*,
　　254*f*, 255*f*, 256*f*, 263*f*
external auditory meatus, 2*f*, 4*f*, 15*f*, 22,
　　25*f*, 31*f*, 54*f*
external capsule, 64*f*
external carotid artery
　branches of, 51*f*
　left, 52*f*
external iliac artery, 250*f*, 255*f*, 257*f*,
　　259–260, 266*f*, 279*f*, 282*f*, 340*f*
　left, 258*f*
external iliac vein, 250*f*, 255*f*, 266*f*, 279*f*,
　　282*f*, 343*f*
external iliac vessels, 254*f*, 277*f*
external jugular vein, 36*f*
external occipital protuberance, 2*f*, 4*f*
external os, 272–273
external sacral neural foramen, 282*f*
external spermatic fasciae, 270
external sphincter, of voluntary muscle,
　　255

external urethral meatus, 264
external urethral orifice, 263
external urethral sphincter, 263–264,
    263f, 265f, 266f
extradural (epidural) haematoma, 88–89
extradural injection, 119
extraocular muscles, 18
extrapleural space, 138, 138b
eye
    anterior segment, 20
    globe of, 19f
    internal anatomy and coverings of, 20
    posterior segment, 20
    radiology of, 19f, 20f, 21–22, 21b, 21f
        computed tomography, 19f, 21
        magnetic resonance imaging, 20f, 21
        plain films, 21
        ultrasound, 19f, 21

F

fabella, 313
facet arthrography, 110
facet joint, 104f, 105f, 109, 109f
    block, 121–122
facial arteries, 48f, 51, 51f, 53f
    left, 52f
    superior labial branch of, 12
facial bones, 1–12
facial (VII) nerve, 23, 24f, 26f, 46f, 71f
    in its bony canal, 25f
    nucleus, 77f
facial vein, 48f, 54, 54f
    common, 54f
    posterior, 46f
faecoliths, 197
falciform ligament, 202–203, 202f, 235,
    236f, 237
fallopian tube, 272f, 273, 273b, 274f, 280
false vocal cords, 29f, 35–36, 35f, 37f
falx cerebelli, 87
falx cerebri, 87
fat lines, 185, 185f
fat pad, 319, 319f, 325f, 336f
    anterior, 297f–298f
    posterior, 297f–298f
fat within muscle cone, 18f
fauces, 24
feeding studies, videofluoroscopic, 33
female reproductive tract, 272–281
female urethra, 264
    radiology of, 264, 265f
femoral artery, 321–322
    descending genicular branch of, 340f
femoral articular cartilage, 325f
femoral condyle, 326f
femoral head, 255f, 265f, 266f, 282f,
    321–322
    cartilage of, 320f
femoral neck version, 313b
femoral nerve, 261, 339f
femoral veins, 282f, 321–322, 343f
femoral vessels, 321f–323f, 339f
femur, 312, 312b, 313f, 319f, 326f, 339f
    blood supply, 313
    bone density, 313–314, 314b
    cortex of, 337f

femur (Continued)
    head of, 247f, 251f, 313f
    intertrochanteric line of, 313f
    lesser trochanter of, 313f
    medullary cavity of, 337f
    neck of, 247f, 313f
    neck version, 313b
    ossification, 313
    radiological features, 313f
    sesamoid bones, 313
    trabecular markings, 313–314, 314b,
        314f
fetal lobulation, 218, 225, 225b
fibrocartilage
    body of, 304f
    posterior bulge of, 324f
fibrous capsule, 224, 292f–293f
    of hip joint, 319f
    of knee joint, 325f
fibrous cartilage, 15f
    on articular surface, 15f
fibrous sheath, 265
fibula, 315, 315f, 317f, 339f
    head of, 315f, 326f
    medulla of, 337f
    neck of, 326f
    ossification of, 315, 315b
    radiological features of, 315
fibular collateral ligament, 327f–329f
fibulocalcaneal ligament, 333f–334f
fimbria, 272f, 275
first extensor compartment syndrome, 305
first metatarsal
    head of, 317f
    shaft of, 317f
fissures, of lungs, 148
fistula, 195
flexor carpi radialis distal muscle belly,
    301f–302f
flexor carpi radialis muscle, 289f,
    297f–298f, 305f, 308f, 309f
    insertion, 301f–302f
flexor carpi ulnaris muscle, 289f,
    297f–298f, 301f–302f, 305f, 308f,
    309f
flexor carpi ulnaris tendon, 301f–302f
flexor digiti minimi muscle, 333f–334f
flexor digitorum brevis muscle, 333f–334f
flexor digitorum longus muscle, 333f–33
    4f, 337f, 339f
flexor digitorum profundus muscle, 289f,
    308f, 309f
flexor digitorum profundus tendon, 301f–
    302f, 306f
    injury, 307
flexor digitorum superficialis muscle, 289f,
    308f, 309f
flexor digitorum superficialis tendon,
    301f–302f, 306f, 307
flexor digitorum tendon, 333f–334f
flexor hallucis longus tendon, 333f–334f,
    336
flexor hallucis muscle belly, 333f–334f
flexor pollicis longus tendon, 289f,
    301f–302f, 305f
flexor retinaculum, 301f–302f, 305f
flexor tendon, 307f
flocculus, 78, 79f

floor of sella, 7f
fluoroscopy, of diaphragm, 134, 134b
focal fatty infiltration, 206b
focal fatty sparing, 206b
folium, 79f
follicles, 276, 277f, 279f
fontanelles, 5–7
foot
    arches of, 316, 316b
    biomechanics, 331–332
    bones of, 312–318, 316f, 317f
        coalition of, 318
        ossification, 317–318, 318b
        radiological features, 316–318, 318f
foramen caecum, 6f
foramen lacerum, 5, 6f, 8t
foramen magnum, 5, 6f, 8t
    anterior limit of, 4f
    posterior limit of, 4f
foramen of Magendie, 80f
foramen of Monro, 63f
foramen ovale, 5, 6f, 7f, 8t, 31f, 32f
foramen rotundum, 5, 5f, 6f, 8t, 32f
foramen spinosum, 5, 6f, 8t, 31f, 32f
foramen transversarium, 36f, 101, 102f,
    103f, 104f
foramina, of skull base, 4–5, 8t
forceps major, 62
forceps minor, 62
forearm, 308
fornix, 59f, 63f, 64f, 65f, 73–74, 74f, 75f,
    82f
    body of, 74f
    crus of, 74f
fossa of Rosenmüeller, 27, 30f, 31f
fourth metatarsal, base of, 317f
fourth ventricle, 61f, 63f, 68f, 77f, 79f,
    80f, 81f, 83, 83b, 83f
fovea, 247f
fracture fragments, vascularity integrity
    of, 306
free fluid, 275f, 279f
frenulum of valve, 197f
frontal bone, 1, 2f, 6f, 18f, 20f
    orbital plates of, 10f
    zygomatic process of, 5f
frontal chest radiograph
    of diaphragm, 131–132, 132f
    of mediastinum, 177–178, 177b, 177f
frontal lobe, 58, 59f, 63f
frontal sinuses, 4f, 5f, 12
frontoethmoidal suture, 6f
frontonasal synchondrosis, 9f
frontopolar artery, 91
functional asplenia, 218
fundus
    of gallbladder, 202f, 209, 209f
    of stomach, 183f, 185, 188f, 189b,
        223f
    of uterus, 272–273, 272f

G

gadoxetate disodium (Primovist), 206
gallbladder, 187f, 192f, 202f, 208–209,
    211b, 213f, 242f
    arterial supply of, 209

gallbladder *(Continued)*
body of, 209*f*
neck of, 209*f*
normal variants of, 209
venous drainage of, 209
gamekeeper's thumb, 307
Gartner's duct cyst, 281
gastric antrum, 185
gastric artery
left, 189*f*, 190*f*, 192*f*, 204
oesophageal branch of, 189*f*, 190*f*
right, 189*f*, 190*f*, 192*f*
splenic, 189*f*
gastric epiploic artery, 190*f*
gastric nodes, 233
gastric vein
left, 190*f*, 220*f*
right, 190*f*, 220*f*
short, 190*f*, 220*f*
gastric vessels, 240*f*
gastrocnemius muscle, 327*f*–329*f*, 336*f*
head of, 339*f*
lateral head of, 327*f*–329*f*, 337*f*
medial head of, 337*f*
gastrocolic ligament, 235–236
gastroduodenal artery, 189*f*, 190*f*, 192*f*, 209*f*, 216*f*, 217*f*, 242*f*
gastroepiploic artery
gastric branches of, 189*f*
left, 189*f*
right, 189*f*, 192*f*, 216*f*
gastroepiploic veins
left, 190*f*, 220*f*
right, 190*f*, 220*f*
gastroesophageal veins, 220*f*
gastrohepatic ligament, 236, 236*f*
gastrohepatic recess, 237
gastro-oesophageal junction, 171*f*, 185, 191*f*
gastropancreatic fold, 236
gastrophrenic ligament, 235
gastrorenal-splenorenal vein, 220*f*
gastrosplenic ligament, 235–236, 236*f*, 238*f*
geniculate body, 69
genioglossus muscle, 24–25, 27*f*, 28*f*, 29*f*, 34*f*
left, 43*f*
geniohyoid muscle, 27*f*, 28*f*
Gerdy's tubercle, 327*f*–329*f*
germinal epithelium, 275
Gerota's fascia, 188*f*, 224
glandular fat, 346*f*
glandular tissue, 346*f*, 351*f*, 352*f*
glans penis, 268*f*, 271
glenohumeral joint capsule, posterior, 292*f*–293*f*
glenohumeral ligament, 294
inferior, 295*f*
middle, 292*f*–293*f*, 295*f*
thickened middle, 295*f*
glenoid, 285*f*, 292*f*–293*f*, 294*f*
glenoid cavity, 285*f*
glenoid labrum, 292*f*–293*f*, 293
absent anterior, 295*f*
glenoid process, 284
globe, 18, 20*f*
globus pallidus, 65*f*, 69*f*

glossoepiglottic folds, 34
lateral, 36*f*
median, 36*f*
glossopharyngeal (IX) nerve, 71*f*, 77*f*
glottis, 34–35
gluteal muscles, 320*f*
gluteus maximus muscle, 223*f*, 250*f*, 251*f*, 253*f*, 254*f*, 255*f*, 266*f*, 269*f*, 282*f*, 321–322, 321*f*–323*f*, 339*f*
gluteus medius muscle, 223*f*, 250*f*, 282*f*, 321–322, 321*f*–323*f*
gluteus minimus muscle, 250*f*, 282*f*, 321–322, 321*f*–323*f*
Golfer's elbow, 299
gracilis muscle, 115*f*, 327*f*–329*f*, 337*f*
conjoined insertion of, 321*f*–323*f*
great cerebral vein, 98, 99*f*, 100*f*
great saphenous vein, 339*f*, 343*f*
great veins, 170
great vessels, 167–170
radiology, 170
greater cornua/horns, 35, 35*f*
greater omentum, 238*f*
greater palatine foramen, 6*f*, 32*f*
greater sciatic foramen, 245, 249*f*
greater sciatic notch, 246*f*
greater trochanter, 247*f*, 251*f*, 313*f*, 321*f*–323*f*
greater tuberosity, 286*f*
greater wing of sphenoid, 2*f*, 6*f*, 10*f*, 19*f*, 20*f*
grey matter, 115*f*, 116
Guyon's canal, 301*f*–302*f*, 305*f*, 306
gyrus rectus, 61*f*

H

habenular commissure, 62, 62*f*, 64*f*
calcification, 7
HAGL injury, 294*b*
hamate, 288*f*, 303*f*
hand
bones of, 288*f*
imaging of, 307
intrinsic muscles of, 307
radiological features of, 300–308
spaces of the palm of, 306–307
hard palate, 4*f*, 17*f*, 28*f*, 29*f*
Hartmann's pouch, 208
haustra, 200–201
head and neck, deep spaces of, 42–45, 42*f*
heart, 153–167
apex of, 154
atria, 154
chambers and valves, 156–158, 157*f*
gross anatomy and orientation, 132*f*, 134*f*, 153–154, 153*f*, 154*b*
radiology, 162–167
chest radiograph, 162–164, 162*f*, 163*f*, 164*b*
computed tomography, 164–166, 164*f*, 165*b*, 165*f*
coronary catheter angiography, 166
echocardiography, 166
magnetic resonance imaging, 166
myocardial viability and perfusion scintigraphy, 166–167

heart *(Continued)*
positron emission tomography CT, 167, 167*f*
veins, 161–162, 161*f*
heel pad thickness, 316, 318*f*
hemiazygos vein, 175*f*, 183*f*, 191*f*, 232*f*
hemiballismus, 70
hemidiaphragm, 106*f*, 132*f*, 134*f*, 183*f*, 188*f*, 223*f*, 240*f*
hemispheres, of cerebellum, 78
hepatic arteries, 190*f*, 192*f*, 202*f*, 207*f*, 209*f*, 216*f*, 217*f*, 241*f*
common, 189*f*, 204
embolization of, 208
left, 189*f*, 240*f*
accessory, 204
phrenic branch of, 189*f*
portal vein and, variations in relationship of, 210*f*
proper, 189*f*
right, 189*f*, 204
accessory, 204
variations in, 209*f*
hepatic duct
accessory, 211
common, 209*f*, 210, 213*f*
double, 211
left, 209*f*, 213*f*
right, 209*f*, 213*f*
hepatic flexure, 185*f*, 187*f*, 198*f*
hepatic nodes, 233
hepatic vein, 183*f*
left, 207*f*
middle, 207*f*, 240*f*
right, 207*f*
hepatorenal space (Morrison's pouch), 237, 237*b*
hepticoduodenal ligament, 236
hilar nodes, 173
hilar point, 132*f*
hilum
of kidney, 222
of spleen, 223*f*, 242*f*
hip joint, 318–319, 319*b*, 319*f*
articular surfaces, 319
capsule, 319
ligaments, 319
radiological features, 319–323
arthrography, 320
computed tomography, 320–321
magnetic resonance imaging, 321–323, 321*f*–323*f*, 322*b*, 323*b*
plain radiographs, 319
radiography, 319
ultrasound, 320, 320*f*
synovium, 319
hippocampus, 68*f*, 73, 75*f*
body, 75*f*
commissure, 62
fimbria of, 75*f*
head, 75*f*
tail, 75*f*
Hoffa's fat pad, 327*f*–329*f*
hook of hamate, 288*f*, 301*f*–302*f*
horizontal fissure, 79*f*, 80*f*, 134*f*
horseshoe kidney, 225
humeral head, 292*f*–293*f*
lesser tuberosity of, 292*f*–293*f*

humeral line, anterior, 286
humeral shaft
    cortex of, 308f
    medullary cavity of, 285f
    humerus, 285f, 286, 297f–298f, 309f
        left, 286f
        medial epicondyle avulsion, 286–287
        nutrient artery to, 310f
        ossification of, 287
        radiological features of, 286–287
        shaft of, 287f
Huntington's disease, 69b
hyaline articular cartilage, 292f–293f
hyaline membrane, 20
hydrocoele, 267f
hyoglossus muscle, 27f, 28f, 34f, 43f
hyoid bone, 17f, 29f, 33f, 35, 35f, 37f, 39f, 48f, 171f
    body of, 29f
    greater cornu of, 35f, 36f
hypoglossal canal, 5, 6f, 7f, 8t
hypoglossal (XII) nerve, 71f, 77f
hypopharynx, 38, 39f
    bucco-fascial lymph nodes, 40, 40f
    central anterior cervical chain, 40, 40f
    lower internal jugular (deep cervical), 39–40, 40f
    medial supraclavicular chain, 39–40, 40f
    middle internal jugular (deep cervical) chain, 39, 40f
    parotid lymph nodes, 40, 40f
    posterior triangle and supraclavicular chain, 40
    posterior wall of, 39f
    retro-auricular and occipital lymph nodes, 40f, 41
    retropharyngeal and retrostyloid lymph nodes, 40, 40f
    upper internal jugular (deep cervical) chain, 39, 40f
hypophyseal arteries, 72
hypothalamus, 70, 71f
    radiological features, 70–71
hypothenar compartment, 306
hypothenar eminence, 301f–302f, 307
hypotympanum, 24f
hysterosalpingography, 281b

ileal loops, 195
ileal vein, 220f
ileocaecal valve, 196–197, 197b, 197f
ileocolic artery, 194f, 195f
ileocolic vein, 220f
ileum, 193–194, 193f, 194t, 197f
    branches of, 194f, 195f
    lower end of, 194f
iliac artery, common, 200f, 220f, 230f
iliac bone, 255f
iliac crest, 245, 246f, 247f
    inner lip of, 246f
    intermediate zone of, 246f
    outer lip of, 246f
    tuberculum of, 246f
iliac tuberosity, 246f

iliac veins, 260, 260b
    common, 111f–112f
iliac vessels, radiology of, 260
    conventional angiography, 260
    CT angiography, 260
    magnetic resonance imaging, 260
    ultrasound, 260
    venography, 260
iliac wing, 320f
iliacus muscle, 245–246, 248f, 250f, 251f, 282f, 321f–323f
iliococcygeus muscle, 248, 252f
iliofemoral ligament, 247f, 319, 321–322
    capsule of, 321f–323f
iliolumbar artery, 257f, 258f, 259
iliolumbar ligament, 245, 247f
iliolumbar vein, 232f
iliopectineal eminence, 245
iliopectineal line, 245–246
iliopsoas muscle, 245–246, 255f, 321–322, 321f–323f
iliopsoas tendon, 321–322
iliopubic eminence, 246f, 252f
iliotibial band, 327f–329f
ilium, 245, 247f
    ala of, 246f, 252f
    auricular surface of, 246f
    body of, 246f
impingement syndromes, 335
incisura, 185, 188f, 191f
incudomallear joint, 22
incus, 22, 24f, 25f
indirect portography, of portal venous system, 222
indusium griseum, 75f
inferior accessory fissure, 144
inferior angle, 285f
inferior brachium, 74
inferior caniculus, 21f
inferior cerebellar peduncle, 79f
inferior constrictor muscle, 35f
inferior dental artery, 52
inferior epigastric vessels, 250f, 282f
inferior gemellus muscle, 321f–323f
inferior gluteal artery, 257f, 258f, 259, 341f
inferior gluteal line, 246f
inferior gluteal vessels, 251f, 282f
inferior hypophysia artery, 93f
inferior meatus, 11f
inferior medullary vein, 98
inferior medullary velum, 82f
inferior mesenteric artery, 258f
inferior nasal turbinate bone, 11f, 21f
inferior ophthalmic veins, 19
inferior orbital fissure, 32f
    lateral aspect of, 10f
inferior petrosal sinus, 97, 98f
inferior pubic ligament, 252f, 269f
inferior pubic ramus, 245, 246f, 247f, 253f, 266f
inferior pulmonary vein
    left, 157f
    right, 157f
inferior rectal artery, 254f
inferior rectus muscle, 18f
inferior sagittal sinus, 96, 98f, 100f
inferior sagittal vein, 99f

inferior tarsal plate, 18f
inferior thyroid artery, 48f
inferior tibiofibular articulation, 333f–334f
inferior turbinate, 21f, 29f
inferior vena cava, 130f, 134f, 153f, 161f, 175f, 183f, 187f, 188f, 192f, 202f, 207f, 216f, 220f, 223f, 230f, 231–232, 232f, 239f, 240f, 242f, 243f
    axial section of, level of pancreatic head and renal hila, 243
    embryology and variants of, 231–232
    persistent left-sided, 231
    radiology of, 231–232
    tributaries of, 231
inferior vermian artery, 92
inferior vermian vein, 98, 99f
inferior vermis, 79f
inferior vesical artery, 257f, 259
inferolateral trunk, 90
infracolic space, 237
inframesocolic mesenteries, 237
infraglenoid tubercle, 285f
infraorbital artery, 52
infraorbital canal, 11
infraorbital foramen, 2f, 10f, 20f
infraorbital groove, 10f, 11
infraorbital nerve, 11
infraspinatus muscle, 180f, 292f–293f, 294f
infraspinous process, 285f
infratemporal fossa, 9–10, 30f, 31f, 42
infratemporal space, 30–31, 30f
infundibular recess, 82f
infundibular stalk, 70
infundibulum, 71f, 73, 222, 222f, 227f, 228, 272f
inguinal canal, 266f
inguinal ligament, 246, 282f
inguinal lymph node, 266f
inner skull table, 4f
innominate bones, 245
innominate line, 5f, 12, 201b
insula (of Reil), 60, 64f, 65f
intercarpal joints, 300, 301f–302f
interclinoid ligaments, 7
intercondylar eminence, tubercles on, 315f
intercondylar fossa, 313
intercondylar notch, 313f, 327f–329f
intercostal arteries, 119f, 127, 131, 345, 347f
    anterior, 127
    posterior, 127
intercostal space, 126–127
intercostal veins, 127, 127b
interhemispheric fissure, 61f, 65f, 68f, 85f
interlobar artery, 132f, 223
interlobar fissures, 137, 144
interlobular arteries, 223
intermediate cuneiform, 317f
intermetacarpal joint, 301f–302f
internal anal sphincter, 255f, 256, 256f
    longitudinal muscle of, 256f
internal auditory meatus, 5, 6f, 7f, 8t, 23, 25f
internal capsule, 62–64, 64f, 65f, 66f, 69f

internal carotid artery, 30*f*, 31*f*, 36*f*, 46*f*,
89*f*, 90, 93*f*, 94*f*
branches of, 90–92
cavernous part of, 94*f*
in cavernous sinus, 72*f*
intracranial part of, 94*f*
left, 52*f*
petrous part of, 94*f*
sinus of right, 52*f*
internal cerebral vein, 98, 99*f*, 100*f*
internal iliac artery, 257*f*, 259, 260*b*
anterior trunk of, 257*f*, 258*f*
left, 258*f*
right, posterior trunk of, 258*f*
superior vesical branches, 257*f*
internal iliac vessels, 253*f*, 255*f*, 275*f*,
282*f*
branches of, 282*f*
internal jugular vein, 30*f*, 31*f*, 36*f*, 56*f*
right, 37*f*
internal mammary lymph nodes, 347*f*
internal mammary lymphatic chain,
contralateral, 347*f*
internal occipital artery, 95*f*
calcarine branch of, 95*f*
parieto-occipital branch of, 95*f*
internal os, 272–273, 280
internal pudendal artery, 259, 341*f*
internal pudendal vessels, 251*f*
internal spermatic fasciae, 270
internal sphincter, of involuntary muscle,
255
internal urethral sphincter, 263–264
internal vertebral venous plexus, 268
interosseous arteries, 310
anterior, 310*f*
posterior, 310*f*
interosseous border, 315
interosseous ligament, 333*f*–334*f*
interosseous membrane, 308, 339*f*
interosseous nerves, 308
interpedicular distance, 103
interpeduncular cistern, 63*f*, 65*f*, 77*f*, 82*f*,
83*f*, 85
interphalangeal joints, 318*f*
intersection syndrome, 305
intersphincteric space, 256*f*
interspinous ligament, 109*f*, 111*f*–112*f*,
113, 113*f*
interthalamic adhesion, 69, 81*f*, 82*f*
intertransverse ligaments, 113
intertrochanteric crest, 313*f*
intertrochanteric femur, 247*f*
intertrochanteric line, of femur, 313*f*
interventricular foramen, 74*f*, 81*f*, 82*f*
interventricular septum, 155*f*, 157*f*, 182*f*
intervertebral disc, 104*f*, 105*f*, 108*f*, 109,
111*f*–112*f*, 113–114, 113*f*, 120*f*
radiological features of, 114
somatic and autonomic nerve supply to,
113–114
vascular supply to, 114*b*
intervertebral disc space, 106*f*
intervertebral foramen, 108*f*, 113*f*, 117*f*
intestinal trunks, 233
intra-atrial septum, 182*f*
intrabulbar fossa, 264
intranuclear cleft, 114

intraoccipital sutures, 9
intravenous injection of contrast, 311
intrinsic tongue muscle, 27*f*
involuntary internal urethral sphincter,
264
iris, 18*f*, 19*f*, 20
ischial spine, 245, 246*f*, 247*f*, 252*f*
ischial tuberosity, 245, 246*f*, 247*f*, 249*f*,
251*f*, 254*f*, 266*f*, 269*f*
ischioanal fossa, 253*f*, 254*f*, 256*f*
ischiocavernosus muscle, 248, 266*f*
ischiopubic ramus, 249*f*
ischiorectal fossa, 248–250, 251*f*, 253*f*,
256*f*, 321–322
ischium, 245, 251*f*, 253*f*, 321*f*–323*f*
body of, 246*f*, 247*f*
cortex of, 282*f*
ramus of, 246*f*, 247*f*
isotope bone scan, 284*b*
isthmus, 45, 48*f*
of fallopian tube, 281*f*
of uterus, 272–273, 272*f*, 280

J

jejunal loops, 195
jejunal vein, 220*f*
jejunum, 193–194, 193*f*, 194*t*
axial section of, below kidneys, 243
branches of, 194*f*, 195*f*
upper end of, 194*f*
Jersey finger, 307
Jones fracture, 317*b*, 318*f*
jugular arch, 54, 54*f*
jugular foramen, 5, 6*f*, 7*f*, 8*t*, 32*f*
jugular fossa, 6*f*
jugular veins
anterior, 35*f*, 48*f*, 54, 54*f*
external, 35*f*, 48*f*, 54, 54*f*, 56*f*
internal, 46*f*, 51*f*, 54, 54*f*, 55*f*, 98*f*, 100*f*
junction lines, 136*f*, 137, 178, 178*f*, 181*f*
junctional cortical defects, 225*b*
junctional parenchymal defects, 225*b*
junctional zone, 265*f*, 279*f*

K

kidney, 188*f*, 222–226, 223*f*, 224*f*, 238*f*,
240*f*, 241*f*, 242*f*, 243*f*
abnormalities and variants of, 225
axial section of
level of pancreatic head and renal
hila, 243
blood supply of, 223
body wall, 243
cortex, 222, 222*f*
development of, 224–225
fascial spaces of, 224, 224*f*
fornix of, 222*f*, 227*f*
hilum of, 188*f*
lymphatic drainage of, 224
radiological features of, 225–226
arteriography, 226
computed tomography, 185*f*, 187*f*,
226
interventional procedures, 226

kidney *(Continued)*
magnetic resonance imaging, 185*f*,
187*f*, 226
plain films, 225
renal venography, 226
scintigraphy, 226
ultrasound, 225–226
relations of, 223
venous drainage of, 224
knee joint, 325, 325*f*
articular surfaces, 325
capsule, 325
collateral ligaments, 329
cruciate ligaments, 329–330, 330*f*
extensor mechanism, 330–331, 330*b*
internal structures, 325, 325*f*
ligaments, 325
radiological features, 325–327, 326*f*
arthrography, 326
magnetic resonance imaging, 326–
327, 327*f*–329*f*
plain radiographs, 325–326
synovium, 325
type, 325

L

L3
inferior articular process, 107*f*
pedicle of, 107*f*
spinous process of, 107*f*
superior articular process of, 107*f*
transverse process of, 107*f*
labia majora, 265*f*
labia minora, 265*f*
labral tears, 294, 294*b*
labyrinthine artery, 92, 93*f*
labyrinths
bony, 22
membranous, 23
lacrimal apparatus, 21–22, 21*f*
lacrimal bone, 2*f*, 10*f*
lacrimal canaliculi, 21–22
lacrimal duct, 11
lacrimal gland, 11, 11*f*, 20*f*, 21, 21*f*
radiology, 22
computed tomography and magnetic
resonance imaging, 22
dacryocystography, 22
lacrimal puncta, 22
lacrimal sac, 11, 21, 21*f*
lactiferous ducts, 346*f*
lambda, 1, 2*f*, 3*f*, 4*f*
lambdoid suture, 1, 2*f*, 3*f*, 4*f*, 6*f*, 25*f*
lamina, 130*f*
lamina dura, 16–18, 16*f*
lamina papyracea, 10–11, 11*b*
lamina terminalis, 82*f*
laminae, vertebral, 102*f*, 104*f*, 106*f*, 108*f*,
111*f*–112*f*, 113*f*
large intestine, 198–201
anterior relations of, 199
arterial supply of, 199
development of, 200
lymphatic drainage of, 200
obstruction, 201*t*
peritoneal relations of, 199

large intestine *(Continued)*
    posterior relations of, 199
    radiological features of, 200–201
        angiography, 200*f*, 201
        computed tomography, 201
        CT colonography, 201
        double-contrast barium enema
            examination, 201
        malrotation, 200, 201*b*
        plain films, 200–201
    venous drainage of, 199
laryngeal airway, 35*f*
laryngeal nerve, recurrent, 51*f*
laryngeal ventricle, 33*f*, 34–35
laryngopharynx, 29*f*, 33*f*, 35*f*, 36*f*
larynx, 33–38, 35*f*
    cross-sectional anatomy of, 35, 35*f*, 36*f*,
        37*f*
    glottic level, 36*f*, 37*f*, 38
    inferior constrictor of, 35*f*
    radiology of, 38
        computed tomography and magnetic
            resonance imaging, 35*f*, 36*f*, 37*f*,
            38, 38*b*
        plain radiography, 38
    sinus of, 34–35
    subglottic level, 38
    supraglottic level, 35–36, 36*f*, 37*f*
    vestibule of, 35*f*
lateral apertures (of Luschka), 83
lateral chest radiograph
    of diaphragm, 132–134, 134*b*, 134*f*
    of lungs, 149–150
    of mediastinum, 178
lateral circumflex femoral artery, 340,
    341*f*
lateral collateral ligament, 332, 332*b*
lateral collateral ligament complex, 329,
    329*b*
lateral conal fascia, 188*f*, 224, 224*f*
lateral condyles, 313*f*
lateral cuneiform, 317*f*
lateral epicondyle, 313*f*
lateral epicondylitis, 299
lateral geniculate body, 71*f*
lateral inferior genicular artery, 342*f*
lateral lenticulostriate artery, 94*f*
lateral ligaments, of ankle joint, 332
lateral malleolus, 333*f*–334*f*
lateral mass, ossification of, 110*f*
lateral meniscus, 325, 325*f*, 327*f*–329*f*
lateral pharyngeal recess, 30*f*
lateral plantar artery, 333*f*–334*f*
lateral plantar nerve, 333*f*–334*f*
lateral plantar vein, 333*f*–334*f*
lateral pterygoid muscle, 15*f*, 31*f*
lateral retinaculum, 327*f*–329*f*
lateral sacral arteries, 257*f*, 258*f*, 259
lateral sacral mass, 247*f*
lateral striate, 91
lateral sulcus, 59*f*
lateral superior genicular artery, 342*f*
lateral supracondylar ridge, 313*f*
lateral thoracic artery, external mammary
    branch from, 347*f*
lateral thoracic vein, external mammary
    branch from, 347*f*
lateral thoracic vessels, 347*f*

lateral tibial plateau, 326*f*
lateral tibial spine, 326*f*
lateral umbilical ligaments, 260
lateral uterine cornu, 272*f*
lateral vaginal fornix, 272*f*
lateral ventricles, 69*f*, 80–81, 81*f*
    anterior horn of, 81*f*, 85*f*
    body of, 68*f*, 80, 81*f*
    choroid plexus of, 81–82, 83*f*
    frontal horn of, 68*f*, 80
    inferior horn of, 81*f*
    occipital horn of, 81, 81*f*
    temporal horn of, 75*f*, 81
latissimus dorsi muscle, 187*f*, 188*f*, 191*f*
    attachments of, 111*f*–112*f*
lens, 18*f*, 21
    anterior aspect of, 19*f*
    posterior aspect of, 19*f*
lenticulostriate artery, 94*f*
lentiform nucleus, 65*f*, 69*b*, 69*f*
lesser cornua/horns, 35
lesser omentum, 238*f*
    free edge of, 221
lesser sac, 212
    associated ligaments, 236, 236*f*, 238*f*
    isolated fluid collections in, 236*b*
    ligaments of, 236–237
    recesses of, 236, 238*f*
    superior recess of, 236
lesser sciatic foramen, 245, 249*f*
lesser sciatic notch, 246*f*
lesser trochanter, of femur, 247*f*, 313*f*
lesser tuberosity, 285*f*, 286*f*
lesser wing of sphenoid, 5*f*, 6*f*
levator ani muscle, 248, 251*f*, 252*f*,
    253*f*, 254*f*, 255*f*, 256*f*, 263*f*, 266*f*,
    269*f*
    lowermost, 251*f*
    puborectalis fibres of, 265*f*
levator muscle, 24
levator palatini muscle, 31*f*
levator palpebrae superioris muscle, 18,
    18*f*, 21–22
levator plate, 248, 266*f*, 280
levator scapulae, 109*f*
levator veli palatini, 27–28, 31*f*
ligament, 235
ligament of Treitz, 193*b*
ligamenta flava, 108*f*, 109*f*, 113, 113*f*
ligamentum denticulatum, 117*f*
ligamentum nuchae, 109*f*, 112
ligamentum teres, 192*f*, 202–203, 202*f*,
    208*b*, 221, 241*f*, 319*f*
ligamentum venosum, 202*f*, 203, 208*b*,
    221, 239
    fissure for, 191*f*, 192*f*, 203, 240*f*
limbic lobe system, 73–74, 74*f*
    fornix, 73–74, 74*f*
    hippocampus, 73, 75*f*
limbus, 18, 18*f*
linea alba, 186*f*, 192*f*, 239
linea aspera, 313*f*
linea semilunaris, 184
lingual artery, 27*f*, 51, 51*f*, 53*f*
    left, 52*f*
    right, 52*f*
lingual septum, 28*f*, 34*f*
lingual tonsils, 33

lingual vein, 54
lingula, 79*f*, 182*f*
    on superior medullary velum, 80*f*
Lister's tubercle, 301*f*–302*f*
liver, 183*f*, 201–208, 202*f*, 213*f*, 216*f*,
    220*f*, 223*f*, 238*f*, 353*f*
    arterial supply of, 204
    axial section of
        level of pancreatic body, 241
        level of pancreatic head and renal
            hila, 241
        level of porta hepatis, 240
        level of upper liver and spleen, 239,
            240*f*
    bare area of, 237
    blood supply of, 204
    body wall, 239
    lymphatic drainage of, 205
    old lobar anatomy of, 204
    radiological features of, 205–208
        computed tomography, 187*f*, 188*f*,
            191*f*, 192*f*, 205–206, 206*f*
        magnetic resonance imaging, 205–
            206
        plain films, 185*f*, 205
        scintigraphy, 207–208
        shear wave elastography, 207
        ultrasound, 206–207, 207*f*
    segmental anatomy of, 202*f*, 203–204,
        203*f*
    venous drainage of, 205
lobular duct, 346*f*
long saphenous vein, 344
long striate artery, 93*f*
longitudinal fold, 213*f*
longitudinal ligament, 111*f*–112*f*
    anterior, 109*f*, 111, 113*f*
    posterior, 112–113, 113*f*
longitudinal ridges, 280
longus capitis, 31*f*
longus colli muscles, 109*f*
lordosis, 101
lower eyelid, 18*f*
lower leg, 337*f*, 338–340, 339*f*
lower limb, 312–344
    arteries of, 340–343, 340*f*, 341*f*, 342*f*,
        343*f*
        radiological features, 341–343
    bones, 312–318
        femur, 312, 312*b*, 313*f*, 314*f*
        fibula, 315, 315*f*
        foot, 315–316, 316*b*, 316*f*, 317*f*,
            318*f*
        patella, 314
        tibia, 314–315, 315*f*
    joints, 318–319
        ankle, 331, 331*f*, 333*f*–334*f*, 336*f*
        hip, 318–319, 319*b*, 319*f*, 320*f*,
            321*f*–323*f*
        knee, 325, 325*f*, 326*f*, 327*f*–329*f*,
            330*f*
        subtalar, 336–337
        symphysis pubis, 323–325, 323*b*,
            324*f*
        tibiofibular, 331
    muscles, 337–340, 337*f*, 338*f*, 339*f*
    veins, 343–344, 343*f*
lower oesophageal sphincter, 185

lower urinary tract, 261–263
  bladder, 261–262
    blood supply, 262
    lymph drainage, 262
    peritoneal reflections, 262
  pelvic ureters, 261
lumbar artery, 230f, 258f
lumbar facet joints, 111
lumbar puncture, for myelography, 113
lumbar rib, 126
lumbar spine, 111f–112f
  myelographic appearance of, 119, 120f
  oblique views of, 107, 107f
  radiographs of, 107
lumbar trunks, 233
lumbar vein, ascending, 232f
lumbar vertebrae, 102, 105f, 109
lumbar vessels, 248f
lumbarization, of sacrum, 246–248
lumbosacral plexus, 261
lumbricals, 307
lunate, 246f, 288f, 301f–302f, 303f, 304f
lungs, 143–152, 143f, 183f, 191f, 238f,
      240f, 351f, 352f
  accessory fissures, 144–145, 144f, 145b
  bronchopulmonary segment, 145,
      145b, 149, 149b
  interlobar fissures, 144
  lower limits at rest, 137t
  lower lobe, 143f
  lymphatics, 147, 147f
  middle lobe, 143f
  radiological features, 148–152
    chest radiograph, 148–149
    computed tomography, 151–152,
        178f, 180f, 181f
    lateral chest radiograph, 149–150
    lymphatics, 149
    magnetic resonance imaging, 152
    pulmonary angiography, 150
    ventilation-perfusion scintigraphy,
        152, 152b
  roots, 147–148, 148f
  upper lobe, 143f
lunotriquetral ligament, 304, 304b
lymph node, 39f, 251f
lymphatic duct, right, 172–173, 173b
lymphatics, of pelvis, 260
  radiology of, 260–261
    cross-sectional imaging, 260–261
    lymphangiography, 260
lymphography, mediastinal lymphatics, 173
lymphoid follicles, 201b

M

macula, 20
magenstrasse, 186, 186b, 191f
magnetic resonance angiography (MRA),
    of lower limb, 342, 343f
magnetic resonance cholangiography,
    212, 213f
magnetic resonance enterography, of small
    intestine, 196, 196f
magnetic resonance imaging
  of ankle joint, 332, 333f–334f
  of basal ganglia, 67–69

magnetic resonance imaging (Continued)
  of breasts, 351–352
  of cerebellum, 79–80, 80b
  of cerebral cortex, 60, 61f
  of cerebral vein, 100
  of corpus callosum, 65–66, 65b, 65f
  of diaphragm, 135
  of elbow joint, 297f–298f, 298–299
  of heart, 166
  of hip, 321–323, 321f–323f, 322b,
      323b
  of intracranial arteries, 94–95
  of kidney, 185f, 187f, 226
  of knee, 326–327, 327f–329f
  of liver, 205–206
  of lungs, 152
  of pancreas, 213f, 216
  of pelvic floor, 250, 253f, 254f
  of sigmoid and rectum, 257–258
  of spinal cord, 109f, 111f–112f, 117f,
      120
  of spleen, 219
  of stomach, 188, 191f, 192f
  of ventricular system, 83–84
  of vertebrae, 107–108, 109f
  of wrist, 302–308, 304b
magnetic resonance tractography, 66, 67f
magnetic resonance urography, of ureter,
    228–229, 228b, 229f
magnetic resonance venography
  of cerebral veins, 98–99, 100f
  of lower limb, 344
male reproductive organs, 264–272
  blood supply, 268
  lymph drainage, 268
  nerve supply, 268
  prostate gland, 264–265, 267f
  seminal vesicles, 268
male urethra, radiology of, 264
malleolus, 315f
mallet finger, 307
malleus, 22, 25f
  head of, 24f
mammary artery, internal, 51f, 55, 55f,
    56f, 347f
mammary lymph node, 347f
mammillary bodies, 63f, 64f, 70, 71f, 74f,
    77f
mammillary gland, 82f
mammography, 347–350, 348f, 349f
  patterns, 353
mandible, 2f, 14, 27f, 29f, 32f, 46f
  angle of, 14, 14f, 17f, 28f, 47f
  body of, 14f, 17f, 28f, 46f
  condylar process of, 17f, 47f
  condyle of, 15f, 46f
  coronoid process of, 47f
  inner aspect, 14f
  neck of, 4f, 14f
  radiology of, 17–18
    dental pantomography, 17–18, 17f
    plain films, 17
  ramus of, 14f, 17f, 28f, 30f, 46f
mandibular alveolus, 28f
mandibular body, right, 43f
mandibular canal, 14
mandibular condyle, 15f
  right, 9

mandibular foramen, 14, 14f
mandibular head, 32f
mandibular notch, 14f, 17f, 47f
manubriosternal joint, 134f
manubrium sterni, 106f, 153f, 180f
marginal artery of Drummond, 159, 199,
    200f
marrow patterns, 294–296, 296b, 296f
massa intermedia, 63f, 69
masseter muscle, 28f, 30f, 46f
  coronoid process of, 30f
masticator space, 42
mastoid air cells, 4f, 25f
mastoid antrum, 25f
mastoid process, 2f, 5f, 15f, 46f
maxilla, 2f, 10f, 18f, 32f
  orbital process, 11
  palatine process, 12
maxillary alveolus, 28f
maxillary antrum, 31f
maxillary artery, 12, 42, 51f, 52, 52f, 53f
maxillary bone
  frontal process of, 2f
  orbital process of, 10f
maxillary infundibulum, 11f
maxillary sinuses, 4f, 5f, 9f, 11f, 12–13,
    17f, 30f, 32f
  floor of, 17f
  medial wall of, 17f
  polyp in, 30f
maxillary tuberosity, 28f
maxillary vein, 54, 54f
McGregor's line, 107
Meckel's cave, 71–72
medial border, 285f
medial circumflex femoral artery, 340
medial collateral ligament, 329, 329b, 333
medial condyles, 313f, 315f
medial cuneiform, 317f
medial epicondyle avulsion, 286–287,
    286f
medial epicondylitis, 299
medial inferior genicular artery, 342f
medial lemniscus, 77f
medial lenticulostriate arteries, 91, 94f
medial ligaments, of ankle joint, 332
medial longitudinal arch angle, 317b
medial longitudinal fasciculus, 77f
medial malleolus, 333f–334f
medial meniscus, 325, 325f, 327f–329f
  anterior horn, 327f–329f
  posterior horn, 327f–329f
medial plantar artery, 333f–334f
medial plantar nerve, 333f–334f
medial plantar vein, 333f–334f
medial pterygoid muscle, 28f, 31f
medial retinaculum, 327f–329f
medial striate, 91
medial superior genicular artery, 342f
medial supracondylar ridge, 313f
medial tibial plateau, 326f
medial tibial spine, 326f
median aperture (of Magendie), 83
median cubital vein, 311f
median glosso-epiglottic fold, 37f
median nerve, 289f, 301f–302f, 305f,
    308, 308f, 309f, 347f
median sacral artery, 258f

median vein, 310, 311f
mediastinal divisions, 152f
mediastinal fat, 181f
mediastinal lines, 166f, 178–179, 178f
mediastinal lymph nodes, 173
mediastinal lymphatics, 172–173
mediastinum, 152–153, 239
　anterior, 152f, 182f
　chest radiograph of, 177–179
　　frontal, 177–178, 177b, 177f
　　lateral, 178
　cross-sectional anatomy, 179–183
　　level T_3, 179, 179f
　　level T_4, 179, 180f, 181f
　　level T_5, 179, 181f, 182f
　　level T_6, 179, 182f
　　level T_8, 181, 182f
　　level T_{10}, 181–183, 183f
　middle, 152f
　nerves of, 175–177
　posterior, 152f, 169f
　superior, 152f
mediastinum testis, 267f, 270
medulla, 222, 282f
medulla oblongata, 63f, 68f, 76–78, 85f, 109f
　small branches to, 92
medullary cavity, 308f
　of femur, 337f
membrana tectoria, 110
membranous labyrinth, 23
membranous urethra, 263, 263f, 266f
membranous urogenital diaphragm, 263
mendosal sutures, 9
meningeal artery, middle, 52f
meningeal layer, 118
meningeal veins, 1
meningeal vessels, middle, 8
　anterior branches, 4f
　posterior branches, 4f
meninges, 87–90, 88f
　arachnoid mater, 87–88
　arterial supply of, 88
　dura mater, 87
　nerve supply of, 88
　pia mater, 88
　radiological features of, 88–90
meningohypophyseal artery, 90
meniscal homologue, 304f
meniscal tears, 327, 329b
menisci, 326–329
　anatomy, 327
　discoid, 329
meniscofemoral ligaments, 325f
mental foramen, 2f, 14, 14f
mental protuberance, 14f
mental tubercle, 14f
mesenteric artery
　inferior, 199, 200f, 230f, 243f
　superior, 187f, 188f, 192f, 194f, 195f, 199, 216f, 217f, 230f, 242f
mesenteric nodes, superior and inferior, 233
mesenteric vein
　inferior, 219–221, 220f
　superior, 187f, 190f, 204–205, 209f, 217f, 219, 220f, 242f
mesenteric vessels, 243f

mesentery, 235
mesometrium, 274–275, 274f
mesorectal fascia, 254–255, 254b, 255f, 266f
mesorectal fat, 255f, 266f
mesosalpinx, 274–275, 274f
mesovarium, 274f, 275
metacarpal, 288f, 289
　fifth, 303f
　first, 303f
　fourth
　　base of, 288f
　　head of, 288f
　　shaft of, 288f
　ossification of, 290
　radiological features of, 289–290
metacarpal base
　fifth, 303f
　third, 303f
metacarpal index, 290
metacarpal sign, 289
metacarpophalangeal joint
　first, 288f
　fourth, 288f
metaphyseal red marrow, 296f
metatarsals, 316f
metatarsophalangeal joints, 318f
metopic suture, 3f, 9
midbrain, 63f, 68f, 74–76, 77f
　crus of, 61f
midcarpal joint, 300, 301f–302f
middle cerebellar peduncle, 61f, 71f, 79f
　left, 77f
middle cerebral artery, 61f, 91–92, 93f, 94f
middle constrictor, 34f
middle-ear cavity, 24f
middle genicular artery, 342f
middle meatus, 11f, 12
middle phalanx, 316f
middle rectal artery, 254f, 257f, 259
middle turbinate, 21f, 29f
midline aperture, 82f
midpalmar space, 306
midthigh, 337f, 338, 339f
Mirizzi's syndrome, 211b
mitochondrial DNA, disorders of, 70b
mitral valve, 157f, 158, 182f
moderator band, 157f
molars, 17f
motor cortex, of frontal lobe, 58
mouth, floor of, 27f
MRA. See magnetic resonance angiography
MRI. See magnetic resonance imaging
mucosal surface, 256f
mucous membrane, 27f
　in anal canal, 255
　in mouth, 46f
muscle cone, fat within, 18f
muscle fibres, 130f
musculocutaneous nerve, 56
myelography, lumbar puncture for, 113
mylohyoid line, 14f, 24
mylohyoid muscle, 24, 27f, 28f, 29f, 34f, 48f
　left, 43f
myometrium, 265f, 273, 279f

N

nabothian cysts, 277, 277f
nares, 32f
nasal bones, 2f, 9f, 10, 10b, 10f, 19f, 30f
nasal cavity, 12–14, 21f
　blood supply of, 12, 12b
nasal septum, 2f, 5f, 10f, 11f, 19f, 21f, 30f
nasal spine
　anterior, 2f
　of frontal bone, 9f
nasal turbinate
　inferior, 5f
　middle, 11f, 29f
nasofrontal suture, 2f, 3f
nasolacrimal canal, 10f
nasolacrimal duct, 12, 21, 21f
　inferior part of left, 21f
　opening of, 21f
　upper end of right, 21f
nasopharyngeal space, 30f
nasopharynx, 27–31, 27b, 29f, 33f
　cross-sectional anatomy of, 28–29, 30f, 31f
　lymphatic drainage of, 28
natal cleft, 321–322
navicular, 316f, 317f, 318
navicular fossa, 263f, 264
neck lymph node levels, 38–41
　submental and submandibular, 38
neck veins, 54, 54f
neck vessels, 50–56
nephron, 222
neural arch, 101
neural foramen, 117–118
neurocentral joints (of Luschka), 101, 109
nipple, 346f, 348f, 352f
nucleus pulposus, 113–114
nutrient arteries, scaphoid, 289

O

obex, 83
oblique epiphyseal line, 318f
oblique fissure, 134f
oblique line, 14f
oblique muscle
　external, 184, 186f, 188f, 191f, 223f, 243f
　internal, 184, 186f, 188f, 223f, 243f
　superior, 20f
obliquus capitis superior muscle, 109f
obliterated umbilical artery, 257f, 259
obturator artery, 257f, 258f, 259, 341f
obturator canal, 252f
obturator crest, 246f
obturator externus muscle, 251f, 253f, 254f, 265f, 266f, 321–322, 321f–323f
obturator fascia, 252f
obturator foramen, 245, 246f, 249f, 266f
obturator groove, 246f
obturator internus muscle, 249f, 250f, 251f, 252f, 253f, 254f, 255f, 265f, 266f, 281, 282f, 321f–323f
obturator nerve, 261

obturator vessels, 251*f*
obtuse marginals, 161*f*
occipital artery, 51, 51*f*, 53*f*
occipital association cortex, 60
occipital bone, 1, 2*f*, 5*f*, 6*f*
    inferior margin of, 85*f*
occipital condyle, 104*f*
occipital lobe, 59*f*, 60, 61*f*, 63*f*
occipital protuberance
    external, 4*f*
    internal, 4*f*
occipital sinus, 98*f*
oculomotor (III) nerve, 71*f*, 75–76
odontoid peg, 109*f*
odontoid process, 63*f*, 101, 104*f*, 108*b*
    ossification of, 110*f*
oesophageal hiatus, 131
oesophageal vein, 190*f*
oesophagogastric junction, 183*f*, 185,
        191*f*
oesophagus, 35*f*, 36*f*, 48*f*, 130*f*, 153*f*,
        155*f*, 157*f*, 169*f*, 170–172, 171*f*,
        178*f*, 180*f*, 181*f*, 182*f*, 183*f*, 188*f*,
        194*f*, 230*f*
    blood supply, 171, 171*b*
    lymph drainage, 171
    radiology, 172, 178*f*, 179*f*, 180*f*, 181*f*
olecranon, 297*f*–298*f*
olecranon fossa, 286, 286*f*, 287*f*,
        297*f*–298*f*
olecranon process, 287*f*, 297*f*–298*f*
olfactory (I) nerve, 71*f*
olivary nucleus, 77*f*
olive, 71*f*
omentum, 235
ophthalmic artery, 10, 19, 90, 93*f*, 94*f*,
        96*f*–97*f*
ophthalmic veins, 98*f*
    inferior, 19
    superior, 19*f*
ophthalmic vessels, 18
opponens abductor pollicis tendons, 289*f*
optic canal, 4, 6*f*, 8*t*, 10, 10*f*, 19*f*, 20*f*
optic chiasm, 61*f*, 63*f*, 70, 71*f*, 72*f*, 82*f*
optic disc, 20
optic foramen, 6*f*, 10
optic (II) nerve, 18*f*, 19, 19*f*, 20*f*, 71*f*
optic tract, 71*f*
ora serrata, 18*f*, 20
oral cavity, 24–26, 28*f*
    boundaries of, 25–26
    lymphatic drainage of, 25
    muscles of, 24
orbit, bony, 10–11, 10*f*, 11*b*
    floor of, 4*f*
    lateral wall of, 19*f*
    radiology of, 11–12
    wall, 10–11
orbital contents, 18–22, 18*f*, 19*b*
    radiology, 21–22
        computed tomography, 19*f*, 21
        magnetic resonance imaging, 20*f*, 21
        plain films, 21
        ultrasound, 19*f*, 21
orbital fissure
    inferior, 2*f*, 8*t*, 10*f*, 11, 32*f*
    superior, 2*f*, 4–5, 8*t*, 10*f*, 11, 19*f*
orbital plates, of frontal bones, 3

orbital process, 12
orbital septum, 18, 18*f*
orbitofrontal artery, 91
oropharyngeal tonsil, 28*f*, 34*f*
oropharynx, 29*f*, 31–33, 33*f*, 34*f*
os peroneum, 318*f*
os supratalare, 318*f*
os tibiale externum, 318*f*
os trigonum, 318*f*
os vesalianum, 318*f*
ossicles, 22
ossification
    of bones of the foot, 317–318, 318*b*
    of femur, 313
    of fibula, 315, 315*b*
    of patella, 314
    of tibia, 315
osteophytes, 171*f*
osteoporosis, 107*b*
ostiomeatal complex, 12–13
ostium, maxillary, 11*f*, 12–13
outer skull table, 4*f*
oval window, 22, 25*f*
ovarian artery, 230*f*, 272*f*, 274*f*
ovarian fimbria, 273
ovarian ligament, 272*f*, 275
ovarian volume, 278, 278*b*
ovaries, 272*f*, 274*f*, 275, 275*f*
    left, 277*f*, 282*f*
    right, 277*f*, 282*f*
    sagittal, 277*f*

P

paired deep dorsal arteries, 271
palatal muscles, 27–28
palatal studies, 33
palatine artery, greater, 12
palatine bone, 31
palatine canal, greater, 11*f*, 31, 32*f*
palatine tonsils, 24, 29*f*
palatoglossus, 24
palatopharyngeal arch, 28
palatopharyngeus, 24, 34*f*
palatopharyngeus constrictor, 34*f*
palmar aponeurosis, 306
pampiniform venous plexus, 267*f*, 270–
        271
pancake kidney, 225
pancreas, 188*f*, 212–218, 224*f*, 238*f*
    arterial supply of, 215, 216*f*
    axial section of
        level of pancreatic body, 241
        level of pancreatic head and renal
            hila, 243
    body of, 187*f*, 212, 216*f*, 217*f*, 241*f*,
        242*f*
    development of, 214*f*
    dorsal, 212
    ectopic, 214
    head of, 187*f*, 212, 217*f*, 238*f*, 242*f*
    lymphatic drainage of, 215
    neck of, 212, 242*f*
    radiological features of, 215–218
        angiography, 218
        computed tomography, 187*f*, 215–
            216, 217*f*

pancreas *(Continued)*
        endoscopic retrograde
            cholangiopancreatography, 216–
            218
        magnetic resonance imaging, 213*f*,
            216
        plain films, 215
        ultrasound, 215, 216*f*
        venography, 218
    tail of, 187*f*, 212, 216*f*, 217*f*, 223*f*,
        238*f*, 242*f*
    venous drainage of, 215
pancreas divisum, 214, 215*b*
pancreatic artery
    dorsal, 189*f*, 215
    transverse, 189*f*
pancreatic body, body wall, 241
pancreatic duct, 213*b*, 213*f*, 217*f*
    development of, 212–214, 214*f*
    variation in anatomy of, 214–215, 214*f*
pancreatic head, body wall, 241
pancreatic rests, 214
pancreatica magna artery, 215, 216*f*
pancreaticoduodenal artery
    inferior, 191, 192*f*, 215, 216*f*
    superior, 189*f*, 190*f*, 191, 192*f*, 215,
        216*f*
pancreaticoduodenal veins, 220*f*
pancreaticosplenic nodes, 233
papilla, pancreatic, 210, 211*b*, 213*f*, 222,
        222*f*, 227*f*
papillary muscle, 157*f*
papillary process, 206*b*, 241*f*
para-aortic nodes, 233
paracolic gutters, 199
paracolic space, right and left, 237
paraglottic fat, 37*f*, 39*f*
parahippocampal gyrus, 74*b*, 75*f*
paralaryngeal space, 35*f*, 38, 42*f*
paranasal sinuses, 12–14
    development of, 13–14, 13*b*, 13*f*
    radiology of, 14
paranasopharyngeal space, 31*f*
parapharyngeal fat, 28*f*, 31*f*
parapharyngeal space, 30*f*, 43, 43*b*
pararectal fascia, 254
pararectal fat, 250*f*
pararectal nodes, 257
paraspinal lines, 106*f*, 107, 178*f*, 179,
        182*f*
parathyroid glands, 48–50
    position of, 48*f*
    radiology of, 50
        cross-sectional imaging, 50
        nuclear medicine studies, 50
paratracheal interface, 132*f*
paratracheal nodes, 147*f*, 173
paratracheal stripe, 132*f*, 178, 178*f*, 179*f*
    right, 148–150
paraumbilical veins, 202–203
parietal association cortex, 59
parietal bones, 1, 2*f*, 6*f*
parietal foramina, 1
parietal lobe, 58–59, 59*f*, 63*f*
    branches, 91
parietal pleura, 135
parietal star, 4*f*
parieto-occipital artery, 93, 95*f*

parieto-occipital sulcus, 58, 59*f*
parotid duct (Stensen's duct), 46, 46*f*, 47*f*
  cannula in, 47*f*
parotid gland, 15*f*, 28*f*, 30*f*, 31*f*, 45–46, 46*f*
  deep lobe of, 30*f*
  left, 43*f*
parotid orifice, cannula in, 47*f*
parotid space, 42–43
pars interarticularis, 105*f*, 107*f*
pars intermedia, 73
Passavant ridge, 28
patella, 314, 325*f*, 326*f*
  articular surface, 313*f*
  dislocation of, 314, 314*b*
  lateral articular facet of, 327*f*–329*f*
  radiological features of, 314, 314*b*
patellar tendon, 325*f*, 327*f*–329*f*
pecten pubis, 246*f*, 252*f*
pectineus muscle, 251*f*, 254*f*, 255*f*, 266*f*, 321–322, 321*f*–323*f*
pectoralis major muscle, 180*f*, 346*f*, 347*f*
pectoralis minor muscle, 180*f*, 347*f*
pectoralis muscle, 348*f*, 351*f*, 352*f*
  fascia of, 346*f*
pedicle, 104*f*, 105*f*, 106*f*, 113*f*, 120*f*
pelvic brim, 247*f*
  plane of, 263*f*
pelvic floor, 248–250, 251*f*
  radiology of, 250, 253*f*, 254*f*
pelvic inlet, 245–246
  margin of, 249*f*
pelvic kidney, 225
pelvic ring, 246–248, 248*b*
pelvic sacral foramina, 105*f*
pelvis, 222*f*, 223*f*, 227*f*, 245–283
  blood supply, 250
  female
    cross-sectional anatomy, 281–283
    differences between male and, 248
    lower sacral level, 283
    mid-sacral level, 281
    radiology of, 276–281, 277*f*
    through the perineum, 251*f*, 283
  lymph drainage, 250
  lymphatics, 258–261
  male, 247*f*
    cross-sectional anatomy, 281–283
    differences between female and, 248
    lower sacral level, 281
    mid-sacral level, 281
    through the perineum, 251*f*, 283
  nerves of, radiology of, 261, 261*b*
penile urethra, 263*f*, 264
penis, 271
  bulb of, 253*f*, 271
  radiology of, 271–272, 272*b*
perforating artery, 341*f*
perforating nerves, 340*f*
perforating veins, 344
periaqueductal grey matter, 82–83
pericallosal artery, 91, 94*f*
pericallosal cistern, 85
pericardial recesses, 154–155
pericardial sinuses, 154–155
pericardium, 154–156, 155*f*, 156*b*, 157*f*, 182*f*
  radiological features, 155*f*, 156, 156*b*

pericranium, 1
perihepatic space, 238*f*
perilymph, 23
perineal body, 248, 250, 253*f*, 263*f*, 266*f*, 269*f*, 276, 276*b*
perineal membrane, 248, 252*f*
perineum, 248
periodontal membrane, 16, 16*f*
periorbita, 11, 18
periorbital fascia, 18*f*
periosteum, 1
peripheral zone, of prostate gland, 255*f*, 265*f*, 266*f*, 267
periprostatic vessels and ligaments, 251*f*
perirectal fascia, 250*f*, 254, 281
perirectal fat, 250*f*, 254, 281, 282*f*
perirenal space, 224, 224*f*, 235–239
  development and terminology, 235–237, 235*f*
  radiological features of, 237, 238*f*
perisplenic space, 237
peritoneal cavity, 224*f*, 236*f*
peritoneal fat, 243*f*
peritoneal fold, 274*f*
peritoneal spill, 281*f*
peritoneum, 186*f*, 253*f*, 263*f*
  covering ovarian vessels, 274*f*
  posterior, 224*f*
perivertebral space, 44, 44*b*
perivesical fat, of pelvis, 250*f*
peroneal artery, 339*f*, 340*f*, 341, 342*f*
peroneal tendons, 335, 335*b*
peroneus brevis tendon, 333*f*–334*f*
peroneus longus muscle, 337*f*, 339*f*
peroneus longus tendon, 333*f*–334*f*
Perthes lesion, 294*b*
pes hippocampi, 74*f*
petiole, 34
petrous bone, 22
petrous ridge, 5*f*
Peyer's patches, 194
phalanx, 289–290
  distal, 288*f*, 307*f*
    thumb, 288*f*
  middle, 288*f*, 307*f*
    middle finger, 288*f*
  ossification of, 290
  proximal, 288*f*
  radiological features of, 289–290
pharyngeal artery, ascending, 51, 51*f*, 53*f*
  left, 52*f*
pharyngeal constrictor muscle, 26, 35*f*, 36*f*
pharyngeal mucosal space, 44
pharyngeal recess, 27
  lateral, fossa of Rosenmüeller, 30*f*
pharyngeal tonsil, 29*f*
pharyngobasilar fascia, 26, 30*f*
pharyngoepiglottic folds, 38
  lateral, 35*f*
  medial, 35*f*
pharyngotympanic tube, groove for, 6*f*
pharynx, 26–27, 26*b*, 29*f*, 46*f*
  radiology of, 32–33
    cross-sectional imaging, 33, 33*b*
    palatal studies and videofluoroscopic feeding studies, 33, 33*b*
    plain films, 32–33, 33*f*

phrenic artery, inferior, 131, 230*f*
phrenic nerves, 55*f*, 131, 153*f*, 175–176, 176*b*
phrenicocolic ligament, 199, 235, 237
phrygian cap, 209
pia mater, 88, 117*f*, 118
pineal gland, 7, 63*f*, 64*f*, 70
  calcification, 7
  radiological features, 70–71
pineal recess, 82*f*
pinna, 22
piriform fossae, 37*f*, 38, 39*f*
piriform sinus, 35*f*
piriformis muscle, 249*f*, 250*f*, 252*f*, 255*f*, 282*f*, 321–322, 321*f*–323*f*
pisiform, 288*f*, 303*f*
pisiform-triquetral joint, 301*f*–302*f*
pituitary fossa, 3, 4*f*, 7*f*
  elongation, 8*b*
  floor of, 5*f*
pituitary gland, 63*f*, 71–73, 72*f*, 82*f*
pituitary stalk, 72*f*
plain films
  of abdomen, 185, 185*f*
  of biliary system, 211
  of kidney, 225
  of large intestine, 200–201
  of liver, 185*f*, 205
  of pancreas, 215
  of pelvic ring, 246–248
  of sigmoid and rectum, 257
  of skull, 64–65
  of small intestine, 195
  of spleen, 218
  of stomach, 185*f*, 188
  of wrist, 302
plantar aponeurosis, 333*f*–334*f*
plantar fascial aponeurosis, 317*b*
plantaris tendon, 331, 331*b*
planum sphenoidale, 4*f*, 5*f*, 7*f*
platysma, 27*f*, 36*f*
  left, 43*f*
pleura, 135–138, 135*b*, 135*f*, 136*f*
  lower limits at rest, 137*t*
  radiological features, 137–138, 137*b*
pleuro-oesophageal line, 178, 179*f*
plicae palmatae, 280
plicae semilunaris, 194
poles, 48
  lower, 48*f*
  upper, 48*f*
polysplenia, 218
pons, 61*f*, 63*f*, 68*f*, 71*f*, 76, 85*f*
pontine artery, 92, 93*f*
pontine cistern, 82*f*, 84–85
pontine vein, 98, 99*f*
popliteal artery, 340*f*, 341, 342*f*
  genicular branches, 340*f*
  muscular branches, 342*f*
popliteal vein, 343*f*
popliteal vessels, 327*f*–329*f*
popliteus insertion, notch, 327*f*–329*f*
popliteus muscle, 339*f*
popliteus tendon, 325*f*, 327*f*–329*f*, 331, 331*b*
porta hepatis, 202*f*, 203
  axial section of, 240–241, 241*f*
  body wall, 240

portacaval node, 233
portacaval space, 221*b*
portal vein, 187*f*, 190*f*, 192*f*, 194*f*, 202*f*, 204–205, 205*f*, 207*f*, 209*f*, 213*f*, 220*f*, 221, 240*f*, 241*f*, 242*f*
  hepatic arteries and, variations in relationship of, 210*f*
  right branch of, 191*f*, 192*f*
portal venous system, 219–222, 220*f*
  portography of, 222
  radiological features of, 221–222
portosystemic anastomoses, 221, 221*t*
portosystemic communications, 220*f*
porus acousticus, 23
positron emission tomography-computed tomography (PET/CT), mediastinal lymphatics, 173
postcentral gyrus, 59*f*, 61*f*
post-cricoid region, 39*f*
postcricoid venous plexus, 171*f*
posterior band of disc, 15*f*
posterior cerebral arteries, 92–93, 93*f*, 95*f*, 96*f*–97*f*
  central perforating branches of, 92
  medial and lateral posterior choroidal arteries of, 93
  multiple cortical branches of, 93
  postcommunicating part of, 93*f*
  precommunicating part of, 93*f*
  thalamoperforate branch of, 95*f*
  thalamostriate arteries of, 92
posterior cervical space, 45
posterior cervix, 277*f*
posterior chamber, 18*f*
posterior commissure, 35*f*, 37*f*, 38, 62, 62*f*, 75*f*
posterior communicating artery, 90, 93*f*
posterior cruciate ligament, 325, 325*f*, 327*f*–329*f*, 330, 330*b*
posterior cusp, of aortic valve, 168*f*
posterior ethmoidal cells, 4*f*
posterior fossa, veins of, radiological features, 98
posterior gluteal line, 246*f*
posterior impingement syndrome, 335
posterior inferior cerebellar artery (PICA), 95*f*, 96*f*–97*f*
posterior inferior iliac spine, 246*f*
posterior mesencephalic vein, 98, 99*f*
posterior myometrium, 277*f*
posterior of joint capsule, 15*f*
posterior pararenal space, 224, 224*f*
posterior parietal artery, 94*f*
posterior perforated substance, 70
  in interpeduncular fossa, 71*f*
posterior pituitary bright spot, 73
posterior spina bifida, 108
posterior spinal artery, 92
posterior subtalar joint, 333*f*–334*f*
posterior superior iliac spines, 245, 246*f*
posterior talofibular ligament, 331, 331*f*, 333, 333*f*–334*f*
posterior temporal artery, 94*f*, 95*f*
posterior tibial artery, 339*f*, 340*f*, 341, 342*f*
posterior tibial nerve, 337*f*, 339*f*
posterior tibial vein, 337*f*, 343*f*
posterior tibiofibular ligament, 333*f*–334*f*

posterior trunk, 257*f*
posteromedial central artery, 93*f*
pouch of Douglas, 272–273, 276*f*
preaortic nodes, 233
precentral cerebellar vein, 98, 99*f*
precentral gyrus, 58, 59*f*, 61*f*
pre-epiglottic space, 37*f*
prefrontal sulcal artery, 91
premotor cortex, of frontal lobe, 58
preoccipital notch, 58, 59*f*
prepatellar bursa, 325*f*
preperitoneal fat, 186*f*
prepontine cistern, 63*f*
prepyloric vein (of Mayo), 192
prepyramidal fissure, 79*f*, 80*f*
prerolandic artery, 91
presacral fat space, 111*f*–112*f*
presacral plexus, 111*f*–112*f*
presacral space, 276*f*
pretracheal fascia, 48
prevertebral fascia, 39*f*, 48*f*
prevertebral muscles, 30*f*, 36*f*, 46*f*, 48*f*, 50
prevertebral space, 33*f*
primary compressive trabeculae, 314*f*
primary fissure, 80*f*
primary tensile trabeculae, 314*f*
primary visual cortex, 60
principal plane, 203
probe skin interface, 277*f*
processus vaginalis, 270
profunda brachii artery, 310*f*
profunda brachii vessels, 309*f*
profunda femoris artery, 340, 340*f*, 341*f*
profunda femoris vessels, 339*f*
projection fibres, 60, 62–64
  radiological features, 64–66
promontory, 22, 24*f*
pronator quadratus, 288, 301*f*–302*f*
pronator teres, 297*f*–298*f*
properitoneal fat, 184, 224*f*
prostate gland, 251*f*, 321–322
  capsule, 266*f*
  median lobe of, 265*f*
  MRI, 269–270, 270*b*
  neurovascular bundles of, 265*f*, 266*f*, 268, 268*b*
  radiology of, 268–270
prostatic urethra, 263, 263*f*, 266*f*, 267*f*
prostatic utricle, 263
prostatic venous plexus, 265, 268
proximal interphalangeal joint, 288*f*, 307*f*
proximal phalanx, 288*f*, 307*f*, 316*f*, 317*f*
  head of, 307*f*
  shaft of, 288*f*
proximal tibia, fused growth plate, 326*f*
psoas major, 248*f*
psoas minor, 248*f*
psoas muscle, 108*f*, 111*f*–112*f*, 130*f*, 185*f*, 188*f*, 223*f*, 227*f*, 242*f*, 243*f*
psoas muscles, 245–246, 250*f*
psoas tendon, 250*f*, 251*f*, 282*f*
pterion, 1, 2*f*, 3*f*
pterygoid bone, 30*f*
pterygoid hamulus, 26
pterygoid muscles
  lateral, 30*f*, 31*f*
  medial, 14, 30*f*, 46*f*

pterygoid plate, 6*f*, 31*f*
  lateral, 2*f*, 30*f*, 32*f*
    left, 9*f*
  medial, 30*f*
    left, 9*f*
pterygomaxillary fissure, 31, 32*f*
pterygopalatine fossa, 6*f*, 30–31, 31*f*, 32*f*
pubic bone, 245, 251*f*, 266*f*, 279*f*
  body of, 245, 247*f*
pubic crest, 252*f*
pubic symphysis, 247*f*, 252*f*, 254*f*, 266*f*, 269*f*, 279*f*, 321*f*–323*f*
pubic tubercle, 245, 246*f*, 249*f*, 252*f*
puboanalis muscle, 252*f*
pubocervical ligaments, 275
pubococcygeal line, 280
pubococcygeus muscle, 248, 252*f*
pubofemoral ligament, 247*f*
puboprostatic ligament, 265
puborectalis muscles, 248, 253*f*, 254*f*, 255*f*, 256*f*, 266*f*, 279*f*
pubourethral ligaments, 275
pubovesical ligaments, 275, 276*f*
pudendal artery, 257*f*
pudendal canal, 261
pudendal nerves, 261
pulmonary angiography, 150
pulmonary arteries, 134*f*, 145–146, 146*b*, 146*f*, 148*f*, 169–170, 181*f*, 182*f*
  left, 153*f*
  left lower lobe, 132*f*
  right, 138*f*, 155*f*
pulmonary fibrosis, 140
pulmonary interstitium, 145
pulmonary ligaments, 148*f*
  inferior, 135–137, 135*b*, 137*b*
pulmonary lobule, secondary, 145, 145*b*, 145*f*
pulmonary outflow tract, 134*f*
pulmonary trunk, 132*f*, 138*f*, 146*f*, 149, 153*f*, 170, 181*f*
pulmonary vasculature, 149, 149*b*
pulmonary veins, 146–147, 146*f*, 147*b*, 148*f*, 157*f*, 182*f*
  left superior, 165*f*
pulp cavity, 16, 16*f*
pupil, 20
putamen, 64*f*, 65*f*, 69*f*
pyloric canal, 185
pyloric stenosis, 189*b*
pylorus, 185, 188*f*, 189*b*
pyramid
  of brainstem, 71*f*, 79*f*
  of kidney, 222*f*

Q

quadratus femoris muscle, 321–322, 321*f*–323*f*
quadratus lumborum, 248*f*
quadratus lumborum muscle, 130*f*
quadratus plantae muscle, 333*f*–334*f*
quadriceps tendon, 325*f*, 326*f*, 327*f*–329*f*
quadrigeminal cistern, 63*f*, 64*f*, 77*f*, 80*f*, 82*f*, 85
quadrigeminal plate, 61*f*, 63*f*, 64*f*, 75
quadrilateral space, 292*f*–293*f*

R

radial artery, 310, 310f
  position of, 308f
radial collateral ligament, 297f–298f
radial fossa, 286f
radial head, 297f–298f
radial nerve, 56, 297f–298f, 308, 309f
radial tuberosity, 287f
radial vein, position of, 308f
radial vessels, 309f
radicular arteries, 118
radiculomedullary arteries, 118, 119f
radiocarpal joint, 288f, 300, 301f–302f
radiography
  femur, 312–313, 313b
  hip joint, 319
  subtalar joint, 337
radioisotope, in tumour, 353f
radiology, of sigmoid and rectum, 257–258
radioulnar joint, inferior, 300, 301f–302f, 303f
radius, 287, 287f, 297f–298f, 301f–302f, 304f, 308f
  head of, 287f
  neck of, 287f
  ossification of, 288
  radial of, 287f
  radiological features of, 287–288, 288b
  shaft of, 287f
  styloid process of, 288f
raphe, 24
raspberry tumour, 195
rectal artery
  middle, 200f
  right, 225b
  superior, 200f
rectal fascia, 276f
rectal vein
  inferior, 220f
  superior, 220f
rectoprostatic fascia, 265
rectovaginal fascia, 275
rectovesical pouch, 262
rectum, 194f, 198f, 200f, 250–255, 250f, 254f, 255f, 256f, 263f, 266f, 276f, 279f, 282f, 321–322
  computed tomography, 257
  contrast enema, 257
  CT colonography, 257
  dynamic imaging, 258, 258b, 259f
  lower, 266f
  magnetic resonance imaging, 257–258
  plain films, 257
  radiology of, 257–258
  wall, 250f
    smooth muscle layers of, 256f
rectus abdominis muscle, 184, 186f, 187f, 188f, 191f, 239, 240f, 250f, 251f, 255f, 266f, 279f, 282f, 321–322
rectus capitis posterior minor, 109f
rectus femoris muscle, 251f, 321f–323f, 337f, 339f
  insertion, 321f–323f
rectus muscles, 243f, 279f, 282f
  inferior, 18, 20f

rectus muscles (Continued)
  lateral, 18, 19f, 20f
  medial, 18, 19f, 20f
  superior, 18, 20f
rectus sheath, 184
recurrent artery of Huebner, 91
recurrent laryngeal nerves, 175–176
red nuclei, 75, 77f
renal artery, 188f, 230f
  left, 242f
  right, 207f, 242f
renal cortex, 187f
renal fascia, 224, 224f
renal hila, body wall, 241
renal lobulation, 242f
renal medulla, renal pyramid in, 187f
renal pelvis, 188f, 189f
renal sinus fat, 222f, 242f
renal vein, 175f, 188f, 217f, 242f
  left, 216f, 232f, 242f
  right, 242f
renal vessel, axial section of, level of pancreatic head and renal hila, 243
rete testis, 267f, 270
reticuloendothelial system, 219b
reticulospinal tract, 115f
retina, 18f, 20
retinal surface, 19f
retroaortic nodes, 233
retrobulbar fat, 19f, 21
retrocrural space, 239
retroglandular fat, 351f
retrograde venography, of lower limb, 344
retromandibular vein, 54, 54f
  anterior branch of, 54f
  posterior branch of, 54f
retromaxillary fat pad, 28f
retromolar trigone, region of, 28f
retroperitoneal paravertebral veins, 220f
retroperitoneum, 224
retropharyngeal space, 44
retropubic fatty space, 261–262
retropubic space, 255f, 266f, 276f
retrosternal airspace, 134f
rheumatoid arthritis, 111b
rhomboid fossa, 83, 286b
ribs, 104f, 123, 126b, 351f
  absent, 125–126
  atypical, 124–125
  bifid, 125, 126f
  cervical, 125, 125f
  eight, 106f
  eleventh, 125, 240f, 241f
  first, 124, 124f, 310f
  lumbar, 126
  second, 124
  seventh, 106f, 346f
  short, 125
  tenth, 125
  twelfth, 125, 185f
  typical, 123–124, 123b, 124b, 124f
  variant anatomy in, 125–126
Riedel's lobe, 208b
rima glottidis, 34–35, 35f
Rolandic arteries, 91
roof of orbit, 4f, 20f
root canal, 16f
rostrum, 62, 62f

rotator cuff, 292
round ligament, 272f, 274f, 276, 279f, 280, 282f
round window, 22, 24f
rubrospinal tract, 115f
rugae, 186, 191f

S

S4 vertebra, lower sacral segment of, 250f
sacculation, of colon, 193f
saccule, 26f
  of larynx, 34–35
  membranous labyrinth, 23
sacral canal, 105f, 245, 252f
sacral flexure, 254f
sacral foramen, dorsal, 105f
sacral foramina, 245, 247f
sacral hiatus, 245
sacral promontory, 102, 105f, 279f
sacral vein, 232f
sacralization, of lumbar spine, 246–248
sacroiliac joint, 110, 245–246, 247f, 252f, 255f
sacroiliac ligaments, 105f, 245
sacrospinous ligament, 245, 247f, 249f
sacrotuberous ligament, 245, 247f, 249f
sacrum, 102, 105f, 245, 252f, 276f, 282f
sagittal band, 306f
sagittal suture, 3f, 5f
salivary glands, 45–47, 46f, 47f, 48f
  radiology, 47–48
    computed tomography and magnetic resonance imaging, 47–48
    nuclear imaging, 48
    sialography, 47–48, 47f
    ultrasound, 48, 48b, 48f
sartorius muscle, 250f, 251f, 282f, 321–322, 327f–329f, 337f, 339f
scalenus anterior muscle, 55, 55f, 57f, 124f, 169
scalenus medius, 109f
scalp veins, 1
scaphoid, 288f, 301f–302f, 303f
  injury, 305
  nutrient arteries of, 289
scapholunate ligament, 301f–302f, 302–304, 304b
scapula, 134f, 179f, 180f, 182f, 284, 285f, 292f–293f
  coracoid process of, 132f, 285f
  glenoid fossa of, 285f
  neck, 285f
  ossification, 284, 284b
  radiological features of, 284, 284b
Scarpa's fascia, 184, 185b
Schatzki ring, 171f
sciatic nerve, 251f, 253f, 255f, 261, 321–322, 339f
  position of, 337f
scintigraphy
  of biliary system, 212
  of kidney, 226
  of liver, 207–208
  of spleen, 219
sclera, 18, 18f, 19f, 20f
scrotal skin, 267f

scrotum, 267*f*
scutum, 22, 24*f*, 25*f*
secondary compressive trabeculae, 314*f*
secondary ductules, 47*f*
sella turcica, 6*f*
semicircular canals, 22
    lateral, 25*f*, 26*f*
    posterior, 25*f*, 26*f*
    superior, 25*f*, 26*f*
semicircular duct
    lateral, 26*f*
    posterior, 26*f*
    superior, 26*f*
semimembranosus muscle, 327*f*–329*f*,
        337*f*, 339*f*
seminal colliculus, 263
seminal vesicles, 250*f*, 262*f*, 265*f*, 266*f*,
        267*f*
    left, 282*f*
    radiology of, 268–270
seminiferous tubules, 270
semispinalis capitis muscle, 109*f*
semispinalis cervicis, 109*f*
semitendinosus muscle, 321*f*–323*f*,
        327*f*–329*f*, 337*f*, 339*f*
sentinel loop, 215*b*
sentinel node mapping, 352–353, 353*b*,
        353*f*
septal vein, 98, 99*f*
septum pellucidum, 61*f*, 63*f*, 65*f*, 74*f*, 82*f*
serosa, 256*f*, 273, 279*f*
serratus anterior muscle, 191*f*, 239
sesamoid bones, 288*f*, 290, 313, 316*f*,
        317, 318*f*
Shenton's line, 312, 319, 320*f*
short ribs, 125
short saphenous vein, 343*f*, 344
shoulder joint, 290, 292*f*–293*f*, 294*f*,
        295*f*, 296*f*
    capsule, 290
    cortex, 285*f*
    ligaments, 290
    radiological features of, 290–294
    stability, 290, 292–294
    synovium, 290
sialography, 47–48, 47*f*
sigmoid arteries, 200*f*
sigmoid colon, 198*f*, 200*f*, 250, 253*f*,
        279*f*, 282*f*
    computed tomography, 257
    contrast enema, 257
    CT colonography, 257
    dynamic imaging, 258, 258*b*, 259*f*
    magnetic resonance imaging, 257–258
    plain films, 257
    radiology of, 257–258
sigmoid groove, 6*f*
sigmoid sinus, 96, 98*f*, 100*f*
sinus artery, 160*f*
sinus tarsi, 317*f*, 333*f*–334*f*, 335
sinuses of Valsalva, 158–159
situs inversus, 149
Skene glands, 281
Skene's tubules, 264
skier's thumb, 307
skin
    of anal canal, 255, 256*f*
    of pelvis, 251*f*, 282*f*

skull, 1–12, 2*f*, 3*f*
    base of, 30*f*
    bony landmarks, 4*f*
    computed tomography of, 3*f*
    growing, 5–7, 7*b*
    neonatal, 5–7, 7*b*
    sinuses/air cells, 4*f*
    soft tissues, 4*f*
    vascular markings, 4*f*
skull base, 1–3
    foramina of, 4–5, 4*b*, 8*t*
    individual bones of, 3
    internal aspect, 6*f*
    radiological features of, 8–9, 8*b*
        cross-sectional imaging, 8–9, 33, 33*b*
        plain films, 32–33
skull radiographs, of cerebral vein, 98
skull vault, 1, 1*b*
    radiological features, 8–9, 8*b*
    thickness of, 9
small bowel, 238*f*, 282*f*
    enema, 195
    loops, 185*f*, 187*f*, 188*f*, 239*f*, 242*f*,
        243*f*, 279*f*
    mesentery, 238*f*, 239*f*
small cardiac vein, 162
small intestine, 193–196
    arterial supply of, 194, 194*f*, 195*f*
    lymphatic drainage of, 194
    Meckel's diverticulum in, 194–195
    obstruction, 201*t*
    peritoneal attachments of, 194*f*
    radiological features of, 195–196
        angiography, 196
        barium studies, 193*f*, 195
        computed tomography, 196
        magnetic resonance enterography,
            196, 196*f*
        plain films, 195
    root of mesentery of, 194*f*
    venous drainage of, 194
soft palate, 4*f*, 28*f*, 29*f*, 33*f*
soleal line, 315*f*
soleus muscle, 337*f*, 339*f*
somatosensory cortex, 59
sonohysterography, 278
spermatic cord, 270, 270*b*
sphenoethmoidal recess, 11*f*, 12
sphenofrontal suture, 2*f*, 6*f*
sphenoid air cells, 12
sphenoid bone, 3
    greater wing of, 1, 2*f*, 4*f*
    lesser wing of, 2*f*, 10*f*
sphenoid sinus, 4*f*, 7*f*, 11*f*, 12, 29*f*, 32*f*,
        63*f*, 71, 72*f*
    pneumatization, 13–14
spheno-occipital synchondrosis, 9
sphenopalatine artery, 12, 52
sphenopalatine foramen, 5, 32*f*
sphenoparietal sinus, 97
sphenoparietal suture, 2*f*, 6*f*
sphenosquamosal suture, 1, 2*f*, 3*f*, 6*f*
sphenotemporal (sphenosquamosal)
        suture, 3*f*
sphincter of Oddi, 210
spina bifida, defect, 109
spinal angiography, 114
spinal artery, 119*f*

spinal canal, 117, 117*f*
    width of, 103
spinal column, 101–122
spinal cord, 63*f*, 103*f*, 109*f*, 114–118,
        130*f*, 180*f*
    blood supply of, 118–122, 119*f*
    cross-section of, 115*f*, 116–118
    radiological features of, 119–122
        computed tomography, 108*f*, 120
        epidural space, 119–120
        magnetic resonance imaging, 109*f*,
            111*f*–112*f*, 117*f*, 120
        myelographic appearance, 119
        myelographic technique, 119
        spinal angiography, 121–122, 122*f*
        spinal ultrasound, 121, 121*f*
    venous drainage of, 118–119
spinal meninges, 118, 118*f*
spinal nerve, 115
    root, 109*f*, 111*f*–112*f*, 120*f*
    trunk of, 118
spine, 285*f*
spinocerebellar tracts, 115*f*
spinotectal tracts, 115*f*
spinothalamic tracts, 115*f*
spinous process, 102*f*, 104*f*, 105*f*, 106*f*,
        108*f*, 109*f*, 111*f*–112*f*, 113*f*, 185*f*
    of first sacral segment, 247*f*
    of L5 vertebra, 247*f*
    of S3 vertebra, 247*f*
spinous tubercle, 105*f*
spiral valves of Heister, 211*b*
splanchnic nerves, 131
spleen, 183*f*, 188*f*, 218–219, 238*f*, 240*f*,
        242*f*
    accessory, 218
    axial section of, 240*f*, 241*f*
        level of porta hepatis, 240
        level of upper liver and spleen, 239
    blood supply of, 218
    body wall, 239
    multiple, 218
    radiological features of, 218–219
        computed tomography, 187*f*, 191*f*,
            192*f*, 219, 219*f*, 223*f*
        magnetic resonance imaging, 219
        plain films, 218
        scintigraphy, 219
        ultrasound, 219
    variants of, 218
    wandering, 218
splenial gyrus, 74*f*
splenic artery, 188*f*, 189*f*, 190*f*, 192*f*,
        216*f*, 218, 241*f*
    dorsal, 216*f*
    transverse, 216*f*
splenic flexure, 185*f*, 191*f*, 192*f*, 193*f*,
        198*f*, 223*f*, 242*f*
splenic hump, 225*b*, 226
splenic vein, 187*f*, 190*f*, 192*f*, 204–205,
        209*f*, 216*f*, 220*f*, 221, 242*f*
splenium, 62, 62*f*
splenius capitis, 109*f*
splenoportography, of portal venous
        system, 222
splenorenal ligament, 235–236, 236*f*,
        238*f*
splenules, 218

splenunculi, 218
squamosal suture, 2*f*
squamosal temporal suture, 6*f*
stapes, 22, 24*f*
Stensen's duct, 46
sternoclavicular joint, 290
sternocleidomastoid muscles, 37*f*, 46*f*, 48*f*, 54*f*, 109*f*
sternomastoid muscle, 36*f*, 46*f*, 48, 57*f*
    abscess in, 36*f*
sternum, 128–129, 128*f*, 129*b*, 134*f*, 152*f*, 181*f*
    body of, 126*f*, 153*f*, 181*f*
    manubrium of the, 124*f*, 126*f*
    ossification, 129
    radiological features, 129, 129*b*, 129*f*
stomach, 185–189, 187*f*, 188*f*, 193*f*, 213*f*, 238*f*, 240*f*, 241*f*, 242*f*
    arterial supply of, 187, 189*f*
    bed, 189
    body of, 185, 188*f*, 227*f*
    bubble, 134*f*
    greater curve of, 188*f*, 191*f*
    lesser curve of, 188*f*, 191*f*
    lymphatic drainage of, 187
    muscle layers of, 186
    orifices, 185
    posterior relations of, 188*f*
    radiological features of, 188–189
        computed tomography, 188, 191*f*, 192*f*
        double-contrast barium-meal examination, 188, 191*f*
        magnetic resonance imaging, 188, 191*f*, 192*f*
        plain film, 185*f*, 188
        ultrasound, 189
    venous drainage of, 187, 190*f*
straight sinus, 96, 98*f*, 99*f*, 100*f*
strap muscles, 35*f*, 36*f*, 37*f*, 48*f*, 49, 49*f*
striate vein, 99*f*
stripe, 178
stroma, 346*f*
styloglossus muscle, 24, 27*f*, 34*f*
stylohyoid ligament, 35
styloid 'diaphragm', 31*f*
styloid foramen, 31*f*
styloid muscle, 30*f*, 46*f*
styloid process, 2*f*, 3, 4*f*, 6*f*, 30*f*, 31*f*, 46*f*, 316*f*, 317*b*, 317*f*
stylomastoid artery, 52
stylomastoid foramen, 6*f*
stylopharyngeus muscle, 34*f*
subacromial bursography, 291, 291*f*
subacromial subdeltoid bursa, 291, 292*f*–293*f*
subarachnoid cistern, 84–86
    radiological features, 86
subarachnoid haemorrhage, 89
subarachnoid septum, 117*f*
subarachnoid space, 18*f*, 117*f*
subarticular recess, 117
subarticular zone, 117
subcapital fracture, 313
subclavian arteries, 55*f*, 119*f*, 124*f*, 138*f*, 153*f*, 169, 179*f*, 180*f*, 309, 310*f*
    branches of, 55–56
    left, 52*f*, 55*f*, 168*f*

subclavian arteries (*Continued*)
    in neck, 55–56, 55*f*
    right, 52*f*
subclavian veins, 51*f*, 54*f*, 55*f*, 56, 56*f*, 124*f*, 175*f*, 310
subcoracoid recess, 291*f*
subcostal groove, 124*f*
subcostal vein, 232*f*
subcutaneous fat, 36*f*, 111*f*–112*f*, 180*f*, 243*f*, 250*f*, 251*f*, 277*f*, 279*f*, 282*f*, 307*f*, 308*f*, 346*f*
subdiaphragmatic fat, 183*f*
subdural haematoma, 89
subdural injection, 119
subdural space, 117*f*
subendometrial halo, 276–277
subglottic larynx, 35*f*
subglottis, 37*f*
subhepatic space, 237
subhyaloid space, 20
subiculum, 75*f*
sublingual gland, 27*f*, 28*f*, 43*f*, 47
sublingual space, 43–44, 43*f*
submandibular duct, 27*f*, 47*f*, 48*f*
    cannula of orifice, 47*f*
submandibular gland, 27*f*, 36*f*, 43*f*, 46, 48*f*
submandibular space, 44
subphrenic space, 236*f*, 237, 238*f*
subscapular artery, 55*f*, 310*f*
subscapularis muscle, 180*f*, 292, 292*f*–293*f*, 294*f*
subscapularis tendon, 292*f*–293*f*
substantia nigra, 75, 77*f*
subtalar joint, 336–337
subthalamic nuclei, 65*f*, 69*b*, 70
sulci, 68*f*
sulcus chiasmaticus, 3, 6*f*, 7*f*
super constrictor muscle, 46*f*
superficial cerebral vein, 97, 98*f*
superficial circumflex iliac artery, 340*f*
superficial cortical veins, 100*f*
superficial epigastric artery, 340*f*
superficial fascia, 346*f*
superficial femoral artery, 340–341, 340*f*, 341*f*
superficial femoral vessels, in adductor canal, 337*f*
superficial middle cerebral vein (of Sylvius), 97, 98*f*, 100*f*
superficial palmar arch, 310*f*
superficial pudendal artery, 340*f*
superficial temporal artery, 51*f*, 52*f*, 53*f*
superficial veins, 344
superior accessory fissure, 144
superior brachium, 74
superior canaliculus, 21*f*
superior cerebellar artery, 92, 93*f*, 95*f*, 96*f*–97*f*
superior cerebellar peduncle, 61*f*, 79*f*
superior colliculi, 77*f*
superior epigastric artery, 130*f*
superior frontal gyrus, 61*f*
superior gluteal artery, 257*f*, 258*f*, 259
superior gluteal vessels, 282*f*
superior horn, 48*f*
superior hypophyseal artery, 72, 90, 93*f*
superior intercostal vein, 56*f*, 175*f*

superior labrum, 292*f*–293*f*
superior longitudinal muscle, 28*f*
superior meatus, 11*f*
superior medullary vellum, 75, 79*f*, 82*f*
superior ophthalmic vein, 19*f*
superior orbital fissure, 5*f*, 10*f*
superior petrosal sinus, 97, 98*f*, 100*f*
superior pubic ramus, 245, 246*f*, 247*f*, 252*f*
superior pulmonary artery, 182*f*
superior pulmonary vein, 182*f*
superior rectal artery, 254*f*
superior rectus muscle, 18*f*
superior sagittal sinus, 61*f*, 65*f*, 96, 98*f*, 99*f*, 100*f*
superior tarsal plate, 18*f*
superior thoracic artery, 310*f*
superior thyroid artery
    left, 52*f*
    origin of, 53*f*
    right, 52*f*
superior turbinate, 11*f*
superior vena cava, 56*f*, 132*f*, 138*f*, 153*f*, 155*f*, 157*f*, 161*f*, 170, 175*f*, 178*f*, 180*f*, 181*f*, 182*f*
superior vermian vein, 98, 99*f*
superior vermis, 79*f*
superior vesical artery, 341*f*
supinator muscle belly, 297*f*–298*f*
supracondylar process, 286*b*, 300
supraoptic recess, 82*f*
supraorbital artery, 8–9
supraorbital foramen, 2*f*
supraorbital notch, 10*f*
supraorbital vein, 19, 54*f*
suprapatellar bursa, 325*f*
suprapineal recess, 82*f*
suprarenal gland, left, 188*f*
suprascapular artery, 55*f*
suprascapular notch, 285*f*, 291*f*, 292*f*–293*f*
suprascapular vein, 54*f*
suprasellar cisterns, 72*f*, 77*f*, 82*f*, 85
supraspinatus muscle, 180*f*, 291, 292*f*–293*f*, 294*f*
supraspinatus tendon, 291*f*, 292*f*–293*f*, 295*f*
    attachment, 291*f*
    insertion, 292*f*–293*f*
supraspinous fossa, 285*f*
supraspinous ligament, 112, 113*f*
supratrochlear vein, 54*f*
supreme intercostal vein, 175*f*
suspensory ligament
    of eye, 18*f*
    of ovary, 272*f*, 275
sustentaculum tali, 317*f*, 333*f*–334*f*
sutures, 3*f*, 7, 9
sylvian fissure, 58, 61*f*, 65*f*, 68*f*
sylvian point, 94, 94*f*
sylvian triangle, 94
sympathetic trunk, 51*f*, 176
symphyseal cleft, normal, 324*f*
symphysial surface, 246*f*
symphysis menti, 14
symphysis pubis, 245, 263*f*, 276*f*, 323–325, 323*b*, 324*f*
symphysography, 325

syndesmosis, 335, 335*b*
syndesmotic impingement syndrome, 335
synovial cover, 292*f*–293*f*
synovial fringe, lateral, 300
synovial lining, 15*f*
synovium, 297*f*–298*f*
  ankle joint, 331
  hip joint, 319, 319*f*
  knee joint, 325, 325*f*

T

T4
  vertebral body, 134*f*
taeniae coli, 198–199
talocalcaneal joint, 336
talocalcaneonavicular joint, 336–337
talus, 315–316, 317*f*, 333*f*–334*f*
  body of, 315
  head of, 315, 316*f*, 317*f*
  inferior surface of, 316
  neck of, 315, 317*f*
  posterior process of, 315, 317*f*
  trochlear surface of, 316*f*
tapetum, 61*f*, 62, 65*f*
tarsal tunnel, 333*f*–334*f*
technetium sulphur colloid scan, 207
tectospinal tract, 115*f*
tectum, 75
teeth
  nomenclature and anatomy, 15–16
  radiology of, 14*f*, 17–18, 17*f*
    plain films, 17
tegmen tympani, 22, 24*f*
tela choroidea, 88
temporal artery, 91
  superficial, 52
temporal association cortex, 59
temporal bone, 2*f*, 15*f*
  petrous part of, 61*f*
temporal fossa, 9–10, 19*f*
temporal gyri, 59*f*
  inferior, 59*f*
  middle, 59*f*
  superior, 59*f*
temporal lobe, 20*f*, 59–60
  parahippocampal gyrus of, 68*f*
  right, 61*f*
temporal veins, superficial, 54, 54*f*
temporalis muscle, 19*f*, 20*f*
temporalis tendon, 28*f*
temporomandibular fossa, 15, 15*f*, 17*f*
temporomandibular joint, 4*f*, 15, 15*f*
  computed tomography of, 17
  head of, 15*f*
  magnetic resonance imaging, 15*f*, 17
  neck of, 15*f*
  radiography of, 15*f*
temporoparietal (squamosal) suture, 3*f*
temporopolar artery, 91
tendinous arch
  of levator ani, 248, 252*f*
  of pelvic fascia, 275, 276*f*
tennis elbow, 299
Tenon's capsule, 18*f*, 19
tensor fasciae latae muscle, 250*f*, 251*f*, 321–322, 321*f*–323*f*

tensor veli palatini muscle, 24, 28, 31*f*
tentorium cerebelli, 63*f*, 87
teres minor muscle, 292*f*–293*f*, 294, 294*f*
terminal ductal lobular unit, 346*f*
terminal ventricle, 116
testicular artery, 230*f*, 267*f*, 270–271
testis, 266*f*, 267*f*, 270
  capsule of, 267*f*
  lobe of, 267*f*
  septum of, 270
  size, 270
thalamic nuclei, 70
thalamoperforating artery, 93*f*
thalamostriate vein, 98, 99*f*, 100*f*
thalamus, 65*f*, 69–70, 74*f*
  radiological features, 70–71
thecal sac, 108*f*, 111*f*–112*f*, 180*f*, 242*f*
thenar compartment, 306
thenar eminence, 301*f*–302*f*, 307
thenar space, 307
thin zone of disc, 15, 15*f*
third ventricle, 63*f*, 65*f*, 68*f*, 72*f*, 81–82, 81*f*, 82*f*, 85*f*
  supraoptic recess of, 63*f*
  suprapineal recess of, 63*f*
thoracic aorta, 132*f*, 153*f*, 167–169
  ascending, 155*f*
  descending, 155*f*
thoracic artery
  internal, 55*f*
  lateral, 55*f*, 310*f*
  superior, 310*f*
thoracic cage, 123–129
  muscles, 127–128, 128*b*, 180*f*
thoracic duct, 56*f*, 169*f*, 172–173
thoracic kidney, 225
thoracic spine
  myelographic appearance of, 119
  radiograph of, 106*f*, 107
thoracic vertebrae, 102, 104*f*
  eleventh, 240*f*
  first, 124*f*
thoracoacromial artery, 55*f*
thymus, 173–174
  left lobe, 175*f*
  radiology, 173–174, 174*f*, 175*f*
    chest radiograph, 173
    CT and MRI, 173–174
  right lobe, 175*f*
  ultrasound, 174
thyrocervical trunk, 55, 55*f*, 309
thyrohyoid ligament, 29*f*
thyrohyoid membrane, 35, 48*f*
thyroid arteries
  inferior, 51*f*, 55*f*
  superior, 49, 51, 51*f*, 53*f*
thyroid cartilage, 29*f*, 34, 35*f*, 36*f*, 37*f*, 39*f*, 48*f*, 109*f*
  inferior cornu of, 35*f*
  superior cornu of, 35*f*
thyroid gland, 38, 48–50, 353*f*
  blood supply of, 49
  cross-sectional anatomy, 48*f*, 49
  development of, 49, 49*b*
  isthmus of, 48*f*
  lobe of
    lateral, 35*f*

thyroid gland (Continued)
  left, 36*f*
  right, 36*f*, 48*f*
  lymph drainage of, 49
  radiology of, 49, 49*f*
    computed tomography, 49
    magnetic resonance imaging, 49
    nuclear medicine studies, 49
    ultrasound, 49
  upper pole of, 36*f*
thyroid isthmus, 138*f*
thyroid notch, 48*f*
  superior, 34
thyroid veins
  inferior, 49, 56*f*
  middle, 49
  superior, 49
thyroidea ima, 49
tibia, 314–315, 315*f*, 317*f*, 333*f*–334*f*, 339*f*
  in adulthood, 315
  cortex of, 337*f*
  medulla of, 337*f*
  radiological features of, 315
tibial articular cartilage, 325*f*
tibial plateau, 326*f*
tibial spine, 326*f*
tibial tuberosity, 315, 315*f*, 327*f*–329*f*
tibialis anterior muscle, 339*f*
tibialis anterior tendon, 333*f*–334*f*, 336, 336*b*
tibialis posterior muscle, 337*f*, 339*f*
tibialis posterior tendon, 333*f*–334*f*, 335–336, 336*b*
tibiocalcaneal fibres, 331*f*
tibiocalcaneal ligament, 333*f*–334*f*
tibiofibular joints, 331
tibionavicular fibres, 331*f*
tibioperoneal trunk, 341, 342*f*
tibiotalar articulation, 333*f*–334*f*
tibiotalar fibres, 331*f*
tongue, 27*f*, 29*f*
  base of, 4*f*, 34*f*, 35*f*, 36*f*
  contrast on superior surface of, 47*f*
  contrasts on surface of, 47*f*
  intrinsic muscle of, 29*f*
tonsils, 78, 79*f*
torus tubarius, 27, 30*f*, 31*f*
trachea, 33*f*, 35*f*, 48*f*, 106*f*, 132*f*, 138–143, 138*f*, 139*f*, 146*f*, 153*f*, 179*f*, 180*f*, 181*f*
  anterior wall, 134*f*
  blood supply, 140, 140*b*
  radiological features, 150–151
  relations of, 138–140
    cervical, 138–139
    thoracic, 139–140
  with right vagus nerve, 153*f*
  rings of, 48*f*
tracheal stripe, posterior, 134*f*, 179
tracheobronchial nodes, 147, 147*f*, 173
tracheo-oesophageal line, 179*f*
transforaminal nerve root block, 122
transition zone, of prostate gland, 255*f*, 265*f*, 266*f*, 267
transumbilical portography, of portal venous system, 222
transversalis fascia, 186*f*

transverse acetabular ligament, 319*f*
transverse arytenoid muscle, 35*f*
transverse cervical artery, 55*f*
transverse cervical ligaments, 275, 276*f*
transverse cervical vein, 54*f*
transverse colon, 188*f*, 193*f*, 194*f*, 198*f*, 200*f*, 227*f*, 238*f*, 239*f*, 241*f*, 242*f*, 243*f*
transverse fissure, 144
    left, 145, 145*b*
transverse fracture, 314*b*, 318*f*
transverse groove, 6*f*
transverse humeral ligament, 292*f*–293*f*
transverse ligament, 325, 325*f*
transverse mesocolon, 188*f*, 194*f*, 238*f*
transverse perineal ligament, 252*f*
transverse perineal muscle, 248, 253*f*, 255*f*
transverse process, 102*f*, 103*f*, 104*f*, 105*f*, 106*f*, 107*b*, 111*f*–112*f*, 185*f*
    of C₆, 55*f*
    persistent epiphyses in, 109*b*
transverse process, of L5 vertebra, 247*f*
transverse sinus, 4*f*, 96, 98*f*, 100*f*
transversus abdominis muscle, 184, 186*f*, 187*f*, 188*f*, 223*f*, 243*f*, 248*f*, 279*f*
trapezium muscle, 288*f*, 303*f*
    distal tubercle of, 301*f*–302*f*
trapezius muscle, 109*f*, 180*f*
trapezoid, 288*f*, 303*f*
triangular cornua, 280
triangular fibrocartilage, 301*f*–302*f*
triangular fibrocartilage complex (TFCC), 304, 304*f*
triceps muscle, 287, 292*f*–293*f*, 299, 299*b*, 309*f*
    lateral head of, 308*f*, 309*f*
    long head of, 308*f*, 309*f*
    medial head, 308*f*
triceps tendon, 297*f*–298*f*, 299, 299*b*
tricuspid valve, 158
trigeminal ganglion, in Meckel's cave, 72*f*
trigeminal (V) nerve, 61*f*, 71*f*, 76, 77*f*
trigone
    of bladder, 261, 266*f*
    of lateral ventricle, 81*f*
trileaflet aortic valve, 165*f*
trimalleolar fracture, 332
triquetral bone, 288*f*, 301*f*–302*f*, 304*f*
triquetrum, 303*f*
triradiate cartilage, 245, 320*f*
triticeal cartilage, 35*f*
trochlea, 18, 286*f*, 287*f*, 297*f*–298*f*
trochlear groove/ridge, pseudodefect of, 300
trochlear (IV) nerve, 71*f*, 75–76
trochlear notch, 297*f*–298*f*
true vocal cords, 29*f*, 35*f*, 37*f*, 38, 39*f*
tuber, 79*f*
tuber cinereum, 70, 82*f*
tubercle
    anterior, 102*f*, 103*f*
    nonarticular part of, 124*f*
    posterior, 103*f*
tuberculum sellae, 4*f*, 6*f*
tuberothalamic artery, 93*f*

tunica albuginea, 270–271, 275
tunica dartos, 270
tunica vaginalis, 267*f*, 270
turbinates, 12
'Twining's line', 144
tympanic annulus, 24*f*
tympanic membrane, 22

U

ulna, 287, 287*f*, 301*f*–302*f*, 303*f*, 304*f*, 308*f*, 309*f*
    radiological features of, 287–288, 288*b*
    shaft of, 287*f*
    styloid process of, 288*f*
ulnar artery, 305*f*, 310, 310*f*
ulnar bursa, 305*f*
ulnar collateral ligament, 297*f*–298*f*, 298, 298*b*, 304*f*
ulnar nerve, 56, 297*f*–298*f*, 309*f*
ulnar vessels, 309*f*
ulnotriquetral ligament, 304*f*
ultrasound
    of ankle joint, 332
    of basal ganglia, 69, 69*b*, 70*b*, 71*b*
    of biliary system, 211
    of CNS, 95
    of duodenum, 193*f*
    of infant hip, 320, 320*f*
    of intracranial arteries, 95
    of kidney, 225–226
    of knee, 327
    of limbic lobe, 74
    of liver, 206–207, 207*f*
    of lower limb, 343
    of pancreas, 215, 216*f*
    of projection fibres, 66, 68*f*
    spinal, 121, 121*f*
    of spleen, 219
    of stomach, 189
    of testis, 271, 271*b*
    of thalamus, 70–71
    of veins of lower limb, 344
    of ventricular system, 84, 84*b*, 85*f*
umbilical ligaments of, 185
    lateral, 185
    medial, 185
    median, 185
umbilicus, 220*f*
uncinate process, 11*f*, 12–13, 212, 217*f*
uncovertebral joints, 101
uncus, 73, 77*f*
unerupted teeth, 17*f*, 32*f*
unmyelinated immature white matter, 65*b*, 66*f*
upper aerodigestive tract, 23–38, 27*f*
upper eyelid, 18*f*
upper left incisor, 17*f*
upper limb, 284–311
    arterial supply of, 309–310, 310*f*
        radiological features, 310
    bones of, 284–290
    joints of, 290–308
    muscles of, 308–309, 308*f*, 309*f*
    veins of, 310–311, 311*f*
        radiological features of, 310–311
upper thigh, 337, 337*f*, 338*f*

ureter, 189*f*, 222*f*, 226–229, 227*f*, 239*f*, 242*f*, 262*f*, 266*f*, 272*f*, 274*f*
    abnormalities and variants of, 228
    blood supply of, 227
    development of, 228
    radiological features of, 228–229
ureteric ectopy, 228
ureterocele, 228
urethra, 251*f*, 262*f*, 263*f*, 265*f*, 266*f*, 268*f*, 269*f*
urethral diverticulum, 281
urethral glands, 264
urogenital diaphragm, 263*f*
urogenital hiatus, 252*f*
uterine artery, 259, 272*f*, 274*f*
    ovarian branch of, 274*f*
uterine cavity, 272*f*
uterine cornu, 281*f*
uterine fundus, 277*f*
uterine veins, 274*f*
uterine vessels, 253*f*
uterosacral ligaments, 275, 276*f*, 280
uterus, 272–273, 282*f*, 321*f*–323*f*
    body of, 253*f*, 263*f*, 272–273, 272*f*, 275*f*, 281*f*
    fundus of, 272–273, 272*f*, 281*f*
    retroflexed, 279*f*
utricle, 23, 26*f*
    filling of, 263*f*
utriculosaccular duct, 23
uveal tract, 20
uvula, 24, 34*f*, 79*f*

V

vagina, 251*f*, 263*f*, 272, 272*f*, 277*f*, 279*f*, 280*b*
    fornices of, 272
vaginal artery, 257*f*, 272*f*
vaginal canal, 279*f*
vaginal fornix
    anterior, 279*f*
    posterior, 279*f*
vaginal wall, 277*f*
    anterior, 254*f*, 279*f*
    posterior, 254*f*, 279*f*
vaginography, 281, 281*b*
vagus (X) nerve, 51*f*, 55*f*, 71*f*, 77*f*, 153*f*, 175–176
vallecula, 34, 35*f*, 36*f*, 37*f*, 79*f*
valve of Hasner, 22
valves of Houston, 198*f*, 250–254, 254*f*
valvulae conniventes, 194
vas deferens, 262*f*, 267*f*, 270
vasculature, of pulmonary arteries, 150–151, 150*b*
vasography, 270
vastus intermedius muscle, 337*f*, 339*f*
vastus lateralis muscle, 251*f*, 321*f*–323*f*, 337*f*, 339*f*
vastus medialis muscle, 327*f*–329*f*, 337*f*, 339*f*
veins, of lower limb, 343–344, 343*f*
velum interpositum, cistern of, 81, 82*f*, 85
venacavography, superior, 310–311

venography
  lower limb, 344
  renal, 226
  upper limb, 310–311
venous angle, 98, 100*f*
venous drainage
  of brain, 95–100, 98*f*, 99*f*, 100*f*
  of cardiac chambers, 273–274
venous sinuses, 96–97, 98*f*
  radiological features, 98–100
ventilation-perfusion scintigraphy, for
    lungs, 152
ventral nerve root, 109*f*, 121*f*
ventral ramus, 117*f*
ventral sacroiliac ligament, 247*f*
ventricles, 35*f*, 80–87, 81*f*, 82*f*, 153*f*,
    155*f*, 157*f*
  left, 134*f*, 158, 158*b*, 175*f*
  right, 158
ventricular outflow tract
  left, 182*f*
  right, 182*f*
ventricular system, radiological features,
    83–84, 84*b*
ventricular vein, 162
  posterior, 161*f*
vermis, 78
vertebra prominens, 101–102
vertebrae
  anterior wedging of, 107
  computed tomography of, 107, 108*f*
  magnetic resonance imaging of, 107–
    108, 109*f*
  occipital, 103–107
  radiological features of, 102–108
  thoracic, 102, 104*f*
  transitional, 103–107, 103*b*
  typical, 101, 108
vertebral artery, 46*f*, 51*f*, 53*f*, 55*f*, 92, 93*f*,
    109*f*, 119*f*
  left, 52*f*, 95*f*
  meningeal branch of, 92
  muscular branch of, 92
  in neck, 55
  right, 52*f*, 95*f*
  spinal branch of, 92

vertebral body, 104*f*, 105*f*, 109*f*,
    111*f*–112*f*, 113*f*, 121*f*, 130*f*
  of L2, 107*f*
vertebral canal, 104*f*, 105*f*, 117*f*
vertebral column, 101, 153*f*
  blood supply of, 114
  joints of, 109–111
  ligaments of, 111–113, 113*f*
    radiological features of, 113
vertebral system, angiography
    of, 93–94
vertebral veins, 46*f*, 54, 56*f*
vertebral venous plexus, 232
vertebrobasilar system, 92, 94*f*, 95*f*
vertex, 4*f*
vertical artery, groove for, 103*f*
verumontanum, 263, 265*f*, 266*f*
vesical artery, 258*f*
vesical fascia, 276*f*
vesicouterine pouch, 273
vestibular aqueduct, 22, 25*f*
vestibular fossa, 265*f*
vestibular vocal cords, 34–35
vestibule, of ear, 22, 25*f*, 29*f*, 34–35
vestibulocochlear (VIII) nerve, 26*f*, 71*f*,
    77*f*
vestibulospinal tract, 115*f*
videofluoroscopic feeding studies, 33
vidian canal, 32*f*
Virchow node, 173
visceral pleura, 135
visceral space, 45
visual cortex, 60
vitellointestinal duct, 195
vitreous body, 19*f*, 20
vocal cords, 29*f*, 35*f*, 36*f*, 109*f*
vocal ligaments, 33, 35*f*
volar plate, 307
volar radioulnar ligament, 304*f*
Von Rosen's view, 319

W

Waldeyer's ring, 33
wandering spleen, 218

watershed area, 199*b*
Weigert-Meyer law, 228
Wharton's duct, 46
white matter, 60–66, 116–117
  commissural fibres, 62
  internal capsule, 62–64
  projection fibres, 60, 62–64
    radiological features, 64–66
Wormian bones, 3*f*, 9
wrist
  biomechanics, 300–302
  extensor tendons of, 305
  flexor tendons of, 305
  imaging of, 305, 307
  radiological features of, 288*f*, 300–308,
    301*f*–302*f*
    arthrography, 302
    magnetic resonance imaging,
      302–308, 304*b*
    plain radiographs, 302
  tendon
    axial diagram of, 289*f*
    injury at, 305–306

X

xiphoid process, 129, 130*f*

Z

Zuckerkandl's fascia, 188*f*, 224
zygoma, 2*f*, 9–10, 10*f*, 30*f*, 31*f*
zygomatic arch, 2*f*, 32*f*
  cut ends of, 32*f*
  right, 9
zygomatic bone, 2*f*
  frontal process of, 5*f*, 19*f*, 20*f*
zygomatic process, 3, 12
zygomaticofrontal suture, 2*f*, 3*f*, 10*f*
zygomaticotemporal suture, 2*f*